# Pituitary
# Microadenomas

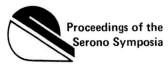

**Proceedings of the Serono Symposia**

---

*At the time of going to press these titles were in preparation.

# Pituitary Microadenomas

Proceedings of the
Serono Symposia, Volume 29

Edited by

## G. Faglia

2nd Medical Clinic,
University of Milan,
35, Via F. Sforza,
20122 Milano, Italy

## M.A. Giovanelli

Department of Neurosurgery,
University of Milan,
35, Via F. Sforza,
20122 Milano, Italy

## R.M. MacLeod

Department of Internal Medicine,
University of Virginia School of Medicine,
Charllottesville,
Virginia, USA

1980

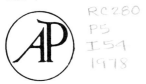

## ACADEMIC PRESS

A Subsidiary of Harcourt Brace Jovanovich, Publishers
London New York Sydney Toronto San Francisco

ACADEMIC PRESS INC. (LONDON) LTD.
24-28 OVAL ROAD
LONDON NW1


U.S. Edition published by
ACADEMIC PRESS INC
111 FIFTH AVENUE
NEW YORK, NEW YORK 10003

*British Library Cataloguing in Publication Data*
International Symposium on Pituitary Microadenomas,
  *Milan, 1978*
  Pituitary microadenomas. –(Proceedings of the
  Serono Foundation symposia; vol.29
  ISSN 0308–5503).
  1.Pituitary body–Tumors–Congresses
  2. Adenoma–Congresses
  I. Title II. Faglia, G III. Giovanelli, M A
  IV MacLeod, Robert Meredith V Series
  616.9'94'47  RC280.P5  79-41478

ISBN 0-12-248150-X


Typeset by Reproduction Drawings Ltd., Sutton, Surrey
Printed by Photolithography in Great Britain by
Whitstable Litho Ltd, Whitstable, Kent

## FOREWORD

The main justification of any International Symposium is the existence of a body of new information in a restricted subject derived from a number of scientific disciplines which may be separated by traditional communication barriers. This International Symposium on Pituitary Microadenomas admirably fulfilled this need. Much new information has been acquired in the past few years about pituitary microadenomas that has changed our concepts on the basic biology, diagnosis and treatment of pituitary microadenomas. The participants in this Symposium represented a wide spectrum of scientific and clinical disciplines.

Initial consideration was given to the basic biology of pituitary tumors including the cellular processes of hormone secretion, their ultrastructural characteristics, and their behavior in tissue failure. Other speakers addressed important problems in etiology of microadenomas and their hypothalamic control. The endocrinologic characteristics and endocrine diagnostic procedures were discussed from several points of view. The usefulness and limitations of the highly developed techniques of radiologic diagnosis and current methods of radiation therapy were presented. The Symposium also included a critical evaluation of the extensive experience of the participating neurosurgeons in transsphenoidal removal of microadenomas and of the clinical endocrinologists in the treatment of prolactinomas and growth hormone-secreting adenomas with bromocriptine and other agents.

The Secretaries and the Organizing Committee are to be commended for their selection of this subject and the participants. This book makes the valuable information exchanged at this Symposium available to those who were not fortunate enough to attend.

WILLIAM H. DAUGHADAY
Co-President, International Symposium on Pituitary Microadenomas

# PREFACE

The papers of this book comprise the series of lectures and communications given during the International Symposium on Pituitary Microadenomas which was held in Milan on October 12-14, 1978.

Though the importance of intrapituitary adenomas has been recognized by Harvey Cushing since 1932, it is only in very recent years that considerable progress has been made in this area. This Symposium was intended to focus upon present knowledge arising from recent morphological contributions and biological advances together with current diagnostic procedures and therapeutic approaches to pituitary microadenomas. The topics covered in this Symposium were:

the role of receptors and neurotrasmitters in the control of pituitary functions; morphological and molecular aspects of hormonal secretion in normal and tumoral cells in the pituitary; immunohistochemical aspects; pathogenesis of pituitary tumors; neuroendocrinology and endocrinology of pituitary microadenomas; diagnostic studies including endocrine function tests and radiology; therapeutic approaches, including microneurosurgery, cryosurgery, alpha particle therapy, neuroactive drugs.

This Symposium could not have taken place without the dedicated efforts of a number of people. In particular we are grateful to Professors W. H. Daughaday and C.B. Wilson for their interest and help with the meeting itself. Thanks are due to the Program and Organizing Committees consisting of V. Bernasconi, H. G. Friesen, G. Guiot, A. M. Landolt, R. M. MacLeod and K. von Verder, and B. Ambrosi, P. Beck-Peccoz, S. M. Gaini, E. D. F. Motti, G. Tomei, P. Travaglini and R. Villani respectively.

Dr. J. T. Nutter, Dr. Betty Rubin, Dr. Anna Spada, Miss Rita Paglino and Miss Cristina Citi merit special mention for their editorial assistance. Also to be commended are the speakers who contributed their manuscripts and Dr. S. Rossetti of Serono Symposia International for his particular interest in the meeting and his valuable help with the management.

February, 1980

G. FAGLIA
M. A. GIOVANELLI
R. M. MACLEOD

# CONTENTS

# PRESIDENTIAL ADDRESS 1

W. H. Daughaday

*Metabolism Division and Diabetes Research and Training Center, Washington University School of Medicine, St. Louis, Missouri 63110, USA*

I was greatly honored to be asked to share the presidency of this symposium with Professor Wilson.

In preparation for this symposium I reread some of the publications of Harvey Cushing. The participants need not be reminded that Cushing combined superb neurosurgical technical skills with penetrations of scientific curiosity which led to discoveries not only in the operating room and at the bedside but also in the experimental laboratory.

Many of Cushing's predictions and ideas about pituitary surgery as expressed to the Medical Society of London in 1927 provided the substance of this symposium.

> Are we entitled to attack a chromophile adenoma while small in the hope of forestalling its future devastating effects on the body? This is the rub, and though another generation will have to answer the question practically, we are at least entitled to consider it theoretically.

He certainly would be at home with the transsphenoidal approach to pituitary, as shown in the familiar drawing by Max Brodel which is almost identical to that from Professor Hardy's paper a half century later. We are indebted to Cushing for his exhaustive clinical description of acromegaly and for recognizing that pituitary adenomata could cause the syndrome which now bears his name. American endocrinologists commonly give credit to Forbes *et al.* (1954) for suggesting that the amenorrhea galactorrhea syndrome was caused by a prolactin-secreting tumor. This hypothesis, however, was clearly enunciated by Cushing (1933) in his classic paper on "'Dyspituitarism': Twenty years later". He commented as follows on a patient with postpartum amenorrhea and persistent lactation:

> Whether the cells of the patient's tumor secreted a lactogenic hormone corresponding to the "Prolactin" of Riddle could only have been deter-

1

mined by testing the effect, on the previously sensitized mammary glands of animals, of implanted tissue taken from the growth. Both Riddle and Evans feel assured that the adenohypophysis provides such a hormone definitely separable from the principles influencing growth and sex.

Turning to the challenges of the present, we still know little about the pathogenesis of the pituitary microadenomata and the possible contribution of the hypothalamus in the development of such tumors. We know that many pituitary tumors are not autonomous but their secretion can be modulated by metabolites such as glucose and arginine, catecholamines and hypothalamic peptides.

Two hypotheses of the genesis of microadenomata exist. First, these secretory tumors are believed to arise as an autonomous neoplastic event. In the second hypothesis, hypothalamic stimulation at first leads to hyperplasia and subsequent neoplastic transformation of a secretory cell type. The strongest evidence of a primary pituitary neoplastic change is the frequent resumption of normal pituitary function after removal of a microadenomata. Nevertheless there is evidence that neoplasia can follow prolonged pituitary hypersecretion caused by hypogonadism and hypothyroidism. Many have speculated that the high incidence of prolactinomas may be the result of lactotroph stimulation by pregnancy and contraceptive pills.

Most intriguing are the morphologic studies of the "uninvolved" pituitary at the time of removal of microadenomata. Saeger (1977) in Hamburg has found cases of lactotroph hyperplasia in the tissue surrounding prolactinomas and corticotroph hyperplasia surrounding corticotroph adenomas. Similar findings from Professor Landolt of Zurich were heard at this meeting. Dr Daniel McKeel of St Louis also has found similar cases of lactotroph hyperplasia (personal communication). As yet the correlation of this type of hyperplasia with hormonal response to adenomectomy is incomplete. The morphological evidence may provide an explanation for the failure of adenomectomy to cure some cases.

If in fact there are two types of cases with microadenomata (i.e. 1. those with autonomous adenomas and suppressed normal pituitary, and 2, those with adenomas and more generalized surrounding hyperplasia), it would be important to distinguish between the two types. To do this it is necessary to separate the effects of pharmacologic agents on the hypothalamus from those exerted by the drug directly on the pituitary. To accomplish this Fine and Frohman (1978) have compared the response of patients with hyperprolactinemia to L-dopa before and after pretreatment with carbidopa.

## REFERENCES

Cushing, H. (1927). Annual oration before Medical Society of London.
Cushing, H. (1933). *Arch. Intern. Med.* **51**. 487.
Fine, S. A. and Frohman, L. A. (1978). *J. Clin. Invest.* **61**, 973.
Forbes, A. P., Henneman, P. H., Griswold, G. C. and Albright, F. (1954). *J. Clin. Endocrinol.* **14**, 265.
Saeger, W. (1977). *Virchows Arch. A Path. Anat. Histol.* **372**, 299.

# PRESIDENTIAL ADDRESS 2

C. B. Wilson

*Department of Neurological Surgery, University of California, San Francisco, California 94143, USA*

I was deeply honored to serve as a Co-President of this symposium. The selection of a surgeon for this honor undoubtedly reflects the contributions neurosurgeons have made in developing our present concepts of endocrine-active pituitary adenomas. Although many surgeons have been active in the field of pituitary tumors, I will take the presidential prerogative to designate four who, in my opinion, have contributed significantly to our understanding and treatment of microadenomas.

In 1914, Harvey Cushing reported his early experience with the transnasal approach to pituitary tumors (Cushing, 1914). With little modification, his sublabial transseptal technique for entering the sella turcica through the sphenoid sinus has become the most widely used operation for pituitary microadenomas (Guiot *et al.*, 1958; Hardy, 1973; Wilson and Dempsey, 1978). Cushing's second contribution was the recognition of basophilic microadenomas as a cause of hypercortisolism—without question one of the most brilliant clinicopathologic correlates in the history of medicine.

Subsequently, the transsphenoidal approach, which was destined to assume a crucial role in the surgical removal of microadenomas, was abandoned by Cushing and others because of the restrictions imposed by limited visibility of the operative field. To Gerard Guiot belongs the credit for reviving the transsphenoidal operation, with his use of magnifying loupes and a lighted retractor (Guiot, 1958). His excellent results and extensive experience have become a legend.

Guiot's pupil, Jules Hardy, refined this operation through the use of radiofluoroscopy and the surgical microscope (Hardy and Wigser, 1965), and his technique has been widely adopted. Exactly ten years ago, Hardy reported the successful removal of a pituitary microadenoma—an accomplishment that revo-

3

lutionized the treatment of the endocrine-active tumor (Hardy, 1969). All later reports of the successful surgical treatment of microadenomas by this technique offer testimony to the importance of Hardy's contribution to pituitary micro-surgery.

Alex Landolt, an acknowledged expert in the transsphenoidal arena, has made his major contribution outside the operating room (Landolt, 1975; Landolt, 1978; Landolt and Rothenbuhler, 1977; Landolt *et al.*, 1978). Landolt's monograph "Ultrastructure of Human Sella Tumors" (1975) brought together morphological, biochemical and clinical information largely derived from his own studies, and through thoughtful analysis, he provided a coherent overview of endocrine-active adenomas. Landolt's perception of the biological behavior of pituitary tumors reflects an insightful synthesis of laboratory and clinical science.

Neurosurgeons are becoming increasingly involved in the treatment of endocrine disorders caused by pituitary adenomas. Until transsphenoidal microsurgery was directed to microadenomas, we were concerned primarily with the subtotal removal, usually by craniotomy, of large pituitary tumors that produced visual impairment and pituitary hypofunction. Today, the large endocrine-inactive adenomas constitute a shrinking minority of tumors that are treated by the transsphenoidal approach. In my own series of pituitary tumors, there has been a rapidly increasing proportion of prolactin-secreting and adrenocorticotropin-secreting microadenomas (Table I). It is not unreasonable to anticipate that we will be encountering a greater number of tumors that are presently considered rare—namely, gonadotropin-secreting tumors in both sexes and prolactin-secreting tumors in men.

*Table I.* Distribution of pituitary adenomas by endocrine activity

| Type of adenoma | No. of cases | % of cases |
|---|---|---|
| *Endocrine-active* | | |
| PRL | 165 | |
| GH | 114 | |
| ACTH | 66 | |
| TSH | 1 | |
| | 346 | (72.4%) |
| *Endocrine-inactive* | | |
| | 104 | (37.6%) |
| Total | 450 | (100%) |

This is an exciting period in the history of pituitary disorders, and I am confident that neurosurgeons will continue to have a role in the acquisition of new knowledge. Just ten years ago, surgical removal of an endocrin-active microadenoma was little more than a conceptual possibility—I hesitate to predict the state of the art ten years hence.

## REFERENCES

Cushing, H. (1914). *J.A.M.A.* **63**, 1515.

Guiot, G. (1958). "Adénomes Hypophysaires". Masson, Paris.

Guiot, G., Rougerie, J., Brian, S. and Hertzog, E. (1958). *Ann. Chir. (Paris)* **12**, 689.

Hardy, J. (1969). *Clin. Neurosurg.* **16**, 185.

Hardy, J. (1973). *In* "Diagnosis and Treatment of Pituitary Tumors" (P. O. Kohler and G. T. Ross, eds) 179. Excerpta Medica, Amsterdam.

Hardy, J. and Wigser, S. (1965). *J. Neurosurg.* **23**, 612.

Landolt, A. M. (1975). *Acta Neurochir. (Wein)* Suppl. 22.

Landolt, A. M. (1978). *In* "Advances and Technical Standards in Neurosurgery" (H. Krayenbuhl, ed) Vol. 5, 4–49. Springer-Verlag, New York.

Landolt, A. M. and Rothenbuhler, V. (1977). *Acta Endocrinol. (Kobenhavn)* **84**, 461.

Landolt, A. M., Rothenbühler, V. and Kistler, G. (1978). *In* "Treatment of Pituitary Adenomas" (R. Fahlbusch and K. V. Werder). Georg Thieme Verlag, Stuttgart.

Wilson, C. B. and Dempsey, L. C. (1978). *J. Neurosurg.* **48**, 13.

# TEN YEARS AFTER THE RECOGNITION OF PITUITARY MICROADENOMAS

J. Hardy

*Service of Neurosurgery, Notre-Dame Hospital, and University of Montreal, Canada*

Ten years ago, in September 1968, at the Congress of Neurological Surgeons held in Toronto, Canada, I presented for the first time the surgical findings of intrapituitary microadenomas in patients suffering from hypersecreting pituitary disorders associated with a normal sized sella turcica (Hardy, 1969).

This presentation was received with scepticism, some criticism, passive and active resistance. Indeed in the past, it was generally assumed that pituitary tumor formation occurred as a diffuse neoplastic adenomatous process within the whole pituitary body. The usual method of removing the tumor did not permit us to distinguish between normal and pathological tissues and both were excised. This problem was well assessed by Guiot (1958). "That the complete removal of pituitary adenoma might restore the previous hormonal deficit one should agree that this is rather exceptional. . . From this point of view, one must say that the patient is rather aggravated since the adenomatous tissue is *not separable* from the normal hypophyseal tissue and the attempt to perform a complete radical excision brings in the curettes the glandular tissue still functionally active. Therefore, this increases the hormonal deficit which can lead to a complete pituitary insufficiency following surgery" (quotation translated). As a consequence, total hypophysectomy or sellar clean-out was recommended as the most effective treatment of hypersecreting diseases, particularly in acromegaly (Ray *et al.*, 1968). Panhypopituitarism was the *sine qua non* condition for a definitive cure.

The revival of the extracranial transsphenoidal open surgical approach (Guiot *et al.*, 1958) has benefited from major technical advances with the introduction of the combined use of televized radiofluoroscopic control (Hardy and Wigser, 1965), the optical magnification with the surgical microscope and the development of microsurgical techniques of dissection (Hardy, 1969a,b; 1971). Optical magnifi-

7

cation permits a clear distinction between normal and pathological tissue: this has opened the field of *histological functional microsurgery*. We were thus able to recognize lesions measuring less than 10 mm in diameter which we have originally called "microadenomas". It then became possible to perform a selective excision of these lesions with preservation of the normal pituitary tissue, resulting in the possibility of achieving clinical and biological cure of hypersecreting pituitary disease with preservation of other pituitary functions (Hardy, 1973).

In our series of over 500 cases of pituitary tumors surgically removed and pathologically verified (Table I), microadenomas occurred in 33% of the cases. They were found in 38/161 cases of acromegaly, 105/195 cases of prolactin adenomas in females, 3/30 cases of prolactin adenomas in males, 22/28 cases of Cushing's disease and 6/9 cases of Nelson's syndrome. The two cases of non-secreting microadenoma were detected by the presence of intrasellar calcification. This presentation will be limited to some particular features of microadenomas as compared with larger sized tumors.

*Table I.*  Pituitary adenomas pathologically verified.

|                     | No. of cases | Microadenomas | Macroadenomas |
|---------------------|:------------:|:-------------:|:-------------:|
| *Secreting*         |              |               |               |
| GH                  | 161          | 38            | 123           |
| Prolactin (female)  | 195          | 105           | 90            |
| Prolactin (male)    | 30           | 3             | 27            |
| ACTH (Cushing)      | 28           | 22            | 6             |
| ACTH (Nelson)       | 9            | 6             | 3             |
| TSH                 | 1            | 0             | 1             |
| *Non-secreting*     | 102          | 2             | 100           |
| Total               | 526          | 176           | 350           |

## RADIOLOGICAL ASPECTS OF MICROADENOMAS

According to our radiological classification (Hardy, 1973; Hardy *et al.*, 1973; Hardy, 1975), grade I sellas were encountered in 154/176 cases (88%) (Table II).

The sella was normal on tomography in twelve cases of Cushing's disease and three cases of Nelson's syndrome.

In patients previously treated with radiation therapy, although the sella turcica may be enlarged and classified grade II the tumor may be shrunken and reduced in size to less than 10 mm (microadenoma), as we have found in four cases of acromegaly. Similar findings occurred in three cases of prolactin adenoma previously treated with bromo-ergocryptine.

In a few cases however, discrepancies were found between radiological and surgical findings. For instance, the finding of an intrasellar arachnoidal invagination has often been misinterpreted in the literature with improper use of the term "empty sella". However, when the patient has a clinical syndrome of pituitary

*Table II.* Radiological aspects in microadenomas.

| Types of microadenomas | No. of cases | Radiological classification | | |
| --- | --- | --- | --- | --- |
| | | Normal | Grade I | Grade II |
| *Secreting* | | | | |
| GH | 38 | 0 | 34 | 4 |
| Prolactin (female) | 105 | 0 | 102 | 3 |
| Prolactin (male) | 3 | 0 | 3 | 0 |
| ACTH (Cushing) | 22 | 12 | 10 | 0 |
| ACTH (Nelson) | 6 | 3 | 3 | 0 |
| *Non-secreting* | 2 | 0 | 2 | 0 |
| Total | 176 | 15 | 154 | 7 |

hypersecretion, the arachnoidal invagination is associated either with a well-defined microadenoma or with adenomatous tissue (Sutton and Vezina, 1974), having a carpetlike appearance which we have called "adenoma en plaques" as an analogy with the well known meningioma "en plaques" of the sphenoid wing.

Ectopic adenomatous tissue can not be correlated with the radiological classification. For example, in a patient with a grade I sella, at surgery tumor tissue was found posteriorly invading the bone corresponding to a localized invasive grade III adenoma. Ectopic tumor tissue may also be found totally outside the pituitary gland or the sella turcica (Fig. 3).

## BIOLOGICAL ASPECTS OF MICROADENOMAS

In Cushing's disease, there seems to be no correlation between the duration, the severity of the disease, the increased level of plasma cortisol and the size of the lesion.

In the group of growth hormone and prolactin-secreting adenomas, there seems to be a clear correlation between the radiological classification of the lesion and the level of hormone hypersecretion. In 72 untreated cases of acromegaly, the mean range of growth hormone levels found were as follows: in grade I—32 ng/ml; grade II—47 ng/ml and 67 ng/ml with suprasellar expansion; in grades III and IV—97 ng/ml. In prolactin-secreting adenomas, a similar correlation has been found with the radiological classification of the tumor. In grade I, the mean level was 116 ng/ml; in grade II, it was 600 ng/ml and in the grade III and IV, the mean level of prolactin was 700 ng/ml; with suprasellar expansion, the mean level was 1160 ng/ml. This correlation between the level of hormone and the size of the tumor is most important to remember in order to establish the prognosis following surgical treatment.

## SURGICAL ASPECT OF MICROADENOMAS

From the therapeutic point of view, I do not need to reemphasize the major advantage of surgery, particularly of the open extra-cranial transsphenoidal approach which turns out to be a relatively benign, non traumatic and rapid

*J. Hardy*

procedure. Microsurgical selective removal of the microadenoma was always attempted and the results will be presented in another paper. The most striking biological event is the immediate reversal of hormone hypersecretion (Hardy, 1975).

The assessment of the size of the microadenoma can be made accurately in several ways: during surgery, by the use of a template such as the tip of the micro-suction tube or the diameter of the ring curettes; after tumor removal, by opaque contrast sponge in the tumor-bed with radiographic picture, and finally, by measuring directly the pathological material.

In Cushing's disease (Fig. 1), 22 microadenomas were all located in the central core of the gland corresponding to the mucoid zone, in the area of concentration of ACTH-MSH cells. In eight cases, the lesions measured from 6 to 9 mm and

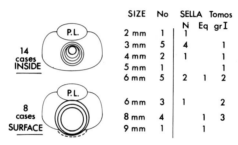

MICROADENOMA
IN
CUSHING'S SYNDROME
( 22 / 28 adenomas)

| | SIZE | No | SELLA N | Eq | Tomos gr I |
|---|---|---|---|---|---|
| P.L. 14 cases INSIDE | 2 mm | 1 | 1 | | |
| | 3 mm | 5 | 4 | | 1 |
| | 4 mm | 2 | 1 | | 1 |
| | 5 mm | 1 | | | 1 |
| | 6 mm | 5 | 2 | 1 | 2 |
| P.L. 8 cases SURFACE | 6 mm | 3 | 1 | | 2 |
| | 8 mm | 4 | | 1 | 3 |
| | 9 mm | 1 | | 1 | 1 |

*Fig. 1.* Localization of ACTH-secreting microadenomas.

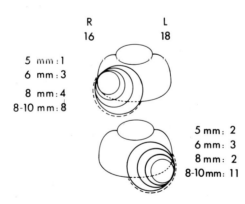

GROWTH HORMONE-SECRETING
MICROADENOMAS

( 34 cases )

R
16

L
18

5 mm : 1
6 mm : 3
8 mm : 4
8-10 mm : 8

5 mm : 2
6 mm : 3
8 mm : 2
8-10mm : 11

ALL SURFACE

ALL SELLA  gr I

*Fig. 2.* Localization of GH-secreting microadenomas.

could be seen readily at the surface of the gland upon opening the dura. In 14 cases where the lesion was smaller than 6 mm in diameter, it was found inside the gland after incision of the surface.

In acromegaly (Fig. 2), there were 34 cases of grade I sella with a microadenoma (four other cases of microadenoma were found in grade II sella previously treated with radiation therapy). Sixteen were located on the right side and 18 on the left side. The smaller ones measured 5 mm and were all readily seen, bulging on the anterior surface of the lateral wing.

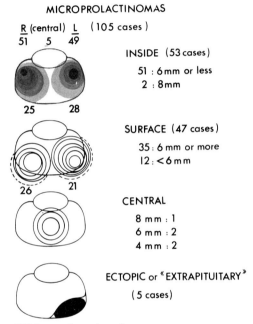

MICROPROLACTINOMAS

R (central) L    (105 cases)
51    5    49

INSIDE (53 cases)
51 : 6mm or less
2 : 8mm

25        28

SURFACE (47 cases)
35 : 6 mm or more
12 : <6mm

26        21

CENTRAL
8 mm : 1
6 mm : 2
4 mm : 2

ECTOPIC or "EXTRAPITUITARY"
(5 cases)

*Fig. 3.* Localization of PRL-secreting microadenomas.

In amenorrhea-galactorrhea and hyperprolactinemia (Fig. 3), there were 105 microadenomas. Five appeared to be predominantly located in the central midportion of the gland. All the others were lateral, 51 on the right side and 49 on the left side. Irrespective of the side of the lesion, 53 microadenomas were inside the gland, which had to be incised before discovering the lesion. All but two cases measured 6 mm or less in diameter. Forty-seven were seen bulging on the surface of the gland and 35 of those measured 6 mm or more in diameter. Thus, the smallest microadenomas are buried in the pituitary parenchyma while larger microadenomas protrude from the surface (Fig. 4).

As the microadenomas do not have a capsule but rather a thin sheath of compressed normal glandular tissue (Hardy, 1969a), it is often mandatory to perform a preoperative biopsy to ascertain the complete removal of adenomatous tissue.

In acromegaly, the texture and consistency of the microadenomas are clearly distinguishable from the normal tissue and most often the biopsy confirms the surgeon's visual impression (Hardy *et al.*, 1973; Hardy *et al.*, 1976). Prolactin microadenomas are presenting a challenging surgical problem because of their peculiar localization, their consistency and their morphological aspect (Hardy *et al.*, 1978). In contrast with GH and ACTH-secreting microadenoma, the pro-

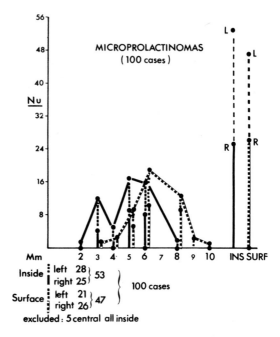

*Fig. 4.* Localization of microprolactinomas according to the tumor size.

lactin lesions are often paler, whitish, creamy or milky, almost similar to the surrounding softened oedematous normal pituitary gland. In those cases where the tumor was not apparent at the surface of the gland, the anterior portion of the lateral wing was excised and this fragment was used as a frozen biopsy to compare with the tumor tissue, resulting practically in a wedge resection.

In Cushing's disease, it is mandatory to obtain biopsies of the surrounding pituitary tissue if one wishes to preserve some pituitary functions. The real challenge is to be able to differentiate between a basophilic adenoma and the posterior neural lobe which appears almost similar in consistency and colour during the surgical dissection.

The pathological studies of our series (Robert, 1973; Robert and Hardy, 1975; Robert *et al.*, 1978; Robert, 1978) have shown that pituitary microadenomas in general do not show cellular features different from those found in larger pituitary tumors. In the growth hormone microadenomas, however, the tumoral cells are heavily granulated, in contrast to larger tumors which may be degranulated (Robert, 1978).

With regard to the concept of hyperplasia versus adenomatous tissue (Ludecke *et al.*, 1976), we may say that in our series, all cases of microadenomas histologically verified were true adenomas in acromegaly and Cushing's disease. In two cases of amenorrhea-galactorrhea with hyperprolactinemia associated with radiological and surgical signs of a pituitary tumor, the pathological examination revealed hyperplasia of thyrotrophic cells. These two cases also suffered from hypothyroidism. On the other hand, in 20 negative explorations (16 cases of hyperprolactinemia, 3 Cushing, 1 Nelson), the biopsies have not shown hyperplasia.

The incidence of microadenomas in routine autopsy cases has been a subject of great concern to us. Ten years ago, we reported a study carried out on 1000 autopsy specimens at the Notre-Dame Hospital and University of Montreal (Hardy, 1969b). We found 56 pituitaries containing a focal area of abnormal tissue. After removing the doubtful cases of hyperplasia or focal infarction, we were left with 27 cases which, according to the criteria of unicellular proliferation, were typical microadenomas. Therefore, the real incidence of microadenomas at autopsy is 2.7%. This incidence is in contrast with that of 22.5% reported by Costello (1936). His criteria may have been different from ours.

## CONCLUSION

The discovery of microadenomas associated with pituitary hypersecreting disorders is of paramount clinical significance and has resulted in a new therapeutic management of pituitary disorders (Hardy, 1975).

After the total selective removal of a hypersecreting pituitary microadenoma, a complete biological and clinical cure can be obtained in acromegaly (Hardy 1973), Cushing's disease and galactorrhea-amenorrhea with infertility syndrome (Hardy *et al.*, 1973; Hardy, 1975; Hardy *et al.*, 1976; Hardy and Vezina, 1976; Hardy *et al.*, 1978). The final evidence is the restoration of normal diurnal variation of growth hormone, cortisol and prolactin now and thereafter under the normal physiological control of hypothalamic factors. A persisting biological cure over a long period of time would support the hypothesis that pituitary hypersecreting disorders are produced by primary pituitary adenomas.

In contrast to the results obtained in the treatment of larger tumors, patients harbouring a microadenoma have a higher incidence of biological and clinical cure. The hypothesis of an hypothalamic disturbance of the releasing factors as the cause of tumor formation (Daughaday *et al.*, 1973) can hardly be supported on the basis of the results in those patients who remain cured following pituitary microadenomectomy. We believe that the persistence of elevated pituitary hormones following surgical treatment is not due to a perturbation of hypothalamic control but rather to the presence of residual adenomatous tissue.

Similar and more recent findings by other colleagues (Ludecke *et al.*, 1976; Salassa *et al.*, 1978; Wilson and Tyrrel, 1977; Wilson and Dempsey, 1978), who have been using our microsurgical technique have led from passive to active acceptance of the reality of pituitary microadenomas as internationally recognized for the first time by the theme of this symposium.

## REFERENCES

Costello, R. T. (1936). *Am. J. Pathol.* **12**, 205.
Daughaday, W. H., Cryer, P. E. and Jacobs, L. S. (1973). *In* "Diagnosis and Treatment of Pituitary Tumors" (P. O. Kohler and G. T. Ross, eds) 26–34. Elsevier, Amsterdam.
Guiot, G. *et al.*, (1958). *In* "Adénomes Hypophysaires", p. 216. Masson et Cie, Paris.
Hardy, J. (1969a). *Clin. Neurosurg.* **16**, 185.

Hardy, J. (1969b). *In* "Microneurosurgery" (R. W. Rand, ed) p. 87. Mosby, St. Louis.

Hardy, J. (1971). *J. Neurosurg.* **34**, 581.

Hardy, J. (1973). Proceedings of a conference held in Bethesda, Md., USA, pp. 18-194, Elsevier, Amsterdam.

Hardy, J. (1975). *In* "Progress in Neurological Surgery" (H. Krayenbühl, E. Maspes and W. H. Sweet, eds) 200-216. Karger, Basel.

Hardy, J. and Vezina, J. L. (1976). *In* "Advances in Neurology" (R. A. Thompson and J. R. Green, eds) 261-274. Raven Press, New York.

Hardy, J. and Wigser, S. (1965). *J. Neurosurg.* **23**, 612.

Hardy, J., Beauregard, H. and Robert, F. (1978). *In* "Progress in Prolactin; Physiology and Pathology" (C. Robyn and M. Harter, eds) Vol. II, 361-370.

Hardy, J., Somma, M. and Vezina, J. L. (1976). *In* "Current Controversies in Neurosurgery" (J. P. Morly, ed) 377-391. Saunders, Philadelphia.

Hardy, J., Robert, F., Somma, M. and Vezina, J. L. (1973). *Neuro-Chirurgie*, T. 19, Suppl. 2, 1. Masson et Cie, Paris.

Ludecke, D., Kautzky, R., Saeger, W. and Schrader, D. (1976). *Acta Neurochir.* **35**, 27.

Ray, B. S., Horwith, M. and Mantalen, C. (1968). *In* "Clinical Endocrinology" (E. B. Astwood and C. E. Cassidy eds) Vol. II, 93-102. Grune and Stratton, New York.

Robert, F. (1973). *Neuro-Chirurgie*, T. 19, Suppl. 2, 117.

Robert, F. (In press). "Electron Microscopy of Pituitary Adenomas". Raven Press, New York.

Robert, F. and Hardy, J. (1975). *Arch. Pathol.* **99**, 625.

Robert, F., Pelletier, G. and Hardy, J. (1978). *Arch. Pathol.* **102**, 448-455.

Salassa, R. M., Laws, E. R., Jr., Carpenter, P. C. *et al.* (1978). *Mayo Clin. Proc.* **53**, 24.

Sutton, T. J. and Vezina, J. L. (1974). *Am. J. Roentgenol.* **122**, 508.

Wilson, C. B., Tyrrel, J. B. (1977). *J. Neurosurg.* **47**, 840.

Wilson, C. B. and Dempsey, L. C. (1978). *J. Neurosurg.* **48**, 13.

# HYPOTHALAMIC MONOAMINE PATHWAYS AND THEIR POSSIBLE ROLE IN DISTURBANCES OF THE SECRETION OF HORMONES FROM THE ANTERIOR PITUITARY GLAND*

K. Fuxe, K. Andersson, L. Agnati, L. Ferland, T. Hökfelt, P. Eneroth[1] and J.-A. Gustafsson[2]

[1] Department of Histology, Department of Obstetrics and Gynecology and
[2] Department of Medical Chemistry, Karolinska Institutet Stockholm, Sweden

## INTRODUCTION

Neuroendocrinological research in recent years has clearly demonstrated that the catecholamine (CA) and 5-hydroxytryptamine (5HT) neurons innervating the hypothalamus, including the median eminence and limbic areas, play an important role in the control of LH, prolactin, GH, TSH and ACTH secretion (Costa and Gessa, 1977; Cox et al., 1978). In this paper special attention will be focused on the role of monoamines in the control of prolactin, GH and ACTH secretion since microadenomas in man produce the following three main types of diseases:

1)  The amenorrhea-galactorrhea syndrome (hypersecretion of prolactin),
2)  acromegaly (hypersecretion of GH) and
3)  Cushing's disease (hypersecretion of ACTH) (see Peillon et al., this symposium).

At the present time it seems possible that hypothalamic mechanisms could be of importance in the development of microadenomas since they exert both inhibitory and facilitatory effects on the secretion of anterior pituitary hormones through modulating the secretion of hypothalamic hormones from the median

*This work has been supported by a grant (04X-715) from the Swedish Medical Research Council and by a grant from Magnus Bergvall's Stiftelse.

eminence into the portal system. Monoamines are of special concern in this respect since they play a major role in the control of prolactin and GH secretion (Müller *et al.*, 1977).


## THE ANATOMY OF THE CENTRAL MONOAMINE SYSTEMS

The dopaminergic systems in the hypothalamus are mainly intrahypothalamic. Thus, the most important system is the tuberoinfundibular dopamine (DA) system which originates in the periventricular hypothalamic and arcuate nuclei and extensively innervates the external layer of the median eminence. Several types of tuberoinfundibular dopamine neurons probably exist. One system probably releases dopamine as a prolactin inhibitory factor (PIF) from the median eminence into the portal vessels (Macleod and Lehmeyer, 1974). In the rat this pathway seems to have a medial location innervating the medial palisade zone (MPZ) of the median eminence (Fuxe *et al.*, 1977a). Another DA system directly innervates the pars intermedia of the adenohypophysis (Björklund *et al.*, 1973) and can thus directly influence the secretion of the ACTH, α-MSH, β-endorphin and β-lipotropin present in these gland cells. Still another DA system may also establish axo–axonic contacts with LHRH-containing nerve terminals in the lateral palisade zone (LPZ). By way of this contact, DA may inhibit the release of LHRH through presynaptic inhibition (Fuxe *et al.*, 1979a). There may also exist within the external layer of the median eminence DA nerve terminals which can influence the secretion of somatostatin, GH releasing factor and TRH via axo–axonic interactions.

The noradrenaline (NA) nerve plexa present within the hypothalamus and the median eminence originate from NA cell bodies located within the medulla oblongata and the pons. The majority of the NA axons originate from non-locus coeruleus NA cell bodies. These give rise to the large and strongly fluorescent noradrenergic nerve terminal plexa of the hypothalamus. They contain a higher NA concentration per viscosity than the fine NA terminals originating from the locus coeruleus. It must be emphasized that each NA nerve terminal plexus present in one nucleus can be independently regulated from other hypothalamic NA plexa via dendro–axonic and axo–axonic interactions. Thus, local circuit neurons (Golgi type II nerve cells) seem to play an important role in the control of noradrenaline release and turnover (Fuxe *et al.*, 1978a). Obviously such neurons may also, through axo–axonic influences, differentially control DA release and turnover in the various parts of the external layer of the median eminence. Thus, some DA terminals in the median eminence may mainly be controlled by GABA terminals while others are controlled by enkephalin-containing terminals. Available evidence indicates that the NA nerve terminal plexa in various hypothalamic nuclei participate in the control of LH, prolactin, GH, TSH and ACTH secretion. It may, for example, be mentioned that the noradrenaline nerve terminal plexa in the preoptic area are involved with the facilitatory control of the phasic secretion of LH (Tyson, 1978) probably through inhibition of inhibitory intraneurons controlling activity in the LHRH pathways projecting to the external layer of the median eminence. By a similar mechanism, NA nerve terminal plexa in the paraventricular hypothalamic nucleus may facilitate activity in the TRH-containing pathways to the median eminence. It should be underlined that a rich NA nerve terminal plexus exists within the subependymal layer (SEL) of the median eminence and some NA terminals are also present within the MPZ.

In recent years evidence has also been obtained that adrenaline (A) pathways participate in the innervation of the hypothalamus. A nerve terminals are present in various hypothalamic nuclei, and A cell bodies seem to be located in the rostral part of the medulla oblongata (Hökfelt *et al.*, 1974). A nerve terminals are, for example, found within the periventricular and paraventricular hypothalamic nucleus and within the arcuate nucleus. Only a few are found within the internal layers of the median eminence. Evidence exists that they may participate in the control of prolactin, LH and GH secretion (Tyson, 1978; Fuxe *et al.*, 1977b, 1979a; Gold *et al.*, 1978).

Another important monoaminergic system to the hypothalamus is the 5HT system. This 5HT system originates mainly from the mesencephalic raphe nuclei and innervates practically all hypothalamic and preoptic nuclei. Available evidence indicates that this system participates in the control of the secretion of all of the anterior hypophyseal hormones (Müller *et al.*, 1977).

When performing experiments with α- and β-adrenergic agonists and antagonists it should be remembered that complex interactions exist between A and NA

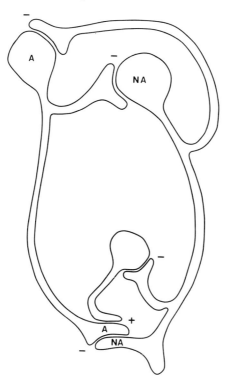

*Fig. 1.* Schematic illustration of interactions between Adrenaline (A) and Noradrenaline (NA) systems in the brain. The two CA systems may exert inhibitory effects on the activity of one another, effects which can be exerted both at the cell body and the nerve terminals.

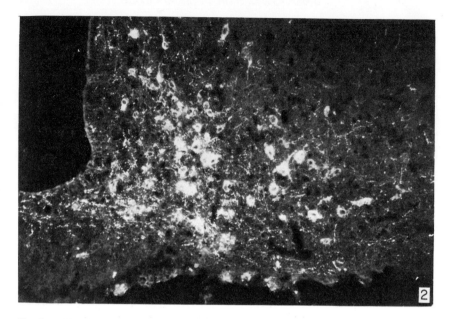

*Fig. 2.* ACTH-like immunoreactivity in nerve cell bodies and nerve terminals of the arcuate and periarcuate nucleus of the hypothalamus and of the subependymal layer of the median eminence. Antibodies against human ACTH 1–39 (Burroughs-Wellcome). Adult male rat. Colchicine treatment 24 h before killing (75 μg intraventricularly). × 120.

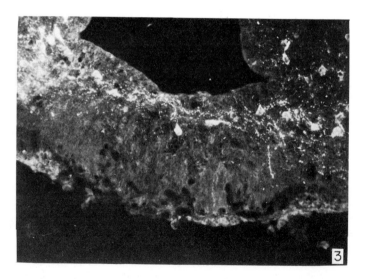

*Fig. 3.* ACTH-like immunoreactivity in nerve cell bodies and nerve terminals of the inner layers of the median eminence. For further details, see text to Fig. 2. × 120.

systems. A pathways seem to exert an inhibitory control of the activity in the NA systems mainly via an action on the cell bodies and dendrites of the NA nerve cells, but action at the NA nerve terminal level is also possible (Fig. 1). This control appears to be inhibitory. It also seems possible that the NA systems, in a similar way, can exert an inhibitory control over the activity in the A pathways.

So far we have described the existence of tubero-infundibular DA neurons and of reticulo-hypothalamic NA, A and 5HT pathways and the existence of peptidergic neurons innervating the external layer of the median eminence (Hökfelt *et al.*, 1978; Fuxe *et al.*, 1978a). Using antibodies against prolactin, ACTH 1–39 β-endorphin and β-lipotropin (Fuxe *et al.*, 1977c, 1978b; Akil *et al.*, 1978) evidence has also been obtained of the existence of nerve cell bodies within the arcuate and periarcuate nucleus and in the SEL of the median eminence, projecting not to the external layer of the median eminence but dorsally into periventricular hypothalamic and preoptic areas and into restricted areas of the thalamus and the limbic cortex (Figs 2 and 3). It is at present unclear to what extent prolactin-like, β-endorphin-like, ACTH-like immunoreactivity exist in one and the same nerve cell system or in different types of neurons. Also, it is unclear whether or not the respective antibodies can crossreact with the various peptides, proteins and possible precursor molecules claimed to exist in such nerve cells. These morphological studies indicate that ACTH-related peptides, β-endorphin-related peptides and prolactin-related proteins could have a role in synaptic functions in the brain. If so, they seem to participate in transmitting information from nerve cells originating in the medial basal hypothalamus. It seems possible that such nerve cells receive collaterals from various types of peptidergic and monoaminergic neurons innervating the medial basal hypothalamus including the external layer of the median eminence. Therefore, these newly discovered systems may represent feedback systems for informing various types of regions of the activity in *inter alia* peptidergic neurons releasing hypothalamic hormones into the primary capillary plexus.

## METHODS USED TO STUDY THE NEUROENDOCRINE FUNCTION OF THE CENTRAL MONOAMINE SYSTEMS

One way to analyze the neuroendocrine role of the monoamine pathways is to study the amine turnover in various endocrine states. In this laboratory amine turnover has over the years been measured by studying the disappearance of the CA and 5HT stores following inhibition of tyrosine hydroxylase and tryptophan hydroxylase respectively. As an inhibitor of CA synthesis, α-methyltyrosine methylester (H44/68) has been used and as an inhibitor of tryptophan hydroxylase, α-propyldopacetamide has been used (Andén *et al.*, 1969). The faster the disappearance of the monoamine stores after inhibition of amine synthesis, the higher the turnover in the system. The CA stores in the present experiments have been measured by means of quantitative microfluorometrical analysis of the CA fluorescence in brain sections processed by the Falck–Hillarp procedure for demonstration of cellular CA stores (Löfström *et al.*, 1976a, b). However, in order to understand the function of the CA systems in neuroendocrine regulation, it was important to evaluate not only presynaptic events but also postsynaptic events at the CA synapses. As an example, it may be mentioned that estrogen treatment of ovariectomized female rats in repeated doses of 25 μg/rat for 3 days (twice daily) results in a marked increase in the dissociation constant for $^3$H-clonidine binding in the hypothalamus (Fuxe *et al.*, 1979b). The $B_{max}$ values are increased by 100% after the estrogen treatment. One of the possible mechanisms for the estrogen-induced changes in receptor characteristics is illustrated in Fig. 4. In this schematic illustration it is suggested that estrogen stimulates estrogen receptors present in neurons innervated by NA terminals. The activation of the cytoplasmic estrogen receptor, following translocation of the receptor estrogen complex into the nucleus, leads to formation of messenger RNA, which in turn induces *de novo* protein synthesis. In this way regulators are formed which can block the action of cyclic AMP on the protein kinase that regulates receptor affinity. It is speculated that a high affinity α-receptor state requires phosphorylation of the receptor. Since the regulator will block the release of the catalytic unit of the protein kinase, no phosphorylation will occur and the α-receptor will exist mainly in the low affinity state, which characterizes the dephosphorylated α-receptor. It is further speculated that the presence of low affinity α-receptors initiates a feedback signal that stimulates receptor synthesis to compensate for the impairment of transmission. The increase in receptor synthesis would explain the increase in the $B_{max}$

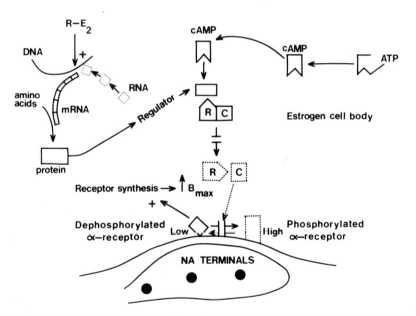

**Fig. 4.** Schematic illustration of a possible mechanism for the estrogen-induced changes in $^3$H-clonidine binding in the hypothalamus and preoptic area of the ovariectomized female rat. Estrogen (25 μg, twice daily, for 3 days) produces a marked lowering of the $K_D$ and an increase in $B_{max}$ for $^3$H-clonidine binding. This action could be due to blockade of a protein kinase which phosphorylates certain α-receptor sites from a low affinity dephosphorylated state into a high affinity phosphorylated state. This initiates a signal leading to increased receptor synthesis and thus to increased $B_{max}$ values.

values observed. Similar changes, but less marked, also occur with the α-adrenergic antagonists WB-4010 as radioligand. It must be emphasized, however, that $^3$H-spiroperidol binding to DA receptors in the striatum is not changed following treatment with estrogen of ovariectomized female rats. The dissociation constant remains the same whether estrogen is given or not. Thus the estrogen-induced changes in receptor characteristics in the α-receptor do not seem to be a general phenomenon, since the DA receptors do not appear to be affected in the same way. Instead, it may be speculated that the estrogen-induced change in the α-adrenergic receptors in the hypothalamus is part of the inhibitory feedback action of estrogen on the hypothalamus, since NA systems are facilitatory pathways for secretion of LHRH. Changes in α-receptor characteristics induced by estrogen are paralleled by a reduced NA turnover in the hypothalamus, which would further reduce NA receptor activity and thus lead to an even further reduction of activity in the LHRH pathways. In view of these findings it becomes important in various hormonal states also to evaluate the changes in the post-synaptic monoamine receptors that can be revealed by studies of the binding of various types of radioligands to the monoamine receptors.

## REGULATION OF PROLACTIN SECRETION BY MONOAMINERGIC SYSTEMS

Several investigations have indicated that DA can be released from the median eminence into the portal system to act as a potent prolactin inhibitory factor on DA receptors located on the prolactin-containing gland cells (MacLeod and Lehmeyer, 1974; Porter *et al.*, 1978). The inhibitory feedback effect of prolactin on its own secretion is probably also mediated by increasing the release of DA from the median eminence (Fuxe *et al.*, 1977d; Moore and Gudelsky, 1977). In the rat it seems that the DA projection to the MPZ is involved in the control of prolactin secretion. However, prolactin injections given in repeated doses or endogenous hypersecretion of prolactin from pituitary transplants not only increases the DA turnover in the MPZ but also in the LPZ where DA terminals *inter alia* may establish axo–axonic contacts with LHRH-containing nerve terminals (Fig. 5). Since DA seems to inhibit the release of LHRH from its nerve terminals, this action of prolactin may at least in part explain its ability to inhibit LH secretion (Fuxe *et al.*, 1977d). In man, hyperprolactinemia is associated with amenorrhea and in view of the above this symptom may be explained on the basis that prolactin can increase the release of DA onto the DA receptors controlling LHRH secretion (Fig. 5). The mechanism for the prolactin-induced increase of DA turnover is not known but could involve the activation of prolactin receptors in the medial basal hypothalamus. It may be mentioned that prolactin-like immunoreactivity has been described within nerve terminals in the arcuate nucleus and in the periventricular hypothalamic regions (Fuxe *et al.*, 1977c). It should be noted that acutely, within the first couple of hours, prolactin does not increase DA turnover (Fuxe *et al.*, 1978b). But it has been reported, based on *in vitro* studies, that prolactin can enhance the potassium-induced release of dopamine from the hypothalamus (Westfall and Perkins, 1978).

It is certainly possible that in some cases the tubero-infundibular DA neurons

GONADOTROPHIN    REGULATION

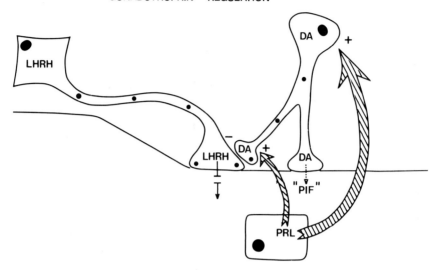

*Fig. 5.* Schematic illustration of the effects of prolactin on tubero-infundibular DA neurons leading to increased release of DA and subsequent inhibition of prolactin and LH secretion. This mechanism may partly explain the amenorrhéa found in hyperprolactinaemia in man.

are involved not only secondarily in pituitary disease processes. It may well be that an underfunctioning DA system controlling prolactin secretion contributes to the pathogenesis of a pituitary microadenoma, especially one which hyper-secretes prolactin. Thus, loss of inhibition by lack of activation of the inhibitory DA receptors located on prolactin-containing gland cells could be a contributory factor to the development of hyperplasia or of microadenomas secreting prolactin. According to such a hypothesis, however, the deficit in DA function in the median eminence should be localized, since one of the explanations for amenorrhea in hyperprolactinemia is based on the assumption that prolactin enhances DA receptor activity in those receptors located on LHRH-containing nerve terminals in the median eminence.

It should also be discussed that the possible deficits existing in certain tubero-infundibular DA systems may not be primarily caused by a malfunction of those systems but be due to malfunction in those neurons controlling the activity in the tubero-infundibular DA neurons. Recently it has been demonstrated that meten-kephalin and β-endorphin can reduce DA turnover in the external layer of the median eminence (Fig. 6). These effects were observed when endorphins were injected into the lateral ventricles of anesthetized or unanesthetized male rats (Fuxe *et al.*, 1978a). These results may reflect the existence of endorphin-containing interneurons in the medial basal hypothalamus that control activity in the tubero-infundibular dopamine neurons. It has in fact been demonstrated that such interneurons exist, and they appear to be of at least two types, one con-taining enkephalin-related peptides and one containing β-endorphin-related peptides (Hökfelt *et al.*, 1978). In the case of the β-endorphin-immuno-reactive neurons, the effects on the DA system are probably exerted at

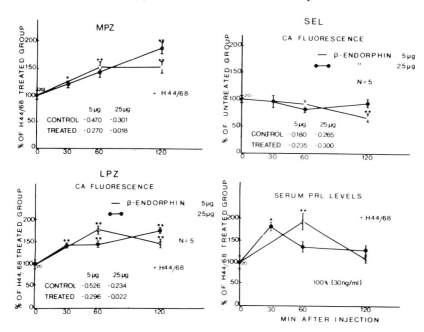

*Fig. 6.* The effects of β-endorphin on the H 44/68-induced CA fluorescence disappearance in the MPZ, LPZ and subependymal layer (SEL), and on serum prolactin levels of normal male rats. β-Endorphin was given intraventricularly to unanesthetized male rats in a dose of 5 or 25 μg/rat. The time after injection of β-endorphin is shown on the x-axis. On the y-axis the fluorescence values and prolactin levels are given in per cent of the values found in the respective H 44/68-alone group. Means ± s.e.m. are shown. All statistical comparisons were made with the H 44/68-alone group. Students' t-test; *; $P < 0.05$; ** $P < 0.01$. The rate constants for the CA disappearance in the various groups are shown in the tables of the figure. (Ferland *et al.*, to be published.)

the level of the nerve cell bodies (Fig. 7), since no β-endorphin-immunoreactive nerve terminals have been demonstrated in the external layer of the median eminence. In the case of the enkephalin immunoreactive interneurons, however, they may also influence the release of DA at the DA nerve terminals, since enkephalin immunoreactive nerve terminals exist not only within the arcuate nucleus but also within the external layer of the median eminence (Fig. 8). Results obtained with iontophoretic application of enkephalins onto arcuate cell bodies indicate that enkephalins can decrease activity in the tubero-infundibular systems by effects on the nerve cell bodies (Carette and Poulain 1978). It is well known that the enkephalins and β-endorphin markedly increase prolactin secretion, and this effect may, thus, partly be caused by inhibition of activity in the tubero-infundibular DA neurons that release DA as PIF into the portal vessels. Overactivity in the endorphin neurons may therefore result in hyperprolactinemia.

As pointed out earlier in this communication, there is a direct DA innervation of the intermediate lobe, where ACTH and β-endorphin related peptides have recently been demonstrated in one and the same gland cell (Akil *et al.*, 1978). It may be speculated that a malfunction of this DA system could lead to increased secretion of e.g. β-endorphins from the intermediate lobe into the circulation.

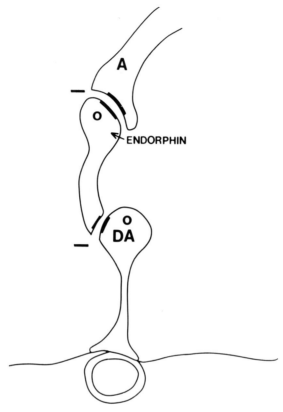

*Fig. 7.* Schematic illustration of the nervous control of the tubero-infundibular DA neurons to the MPZ of the rat. Adrenergic nerve terminals may increase activity in the DA neurons by inhibiting activity in endorphin-immunoreactive neurons (enkephalin- or β-endorphin-immunoreactive nerve cells) inhibiting activity in these DA systems.

ENK.–DA INTERACTION IN CONTROL OF PROLACTIN SECRETION

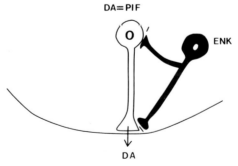

*Fig. 8.* Schematic illustration of interactions between enkephalin-immunoreactive and tubero-infundibular DA neurons involved in central control of prolactin secretion.

Available evidence indicates that the DA system exerts an inhibitory control over the secretion of hormones from gland cells in the intermediate lobe. Therefore, under these conditions β-endorphins and their fragments may reach the median eminence through retrograde flow in the infundibular stalk (Porter *et al.*, 1978), and there they can turn off the DA systems in the median eminence, leading to decreased release of DA and increased secretion of prolactin (Fig. 16). In this way, secretion of opioid peptides from pituitary gland cells may seriously disturb the hypothalamic control of *inter alia* secretion of prolactin from the unaffected gland cells and will in this way worsen the endocrinological disturbance in these patients.

The adrenergic nerve terminals in the medial basal hypothalamus also seem to exert important control over the tubero-infundibular DA neurons controlling the secretion of prolactin (Fig. 7). Clonidine, which in low doses may preferentially activate A receptors, selectively increases CA turnover in the MPZ and decreases prolactin secretion (Fuxe *et al.*, 1977a, b). On the other hand, the α-adrenergic blocking agents piperoxane and yohimbine, which may preferentially block A receptors, markedly increase prolactin secretion. Also inhibitors of the enzyme phenylethanolamine-*N*-methyltransferase markedly increase prolactin secretion, and this increase is associated with a depletion of the catecholamine stores in the MPZ of the median eminence (Fuxe *et al.*, 1979b). This depletion may be related to reduced activity in the tubero-infundibular DA neurons to the MPZ. In view of the fact that A mainly exerts inhibitory effects on the nerve cells it innervates (Cedarbaum and Aghajanian, 1976), it seems likely that the adrenergic nerve terminals may increase activity in the tubero-infundibular DA neurons via inhibiting the activity in inhibitory interneurons controlling the tubero-infundibular DA systems. This possibility is illustrated in Fig. 7. In this figure it is also endorphin-containing interneuron. From the above it is clear that malfunction of the adrenergic systems can lead to increased secretion of prolactin, probably related to decreased activity in the tubero-infundibular DA system. Thus, blockade of A receptors or increased activity at certain types of opiate receptors will produce hyperprolactinemia probably by turning off activity in one of the tubero-infundibular DA systems. Obviously, in patients with hyperprolactinemia caused by a functional disturbance in the tubero-infundibular DA neurons, treatment with certain types of α-adrenergic receptor agonists and with certain types of opiate receptor blocking agents may prove to be of therapeutic significance.

In contrast, NA nerve terminals in the hypothalamus seem to exert a facilitatory influence on the secretion of prolactin. Lesions of the ascending NA pathways to the hypothalamus diminish the increases in prolactin secretion observed in proestrous during the ovarian cycle (Martinovic and McCann, 1977). It seems possible that increased activation of NA receptors may contribute to the increases in prolactin secretion observed in relation to stress. Stress-induced increases in prolactin secretion can be mediated by reduced activity in the DA systems to the median eminence. Immobilization stress does reduce DA turnover in the external layer of the median eminence (Lidbrink *et al.*, 1972). NA nerve terminals within the paraventricular hypothalamic nucleus may also be involved in the facilitatory effects of NA pathways on prolactin secretion. NA receptor activity in this region seems to facilitate activity in the TRH bodies located in this area and which seem to project to the external layer of the median eminence. It is well known that TRH can increase prolactin secretion.

The work of Kordon and collaborators (Kordan *et al.*, 1976) has demonstrated that 5HT nerve terminals in the hypothalamus exert a facilitatory control over prolactin secretion, especially with relation to suckling-induced increases of prolactin secretion. It seems possible that the facilitatory effects are produced via an increased activity in neurons that release a prolactin releasing factor. The 5HT-receptor blocking agent metergoline does not influence the DA turnover in the various tubero-infundibular systems (Fuxe *et al.*, 1975). In this laboratory evidence has also been obtained that 5HT terminals participate in the facilitatory control of prolactin secretion, since highly selective 5HT-uptake blocking agents produce dose-related increases of prolactin secretion (Fuxe *et al.*, 1978b).

Taken together the above findings demonstrate that endorphins and various types of monoamines in the medial basal hypothalamus play an important role in the control of prolactin secretion. In fact the present treatment of hyperprolactinemia is based on activating the inhibitory dopamine receptors located on the prolactin-containing gland cells. The dopaminergic ergot derivative Bromocriptine has proved to be highly effective in lowering prolactin secretion in patients with hyperprolactinemia.

The prolactin-containing gland cells may, however, also contain other types of receptors which may inhibit the secretion of prolactin. Thus, in this laboratory, it has recently been discovered (Fuxe *et al.*, 1978c) that the androgenic steroid methyltrienolone (R1881) can markedly inhibit the secretion of prolactin in castrated male rats (Fig. 10). As can be seen in the figure, these animals did not respond with hypersecretion of prolactin after treatment with the tyrosine hydroxylase inhibitor α-methyl-tyrosine methylester (H44/68) 4 h after R1881. As a matter of fact, 12–48 h following the injection, R1881 in a dose of 1 mg/rat markedly prevented the prolactin hypersecretion induced by H44/68. As seen in Fig. 11, R1881 can increase DA turnover within the MPZ and LPZ, as evidenced by the enhanced disappearance of the CA fluorescence following treatment with H44/68 plus R1881. However, this action is probably not responsible for the marked inhibition of prolactin secretion, since similar increases in DA turnover are also observed following treatment with testosterone propionate or 5α-dihydro-testosterone propionate, which do not cause any significant inhibition of prolactin

R 1881 (ANDROGEN)

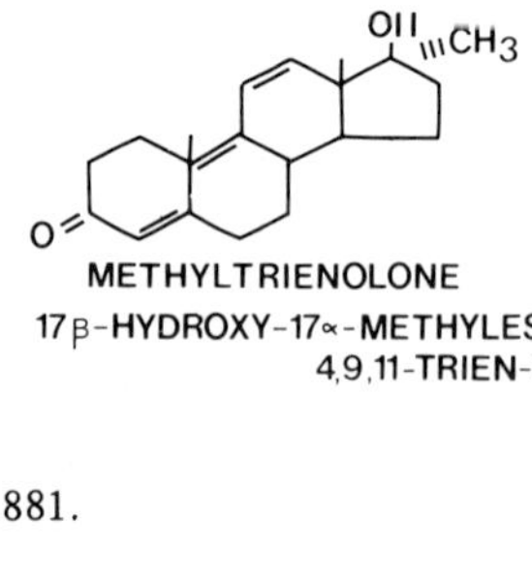

METHYLTRIENOLONE
17β-HYDROXY-17α-METHYLESTRA-
4,9,11-TRIEN-3-ONE

*Fig. 9.* The formula of R1881.

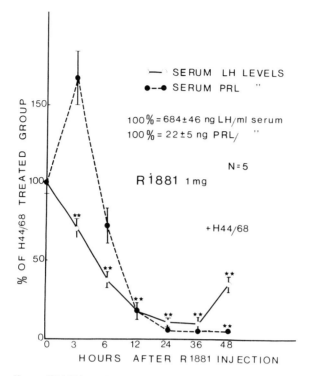

*Fig. 10.* The effects of R1881 on the serum levels of LH and prolactin in the castrated male rat (4 weeks). The dose of R1881 was 1 mg/rat, and the rats were killed at various time intervals after the injection. Two hours before killing all rats received an injection of H 44/68, a tyrosin hydroxylase inhibitor. Means ± s.e.m. are shown for 4-5 rats. The values are given in per cent of the H 44/68-alone group mean value. Students' *t*-test ** : $P < 0.01$. All comparisons were made with the H 44/68-alone group.

secretion, and since TH inhibition does not increase prolactin levels after R1881 treatment. Therefore, the existence of an androgen steroid receptor on the prolactin gland cells may be postulated. Activation of this receptor by R1881 seems to lead to a dramatic reduction in prolactin secretion. It will be of interest to evaluate whether activation of this receptor can be an important new principle for the treatment of hyperprolactinemia in man.

Finally, it should be emphasized that hypersecretion of prolactin from the pituitary gland does not only influence neuron systems within the hypothalamus but changes in dopamine turnover following injections of prolactin have also been observed within the ascending mesoaccumbens DA systems and in certain types of mesostriatal DA systems. In patients with hyperprolactinemia, behavioral and mental changes may be produced by prolactin. In animals the importance of prolactin for various aspects of maternal behavior has been demonstrated.

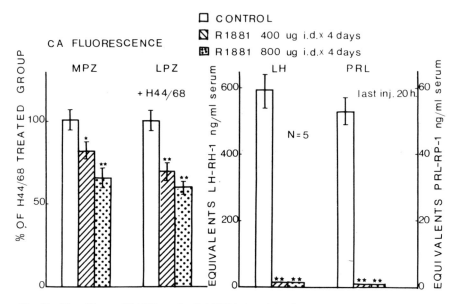

*Fig. 11.* The effects of R1881 on the H 44/68-induced CA fluorescence disappearance in the external layer of the median eminence and on the serum LH and prolactin levels of the castrated male rat. The control rats received solvent. The rats were killed 20 h after the last R1881 injection and 2 h after the H 44/68 injection (250 mg/kg i.p.). Means ± s.e.m. are shown for 4–5 rats. All comparisons were made with the respective control groups (H 44/68-alone group + solvent). Students' $t$-test *: $P < 0.05$; ** $P < 0.01$.

## REGULATION OF GH SECRETION BY MONOAMINE SYSTEMS

GH-secreting microadenomas in the anterior pituitary gland produce acromegaly. It is, therefore, relevant to discuss a possible involvement of the monoamine systems in the pathogenesis of this disease. First, the role of monoamines in the regulation of growth hormone secretion in intact animals will briefly be summarized.

Studies in the rat indicate that noradrenergic and adrenergic pathways have a facilitatory influence on the secretion of GH (Müller, 1976). The fact that injections of GH into the hypophysectomized rat (Andersson *et al.*, 1977) selectively decrease NA turnover in the posterior periventricular hypothalamic region has been interpreted to suggest that NA terminals in this region can facilitate activity in growth hormone releasing factor (GRF)-containing nerve cells present in this area. As already pointed out in this article, clonidine in low doses can preferentially increase A receptor activity. It is also known that clonidine can increase GH secretion and as reported above it can increase DA turnover in the MPZ of the median eminence of the rat. In view of this, it is possible that the facilitatory effects of adrenergic neurons on GH secretion can in part be mediated by increasing activity in DA terminals that establish inhibitory axo–axonic synapses with somatostatin-containing nerve terminals in the MPZ. This hypothesis however seems to be contradicted by the fact that dopaminergic drugs can decrease GH secretion in the rat (Müller, 1976; Müller *et al.*, 1979), and DA can increase somatostatin levels in the portal vessels (Chihara and Arimura, 1978). These results may, however, be explained on the basis of either preferential DA auto-receptor activation and/or depolarization-induced release of somatostatin when the activity of the somatostatin neurons is low (Müller *et al.*, 1979). It may also be speculated that inhibitory axonic DA receptors also exist on the GRF-containing nerve terminals in the median eminence (Fig. 12). If the last speculation is accepted, the final effect of dopaminergic drugs on GH regulation will depend upon the sensitivity of the DA receptors located on the somatostatin- and GRF-containing nerve terminals and on the activity in the somatostatin- and GRF-containing neurons. It may be that when dopaminergic drugs are given to rodents, the activation of DA receptors located on GRF-containing terminals will dominate,

Dopamine mediated GH-feedback in the normal male

Predominant pathway
in normal man

Predominant pathway
in normal rat

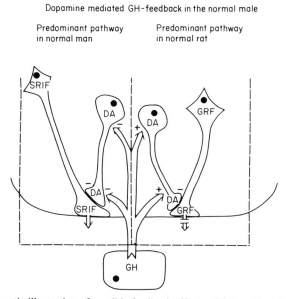

*Fig. 12.* Schematic illustration of possible feedback effects of GH on the tubero-infundibular DA systems controlling somatostatin and GRF containing systems.

while in man the activation of DA receptors located on somatostatin terminals will dominate and cause the increases in GH secretion observed in normal subjects following treatment with dopaminergic drugs.

It should again be mentioned that in the hypophysectomized rat, GH given intravenously acutely reduces DA turnover within the MPZ and LPZ of the median eminence (Fig. 13). These results can be interpreted as suggesting that part of the inhibitory feedback action of GH on its own secretion involves blocking of DA release onto DA receptors located on somatostatin-containing nerve terminals, allowing the somatostatin release to increase in order to reduce the GH secretion. It seems likely that in the hypophysectomized animal the release of GRF from the median eminence is maximal and therefore further reduction of DA release onto the GRF-containing nerve terminals would have little significance.

The present hypothesis may also in part explain how β-endorphin can increase GH secretion while at the same time reducing DA turnover in the MPZ and LPZ of the median eminence of the rat. Under the influence of β-endorphin the reduction in DA receptor activity at the GRF-containing terminals will dominate over the reduction of DA receptor activity at the somatostatin-containing nerve terminals. The reason for this may be that β-endorphin can increase NA turnover in the posterior periventricular hypothalamic region, where GRF-containing nerve cell bodies may be located, while leaving NA turnover unaffected in the anterior periventricular hypothalamic region, where somatostatin-containing nerve cell bodies are located.

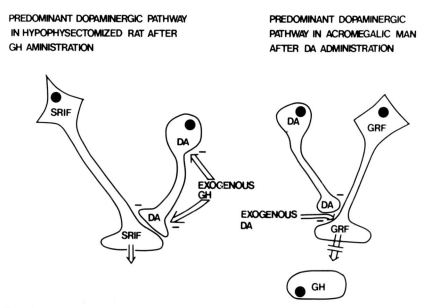

PREDOMINANT DOPAMINERGIC PATHWAY IN HYPOPHYSECTOMIZED RAT AFTER GH AMINISTRATION

PREDOMINANT DOPAMINERGIC PATHWAY IN ACROMEGALIC MAN AFTER DA ADMINISTRATION

*Fig. 13.* Schematic illustration of possible hypothalamic DA involvement after exogenous GH and DA administration to hypophysectomized rats and acromegalic man.

In this context, it should be discussed why dopaminergic agents inhibit GH secretion in acromegalic patients while increasing it in normal volunteers. The most common explanation offered is that the abnormal GH-secreting gland cells, in contrast to the normal GH-containing gland cells, possess DA receptors that are inhibitory with regard to release of GH (Müller *et al.*, 1977). However, the present hypothesis offers a complementary explanation for this paradoxical effect seen in acromegalic patients. If the hypersecretion of GH is mainly due to increased activity in GRF neurons, the inhibitory effects of a DA agonist at GRF terminals will dominate over those at somatostatin terminals and a reduction in GH secretion will occur (Fig. 13). The unmasking of inhibitory DA receptors on the GH-containing gland cells in the microadenomas may, however, be the major mechanism by which DA agonists reduce GH secretion, especially since the concentrations of hypothalamic hormones reaching the gland cells of the microadenomas, once developed, may be considerably lower than in normal pituitary glands.

It should be mentioned that somatostatin, at least in the thyroidectomized animal, seems capable of reducing prolactin secretion. In the four-week thyroid-ectomized rat, the prolactin secretion induced by a tyrosine hydroxylase inhibitor is less. Also the pulsatile secretion of GH appears to be counteracted. At the same time a decreased DA turnover exists in external layer of the median eminence (Fig. 14). All these findings can be explained on the basis of an increased secretion

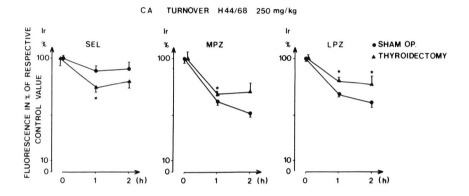

*Fig. 14.* Effects of thyroidectomy (one month) on the H 44/68-induced CA fluorescence disappearance in the male rat. The fluorescence values are given in per cent of the respective control group's mean value. H 44/68 was given in a dose of 250 mg/kg 1 and 2 h before killing. Means ± s.e.m. are shown for 6-8 rats. Mann-Whitney *U* test. All comparisons are made with the respective control group value.

of somatostatin, in part induced by a decreased DA activity in the external layer of the median eminence. These results indicate the potential importance of testing somatostatin as an inhibitor of prolactin and GH secretion in man. In Fig. 15, possible monoaminergic mechanisms operating in the four-week thyroidectomized male rat in the control of GH prolactin and TSH secretion are schematically illustrated. As can be seen, a facilitatory noradrenergic mechanism seems to operate in the paraventricular hypothalamic nucleus to facilitate the activity in TRH neurons projecting to the external layer of the median eminence. In the median eminence some DA synapse also seem to be involved in the inhibitory control of TRH release.

Finally, it should be mentioned that not only facilitatory 5HT mechanisms may exist in the control of GH secretion, but there may also be inhibitory 5HT mechanisms, since specific 5HT-uptake blocking agents produce dose-dependent inhibitions of GH secretion (Fuxe *et al.*, 1978b; de Wied and de Jong, 1974).

32                 *K. Fuxe et al.*

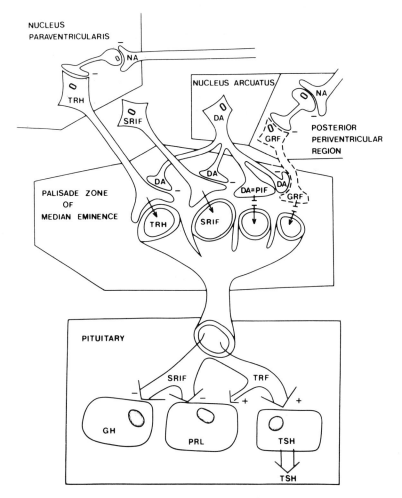

*Fig. 15.* Schematic illustration of the dopaminergic and noradrenergic mechanisms involved in the control TRH, PIF, GRF and somatostatin (SRIF) secretion in the thyroidectomized male rat.

## REGULATION OF ACTH SECRETION BY MONOAMINERGIC SYSTEMS

Microadenomas that secrete ACTH induce Cushing's disease. Immunohisto-chemistry indicates that these microadenomas contain in the gland cells not only ACTH but also α-MSH, β-MSH and β-endorphins (Peillon *et al.*, 1978, this sympo-sium). Noradrenergic and adrenergic pathways to the hypothalamus seem to exert an inhibitory effect on the secretion of ACTH. Injections of PMNT inhibitors increase corticosterone secretion (Fuxe *et al.*, 1979a) and ACTH (100 $\mu g/kg$) given intravenously to hypophysectomized animals will acutely preferentially increase NA turnover within the SEL and the MPZ of the median eminence (Andersson, Fuxe, Eneroth, Gustafsson and Skett, to be published). Therefore, ACTH may exert an inhibitory feedback effect on its own secretion by increasing NA receptor activity in these parts of the median eminence, in this way perhaps inhibiting activity in putative CRF-containing neurons projecting from the SEL into the MPZ. Also $\beta$-endorphin increases NA turnover in SEL (Fig. 16). It is at present unclear whether DA in the median eminence plays any role in the control of the secretion of CRF. 5HT systems may exert both inhibitory and facilitatory effects on the secretion of CRF (Müller *et al.*, 1977; Fuxe *et al.*, 1978d). In view of the above, activation of hypothalamic $\alpha$-adrenergic mechanisms should be helpful for inhibiting activity in CRF-containing pathways and in this way diminishing the hypersecretion of ACTH. Furthermore, a deficit in the activity of the noradrenergic systems projecting into the median eminence should contribute to the development of hypersecretion of ACTH.

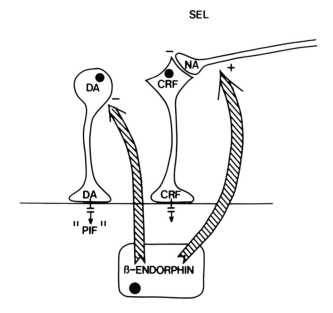

*Fig. 16.* Schematic illustration of the effects of $\beta$-endorphin on NA and DA mechanisms involved in control of CRF and prolactin secretion.

The prolactin-induced reduction of LH secretion seems to be the result, at least in part, of an activation of the dopaminergic receptors localized on the LHRH-containing nerve terminals that inhibit the release of LHRH.

The existence of facilitatory noradrenergic and adrenergic control of GH secretion is suggested as well as a complex regulation of somatostatin and GRF secretion by dopaminergic mechanisms in the external layer of the median eminence. It is emphasized that β-endorphin and its fragments may be secreted in increased amounts in the diseased pituitary gland. By influencing DA turnover within the median eminence, these opiate peptides can further aggravate the endocrine disturbances found in patients with microadenomas. In the case of ACTH regulation, the importance of inhibitory noradrenergic nerve terminals in the MPZ and the SEL of the median eminence is emphasized and their preferential activation of ACTH 1-24 is shown.

## REFERENCES

Akil, H., Watson, S. J., Levy, R. M. and Barchas, J. D. (1978). *In* "Characteristics and Function of Opioids" (J. M. van Ree and L. Terenius, eds) 123–134. Elsevier, Amsterdam.

Andén, N.-E., Corrodi, H. and Fuxe, K. (1969). *In* "Metabolism of Amines in the Brain" (G. Hooper, ed) 38–47. Macmillan, London.

Andersson, K., Fuxe, K., Eneroth, P., Gustafsson, J.-A. and Skett, P. (1977). *Neuroscience Letter* **3**, 83–89.

Björklund, A., Moore, R. Y., Nobin, A. and Stenevi, U. (1973). *Brain Res.* **51**, 171.

Carette, B. and Poulain, P. (1978). *Neuroscience Letter* **7**, 137.

Cedarbaum, J. M. and Aghajanian, G. K. (1976). *Brain Research* **112**, 413.

Chihara, K. and Arimura, K. (1978). Proc. 60th Ann. Meeting, Endocrine Society, Americana Hotel, Miami, Florida, A241, p. 195 (abst.).

Costa, E. and Gessa, G. L. (1977). "Advances in Biochemical Psychopharmacology", Vol. 16, 1–709. Raven Press, New York.

Cox, B., Morris, I. D. and Weston, A. H. (1978). "Pharmacology of the Hypothalamus", 1–277. Macmillan, London.

Fuxe, K., Agnati, L. and Everitt, B. (1975). *Neuroscience Letter* **1**, 283.

Fuxe, K., Agnati, L., Eneroth, P., Gustafsson, J.-Å., Hökfelt, T., Löfström, A., Skett, B. and Skett, P. (1977a). *Medical Biology* **55**, 148.

Fuxe, K., Pérez de la Mora, M., Agnati, L., Eneroth, P., Gustafsson, J.-Å., Skett, P. and Ögren, S.-O. (1977b). *Acta Endocrinologica*, Suppl. 212, p. 15.

Fuxe, K., Hökfelt, T., Eneroth, P., Gustafsson, J.-Å. and Skett, P. (1977c). *Science* **196**, 899.

Fuxe, K., Löfström, A., Agnati, L., Hökfelt, T., Johansson, O., Eneroth, P., Gustafsson, J.-Å., Skett, P., Jeffcoate, S. and Fraser, H. (1977d). *In* "Progress in Reproductive Biology, Volume 2, Clinical Reproductive Neuroendocrinology" (P. O. Hubinont, M. L'Hermite and C. Robyn, eds) 41–53. Karger, Basel.

Fuxe, K., Ferland, L., Andersson, K., Eneroth, P., Gustafsson, J.-Å. and Skett, P. (1978a). *In* "Brain-Endocrine Interaction" (D. Scott, ed) Vol. III, 172–182. Karger, Basel.

Fuxe, K., Ögren, S.-O., Everitt, B. J., Agnati, L. F., Eneroth, P., Gustafsson, J.-Å., Jonsson, G., Skett, P. and Holm, A. C. (1978b). *In* "Depressive Disorders" (F. K. Garattini, ed) 67–94. Schattauer Verlag, Stuttgart and New York.

Fuxe, K., Andersson, K., Löfström, A., Hökfelt, T., Ferland, L., Agnati, L. F., Pérez de la Mora, M., Schwarcz, R., Eneroth, P., Gustafsson, J.-Å and Skett, P. (1979a). *In* "Principles for the Central Regulation of the Endocrine System", Nobel Symposium 42 (K. Fuxe, T. Hökfelt and R. Luft, eds). Plenum, New York (in press).

Fuxe, K., Andersson, K., Agnati, F., Ferland, L., Hökfelt, T., Eneroth, P., Gustafsson, J.-Å. and Skett, P. (1979b). *In* "Catecholamines: Basic and Clinical Frontiers", Pergamon Press, Oxford (in press).

Gold, M. S., Donabedian, R. K. and Redmond, D. E. (1978). *Psychoneuroendocrinology* **3**, 187.

Hökfelt, T., Fuxe, K., Goldstein, M. and Johansson, O. (1974). *Brain Research* **66**, 235.

Hökfelt, T., Elde, R., Fuxe, K., Johansson, O., Ljungdahl, Å., Goldstein, M., Luft, R., Efendic, S., Nilsson, G., Terenius, L., Ganten, D., Jeffcoate, S. L., Rehfeld, J., Said, S., Pérez de la Mora, M., Possani, L., Tapia, R., Teran, L. and Palacios, R. (1978). *In* "The Hypothalamus" (S. Reichlin, R. J. Baldessarini and J. B. Martin, eds) 69–135. Raven Press, New York.

Kordon, C., Epelbaum, J., Enjalbert, A. and McKelvy, J. (1976). *In* "Subcellular Mechanisms in Reproductive Neuroendocrinology" (F. Naftolin, K. J. Ryan and J. Davies, eds) 167–184. Elsevier, Amsterdam.

Lidbrink, P., Corrodi, H., Fuxe, K. and Olson, L. (1972). *Brain Research* **45**, 507.

Löfström, A., Jonsson, G. and Fuxe, K. (1976a). *Journal of Histochemistry and Cytochemistry* **24**, 415.

Löfström, A., Jonsson, G., Wiesel, F.-A. and Fuxe, K. (1976b). *Journal of Histochemistry and Cytochemistry* **24**, 430.

MacLeod, R. M. and Lehmeyer, J. E. (1974). *Endocrinology* **94**, 1077.

Martinovic, J. V. and McCann, S. M. (1977). *Endocrinology* **100**, 1206.

Moore, K. E. and Gudelsky, G. A. (1977). *Advances in Biochemical Psychopharmacology* **16**, 227.

Müller, E. E. (1976). *In* "Proceedings of the Sixth International Congress of Pharmacology" (J. Tuomisto and M. K. Paasonen, eds) Vol. 3 (M. Airaksinen, ed) 131–145. Pergamon ⌐ress, New York.

Müller, E. E., Nisticò, G. and Scapagnini, U. (1977). "Neurotransmitter and Anterior Pituitary Function". Academic Press, New York and London.

Müller, E. E., Cocchi, D., Locatelli, V., Parati, E. A. and Mantegazza, P. (1979). *In* "Principles for the Central Regulation of the Endocrine System", Nobel Symposium 42 (K. Fuxe, T. Hökfelt and R. Luft, eds). Plenum, New York.

Porter J. C., Barnea, A., Cramer, O. M. and Parker, C. R. Jr. (1978). *Clinics in Obstetrics and Gynaecology* **5**, 271.

Tyson, J. E. (1978). *Clinics in Obstetrics and Gynaecology* **5**, 1.

Westfall, T. C. and Perkins, N. A. (1978). *In* "Catecholamines: Basic and Clinical Frontiers", Abstract 78.

de Wied, D. and de Jong, W. (1974). *Ann. Rev. Pharmacol.* **14**, 389.

# SUPPRESSION OF PROLACTIN SECRETION BY THE PHYSIOLOGICAL AND PHARMACOLOGICAL MANIPULATION OF PITUITARY DOPAMINE RECEPTORS*

R. M. MacLeod, S. W. J. Lamberts, I. Nagy, I. S. Login and C. A. Valdenegro

*Department of Medicine, University of Virginia School of Medicine, Charlottesville, Virginia 22908, USA*

## INTRODUCTION

Recently extraordinarily productive studies of the neuroendocrine mechanisms regulating pituitary hormone secretion have generated results which have been widely applied in the clinical management of pituitary disorders. Prolactin, whose very existence was occasionally denied several years ago, has emerged as the pituitary hormone most extensively studied (MacLeod, 1976; Thorner, 1977; Lamberts and MacLeod, 1977). There are several reasons for this, First, hypersecretion of prolactin by a hyperplastic gland or microadenoma is the most frequently documented pituitary disease. Second, the ease with which prolactin secretion can be physiologically and pharmacologically manipulated has encouraged a broad spectrum of investigations.

## DOPAMINE AS A PHYSIOLOGICAL INHIBITOR OF PROLACTIN SECRETION

Dopamine is now acknowledged to be the principle regulator of prolactin secretion. Such a role for this neurotransmitter was initially suggested by its abundance in the median eminence, and especially by its concentration near

---

*This work was supported by USPHS Research Grant CA-07535-15 from the National Cancer Institute.

the vasculature draining that region of the hypothalamus and ultimately leading into the anterior pituitary. The identification of dopamine in portal plasma and in semi-purified hypothalamic preparations capable of inhibiting prolactin secretion contributed to the recognition of dopamine's importance in this system (Ben-Jonathan et al., 1977; Gibbs and Neill, 1978; Shaar and Clemens, 1974; Schally et al., 1976).

The anterior pituitary is known to secrete significantly increased prolactin following the removal of the gland from the sella turcica. Thus physiological substance(s) external to the tissue normally inhibit secretion of the hormone. When anterior pituitary tissue is incubated in vitro, copious prolactin release begins almost instantly and continues for prolonged periods. Hence the removal of the physiological inhibitor permits increased prolactin secretion without the aid of stimulating factor(s).

Ten years ago, catecholamines were demonstrated to inhibit prolactin secretion in vitro (MacLeod and Lehmeyer, 1969). Numerous other investigators have confirmed dopamine's inhibition of prolactin secretion (MacLeod, 1976). Studies conducted in our laboratory have used the traditional radioimmunoassay for prolactin and the more sensitive technique of measuring the isotopically labeled prolactin synthesized by the tissues incubated in vitro with $^3$H-leucine. The data in Table I show that 500 nM dopamine blocks the pituitary secretion of $^3$H-prolactin almost completely during a six hour incubation. During this time $^3$H-prolactin accumulates in the pituitary, but over long periods of incubation,

Table I.   The effect of dopamine on the in vitro synthesis of prolactin.

| Incubation time | Control incubation prolactin c.p.m./mg pituitary | | | Dopamine incubation prolactin c.p.m./mg pituitary | | |
|---|---|---|---|---|---|---|
| | Pituitary gland | Incubation medium | Total | Pituitary gland | Incubation medium | Total |
| 60 min | 210 | 20 | 230 | 250 | 0 | 250 |
| 120 min | 300 | 190 | 490 | 520 | 20 | 540 |
| 240 min | 360 | 2000 | 2360 | 1180 | 50 | 1230 |
| 360 min | 600 | 4400 | 5000 | 1500 | 200 | 1700 |

Three hemipituitary glands from female rats incubated in Medium 199 containing 500 nM dopamine and 10 µCi $^3$H-leucin. Following incubation aliquots of pituitary homogenates and incubation medium were subjected to polyacrylamide gel electrophoresis and the radioactive prolactin in the discs was measured.

prolactin synthesis is eventually curtailed. It is presumed that the accumulation of prolactin in the lactotroph initiates a signal in the tissue which depresses the continued synthesis of the hormone. That these effects are only transient is indicated by the rapid release of prolactin from the gland upon replacement of the incubation medium with medium which does not contain dopamine.

Since these early observations, several dopaminergic drugs have been identified as potent prolactin secretion inhibitors. The data in Table II show that

*Table II.*　*In vitro* inhibition of prolactin secretion by
dopaminergic drugs.

| Drug | Concentration (nM) | Inhibition of prolactin secretion (%) |
|---|---|---|
| Control | 0 | — |
| Dopamine | 100 | 85 |
| Apomorphine | 50 | 62 |
| Bromocriptine | 2 | 94 |
| Bromocriptine | 1 | 84 |
| Bromocriptine | 0.5 | 24 |
| Lisuride | 1 | 93 |
| Piribedil | 50 | 66 |

Experiments conducted as described in Table I.

dopamine and apomorphine are among the least potent compounds which inhibit prolactin release, whereas extremely low concentrations of bromocriptine and lisuride are effective. None of these drugs significantly influence the *in vitro* secretion of growth hormone. Various other ergot alkaloids, such as ergocryptine and ergocornine, are also capable of decreasing prolactin secretion. Several anti-parkinsonian drugs have appeared which are dopamine agonists and inhibit the secretion of prolactin. Among these, piribedil was found to have approximately the same activity as dopamine to block hormone release. Many years ago we found that norepinephrine and epinephrine were capable of blocking prolactin release; however, they are somewhat less potent than dopamine. None of the metabolic methylated or deaminated products of the catecholamines are able to inhibit prolactin secretion (MacLeod and Lehmeyer, 1969).

In order to confirm that dopamine is a physiologic inhibitor of prolactin, it was necessary to show that its presence blocks release of the hormone rapidly and that the release resumes promptly upon removal of the catecholamine. We have recently addressed this problem using dispersed pituitary gland cells suspended in Bio-Gel P-2 and perfused in a chromatographic column, as described by Lowry (1974). Details of the method are given in Fig. 1.

A dispersed pituitary gland cell column was perfused for two hours with 500 nM dopamine. During this time the concentration of prolactin in the eluate decreased gradually to low levels (Fig. 1). The dopamine in the perfusate was then removed, and within ten minutes the pituitary cells resumed their normal rate of prolactin secretion, more than five-fold greater than that observed in the presence of dopamine. The cells maintained this rate until dopamine was introduced again into the perfusate and, as before, prolactin secretion decreased markedly. Removal of the dopamine permitted the cells to secrete prolactin normally. Although not shown in this study, this phenomenon can be repeated many times.

It is known that dibutyryl cAMP stimulates the *in vitro* secretion of prolactin

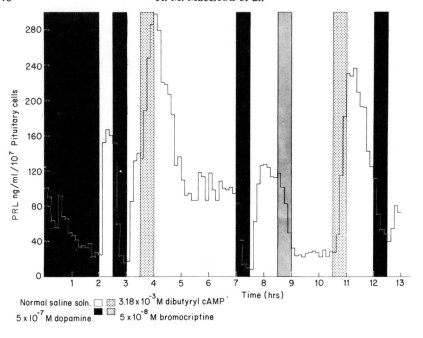

Normal saline soln. □ ▦ 3.18 x 10$^{-3}$ M dibutyryl cAMP

5 x 10$^{-7}$ M dopamine ■ □ 5 x 10$^{-8}$ M bromocriptine

*Fig. 1.* Perfusion of dispersed pituitary cells *in vitro*. Anterior pituitary glands from 12 female rats were quartered and placed in a Teflon® beaker containing 10 ml of Eagle Basal Solution (EBS), 5 μM dopamine (DA), 57 μM ascorbic acid (ASC) and 10 mg trypsin. The tissue was incubated at 37°C, stirring constantly with a Teflon® paddle at 350–400 r/min for 20 min. The cell suspension supernatant was removed and the residue was treated again. The dispersion was increased by gently drawing the remaining tissue with a disposable plastic pipette. The overall procedure was carried out four times, after which no appreciable large fragments of the glands were seen. The cell suspensions were centrifuged at room temperature at 32g (400 r/min) for 45 min. The supernatant was discarded and the cells suspended in 0.5 ml of a solution of 0.4 mg/ml lima bean trypsin inhibitor, 0.25% bovine serum albumin (BSA), 5 μM DA and 57 μM ASC in EBS. Debris were removed by filtration through a nylon gauze, and the cells were counted in a Newbauer counting chamber. Viability was determined by trypan blue exclusion. Cells (10$^7$) were mixed with 0.5 g Bio-Gel P-2 (Bio-Rad, 200–400 mesh) which was swollen overnight in normal saline solution. This suspension was placed in a 2 ml plastic disposable syringe and Medium 199 with Earle's balanced salt solution and L-Glutamine containing 5 μM DA, 5 mg/ml ASC. Prior to beginning the experiment 0.25% BSA, 75 μg/l streptomycin and 75 μg/l penicillin G were pumped through for 1.5 h.

Cells were subsequently exposed to pulses of DA (500 nM), bromocriptine (50 nM) and dibutyryl cAMP (3.18 mM). The solutions also contained 0.28 mM ascorbate, which continued to be perfused throughout the entire period of the experiment. Fractions of the eluant of the cell column were collected every 7.5 min, accounting for a volume of approximately 3.5 ml each. Concentration of prolactin in each sample was determined by the standard radioimmunoassay technique.

greatly (Hill *et al.*, 1976). That the nucleotide is also capable of stimulating prolactin secretion by dispersed cells is indicated in Fig. 1. It should be noted that the rate of prolactin release increased gradually throughout dbcAMP perfusion. Removal of the dbcAMP results in a gradual decrease in prolactin secretion which reached a steady state below the previous basal rate. A probable explanation for this finding is the partial exhaustion of prolactin stores within the tissue. Seven hours after beginning the study the cells again showed sensitivity to dopamine, and upon withdrawal of the catecholamine basal secretion rates were observed.

At this point bromocriptine, 50 nM, was added to the perfusion medium for 30 min. Prolactin secretion decreased, but its rate of decrease was much slower than that produced by dopamine. However, unlike dopamine, the bromocriptine-inhibited cells did not resume spontaneous prolactin secretion even when perfused for 90 min in the absence of the ergot derivative. Thus bromocriptine has a much longer duration of action than dopamine on prolactin secretion. Introduction of dbcAMP into the perfusate at this point completely reversed bromocriptine's inhibitory action and prolactin secretion resumed vigorously. Finally, it was demonstrated that dopamine was still capable of reducing prolactin secretion by the cells 12 hours after the beginning of the study.

These data conclusively demonstrate that prolactin secreting pituitary cells are reversibly sensitive to dopamine and its agonists, and strongly support the thesis that the dopaminergic system mediates a major physiological mechanism for regulating prolactin secretion.

## PITUITARY DOPAMINE RECEPTORS

Three groups of investigators using different sources and preparation techniques have independently identified the characterized anterior pituitary dopamine receptors (Calabro and MacLeod, 1978; Caron *et al.*, 1978; Cronin *et al.*, 1978). The data produced by studies of the binding of dopaminergic

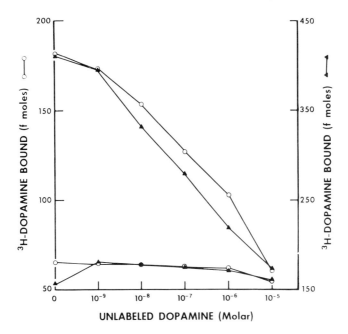

*Fig. 2.* Blockade of [3]H-dopamine binding by non-radioactive dopamine to bovine anterior pituitary gland membranes. Data reproduced from Calabro and MacLeod (1978) with permission of the publisher.

ligands to pituitary receptors are in excellent agreement. Our system investigated the binding of [3]H-dopamine to a washed bovine microsomal preparation (Calabro and MacLeod, 1978). Total and non-specific binding were determined by appropriate methods; their difference was taken to represent specific binding. The data in Fig. 2 show that the total binding of [3]H-dopamine to pituitary membranes stands in inverse proportion to the quantity of non-radioactive dopamine present. The specific binding of [3]H-dopamine to pituitary receptors was saturable, and graphic representation of the results (Fig. 3) suggests that bovine membranes have two dopamine binding sites corresponding to $K_d$ values of 0.44 nM and 47 nM. The corresponding total receptor concentrations in the pituitary were calculated to be 336 and 3340 fmol/mg protein. The lower affinity receptor site described in our study ($K_d$ = 47 nM) corresponds well with that reported by

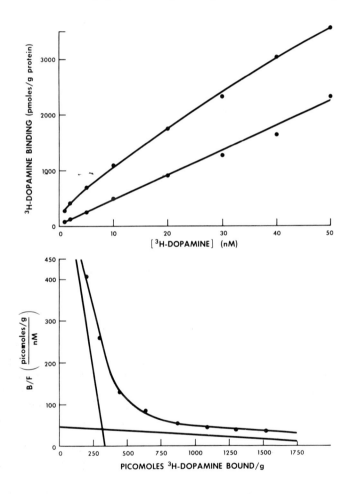

*Fig. 3.* Binding characteristics of [3]H-dopamine to pituitary gland membrane fraction. Data reproduced from Calabro and MacLeod (1978) with permission of the publisher.

Cronin *et al.* (1978), $K_d$ = 50 nM in rat and 80 nM in sheep membranes, and by Caron *et al.* (1978), $K_d$ = 490 nM in bovine pituitary membranes using [3]H-dihydroergocryptine as the dopaminergic ligand.

Several dopaminergic agonists known to inhibit prolactin secretion were examined for their ability to compete for the pituitary dopamine receptor site. The data presented in Table III show that apomorphine, bromocriptine and ergocryptine exhibit progressively greater binding than does dopamine to the membrane receptors. These data agree well with their relative potency to inhibit prolactin secretion. Thus in terms of ability both to bind to the pituitary receptor and to inhibit prolactin secretion, independent studies conclude that ergocryptine > bromocriptine > apomorphine > dopamine > norepinephrine.

*Table III.* Relative potency of dopamine agonists for pituitary receptor sites.

| Agonist | Groups of Investigators | | |
| --- | --- | --- | --- |
| | Calabro and MacLeod (1978) | Cronin *et al.* (1978) | Caron *et al.* (1978) |
| Ergocryptine | 15.5 | — | 75.4 |
| Bromocriptine | — | 9.7 | 20.4 |
| Apomorphine | 4.3 | 8.2 | 6.3 |
| Dopamine | 1 | 1 | 1 |
| Norepinephrine | 0.14 | 0.15 | 0.15 |
| Epinephrine | — | 0.15 | 0.29 |

Data adapted from material published in the above listed references.

## STIMULATION OF PROLACTIN SECRETION

There is extensive literature describing the ability of pharmacological agents to stimulate prolactin secretion (Del Pozo *et al.*, 1976; Frantz, 1973; L'Hermite *et al.*, 1978). Several phenothiazine derivatives and tricyclic neuroleptics are recognized as producing potent and in some cases prolonged increases in serum prolactin. We have shown that administering them to rats makes the pituitary gland refractory to the inhibitory action of dopamine and dopamine agonists when incubated *in vitro* (MacLeod, 1976). It was further demonstrated that these drugs act directly on the pituitary gland to block the inhibitory action of dopamine. It should be emphasized, however, that these drugs can not stimulate prolactin secretion directly or independently.

The results presented in Table IV summarize these findings. Dopamine, 500 nM, inhibited the *in vitro* secretion of radioimmunoassayable prolactin 50% and of newly synthesized prolactin 65% (100%-35%). Low concentrations (5 nM) of perphenazine or haloperidol partially blocked the action of dopamine, increasing prolactin secretion toward control values. The other drugs tested are apparently

*Table IV.* Blockade of the dopamine-mediated inhibition of prolactin secretion by dopamine antagonists.

| Agonist concentration | Antagonist concentration | Prolactin secretion % on control | |
|---|---|---|---|
| | | RIA-PRL | [3]H-PRL |
| 0 | 0 | 100 | 100 |
| 500 nM dopamine | 0 | 50 | 35 |
| 500 nM dopamine | 500 nM haloperidol | 87 | 104 |
| 500 nM dopamine | 50 nM haloperidol | 87 | 95 |
| 500 nM dopamine | 5 nM haloperidol | 70 | 52 |
| 500 nM dopamine | 50 nM perphenazine | 88 | 94 |
| 500 nM dopamine | 5 nM perphenazine | 73 | 69 |
| 500 nM dopamine | 500 nM sulpiride | 103 | 106 |
| 500 nM dopamine | 50 nM sulpiride | 85 | 85 |
| 500 nM dopamine | 50 nM pimozide | 90 | 89 |
| 500 nM dopamine | 50 nM tiapride | 105 | 93 |
| 500 nM dopamine | 50 nM metoclopramide | 97 | 100 |
| 500 nM dopamine | 5 $\mu$M (D)-butclamol | 102 | 100 |
| 500 nM dopamine | 5 $\mu$M (L)-butclamol | 50 | 29 |

not as active, although several are used clinically. In this regard, the high frequency of amenorrhea and galactorrhea observed in patients receiving these drugs can be viewed as a manifestation of the drugs' action to block dopamine's effect on the lactotrophs.

Recently L'Hermite *et al.* (1978) have shown that in human subjects, two new benzamides, tiapride and sultopride, stimulate prolactin secretion beginning 5 min after administration and peaking in about 30 min. Serum prolactin in these patients remained elevated for more than 6 h (Fig. 4). During this time no significant change was observed in serum LH and FSH. Hence the absence of midcycle surge of LH or FSH observed in individuals receiving chronic administration of tiapride may result from increased serum prolactin levels.

Table V presents an example of the ability of these neuroleptics (in this case, tiapride) to block dopamine's inhibitory action on prolactin secretion. These data suggest that tiapride and other dopamine antagonists bind to the dopamine receptor or to a site on the pituitary which affects dopamine binding and biological action. Calabro and MacLeod (1978) and Caron *et al.* (1978) give results which support this suggestion. The latter group showed that several dopamine antagonists are potent agents which compete for the [3]H-DHEC binding sites on

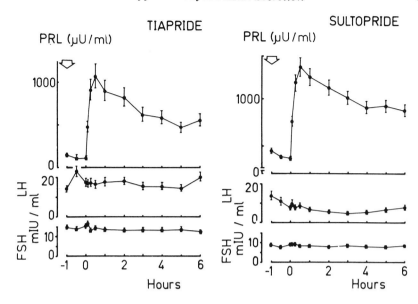

*Fig. 4.* Serum prolactin, LH, and FSH levels in six normal men and women following the i.m. injection of 200 mg tiapride or 100 mg sultopride.

*Table V. In vitro* blockade b y tiapride of the dopamine-mediated inhibition of prolactin secretion.

| | Incorporation of [3]H-leucine into prolactin (c.p.m./mg pituitary) | | Radioimmunoassayable prolactin in medium ($\mu$g/mg pituitary) |
|---|---|---|---|
| | Pituitary | Medium | |
| Control | 8000 ± 320 | 6050 ± 350 | 6.61 ± 0.47 |
| 500 nM dopamine | 10 780 ± 920 | 2290 ± 710[a] | 3.54 ± 0.64[a] |
| 500 nM tiapride | 8270 ± 640 | 7060 ± 810 | 6.65 ± 0.28 |
| DA + tiapride | 9310 ± 600 | 5410 ± 370[b] | 6.69 ± 0.24[b] |

[a]$P < 0.01$ *vs* control.
[b]$P < 0.01$ *vs* dopamine.

pituitary membranes. Our studies show that these drugs compete for pituitary [3]H-dopamine binding sites less well than dopamine and lead us to postulate the existence of sites on the gland which bind neuroleptics. The work of Creese *et al.* (1976; 1978) provides a precedent for such a phenomenon.

One should exercise extreme care when describing the pharmacological action of neuroleptic drugs, especially in neuroendocrine terms. Haloperidol and pimozide were once viewed as highly specific dopamine antagonists. At low concentrations, they do block dopamine's *in vitro* inhibition of prolactin secretion very effectively. At higher concentrations, however, both haloperidol and pimozide themselves inhibit prolactin potently (MacLeod and Lamberts, 1978). Hence these dopamine antagonists can also function as dopamine agonists. These findings have also been reported by Caron *et al.* (1978) and may contribute to the observations of Lawson and Gala (1975) and Langer (1977), who found that graded doses of haloperidol and pimozide progressively stimulate serum prolactin levels up to a maximum, but that further increases in neuroleptic dosage seemed to inhibit prolactin secretion. Although the precise interpretation of these findings is difficult at present, one should view the results of experiments using large concentrations of haloperidol or pimozide with caution.

## EXPERIMENTAL PITUITARY TUMORS

There are several lines of transplantable pituitary tumors in rats which synthesize and secrete various combinations of pituitary hormones, including prolactin, growth hormone, and ACTH. These tumors have been used as convenient sources of *in situ* rat hormones and as models of pituitary adenoma in man. Our work has centered on three mammosomatropic tumors, MtTW5, MtTW15 and 7315a, all of which secrete large quantities of prolactin. Some time ago, we demonstrated that ergotamine, ergocornine and ergocryptine suppress the growth of these tumors in rats (MacLeod and Lehmeyer, 1971; 1973). Other workers have also

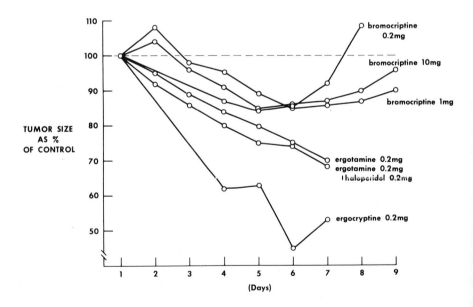

*Fig. 5.* Response of pituitary tumor growth to the injection of ergot alkaloid derivatives. Rats were injected daily s.c. with the indicated amounts of drug and the size (length + width) of the tumor determined.

shown that the drugs decrease the pituitary and serum prolactin concentrations (Amenomori *et al.*, 1970; Quadri *et al.*, 1972).

Recently we have reinvestigated this phenomenon and studied the effect of bromocriptine on experimental pituitary tumor growth and on prolactin secretion (Lamberts and MacLeod, 1979). The effect of semi-chronic administration of 0.2 mg ergocryptine, 0.2 mg ergotamine and 0.2–10 mg bromocriptine daily to female rats bearing the prolactin- and ACTH-secreting tumor 7315a and the prolactin- and growth hormone-secreting tumor MtTW15 was studied. The data in Fig. 5 show that although ergotamine and ergocryptine cause a progressive decrease in pituitary tumor size, bromocriptine was without sustained effect. Bromocriptine's ineffectiveness against these pituitary tumors can again be seen in the data presented in Table VI. It should be noted that very large quantities of prolactin were detected in the serum of tumor-bearing rats. Injection of these rats with ergotamine or ergocryptine caused a significant decrease in the circulating hormone levels. Bromocriptine treatment, however, was without effect on serum prolactin, regardless of the amount of the drug used.

*Table VI.* Effect of ergot alkaloid derivatives on serum prolactin levels in tumor-bearing rats.

| Treatment | $\mu$g prolactin/ml serum | |
|---|---|---|
| | Before treatment | After treatment |
| *Experiment 1* | | |
| Tumor control saline (8 days) | $3.09 \pm 0.71$ | $6.49 \pm 1.46$ |
| Ergotamine 0.2 mg (8 days) | $3.19 \pm 0.79$ | $2.69 \pm 0.93$[a] |
| Bromocriptine 0.2 mg (8 days) | $3.06 \pm 0.51$ | $8.31 \pm 2.17$ |
| *Experiment 2* | | |
| Tumor control saline (5 days) | $11.71 \pm 1.71$ | $13.90 \pm 2.69$ |
| Ergocryptine 0.2 mg (5 days) | $12.52 \pm 1.24$ | $0.37 \pm 0.06$[a] |
| *Experiment 3* | | |
| Tumor control saline (9 days) | not assayed | $6.57 \pm 2.29$ |
| Bromocriptine 1 mg (9 days) | not assayed | $6.45 \pm 0.90$ |
| Bromocriptine 10 mg (9 days) | not assayed | $6.97 \pm 1.02$ |

[a]$P < 0.01$.

The effectiveness of other ergot alkaloids makes bromocriptine's failure to inhibit tumor growth or decrease serum prolactin levels surprising. One explanation may be that in this case, the other ergot alkaloids act through a mechanism other than the dopaminergic system. Haloperidol's failure to block ergocryptine's suppressive effect supports this conjecture. Furthermore, most ergot derivatives have considerable vasopressor activity, which bromocriptine lacks. Transplanted subcutaneously between the scapulae of rats, these tumors are fed only by small capillaries. So in this case the ergot alkaloids may suppress tumor growth and activity by further restricting the already limited blood supply.

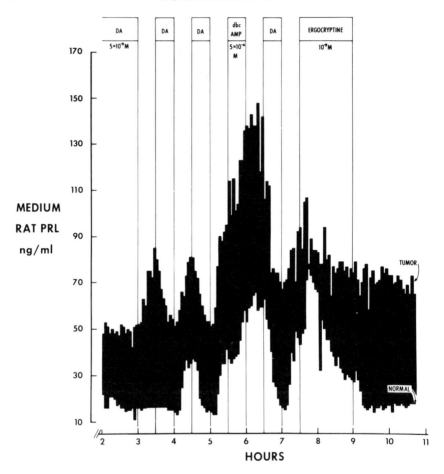

**Fig. 6.** Effects of dopamine, dbcAMP, and ergocryptine on isolated pituitary cells from normal female rats and from pituitary tumor MtTW15. Perfusion of $10^7$ dispersed cells accomplished as described in Fig. 1.

Figure 6 provides data on the relative refractoriness of rat pituitary tumor cell response to dopamine and its agonist ergocryptine. Dispersed pituitary cell preparations made from normal rat pituitary glands and from pituitary tumor 7315a were initially perfused with medium containing a relatively high concentration of dopamine, 5 $\mu$M. Subsequently each column, containing $10^7$ cells, was alternately perfused with medium with and without 500 nM dopamine. Prolactin release from normal cells was inhibited approximately by 65%, whereas cells of pituitary tumor origin were much less responsive to the inhibitory action of dopamine. Interestingly, cells of normal and tumor origin both increased prolactin release following the addition of dbcAMP to the perfusion medium. Likewise the dbcAMP-mediated increase in prolactin secretion was inhibited by dopamine perfusion in both cases. Perfusion of normal cells with 10 nM ergocryptine drastically reduced prolactin secretion, whereas pituitary tumor cells were refractory to the inhibitory effects of the ergot alkaloid. In other unreported studies, 50 nM bromocriptine was virtually without effect on prolactin secretion by cells of tumor origin despite perfusion for several hours. These data are consistent with those reported by others who showed that pituitary tumor cells are less sensitive than normal pituitary cells to the inhibitory action of dopaminergic agents (Malarkey *et al.*, 1977).

These data suggest that rat pituitary tumor cells have fewer or defective dopamine sites. This hypothesis was directly tested by preparing membranes from 7315a and MtTW15 pituitary tumors and studying the binding of [3]H-dopamine according to the method of Calabro and MacLeod (1978). These studies showed that tumor membranes contained less than 10% of the dopamine receptor sites found in pituitary cells of non-tumor origin.

## THE AUTOREGULATION OF PROLACTIN SYNTHESIS AND RELEASE

The implantation of prolactin-secreting pituitary tumors into rats greatly increases serum prolactin levels, and the pituitary glands of the host become partially atrophied, synthesizing and secreting decreased quantities of prolactin

*Table VII.* Restoration of prolactin production in pituitary glands of rats bearing prolactin secreting tumors.

| Treatment | Incorporation of [3]H-leucine into prolactin c.p.m./mg pituitary | | |
|---|---|---|---|
| | Pituitary | Medium | Total |
| *Experiment 1* | | | |
| Non-tumor control | 750 | 5050 | 5800 |
| MtTW15 control | 150 | 600 | 750 |
| MtTW15 + haloperidol 0.1 mg daily for four days | 350 | 3700 | 4050 |
| *Experiment 2* | | | |
| Non-tumor control | 450 | 4100 | 4550 |
| MtTW15 control | 50 | 300 | 350 |
| MtTW15 + haloperidol 0.5 mg 8 h before sacrifice | 100 | 1250 | 1350 |
| *Experiment 3* | | | |
| Non-tumor control | 2520 | 2150 | 4670 |
| MtTW15 control | 170 | 160 | 330 |
| MtTW15 + pimozide 0.7 mg daily for three days | 1430 | 2360 | 3790 |
| *Experiment 4* | | | |
| Non-tumor control | 1100 | 2700 | 3800 |
| 7315a control | 100 | 750 | 850 |
| 7315a + perphenazine 2 mg 8 h before sacrifice | 250 | 1300 | 1550 |
| *Experiment 5* | | | |
| Non-tumor control | 4310 | 4660 | 8970 |
| 7315a control | 140 | 780 | 920 |
| 7315a + reserpine 1.0 mg daily for two days | 2000 | 5740 | 7740 |

*in vitro* (MacLeod and Abad, 1968). *In situ*, it is believed that prolactin release from the pituitary gland is regulated by the dopaminergic system. Increasing the hypothalamic dopaminergic turnover results in a decrease in prolactin secretion (Fuxe *et al.*, 1969), whereas blockade of dopamine turnover results in increased secretion.

Some time ago we showed that the injection of dopamine receptor blocking agents reverses the suppression of prolactin synthesis and release by host pituitary glands in rats bearing prolactin-secreting pituitary tumors (MacLeod and Lehmeyer, 1974). These data are summarized in Table VII. Rats bearing pituitary tumors MtTW15 and 7315a had serum prolactin levels of 5000 to 10 000 ng/ml, and the pituitary glands of these rats produced 75 to 85% less prolactin than did those of non-tumor controls. Administration of the dopamine receptor blocking agents haloperidol, pimozide and perphenazine each caused a prompt increase in prolactin synthesis and secretion rates. Because the administration of these drugs did not affect the exceedingly high serum prolactin levels in these rats, the signal to activate the hypothalamic mechanism which causes a decrease in pituitary gland prolactin production presumably remained operative. In these tumor-bearing animals, we suggest that the elevated levels of serum prolactin activate the tuberinfundibular dopamine neurons, as demonstrated by Fuxe *et al.* (1969) and Eikenburg *et al.* (1977), thereby decreasing prolactin synthesis and release. Treatment of these rats with the neuroleptic drugs, however, blocks the effect of the hypothalamic dopamine at the pituitary gland level, resulting in restoration of prolactin production. This concept is supported by the work of Gudelsky and Moore, who failed to find a change in the median eminence turnover of dopamine following haloperidol injection (Gudelsky and Moore, 1976).

Further support for this concept is provided in Table VII, Experiment 5. As before, the presence of the prolactin-secreting pituitary tumor 7315a markedly decreased the ability of the host's pituitary gland to synthesize and release prolactin. Treatment of these rats with reserpine decreases the hypothalamic stores of catecholamines and thereby presumably interrupts the serum prolactin-mediated signal which causes a suppression of pituitary hormone production.


## INTERACTION OF ESTRADIOL WITH THE DOPAMINERGIC SYSTEM

The stimulatory effect of estradiol on prolactin secretion and synthesis is well established. It is probable that estradiol exerts these actions at both the hypothalamic and the pituitary levels. The association between the proestrus surge of prolactin and the increase in dopaminergic turnover has been made (Fuxe *et al.*, 1969). More recently Eikenburg *et al.* (1977) observed that estradiol treatment failed to alter dopamine turnover in the median eminence of hypophysectomized rats. They concluded that estradiol does not appear to influence the tuberoinfundibular neurons directly, but that this effect is produced by the increased serum prolactin concentration in estradiol-treated rats. Nicoll and Meites (1962) demonstrated the direct effect of estradiol at the pituitary level. More recently Labrie *et al.* (1978) demonstrated that preincubation of pituitary cultures with 17β-estradiol almost completely blocked the inhibitory action of dihydroergocornine on prolactin secretion. These data are consistent with the observations shown in

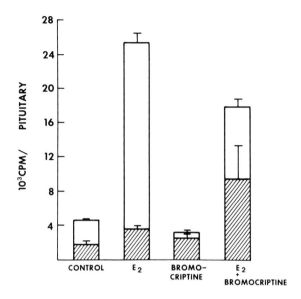

*Fig. 7.* Blockade of the bromocriptine-mediated inhibition of prolactin secretion by the injection of estrogen. Male rats were injected s.c. with 1.0 μg estradiol and 100 μg polyestradiol phosphate 72 h before sacrifice. Non-treated and estradiol-treated pituitary glands were incubated in medium containing $^3$H-leucine and 2 nM and bromocriptine. The newly-synthesized $^3$H-prolactin present in the pituitary (hatched bar) and in the incubation medium (open bar) was measured following PAGE.

Fig. 7. Male rats were injected with estrogens 72 h before sacrifice, and their pituitaries were incubated in the presence and absence of 2 nM bromocriptine in medium containing $^3$H-leucine. Estradiol caused a marked increase in the synthesis and release of prolactin, and bromocriptine inhibited release of the hormone. The ergot alkaloid was, however, only partially capable of inhibiting prolactin secretion by pituitary glands from estradiol-treated rats. However, the amount of newly-synthesized prolactin retained in the gland was much greater than in controls. These data suggest that estradiol acts primarily to increase prolactin synthesis and secondarily to increase release of the hormone.

In a previous section we showed that the pituitary glands of tumor-bearing rats synthesized and released less prolactin than did controls (Fig. 8). The administration of estradiol to these rats produced a significant increase in prolactin synthesis and release. It is tempting to speculate that this steroid effect is mediated directly at the pituitary gland and blocks the inhibitory action of the dopaminergic system on prolactin production. This possibility would not preclude estradiol from acting centrally to stimulate the release of a prolactin stimulating hormone. Further work must be conducted to determine whether estrogens influence the binding agents to the dopamine receptor or whether two competing biological systems act in opposition to one another.

We have initiated efforts towards this goal by studying the action of anti-estrogens on pituitary hormone synthesis and release. Our initial work was done with the catechol estrogen 2-hydroxyestradiol (for review see Nagy *et al.*, 1979).

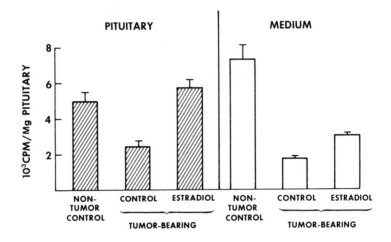

*Fig. 8.* Restoration of prolactin synthesis and release by the anterior pituitary in rats bearing a transplanted pituitary tumor following the injection of estradiol. Female rats bearing pituitary tumor 7315a received 1 μg estradiol and 100 μg polyestradiol phosphate 72 h before sacrifice. The incubation procedure was as described in Fig. 7.

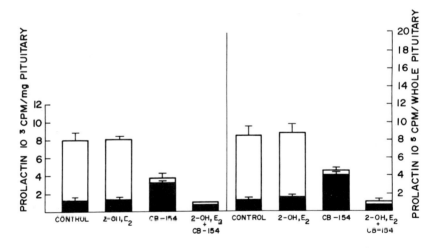

*Fig. 9.* Augmentation of the bromocriptine-mediated inhibition of prolactin synthesis and release by 2-hydroxyestradiol. For four days 20 μg of the catechol estrogen was injected daily and the rats were sacrificed 24 h after the last injection. Added to control and treated pituitary glands was 2 nM bromocriptine; incubation followed the procedure described in Fig. 7.

Because 2-hydroxyestradiol evokes an estrogen-like response when administered in large amounts, we chose to inject 20 μg per day for 4 days, the last injection 24 h before sacrifice. This schedule produced no increase in serum prolactin levels. The data presented in Fig. 9 demonstrated that the catechol estrogen produced no change in the *in vitro* synthesis and release of prolactin. As seen earlier, 2 nM bromocriptine in non-treated rats greatly inhibited release of the hormone and it accumulated in the pituitary gland. Addition of bromocriptine to pituitary glands obtained from 2-hydroxyestradiol-treated rats produced a further decrease in the synthesis and release of prolactin. Thus 17$\beta$-estradiol stimulates the synthesis of prolactin and the antiestrogen inhibits synthesis of the hormone. At a concentration of 0.5 nM, bromocriptine caused only a slight decrease in the *in vitro* release of prolactin from normal rat pituitary glands. However the drug produced a 40% fall in secretion by pituitary glands from 2-hydroxyestradiol-treated rats. It should be noted that the 2-hydroxyestradiol used in these studies was presumably of high quality but the stability of catechol estrogens is tenuous. It appears that the antiestrogen has augmented the prolactin inhibiting action of bromocriptine. If this observation is substantiated in studies using other more stable antiestrogens, it may be a useful modality for the treatment of hyperprolactinemia.

## SUMMARY

There is strong evidence that anterior pituitary membranes have dopamine receptors and that their activation inhibits prolactin release from the lactotrophs. The systemic administration of a broad spectrum of neuroleptic agents stimulates prolactin secretion directly by blocking the dopamine receptor site or indirectly by binding to an adjacent site, thereby blocking the biological effect of the catecholamine. Although most dopamine receptors are closely coupled to the adenylate cyclase system, no activation of the anterior pituitary adenylate cyclase system by dopamine or its agonists is observed. Indeed, exogenously administered dbcAMP is stimulatory to prolactin.

It is interesting to note that prolactin secretory activity is most frequently associated with experimental and human pituitary tumors. Hence the inability of dopamine and its agonist bromocriptine to block release of the hormone from our transplanted tumors was unexpected. Subsequently it was learned that the tumors have fewer than 10% of the dopamine receptors found in the normal anterior pituitary. This phenomenon, however, probably does not pertain to all human pituitary tumors, because most are responsive to dopamine agonist therapy as reflected by inhibition of prolactin secretion and tumor size reduction.

The role of estrogens to stimulate prolactin synthesis and release needs to be reinvestigated more thoroughly. Evidence is accumulating which suggests that the ovarian steroids are inhibitory to the action of the dopaminergic system. Conversely, it appears that antiestrogen drugs have certain activities which mimic those of the dopamine system. Preliminary studies show that tamoxifen and CI-628 inhibit the synthesis and release of prolactin by the anterior pituitary gland (36). Administration of these antiestrogens caused a significant decrease in the size of transplanted prolactin-secreting tumors. These findings may be of significance in the treatment of women with dopamine agonist-resistant microadenomas.

## REFERENCES

Amenomori, Y., Chen, C. L. and Meites, J. (1970). *Endocrinology* **86**, 503.
Ben-Jonathan, N., Oliver, C., Weiner, H. J., Mical, R. S. and Porter, J. C. (1977). *Endocrinolgy* **100**, 452.

54          *R. M. MacLeod et al.*

Calabro, M. A. and MacLeod, R. M. (1978). *Neuroendocrinology* 25, 32.
Caron, M. C., Beaulieu, M., Raymond, V., Gagne, B., Drouin, J. Lefkowitz, R. J. and Labrie, F. (1978). *J. biol. Chem.* 253, 2244.
Creese, I., Burt, D. R. and Snyder, S. H. (1975). *Life Science* 17, 993.
Creese, I., Burt, D. R. and Snyder, S. H. (1976). *Science* 192.
Cronin, M. J., Roberts , J. M. and Weiner, R. I. (1978). *Endocrinology* 103, 302.
Del Pozo, E., Flückiger, E. and Lancranjan, I. (1976). *In* "Basic Applications and Clinical Use of Hypothalamic Hormones" (A. Charro Salgdado, R. Fernandez Durango and J. G. López del Campo, eds) 137–150. Excerpta Medica, Amsterdam.
Eikenburg, D. C., Ravitz, A. J., Gudelsky, G. A. and Moore, K. E. (1977). *J. Neural Transmission* 40, 235.
Fishman, J. (1976). *Neuroendocrinology* 22, 363.
Frantz, A. G. (1973). *In* "Frontiers in Neuroendocrinology" (W. F. Ganong and L. Martini, eds) Vol. 3, 337–374. Oxford University Press, New York.
Fuxe, K., Hökfelt, T. and Nilsson, O. (1969). *Neuroendocrinology* 5, 257.
Gibbs, D. M. and Neill, J. D. (1978). *Endocrinology* 102, 1895.
Gudelsky, G. A. and Moore, K. E. (1976). *J. Neural Transmission* 38, 95.
Hill, M. K., MacLeod, R. M. and Orcutt, P. (1976). *Endocrinology* 99, 1612.
Labrie, F., Beaulieu, M. Caron, M. C. and Raymond, J. V. (1978). *In* "Progress in Prolactin Physiology and Pathology" (M. Harter and C. Robyn, eds) 121–136. Elsevier, Amsterdam.
Lamberts, S. W. J. and MacLeod, R. M. (1977). "Physiological and Pathological Aspects of Prolactin Secretion", Vol. 1. Eden Press, Montreal.
Lamberts, S. W. J. and Macleod, R. M. (1979). *Endocrinology* 104, 65.
Langer, G., Sachar, E. J., Halpern, F. S., Gruen, P. H. and Solomon, M. (1977). *J. Clin. Endocrinol. Metab.* 45, 996.
Lawson, D. M. and Gala, R. R. (1975). *Endocrinology* 96, 313.
L'Hermite, M., Macleod, R. M. and Robyn, C. (1978). *Acta Endocrinol.* 89, 29.
Lowry, P. J. (1974). *J. Endocrinology* 62, 163.
MacLeod, R. M. (1976). *In* "Frontiers in Neuroendocrinology" (L. Martini and W. F. Ganong, eds) Vol. 4, 169–194. Raven Press, New York.
MacLeod, R. M. and Abad, A. (1968). *Endocrinology* 83, 799.
MacLeod, R. M. and Lamberts, S. W. J. (1978). *Endocrinology* 103, 200.
MacLeod, R. M. and Lehmeyer, J. E. (1969). *Endocrinology* 94, 1077.
MacLeod, R. M. and Lehmeyer, (1971). *In* "Lactogenic Hormones" (G. E. W. Wolstenholme and J. Knight, eds), 52–83. Churchill Livingston, London.
MacLeod, R. M. and Lehmeyer, J. E. (1973). *Cancer Research* 33, 849.
MacLeod, R. M. and Lehmeyer, J. E. (1974). *Cancer Research* 34, 345.
Malarkey, W. B., Groshong, J. C. and Milo, G. E. (1977). *Nature* 266, 640.
Nagy, I., Valdenegro, C. A., Login, I. S. and MacLeod, R. M. (1979). Abstracts of the 61st meeting of the Endocrine Society.
Nicoll, C. S. and Meites, J. (1962). *Endocrinology* 70, 272.
Quadri, S. K., Lu, K. H. and Meites, J. (1972). *Science* 176, 417.
Schally, A. V., Dupont, A., Arimura, A., Takahara, S., Redding, T. W., Clemens, A. and Shaar, C. (1976). *Acta Endocrinology* 82, 1.
Shaar, C. J. and Clemens, J. A. (1974). *Endocrinology* 95, 1202.
Thorner, M. O. (1977). *In* "Clinical Neuroendocrinology" (L. Martini and G. M. Besser, eds) 295–308. Academic Press, New York and London

# SYNTHESIS, INTRACELLULAR TRANSPORT, PACKAGING AND RELEASE OF GROWTH HORMONE AND PROLACTIN IN NORMAL AND TUMORAL PITUITARY CELLS

P. De Camilli, A. Zanini, G. Giannattasio and J. Meldolesi

*Department of Pharmacology and CNR Centre of Cytopharmacology,
University of Milan, Italy*

## INTRODUCTION

During the past few years considerable information has been accumulated on the structural organization and functioning of pituitary somatotroph and mammotroph cells. The results obtained so far clearly indicate that secretion of growth hormone (GH) and prolactin (PRL) is carried out by means of a number of sequentially interconnected events analogous in many respects to those operating in all other protein-secreting tissues (for recent reviews see Palade, 1975; Farquhar, 1977; Meldolesi *et al.*, 1978). A comprehensive account of these events in the pituitary gland will be provided in the first part of this article, while in the second part the corresponding knowledge will be reviewed concerning pituitary adenomas and it will be discussed whether, and to what extent, the functioning of these tumors deviates from that of their normal cell counterparts. In the final section the potentialities of adenomas as experimental models for investigation of the physiology of individual pituitary cell types will be considered.

---

Dr. D. Camilli's present address is Department of Pharmacology, Yale University, Medical School, New Haven, Connecticut 6510, USA.

## SECRETION OF GH AND PRL IN NORMAL PITUITARY CELLS

### Biosynthesis

The rate of synthesis of GH and PRL exceeds by far that of any other pituitary protein. Thus, in rat and cow gland fragments incubated *in vitro* with radioactive amino acids, the two hormones together account for over 40 and 20% of the total TCA-insoluble radioactivity, respectively (Zanini *et al.*, 1974a and in preparation). Even higher values were found for the cell-free protein synthesis of bovine pituitary microsomes (Lingappa *et al.*, 1977). Like all other secretory proteins, GH and PRL are also synthesized only on bound polyribosomes, i.e. on polyribosomes attached by their large subunits to the outer surface of the rough-surfaced endoplasmic reticulum (ER) membranes (Sussman *et al.*, 1976; Lingappa *et al.*, 1977). Considerable information exists now about both the mechanisms and the functional significance of this ribosome–membrane link. The attachment to the : membrane does not occur at random but is restricted to specific binding sites, or receptors, structured to allow an easy vectorial transmembrane passage of the growing polypeptide chains synthesized by their bound ribosomes. So far, the organization of these receptors has been investigated only in liver cells and has been found to be very complex. In fact, each single receptor seems to be composed of at least two different glycoproteins, integral to the ER membrane; in addition, all the ribosome receptors appear to be linked to each other in a sort of network organization, parallel to the plane of the membrane, with consequent restriction of their freedom of lateral displacement (Kreibich *et al.*, 1978a,b).

The striking selectivity of the GH and PRL transcription for bound ribosomes has also been recently explained. It has been demonstrated that the mRNAs coding for the two hormones (as well as those of many, and maybe all, secretory proteins) contain peculiar base sequences which are translated as corresponding sequences of amino acids located at the *N*-terminal region. These *N*-terminal sequences (designated as signal peptides) are cleaved from the overall translation product (designated by the prefix pre-, thus preGH and prePRL) before chain termination by a specific proteolytic enzyme (the signal peptidase) located on the inner surface of the ER membrane. The consistent finding of signal peptides for practically all of the secretory proteins so far investigated has fostered the suggestion that the ribosome-ER attachment is initially indirect, triggered by the interaction of signal peptides with the ribosomal receptors of the ER membrane. Thus, the attachment would occur not before, but during the synthesis of the secretory proteins (Blobel and Dobberstein, 1975; Lingappa *et al.*, 1977; Sussman *et al.*, 1976; review: Campbell and Blobel, 1976).

The restriction of the biosynthesis of GH and PRL to bound polyribosomes has an important functional consequence. In fact, during their synthesis the two hormones are able to cross the ER membrane in the form of extended growing polypeptide chains. Eventually, however, once processed by the signal peptidases and discharged from ribosomes, the completed hormone molecules fold, acquire their tertiary configurations and thereafter remain segregated within the ER lumen, while the proteins synthesized by free polyribosomes form a separate pool in the surrounding cytoplasm. By this procedure, therefore, the separation of the two hormones from at least most of the proteins destined to run over within the cells is achieved in pituitary mammotrophs and somatotrophs during the course of their biosynthesis (Sussman *et al.*, 1976; Lingappa *et al.*, 1977).

### Intracellular transport and packaging

As for other secretory systems, the pituitary intracellular hormone transport has been investigated by labeling the cells with a short pulse incorporation of radioactive amino acids and by following the redistribution of labeled hormones, either by cell fractionation or electron microscopic radioautography (Racadot *et al.*, 1965; Tixier-Vidal and Picart, 1967; Howell and Whitfield, 1973; Meldolesi *et al.*, 1972; Zanini *et al.*, 1974a; Farquhar *et al.*, 1975; 1978).

The results of these studies clearly indicate that the newly synthesized hormone molecules, once segregated within the lumen of the ER cisternae, are transported vectorially throughout the cells along a discontinuous, membrane-bounded pathway (which includes the ER, the Golgi complex and the secretory granules), to be ultimately discharged into the extracellular space by exocytosis. Even though this general framework has now been well demonstrated, the cellular mechanisms involved in the transport operations are still incompletely understood. Thus, in this section a number of reasonable speculations will be used to fill the gaps between the relatively few established facts. Beforehand, however, it should be stressed that, at variance with the situation existing for other hormones and secretory proteins, the finished GH and PRL molecules are not subjected to proteolysis in the course of intracellular transport. Therefore, the two hormones are molecularly unchanged in all their cellular locations (Zanini *et al.*, 1974a).

In both somatotrophs and mammotrophs the whole ER is essentially accounted for by a system of frequently anastomosed, flat, rough-surfaced cisternae. In contrast, smooth ER tubules are quite rare. The newly synthesized hormone molecules equilibrate rapidly with those preexisting within the cisternal cavities, and the whole ER-segregated pool is then drained slowly to the Golgi complex. Nothing is known about the mechanisms of this drainage, except that it is energy-dependent (Howell and Whitfield, 1973).

Transfer of hormones from the ER to the Golgi complex is not a fast phenomenon. As shown by the recent radioautographical results of Farquhar *et al.* (1978) in dissociated rat mammotrophs pulse-labeled with $^3$H-L-leucine, radioactive PRL already appears in the Golgi complex five minutes after the beginning of the pulse and reaches a peak at 30 min. Thereafter the hormone accumulates in immature granules (peak at 120 min) and finally in mature granules. Transport from the Golgi to the granules of considerable quantities of labeled hormone continues for at least three hours. We have recently reached similar conclusions by cell fractionation, working with cow pituitary slices (Giannattasio *et al.*, in preparation). Within the Golgi complex, GH and PRL undergo a progressive concentration. By this process the hormone molecules, which are soluble and diluted while in the ER lumen, are turned into small, dense masses, thread-like in texture, which accumulate within the trans-Golgi cisternae as secretory granule cores. The subsequent stages of granule maturation have been studied in detail in rat mammotrophs by Farquhar *et al.* (1978): the PRL granule cores bud off the trans-

Golgi cisternae giving rise to small discrete PRL granules (type I); the latter fuse into polymorphous forms (type II), which round up and assume first a simpler, yet still irregular contour (type III) and finally a spherical or ovoid shape (type IV). A similar heterogeneity of PRL granules, less pronounced than that in the rat, can be observed in other animal species. PRL granules of all types can be discharged by exocytosis (see below).

What about the mechanisms of hormone concentration and packaging in secretory granules? For quite some time these processes were believed to occur by active ion pumping at the granule membrane. More recently, however, it has become clear that within mature secretory granules the segregated hormones are not only concentrated but also assembled to yield solid-state structures devoid of osmotic activity. This phenomenon is particularly striking for the PRL granules, whose internal organization is so stable that it is maintained even after solubilization of the limiting membrane by mild detergent treatment (Giannattasio *et al.*, 1975). That this surprising stability of interaction among the components of the granule content is established in the Golgi complex is shown by the fact that it develops progressively; i.e. the recently assembled granules are far less stable than the older ones (unpublished observation). These findings with mature granules have fostered the view that the concentration of hormones into the granule cores is not due to ion pumping but to self-assembly of the granule components. What makes these granule components associate within the Golgi cisternae is not yet understood. On the basis of studies carried out in a variety of cell systems, essentially two hypotheses have been proposed. According to the first, divalent cations, especially $Ca^{2+}$, may play a major role by bridging negative charged groups in adjacent molecules (review: Meldolesi *et al.*, 1978). This hypothesis rests on the observations that many granules contain considerable concentrations of $Ca^{2+}$ and that $Ca^{2+}$ pumps have been described in Golgi fractions. However, the concentration of $Ca^{2+}$ in PRL granules is relatively low [$\sim$ 20 nmole/mg protein (Zanini and Giannattasio, 1974)] and moreover, in another system, the *in vitro* removal of $Ca^{2+}$ from isolated granules by incubation in the presence of EGTA and the $Ca^{2+}$ ionophore A23187 had no apparent effect on granule stability and organization (Flashner and Schramm, 1977). The second hypothesis involves organic polyanions, especially complex carbohydrates such as glycosaminoglycans and sulfated glycopeptides, that might act by establishing ionic interactions with positively charged groups of many hormone molecules (review: Giannattasio *et al.*, 1979). Recently we have demonstrated that a heterogeneous mixture of complex carbohydrates exists in the segregated contents of rat and cow PRL granules (Giannattasio and Zanini, 1976; Zanini *et al.*, in preparation). The protein moieties of these molecules are probably synthesized on polyribosomes bound to ER membranes (by mechanisms analogous to those described for the hormone) while completion of their saccharide chains and sulfation occur in the Golgi complex. However, the quantity of complex carbohydrates within PRL granules is small and appears to be insufficient to bind directly all the segregated hormone molecules. Small amounts of sulfated macromolecules, as yet uncharacterized, have also been found by others in the contents of GH granules (Slaby and Farquhar, personal communication).

In conclusion, it should be stressed that, contrary to common belief, GH and PRL are not the sole constituents of the corresponding secretory granules. Other components (complex carbohydrates, inorganic ions) are co-packed with the hormones and discharged concomitantly by exocytosis. However, the functional significance of these minority components, both within the cell and after discharge, still remains to be clarified.

Another important aspect of the intracellular transport concerns the membranes involved. In fact, during transport the ER membrane (which is known to be very leaky) is the first barrier which segregates the newly synthesized hormone molecules; this is replaced by the Golgi membrane, which is characterized by a much lower degree of permeability. This implies the possibility that the ionic milieu within the Golgi complex is quite different from that of the surrounding cytoplasm. As already mentioned, this situation may be of great importance in the assembly of hormone molecules into structured granule cores. On the other hand, the subsequent evolution of these cores contained within Golgi cisternae into discrete secretory granules is also exceedingly important because only granule membranes are endowed with the potentiality to fuse with the plasmalemma and discharge their contents by exocytosis (see below) (reviews: Palade, 1975; Meldolesi *et al.*, 1978).

### Release

Release of radioactive GH and PRL into the extracellular environment from pulse-labeled pituitary tissue begins 45–60 min after the end of the pulse (the time needed for intracellular transport and packaging). Release of both hormones occurs by exocytosis, i.e. by fusion of the limiting membrane of the secretion granules with the plasma membrane, followed by fission of the fused region and incorporation of the everted granule membrane into the plasma membrane. Several mechanisms of hormone discharge [especially the molecular leakage from soluble cytoplasmic pool(s)] have been proposed in the past. However, no adequate supportive evidence has ever been reported (for details see Meldolesi *et al.*, 1978). Exocytosis can occur over the entire cell surface of both mammotrophs and somatotrophs. In the latter, however, it occurs much more frequently at the cell processes facing the blood capillaries. As an alternative to exocytosis, secretory granule discharge can also occur by crinophagy (Farquhar, 1977); a process by which the granule content is delivered within lysosomes by fusion-fission of the limiting membranes of the two organelles. Crinophagy is a control process for the size of the intracellular hormone pool and occurs massively in mammotrophs when lactation is suddenly interrupted. In other conditions it is relatively rare.

From pituitary slices incubated *in vitro* release of the two hormones is carried out according to first order kinetics, suggesting that released hormones originate from one single intracellular pool (Meldolesi *et al.*, 1972). This means that each secretory granule, whether it has just emerged from the Golgi apparatus or has remained for quite some time within the cell, has an equal opportunity to discharge its contents by exocytosis. In this respect it should be mentioned that, when analysed under dissociating conditions (SDS-polyacrylamide gel electrophoresis (SDS-PAGE)), the discharged GH and PRL molecules were indistinguishable from those present in the various intracellular locations (Zanini *et al.*, 1974b). These findings rule out the possibility, previously suggested, that GH and PRL present within pituitary cells in heterogeneous pools was different both in molecular composition and turnover (Swearingen, 1971; Stachura and Frohman, 1975). It appears now that these previous results were due to solubilization and adsorption artifacts occurring during the preparation of the samples. As discussed in detail in other articles in this book and elsewhere, secretion of GH and PRL occurs *in vivo* under the control of a variety of hormones and neurotransmitters, acting directly (on the pituitary cells) and/or indirectly [through the influence of the central nervous sytem (CNS)]. In this respect the major difference between the two hormones concerns the overall regulatory tone with dopamine (DA) playing a major inhibitory role for PRL and stimulatory for GH. It is therefore not surprising that in pituitary fragments incubated *in vitro* mammotrophs are derepressed, and therefore secrete PRL at a high rate (*t* 0.5 of ~60 and ~300 min in rats and cows, respectively) (Meldolesi *et al.*, 1972; Giannattasio *et al.*, in preparation), while GH cells function at much lower rates.

How are hormonal signals transduced within pituitary cells to yield changes in GH and PRL secretion? As in other secretory systems, essentially two mechanisms have been detected. On the one hand, considerable evidence indicates that a rise in intracellular cAMP results in the activation of secretion from both cell types. However, whether the regulatory hormones really operate through cAMP-dependent mechanism(s) is still a matter of debate. In particular, it has been observed that secretagogues, such as TRH and LHRH, elevate the levels of cAMP in pituitary tissue slices (Bowers, 1971; Borgeat *et al.*, 1972, 1974; Labrie *et al.*, 1973, 1976; Hinkle and Tashjian, 1977). However, clear modification of the pituitary adenylate cyclase (AC) has been reported for neither one of these hormones. Moreover, as will be discussed further in the section on "Pituitary Adenomas as Experimental Models", the situation is particularly confused for DA which in other systems is known to be a potent AC activator, whereas in homogenates of normal pituitary it has no detectable effect on the enzyme, although it displays a strong inhibitory action on PRL secretion from intact tissue. The link between cAMP rise and secretion stimulation is also unclear. A few years ago the group of Labrie (Labrie *et al.*, 1971; Lemay *et al.*, 1974) reported the cAMP-dependent phosphorylation of pituitary plasmalemma and granule membrane proteins. However, the physiological importance of these findings has never been assessed.

The other means by which pituitary cells can control their functional activity in response to receptor activation is through changes in their internal ionic environments. Electrophysiological and biochemical results showing $Ca^{2+}$ dependency of pituitary responses, depolarization and even the appearance of action potentials in cultured PRL-producing cells after TRH exposure have been reported (Parsons, 1970; Milligan and Kraicer, 1974; 1979; York *et al.*, 1975; Borgeat *et al.*, 1975; Kidokoro, 1975; Douglas and Taraskevich, 1977; Moriarty, 1977; 1978; Bickwell and Schofield, 1977; Tashjian *et al.*, 1978).

Several hypotheses have been proposed to explain the mechanism of action of $Ca^{2+}$. One suggests that it might elicit exocytosis through the phosphorylation of yet unknown proteins, either by a direct action (Krueger *et al.*, 1977; Greengard, 1978) or activation of guanylate cyclase and therefore through an increase of the intracellular level of cyclic GMP (Schultz and Hardman, 1975; Gautwick *et al.*, 1978).

In conclusion, both $Ca^{2+}$ and cAMP might act in concert as second messengers of GH and PRL secretion. According to the nomenclature of Goldberg *et al.* (1974), somatotrophs and mammotrophs should therefore be classified as mono-directional systems. However, large uncertainties still exist about the relationships of individual hormones and neurotransmitters with the second messenger systems as well as about the mechanisms whereby activation of the latter is finally elaborated into the physiological response. Some of these problems will be further discussed in the section on "Pituitary Adenomas as Experimental Models".

## GH AND PRL SECRETION IN HUMAN PITUITARY ADENOMAS

### Functional organization

Although the structure of different human adenomas secreting GH and PRL can be extremely variable (see Olivier *et al.*, 1975; Kovacs, this volume; Landolt, 1975, and this volume), many of the differences from normal pituitary tissue are common to most of them. First of all, in individual adenomas, cells are often very homogenous, as would be expected of elements originating from a single pro-liferating cell type. The rough-surfaced ER is well developed, while the smooth ER is sparse (Fig. 1). Free polyribosomes lying in the cytoplasmic matrix are often numerous (Fig. 1). The size and complexity of the Golgi complex can be well appreciated in freeze-fractured preparations (Fig. 2). In different tumors secretory granules are extremely variable in size, shape, density and number. As a whole, this picture bears relatively little resemblance to that of normal somato-trophs and mammotrophs and therefore the morphological identification of adenomas is difficult. On the other hand, it should be acknowledged that the criteria available for the identification of pituitary cell types rely primarily on the features of secretory granules; these granule features are grossly modified not only in tumors but also in a variety of other physiological, pathological and experi-mental conditions, for instance, in the fetal tissue as well as in glands removed from the control of the CNS (Zanini *et al.*, 1979).

In contrast, the pattern revealed by the analysis of the adenoma tissue proteins by SDS-PAGE is typical (Fig. 3). While in the normal human pituitary, both GH and PRL appear as prominent bands, in most adenomas only one or another of these two bands is present. This conclusion is reinforced by the results of experi-ments in which adenoma fragments were labeled *in vitro* with [3]H-L-leucine. In all cases we examined, the homologous hormone bands were the most labeled of the tissue pattern. The percentage of total protein radioactivity recovered in these bands was variable, probably in relation to the variable secretory and proliferative capacities of the different adenomas. For instance, in GH tumors from 8 to 30% of the radioactivity was recovered in the GH band (De Camilli *et al.*, 1978). Finally, when pulse-labeled adenoma fragments were chased *in vitro*, the only radioactive protein released to a detectable extent was the homologous hormone (Fig. 4).

Are the intracellular mechanisms of secretion the same in normal and adeno-matous somatotrophs and mammototrophs? Even though this problem has not been investigated in detail so far, the available evidence suggests that, at least in

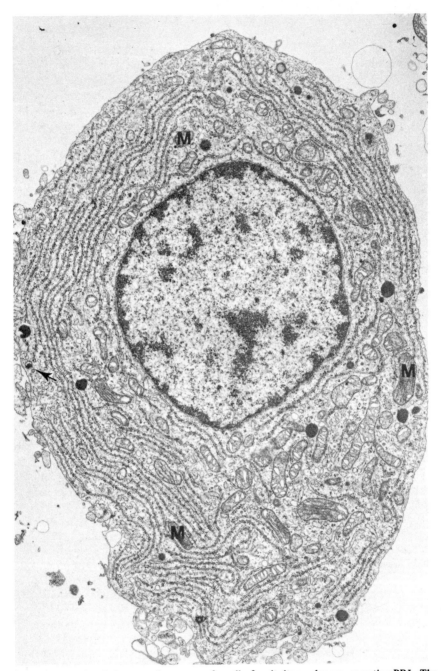

***Fig. 1.*** Conventional electron microscopy of a cell of a pituitary adenoma secreting PRL. The rough-surfaced endoplasmic reticulum is well developed, but the attached ribosomes are irregularly distributed and less numerous than in normal cells. Many free polysomes lie in the cytoplasm. Some mitochondria (M) are irregularly shaped.

In this tumor the secretory granules are few. The arrow indicates a granule core surrounded by a clear space. This image suggests that the granule had already been discharged even though the exocytotic opening is out of the section plane. ($\times$ 93 600).

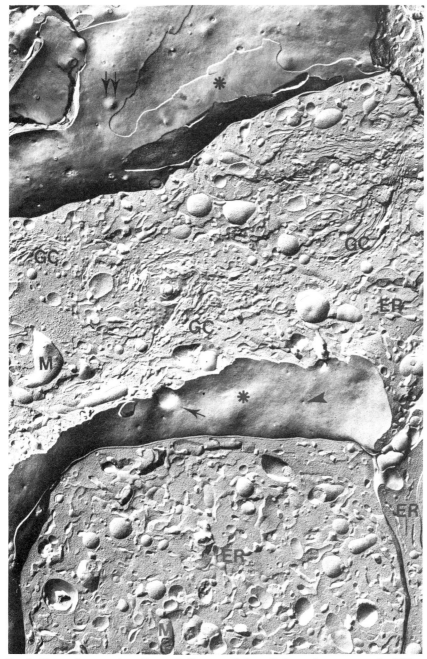

**Fig. 2.** Freeze-fracture view of several adjacent cells in a pituitary adenoma secreting PRL. Large expanses of plasma membrane (*) showing pits (arrowheads), infoldings (arrow) and bulges (double arrows), which might be related to exocytosis, are visible on the P fracture faces (see also Figs 6 and 7).

The fenestrated Golgi complex (GC) of the cell shown in the middle of the picture is very well developed and contains several forming granules. (× 14 560).

ER = endoplasmic reticulum. M = mitochondria.

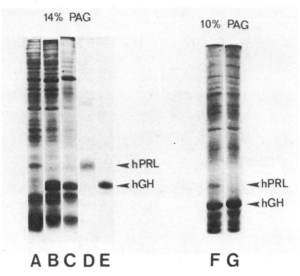

*Fig. 3.* SDS-polyacrylamide gel electrophoresis of homogenates of pituitary tissue. In gels A–E acrylamide concentration was 14%; in gels F–G, 10%.

A = PRL adenoma; B = glandular tissue adjacent to the PRL adenoma; C = autoptic specimen of human anterior pituitary; D = human PRL standard, E = human GH standard, F = glandular tissue adjacent to a GH adenoma; G = human GH adenoma.

Note that the electrophoretogram of the normal tissue shows both the GH and PRL bands, whereas those of the tumors show only one or the other of them.

its broad outline, the general scheme that we have described for normal cells might also apply to adenomas. Thus, the development of the rough-surfaced ER suggests that hormone biosynthesis takes place on bound polyribosomes. Moreover, in adenomas too, hormone molecules begin to accumulate in the extracellular space only several minutes after the completion of their synthesis (De Camilli, unpublished observation), probably because they had to undergo intracellular transport along the ER-Golgi-granules route in order to become available for discharge. We have recently obtained radioautographical evidence of the coexistence of complex carbohydrates with PRL within secretory granules in a PRL adenoma labeled with $^3$H-glucosamine (Fig. 5), as is found in normal mammotrophs (see the section on "Intracellular Transport and Packaging"). In some GH and PRL adenomas images of exocytosis are relatively rare. In this respect it should be pointed out that the occurrence of these images depends not only on the frequency of the process, but also on the persistence of the granule cores in the extracellular environment. The latter is not necessarily the same for normal and tumoral granules. The large and stable PRL granule cores are known to remain aggregated for quite some time after discharge; in contrast, no information exists for their adenomatous counterparts. In addition, it should be pointed out that when adequately sought (for instance by freeze-fracture, a morphological technique which allows one to view large plasmalemma expanses), exocytoses can be easily detected in adenomas also. Figure 6 is a low power view of a tumoral

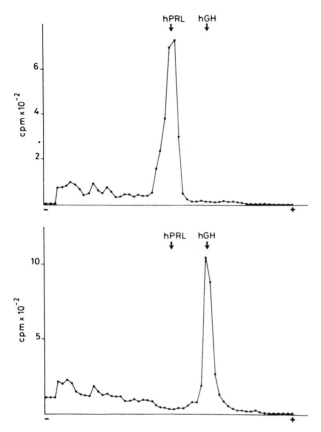

*Fig. 4.* SDS-polyacrylamide gel electrophoresis (gel concentration = 14%) of the radioactive proteins released from human adenomas secreting either PRL (top) or GH (bottom). Tissue fragments were first labeled *in vitro* for 60 min with $^3$H-L-leucine, then transferred to a superfusion apparatus containing non-radioactive medium, operated at a flow rate of 0.8 ml/min. The data shown refer to five-minute fractions collected from the 60th to the 65th min of superfusion. The positions of authentic standards are indicated by arrows.

mammotroph; the small particle-free bulges probably correspond to an initial stage of granule–plasmalemma fusion, while the large irregular dimples are the openings of exocytosis pits. A more advanced stage of this process is shown at higher power in Fig. 7: the granule membrane, recognizable by its lower complement of *P*-face particles, forms a pocket indentation in the plasmalemma.

Finally, we will deal with the regulation of PRL and GH secretion in pituitary adenomas. It is well known that these tumors display an altered pattern of response to a variety of regulatory factors. The responses to agents which induce sharp stimulatory or inhibitory responses in the normal pituitary tissue can be blunted or absent in adenomas; on the other hand, the secretory activity of adenomatous cells can be modified by factors which are totally inactive in their

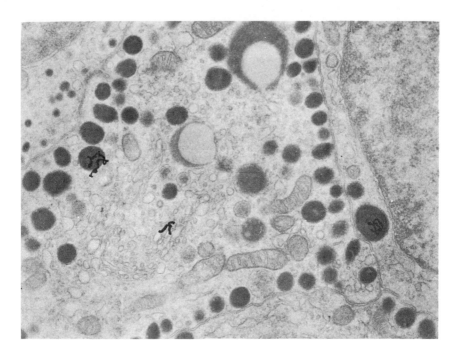

*Fig. 5.* Electron microscopic radioautography of a PRL-reacting pituitary ademona pulse-labeled *in vitro* for 30 min with D [6-³H] -glucosamine (80 μCi/ml; SA = 20 mCi/μmole) and then transferred to non-radioactive medium for 15 min. Note the presence of silver grains over the Golgi complex and secretory granules. This finding indicates that the granules contain macromolecular carbohydrates, which are probably synthesized in the Golgi complex. Unpublished results obtained in collaboration with Dr G. Nussdozfer (× 18 400).

normal counterparts. In some cases, however, it has been demonstrated that a pattern of response similar to that observed in adenomas can also be found in normal tissue under particular experimental conditions. For instance, it has been demonstrated that the somatotrophs of normal pituitaries grafted under the kidney capsule in homologous hypophysectomized animals acquire a responsivity to TRH (Giannattasio *et al.*, 1979) like that observed in adenomatous somatotrophs (Irie and Tsushima, 1972; Faglia *et al.*, 1973a, b). These findings seem to indicate that at least some of the differences in functional regulation which exist between adenomatous and normal pituitary cells are due to modified expression rather than to *de novo* appearance of specific features. A problem that deserves special attention is the sensitivity of PRL adenomas to dopaminergic inhibition, since it has been reported that some tumoral cell lines secreting PRL are insensitive to DA (Malarkey *et al.*, 1977). However, this is by no means the rule, at least for human PRL adenomas. Figure 8 concerns a superfusion experiment in which release of PRL from a human adenoma was stimulated by theophylline (which increases cyclic AMP through the inhibition of phosphodiesterases) and abolished by DA, analogously to what occurs in normal mammotrophs.

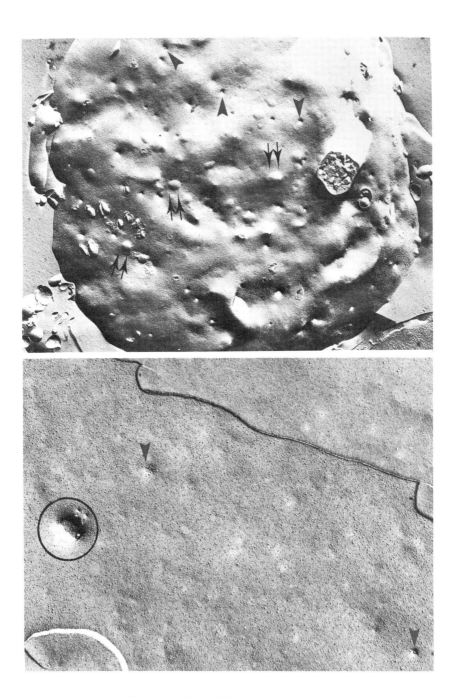

*Figs 6 and 7.* Low and high power views of P-fracture faces of plasmalemma of PRL secreting adenoma cells. The pits and bulges, indicated by arrowheads and double arrows respectively, may correspond to initial stages of granule–plasmalemma interaction leading to exocytosis. The full view of an exocytosis is encircled in Fig. 7. Note that the membrane of the
discharged granule, which is continuous with the surrounding plasmalemma, is characterized
by a lower complement of intramembrane particles (× 15 040 and × 27 920).

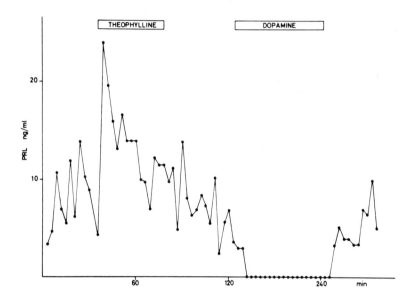

*Fig. 8.* *In vitro* release of PRL from a human prolactinoma. Tissue fragments were incubated at 37°C in a superfusion apparatus operated at a flow rate of 1 ml/min. Fractions were collected every 3 min. Concentrations of theophylline and dopamine were $5.5 \times 10^{-3}$ M and $1 \times 10^{-5}$ M, respectively. Measurements of PRL were carried out by radioimmunoassay.

### Pituitary adenomas as experimental models

The marked heterogeneity of the pituitary tissue can cause major problems in secretion studies. Important phenomena which occur in one single cell type, when studied biochemically in gland homogenates or in cell fractions isolated therefrom, can be blurred or even obscured completely by the contribution of the other cells. One such phenomena is the action of DA on mammotroph cells. In other systems such as various nuclei of the CNS (Kebabian *et al.*, 1972; Clement-Cornier *et al.*, 1974; Greengard, 1976), DA receptors are coupled to AC and the physiological effects of the neurotransmitter are believed to be mediated through the activation of this enzyme. In the pituitary there is no doubt that at least part of the strong inhibition of PRL secretion by DA is due to a direct effect on mammotroph cells (MacLeod, 1976; Fuxe, this volume). Yet numerous laboratories, including ours, have failed to demonstrate any effect of DA on the AC activity of normal pituitary homogenates (Kebabian, 1978). We reasoned that these negative results may be due not totally to different mechanisms of DA action on mammotrophs and neurons, but to the influence of the other cell types, whose AC activity might be modified by DA in the opposite direction or even unaffected. In collaboration with our colleagues of the Medical and Neurosurgical Clinics, we turned therefore to the study of human adenomas, which are constituted by homogeneous cell populations. The results, which are reported in detail in another article in this same book (De Camilli *et al.*, 1979), demonstrate a strict correlation between the ability of DA to inhibit PRL secretion from intact cells and produce changes in AC activity. Similar results have been reported by Kimura *et al.* (1976). Moreover, the pharmacological characterization of this DA-dependent AC agrees well with that of the corresponding DA receptor, as studied clinically in the patients before surgery. The inhibition of AC, which is not unique for DA, but has been observed in other systems for other hormones also (Traber *et al.*, 1975; Jakobs *et al.*, 1978; Nathanson *et al.*, 1978) might account for the effect of DA on mammotrophs since, as already mentioned in the section on "Release", strong evidence indicates that cAMP is a stimulator of PRL secretion.

In conclusion, it is therefore possible that DA receptors are coupled to AC in mammotrophs as in brain neurons. However, in the former case, receptor activation would cause inhibition and in the latter, stimulation of the enzyme. Of course, no proof exists that a similar mechanism operates in normal mammotrophs as well. However, that this might indeed be the case is suggested (a) by the similar effect of the neurotransmitter on PRL secretion and (b) by the similarities of the DA receptors in both systems. DA was also able to modify AC in GH adenomas (De Camilli *et al.*, 1979). However, at variance with the situation found with PRL adenomas, the results differed from case to case, and no agreement was found between the pharmacological features of DA-sensitive AC and the features of DA receptors revealed by clinical studies or between the effects of DA on the enzyme and on hormone secretion. Therefore, the functional role of DA-sensitive AC in GH adenomas is still unclear.

## CONCLUSIONS

Although secretion of GH and PRL are among the favourite subjects for investigation of both endocrinologists and cell biologists, and although individual details of these processes are now reasonably well understood, the available picture is still far from complete. In writing this article we have intended to show that studies of normal and tumoral somatotrophs and mammotrophs can be profitably considered to be complementary to each other. In a sort of feedback interaction, people studying adenomas can take advantage of what is known about normal cells, while results obtained with adenomas can help to fill gaps in the physiological knowledge. The final aim of this effort is the integration of multiple, individual pieces of information into a comprehensive understanding of pituitary hormone secretion.

## REFERENCES

Bickwell, R. J. and Schofield, J. G. (1977). *J. Endocrin.* **72**, 31P.
Blobel, G. and Dobberstein, B. (1975). *J. Cell Biol.* **67**, 835–851.
Borgeat, P., Chavency, G., Dupont, A., Labrie, F., Arimura, A. and Schally, A. V. (1972). *Proc. Natl. Acad. Sci., USA* **69**, 2677–2681.
Borgeat, P., Labrie, F., Drouin, F., Belanger, A., Immer, I., Sestanj, K., Nelson, V., Gotz, M., Schally, A. V., Coy, D. H. and Coy, E. J. (1974). *Biochim. Biophys. Res. Comm.* **56**, 1052–1059.

Borgeat, P., Garneau, P. and Labrie, F. (1975). *Molec. Cell. Endocrin.* **2**, 117–124.
Bowers, C. Y. (1971). *Ann. N. Y. Acad. Sci.* **185**, 263–290.
Campbell, P. N. and Blobel, G. (1976). *FEBS letters* **72**, 215–226.
Clement-Cornier, Y. C., Kebabian, J. W., Petzold, G. L. and Greengard, P. (1974). *Proc. Natl. Acad. Sci., USA* **71**, 1113–1119.
De Camilli, P., Tagliabue, L., Paracchi, A., Faglia, G., Beck Peccoz, P. and Giovannelli, M. (1978). *In* "Treatment of Pituitary Adenomas" (R. Fahlbusch and K. van Werder, eds) 172–179. G. Thieme, Stuttgart.
Douglas, W. W. and Taraskevich, P. S. (1977). *J. Physiol. Lond.* **272**, 41P–42P.
Faglia, G., Beck Peccoz, P., Ferrari, C., Travaglini, P., Ambrosi, B. and Spada, A. (1973a). *J. Clin. Endocrin. Metab.* **36**, 1259–1262.
Faglia, G., Beck Peccoz, P., Travaglini, P., Paracchi, A., Spada, A. and Lewin, A. (1973b). *J. Clin. Endocrin. Metab.* **37**, 338–341.
Farquhar, M. G. (1977). *In* "Comparative Endocrinology of Prolactin" (H. D. Dallmann, J. A. Johnson and D. M. Klachko, eds) 37–94. Plenum Press, New York.
Farquhar, M. G., Skutelky, E. H. and Hopkins, C. R. (1975). *In* "The Anterior Pituitary" (A. Tixier-Vidal and M. G. Farquhar, eds) 83–135. Academic Press, New York and London.
Farquhar, M. G., Reid, J. J. and Daniell, L. W. (1978). *Endocrinology* **102**, 296–311.
Flashner, Y. and Schramm, M. (1977). *J. Cell Biol.* **74**, 789–793.
Gautwick, K. M., Huang, E. and Kriz, M. (1978). *Biochim. Biophys. Acta* **538**, 354–365.
Giannattasio, G. and Zanini, A. (1976). *Biochim. Biophys. Acta* **439**, 349–357.
Giannattasio, G., Zanini, A. and Meldolesi, J. (1975). *J. Cell Biol.* **64**, 246–251.
Giannattasio, G., Zanini, A., Panerai, A. E., Meldolesi, J. and Müller, E. E. (1979). *Endocrinology* **104**, 237–242.
Giannattasio, G., Zanini, A. and Meldolesi, J. (in press). *In* "Complex Carbo-hydrates of the Nervous Tissue" (R. V. Margolis and R. K. Margolis, eds). Plenum Press, New York.
Giannattasio, G., Zanini, A., Rosa, P., Margolis, R. K., Margolis, R. U. and Meldolesi, J. (in preparation).
Goldberg, N. D., Haddox, M. K., Dunham, E., Lopez, C. and Hadden, J. W. (1974). *In* "Control of Proliferation in Animal Cells" (B. Clarkson and R. Baserga, eds) 609–625. Cold Spring Harbor Labs., New York.
Greengard, P. (1976). *Nature* **260** 101–108.
Greengard, P. (1978). *Science* **199**, 146–152.
Hinkle, P. M. and Tashjian, A. H. Jr (1977). *Endocrinology* **100**, 934–944.
Howell, S. L. and Whitfield, M. (1973). *J. Cell Sci.* **12**, 1–21.
Irie, M. and Tsushima, T. J. (1972). *J. Clin. Endocrin. Metab.* **35**, 97 100.
Jakobs, K. H., Saur, W. and Schültz, G. (1978). *N. S. Arch. Pharmacol.* **302**, 285–291.
Kebabian, J. W. (1978). *Life Sci.* **23**, 479–484.
Kebabian, J. W., Petzold, G. L. and Greengard, P. (1972). *Proc. Natl. Acad. Sci., USA* **69**, 2145–2151.
Kidokoro, Y. (1975). *Nature* **258**, 741–742.
Kimura, H., Calabro, M. A. and MacLeod, R. M. (1976). *Federation Proceedings* **35**, 305.
Kreibich, G., Ulrich, B. L. and Sabatini, D. D. (1978a). *J. Cell Biol.* **77**, 464–487.
Kreibich, G., Freinstein, C. M., Pereyra, B. N., Ulrich, B. L. and Sabatini, D. D. (1978b). *J. Cell Biol.* **77**, 488–506.

Kreuger, B. K., Forn, J. and Greengard, P. (1977). *J. Biol. Chem.* **252**, 2764–2773.

Labrie, F., Lemaire, S., Poirier, G., Pellettier, G. and Boucher, R. (1971). *J. Biol. Chem.* **246**, 7311–7317.

Labrie, F., Pellettier, G., Lemay, A., Borgeat, P., Bardeu, N., Dupont, A., Savary, M., Coté, J. and Boucher, R. (1973). *Acta Endocr. suppl.* **180**, 301–340.

Labrie, F., Pellettier, G., Borgeat, P., Drouin, J., Ferland, L. and Belanger, A. (1976). *In* "Frontiers in Neuroendocrinology" (L. Martini and W. F. Ganong, eds) Vol. IV, 63–93. Raven Press, New York.

Landolt, A. M. (1975). *Acta Neurochir.* suppl 22.

Lemay, Q., Deschenes, M., Lemaire, S., Poirer, G., Poulin, L. and Labrie, F. (1974). *J. Biol. Chem.* **249**, 323–331.

Lingappa, V. R., Devillers-Thiery, A. and Blobel, G. (1977). *Proc. Natl. Acad. Sci., USA* **74**, 2432–2436.

MacLeod, R. M. (1976). *In* "Frontiers in Neuroendocrinology" (L. Martini and W. F. Ganong, eds) 169–194. Raven Press, New York.

Malarkey, W. B., Groshong, J. C. and Milo, G. E. (1977). *Nature* **266**, 640–641.

Meldolesi, J., Marini, D. and Demonte-Marini, M. L. (1972). *Endocrinology* **91**, 802–808.

Meldolesi, J. Borgese, N., DeCamilli, P. and Ceccarelli, B. (1978). *In* "Cell Surface Reviews" (G. Poste and G. N. Nicolson, eds) Vol. V, 509–627. Elsevier, Amsterdam.

Milligan, J. V. and Kraicer, J. (1971). *Endocrinology* **89**, 766–773.

Milligan, J. V. and Kraicer, J. (1974). *Endocrinology* **94**, 435–443.

Moriarty, C. M. (1977). *Mol. Cell. Endocrinol.* **6**, 349–358.

Moriarty, C. M. (1978). *Life Sci.* **23**, 185–194.

Nathanson, N. M., Klein, W. and Noremberg, M. (1978). *Proc. Natl. Acad. Sci., USA* **75**, 1788–1791.

Olivier, L., Vila-Porcile, E., Racadot, O., Peillon, F. and Racadot, J. (1975). *In* "The Anterior Pituitary" (A. Tixier-Vidal and M. G. Farquhar, eds) 231–276. Academic Press, New York and London.

Palade, G. E. (1975). *Science* **189**, 347–358.

Parsons, G. A. (1970). *J. Physiol., Lond.* **210**, 973–987.

Racadot, J., Olivier, L., Porcile, E. and Droz, B. (1965). *C. R. Acad. Sci., Paris* **261**, 2972–2974.

Schultz, G. and Hardman, J. G. (1975). *In* "Advances in Cyclic Nucleotide Research" (P. Greengard and G. A. Robison, eds) Vol. V, 339–355. Raven Press, New York.

Slaby, F. and Farquhar, M. G. (in preparation).

Stachura, M. E. and Frohman, L. A. (1975). *Science* **187**, 447–449.

Sussman, P. M., Tushinski, R. J. and Bancroft, F. C. (1976). *Proc. Natl. Acad. Sci., USA* **73**, 29–33.

Swearingen, K. C. (1971). *Endocrinology* **89**, 1380–1388.

Tashjian, A. H., Lomedico, M. E. and Majna, D. (1978). *Biochim. Biophys. Res. Comm.* **81**, 798–806.

Tixier-Vidal, A. and Picart, R. (1967). *J. Cell Biol.* **35**, 501–519.

Traber, J., Reiser, G., Rischer, K., Hamprecht, B. (1975). *FEBS letters* **52**, 327–332.

York, D. H., Baker, F. L. and Kraicer, J. (1975). *Canad. J. Physiol. Pharmacol.* **53**, 777–786.

Zanini, A. and Giannattasio, G. (1974). *In* "Cytopharmacology of Secreton" (B. Ceccarelli, F. Clementi and J. Meldolesi, eds) 329–339. Raven Press, New York.

Zanini, A., Giannattasio, G. and Meldolesi, J. (1974a). *Endocrinology* **94**, 104–111.
Zanini, A., Giannattasio, G. and Meldolesi, J. (1974b). *Endocrinology* **94**, 594–598.
Zanini, A., Giannattasio, G., DeCamilli, P., Panerai, A. E., Müller, E. E. and Meldolesi, J. (1979). *Endocrinology* **104**, 226–236.
Zanini, A., Giannattasio, G., Margolis, R. U., Margolis, R. K., Nussdorfer, G. and Meldolesi, J. (in preparation).

# MORPHOLOGICAL AND MOLECULAR ASPECTS OF PROLACTIN AND GROWTH HORMONE SECRETION BY NORMAL AND TUMORAL PITUITARY CELLS IN CULTURE*

A. Tixier-Vidal, N. Brunet, C. Tougard and D. Gourdji

*Groupe de Neuroendocrinologie Cellulaire, Chaire de Physiologie Cellulaire, College de France, 11 Place Marcelin Berthelot 75231, Paris 05, France*

## INTRODUCTION

The prolactin (PRL) and growth hormone (GH) secreting pituitary tumor cells differ from their normal counterparts in two aspects which are of fundamental importance because of their biological and clinical consequences: the ultrastructural organization and the ability to continuously divide. The analysis at the individual cell level of the functional properties of such tumor cells is easier in a cell culture system than in tumor tissue fragments, where the homogeneity of the cell population is questionable and where the cell exposure to regulatory molecules may be rather heterogeneous. Indeed, the pioneer work of Gordon Sato and his colleagues demonstrated the possibility of isolating functional cell lines from tumors, using the technique of alternate animal and cell culture passage (Buonassisi *et al.*, 1962). Starting from an estrogen-induced mammosomatotropic rat pituitary tumor (MtT/W5) several clonal cell lines which secrete PRL and GH have been isolated (Yasumura *et al.*, 1966; Tashjian *et al.*, 1968, 1970; Bancroft *et al.*, 1969). Their usefulness for studies of control mechanisms of PRL and GH secretion has been extensively demonstrated during the last decade (see review by Tashjian and Hoyt, 1972; Tixier-Vidal *et al.*, 1975a, 1978). In order to compare

*This work was supported by grants from INSERM (ATP No. 24 75 47 and 76 4 496) and from the DGRST (No. 77 7 0 492) and from the CEA (No. 73 09).
We are grateful to Mrs. M. F. Moreau, R. Picart, MM. D. Grouselle and C. Pennarun for their excellent technical assistance.

the properties of these tumor cells in culture with those of normal anterior pituitary cells a cell culture system has to be chosen. The best counterpart will therefore be offered by primary cultures of normal rat anterior pituitary cells which have been shown to retain the ultrastructural organization of normal anterior pituitary cells in culture for at least 5–7 days (Tixier-Vidal, 1975; Tixier-Vidal *et al.*, 1975a). Our purpose here will be to compare, when possible, normal and tumoral PRL and GH secreting cells in culture, from several points of view: ultrastructural organization and subcellular distribution of hormonal antigenicity, kinetics of hormonal secretion, regulation of hormonal secretion by thyroliberin, estrogens and dopamine.

## ULTRASTRUCTURAL ORGANIZATION

### Primary cultures

Primary cultures of normal rat anterior pituitary cells previously dispersed by enzymatic treatment have been shown to retain at least for the first week in culture the various pituitary cell types, which were identified either by electron microscope observation (Tixier-Vidal, 1975) or by immunocytochemical staining (Baker *et al.*, 1974; Tougard *et al.*, 1977, Bácsy *et al.*, 1976).

In this heterogeneous population most of the PRL cells display ultrastructural features of actively secreting prolactin cells as described *in vivo* in the lactating rat (Pasteels, 1963). They generally contain large polymorphic secretory granules. The Golgi zone is large, limited by stacks of saccules and displays in its core large and irregular masses of condensing secretory material. In addition, the rough endoplasmic reticulum presents the typical organization of protein-secreting glandular cells, that is, parallel rows of linear cisternae (Fig. 1). After immuno-cytoenzymatic treatment, using an anti-rat PRL serum which does not cross react with rat GH, the secretory granules were the most antigenic sites. In the core of the Golgi zone masses of condensing secretory material were also sometimes immunoreactive. In addition, the cytoplasm also displayed a positive reaction which was possibly located on free polysomes. In some cells, some RER cisternae were underlined with reaction product, although their contents were always negative. The smooth membrane and the contents of the Golgi stacks of saccules were also always negative (Fig. 2) (Tixier-Vidal *et al.*, 1976). The immunochemical staining therefore shows that in normal prolactin cells in culture the hormone is mainly concentrated in the secretory granules, but also suggests that an extra-granular pool of hormone might exist.

GH-secreting cells are relatively numerous in six-day-old cultures, where they retain an ovoid shape, as can be seen after specific immunocytochemical staining with an anti-human GH. When the cultures were doubly stained for GH and PRL, the hormones were located in separate cells (Baker *et al.*, 1974), which is also observed *in vivo* (Martin-Comin and Robyn, 1976). At the electron microscope level, GH cells in culture are characterized by an accumulation of round secretory granules, a small Golgi zone and an almost total absence of RER linear cisternae. Without the help of the immunocytoenzymatic technique, it is sometimes difficult to differentiate them from PRL cells, when the latter are in a storage phase, or in certain planes of section.

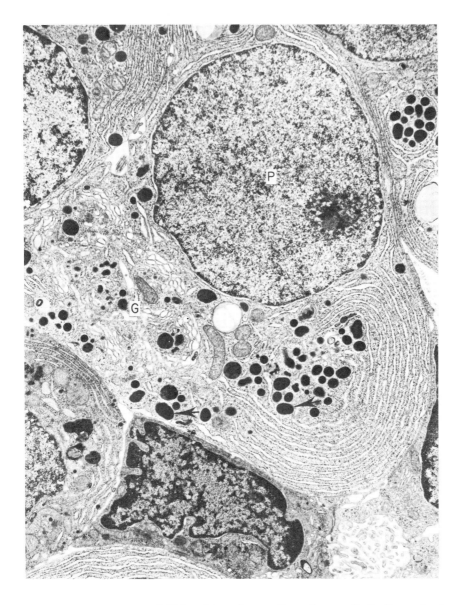

*Fig. 1.* A normal prolactin cell (P) in a 5-day primary culture of enzymatically dispersed male rat anterior pituitary cells treated by conventional methods for electron microscope study. It displays the classical ultrastructural features of actively secreting cells: a large Golgi zone (G), with condensing secretory material, and parallel rows of linear rough endoplasmic reticulum cisternae. One notices the large size of the secretory granules (→) (× 7500).

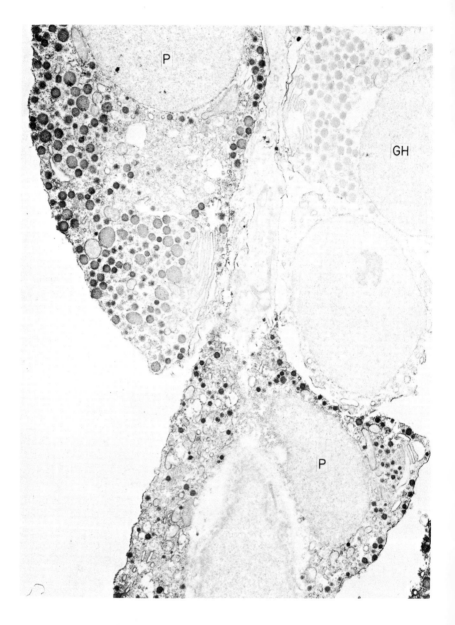

*Fig. 2.* Normal prolactin cells (P) in the same culture as described in Fig. 1. They were immunocytochemically stained, using an anti-rat PRL serum prepared against purified rat PRL (a gift from NIAMDD) dilution: 1/100. The positive reaction presents its maximum intensity on secretory granules. A positive reaction is also found in the cytoplasm. Nucleus, mitochondria and the content of RER cisternae are negative. A GH cell (GH) is totally unstained (× 7500).

## GH3 cells

After their isolation from the MtT/W5 tumor the various "GH" cell lines were found to secrete either GH (Bancroft *et al.*, 1969) or PRL or both GH and PRL (Tashjian *et al.*, 1970). Depending on the GH3 subclones, the ratio of PRL/GH secreted in the medium varies widely. Our morphological and biological studies are performed on GH3 cells or on GH3 subclones which produce more PRL than GH (see the section on "Kinetics of PRL and GH Secretion in Culture").

GH3 cells differ from normal prolactin cells greatly in their ultrastructural organization (Gourdji *et al.*, 1972; Tixier-Vidal *et al.*, 1975a) (Fig. 3). They possess a high nucleus–cytoplasm ratio. The secretory granules are sparse or even absent. In a small proportion of cells they may nevertheless be more numerous. Their diameters vary from 50 to 150 nm and they generally are localized near the cell membrane. They are either polymorphic and small or rounded and large (150–250 nm). The Golgi zone is made of several units scattered within the cytoplasm. Each Golgi unit consists of large dilated and elongated smooth cisternae which are associated with small vesicles and, in some cases, with small condensing secretory granules. The cytoplasm contains many free polysomes and ribosomes, but linear cisternae of rough endoplasmic reticulum were far less developed than in normal PRL cells in culture. The ultrastructural organization of GH3 cells is very similar to that of tumor cells *in vivo*, such as in estrogen-induced rat pituitary tumor (Waelbroeck-Van Gaver and Potvliège, 1969) or in human pituitary chromophobe adenoma (Olivier *et al.*, 1975). In addition, the absence of the normal pattern of ultra-structural organization does not permit one to identify separate PRL-secreting and GH-secreting cell types in the GH3 cell population. This distinction remains difficult even after immunocytochemical staining. Indeed, at the light microscope level the GH3 cells display anti-rat PRL serum used for normal cells. A higher intensity of the reaction was obtained in another cell line, SD1, which was isolated in our laboratory after spontaneous transformation of a primary culture of normal rat pituitary cells and was found capable of producing tumors after *in vivo* passage. The ultrastructural organization of SD1 cells is very similar to that of GH3 cells, but after immunocytochemical staining with anti-rat PRL serum the intensity of the positive reaction permitted electron microscope observations (Tixier-Vidal *et al.*, 1976) (Fig. 4). The secretory granules, although very few and small, were always strongly positive whatever their localization in the cytoplasm. In addition, a cytoplasmic specific staining was always found, even in cells which apparently lacked secretory granules. The particulate feature of the cytoplasmic deposit suggested that the antigenic sites might be located on polysomes, which is consistent with an increased reaction at the border of some RER cisternae. In contrast, no reaction was found within the RER cisternae or in the smooth cisternae of the Golgi zone. As compared to normal PRL cells in primary cultures, SD1 cells display therefore, a similar distribution of the antigenicity among subcellular structures. In both cases, the secretory granules are the most antigenic sites. This suggests the existence of a storage compartment which is larger in normal cells than in tumor-derived cells. The difference between them therefore appears to be more quantitative than qualitative.

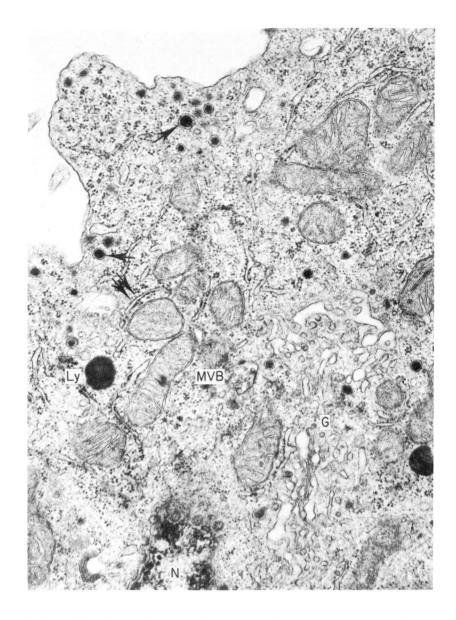

*Fig. 3.* A GH3 cell treated by conventional methods for electron microscope study. As compared to a normal prolactin cell in culture (Fig. 1), one notices the small size and the paucity of secretory granules (→), the very short rough endoplasmic cisternae (⇉) and the presence of numerous free polysomes and ribosomes. The cell also contains a well-defined Golgi zone (G) with small condensing secretory granules. N : nucleus, Ly : lysosome, MVB : multivesicular body (× 30 000).

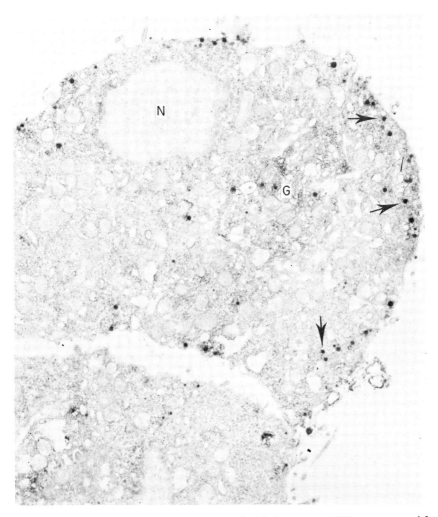

*Fig. 4.* A SD1 cell immunocytochemically stained with the same anti-PRL serum as used for primary cultures (Fig. 2). Again, the small secretory granules display an intensely positive reaction (→). In addition, the cytoplasm also displays an important positive reaction. The nucleus, mitochondria and the contents of the Golgi cisternae are negative. G : Golgi zone, N : nucleus (× 7500).

Although GH has been immunocytochemically localized at the electron micro-scope level in subclones of the GH3 strain which produce GH (Masur *et al.*, 1974), no successful attempt to simultaneously localize GH and PRL within the same cells has been reported so far. The immunocytochemical approach does not permit us therefore, to decide whether PRL and GH are simultaneously secreted by the same cell or by different cells in the GH3 cell population. The situation seems to be different *in vivo*, in rat mammosomatotropic tumors, where GH and PRL have been immunocytochemically identified within the same cells (Ueda *et al.*, 1973).

## KINETICS OF PRL AND GH SECRETION IN CULTURE

In order to understand the functional significance of the difference in the patterns of ultrastructural organization between normal and tumor cells, a kinetic analysis of the secretory cycle in cultured cells was performed. For that purpose cells were plated at the same initial density within plastic tissue culture dishes (35 mm diam., Falcon) and grown for 5 days in regular culture medium (Ham F 10, 15% horse serum, 2.5% fetal calf serum). The distribution of the hormone within cells and medium was measured by radioimmunoassay at increasing time intervals over a 24-hour period following medium withdrawal and cell washing.

### Primary cultures

*PRL secretion (Fig. 5a)*
The amount of PRL released into the medium increased fairly linearly from 1 h to 24 h. A much steeper increase occurred within the first hour, which may represent a rapid cell response to the medium change, just before time 0. During the same 24-hour period the PRL cell content remained the same at time 0 (820 ± 65.6 ng/dish) and after 24 h (780 ± 20.8 ng/dish), if one excepts the variations which were observed after 1 h (682 ± 38.7 ng/dish) and 2 h (1033 ± 72.6 ng/dish). These variations are most probably related to the rapid release which happens within the first hour. During the 24-hour period of observation, the ratio of extracellular PRL to intracellular PRL increased from 36% at 15 min to 200% after 24 h. Assuming that there is no PRL degradation in the system, one might calculate that the cells renew their contents each 12 hours.

*GH (Fig. 5b)*
During the same 24-hour period the amounts of GH released into the medium at the same time as PRL followed a very different curve. It increased steeply during the first 15 min (0 to 245 ±30 ng/dish) but thereafter it remained roughly constant over the rest of the 24-hour period of investigation. After 24 h, the medium contained 7 times more PRL than GH.

The striking differences between the kinetics of PRL and GH secretion are consistent with previous data on the secretory capacity of primary cultures of normal anterior pituitary cells. Indeed it has been previously shown that such cultures secrete large amounts of PRL for several weeks, whereas the other anterior pituitary hormones are released at a dramatically decreasing level and even become undetectable (see review by Tixier-Vidal, 1975; Tixier-Vidal *et al.*, 1975a). The autonomy of PRL secretion in culture as well as the absence of autonomy of GH secretion are well reflected by the difference in their respective short-term kinetics of release. In addition this difference is compatible with the existence in primary cultures of a different cell type for each of these two hormones.

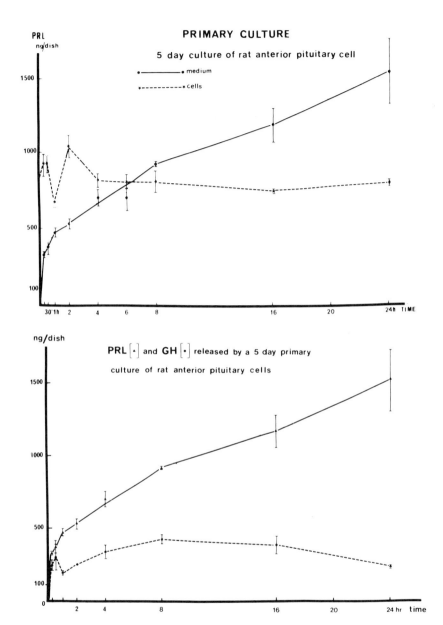

*Fig. 5.* Time-course of prolactin and growth hormone secretion by normal male rat anterior pituitary cells previously dissociated by enzymatic treatment and grown as a monolayer for 5 days before the experiment in Ham F 10 solution supplemented with 15% horse serum and 2.5% fetal calf serum (5.10$^5$ cells/2 ml medium/dish). Before the experiment the medium was withdrawn and the cells were washed with cold F 10 solution. At time 0 of the experiment 1.5 ml of fresh serum-supplemented medium was introduced and the cells were then incubated at 37°C for up to 24 h. At each time interval, 3 dishes were used for measurement of hormone secretion. (a) PRL content in medium (●——●) in cell extracts (x- - -x) as measured by RIA using the NIAMDD kit. (b) PRL (▲——▲) and GH (●- - -●) content in medium of the same dishes. GH was measured by RIA using the NIAMDD kit.

### GH3 cells

The experiments were performed on a GH3 subclone (GH3/B6) which was isolated in our laboratory.

*PRL secretion (Fig. 6a)*

Following medium renewal and washings, the amount of PRL released into the medium increased at a strictly linear rate from time 0 to 16 h. The PRL medium content increased 150 times between 15 min and 16 h. During the same period, the PRL cell content increased 5–6 times, from 37.3 ± 6.9 ng/dish to 216 ± 4.4/dish, and the ratio of extracellular PRL to intracellular PRL displayed a dramatic increase, from 22 to 1170%. Assuming that there is no PRL degradation in the system and given a mean value of 150 ng/dish for the PRL cell content, it may be roughly estimated that the cells renew their PRL content each hour.

*GH secretion (Fig. 6b)*

The amount of GH released into the medium at the same time as PRL by GH3/B6 cells increased very slowly from 15 min (105 ± 21.2 ng/dish) to 24 h (260 ± 25 ng/dish) following medium renewal. During the same period the GH cell content also increased slightly, from 48 ± 6.9 ng/dish to 113.3 ± 8.8 ng/dish. The ratio of extracellular GH to intracellular GH remained roughly the same during that period.

The comparison of the features of GH secretion with those of PRL secretion by the same cell population reveals some similarities and important differences.

(1)   The initial PRL and GH cell contents, at time 0, are identical (PRL: 37.3 ± 6.9 ng/dish; GH: 48.3 ± 6.9 ng/dish); the GH cell content increased thereafter 2 times whereas the PRL cell content increased 6 times.

(2)   The PRL medium content increased by 168 times whereas that of GH increased only about 2 times. If one assumes that GH degradation is not greater than PRL degradation in the system, it appears that, at least under our culture conditions, the GH3/B6 cell capacity for hormonal release is considerably higher for PRL than for GH. This suggests that PRL turnover is higher than that of GH in those cells.

As compared to normal PRL and GH cells in culture, the PRL turnover is obviously faster in GH3 cells than in normal cells. This conclusion is consistent with the above-described differences in their patterns of ultrastructural organization. The interference of cell division with cell secretion seems to be limited in our experiments. Indeed no conclusive evidence has been reported so far for PRL cell division in primary cultures (Tixier-Vidal *et al.*, 1975a). As concerns the GH3 cells, their doubling time was estimated to be around 28–30 h in synchronized cells (Faivre-Bauman *et al.*, 1975). Our experiments were performed on non-synchronized cells. Nevertheless, the thorough washing which preceded the 24 hour-period of investigation may have interfered with the cell cycle. In that respect, the very low increase of PRL medium content between 16 h and 24 h (Fig. 5a) might be related to a partial synchronization since we already found that in synchronized cells the rate of PRL accumulation into the medium decreased and tended to plateau during the *S* phase (Faivre-Bauman *et al.*, 1975).

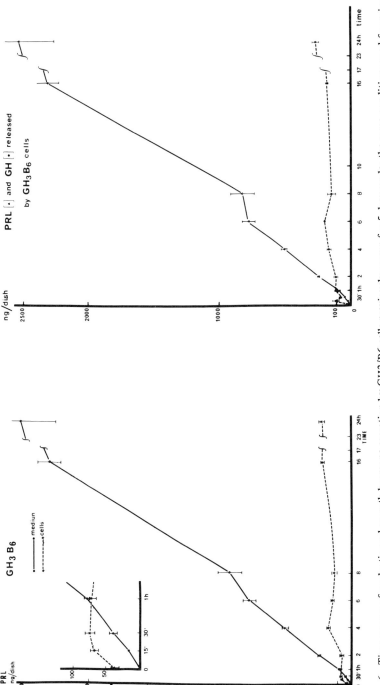

*Fig. 6.* Time-course of prolactin and growth hormone secretion by GH3/B6 cells previously grown for 5 days under the same conditions used for primary cultures (Fig. 5) (2 × 10⁵ cells/2 ml medium/dish). Before the experiment the cells were treated as described in legend of Fig. 5. At the time 0 of the experiment 1 ml of fresh serum-supplemented medium was introduced and the cells were then incubated at 37°C for up to 24 h. At each time interval 4 dishes were used for measurement of the hormonal secretion, as described in the legend of Fig. 5. (a) PRL content in medium (●——●) and cell extracts (x- - -x). (b) PRL (▲——▲) and GH content (●- - -●) in medium.

An interesting similarity between GH3 cells and primary culture resides in the very low level of GH release which is observed in both cases, in spite of the fact that in GH3 cells the initial cell content was the same for both GH and PRL. This surprising observation suggests that PRL and GH secretion are regulated independently in GH3 cells. A similar conclusion was suggested by studies on synchronized GH3 cells where the GH accumulation into the medium during the cell cycle did not parallel that of PRL (Faivre-Bauman et al., 1976). This, of course, raises the question of whether they are produced in the same cell or in separate cells. Although we used a subclone of GH3 cells, the GH3/B6, which was derived from a single cell, the possibility that in mass culture two types of cells can differentiate from a parental cell cannot be excluded (Tashjian and Hoyt, 1972). In addition, one must keep in mind that tumor-derived cell lines retain the features of tumor cells, that is both enhanced cell replication and chances for spontaneous mutations. Indeed, estrogen-induced pituitary tumors have been shown to secrete not only PRL but also GH and upon transplantation the GH production increased and PRL production was even lost (see review of Furth, 1973). The cell culture approach permits one to eliminate the cell heterogeneity of the tumor by cloning, but the stability of the clone may not be better *in vitro* than *in vivo*. Such stability must therefore be repeatedly checked for and maintained, which is possible only in culture.

## REGULATION OF PRL AND GH SECRETION IN CULTURE

Studies on the regulation of PRL and GH secretion in culture have been performed mainly with the various tumor-derived "GH" cell lines, taking advantage of the fact that they offer homogeneous populations of target cells. That permitted considerable progress to be made in knowledge of the molecular mechanisms which regulate GH and PRL synthesis. A complete analysis of these works would exceed the purpose of this brief review, which is to compare regulation of PRL and GH secretion in normal and tumor cells in cultures. The main effects of the three most powerful regulators of PRL secretion will be successively reviewed.

## THYROLIBERIN

The first evidence of a stimulating effect of thyroliberin (Glu-His-ProNH$_2$, TRH) on PRL secretion was obtained in GH3 cells (Tashjian et al., 1971). This unexpected effect of TRH was thereafter observed *in vivo* in several species, including the human (see review of Tixier-Vidal et al., 1975b; Vale et al., 1977). In the normal rat, TRH has only a minor effect or no effect on PRL release *in vivo*, as well as *in vitro* in primary culture. Nevertheless it consistently stimulates PRL release *in vitro* by cultured pituitary cells taken from hypothyroid rats (Vale et al., 1973) as well as *in vivo* in lactating and pregnant or diestrus female rats and estrogen-pretreated male rats (see review by Vale et al., 1977). This suggests the existence of interaction of thyroid hormones and steroid hormones in the response to TRH, which has been indeed analysed at the molecular level using cells in culture (see below).

TRH exerts a biphasic stimulating effect on PRL secretion by SD1 cells: a short-term effect on the release of preformed intracellular PRL and a long-term effect on PRL synthesis (see review in Tixier-Vidal *et al.*, 1978). This model of action, which is compatible with the existence of a storage compartment in tumor cells, is also valid for normal cells in culture (Vale *et al.*, 1973).

The binding of $^3$H-TRH was extensively studied in intact GH3 cells as well as in GH3 cell homogenates. It is time-dependent and dose-dependent (see review of Tixier-Vidal *et al.*, 1975b, 1978). Two families of binding sites were found: high affinity sites ($Kd_1$ : $4.10^{-8}$M) for physiological doses and low affinity sites (Kd: $3.10^{-7}$ M) for high doses (100–1000 nM). Dual sites for TRH binding with similar affinities were also observed in cultured TSH-secreting mouse tumor cells and the same high affinity component was also found in a plasma membrane preparation from bovine pituitary glands (see review by Tixier-Vidal *et al.*, 1975b). These similarities suggest that the TRH receptors in GH3 cells possess features similar to those of normal TSH or PRL secreting cells. This is strongly supported by comparison of the receptor binding affinities and biological activities *in vitro* and *in vivo* of numerous structural analogues of TRH (Hinkle *et al.*, 1974; Vale *et al.*, 1973).

The mechanism of the interaction of 17β-estradiol in the TRH effect on PRL secretion was found to be the same in GH3 cells (Tixier-Vidal *et al.*, 1978) and in normal rat pituitaries *in vivo* (De Léan *et al.*, 1977): 17β-estradiol pretreatment increases the number of TRH-binding sites without modifying their apparent affinity and potentiates the TRH-induced stimulation of PRL release, the apparent $K_m$ of which is lowered. Reciprocally, the inhibitory effect of L-triiodothyronine on TRH-induced stimulation of PRL secretion corresponds to a decrease in the number of TRH receptors, without alteration of their affinity (Perrone and Hinkle, 1978).

The stimulating effect of TRH on GH secretion which was described *in vivo* in cattle, and under the same conditions in rats and humans (see review Vale *et al.*, 1977) is also observed *in vitro* in GH3 cells (Faivre-Bauman *et al.*, 1976), but this is only a short-term effect on GH release which is followed by a decrease in GH synthesis (Tashjian *et al.*, 1971). To our knowledge such a long-term inhibiting effect of TRH on GH secretion *in vivo* has not been reported.

## Estrogens

In view of the importance of the role of estrogens in PRL regulation *in vivo*, the analysis in culture of their mechanisms of action is of particular interest. Indeed it is well known that estradiol exerts two types of action *in vivo* in the rat: a stimulation of PRL secretion (Meites and Nicoll, 1965) and a stimulation of mitotic activity of PRL secreting cells (Furth and Clifton, 1958).

A direct action of 17β-estradiol on PRL secretion has been demonstrated *in vitro* not only in organ cultures (Meites and Nicoll, 1965) but also on GH3 cells where $10^{-4} - 10^{-6}$ M concentrations of estradiol induced an increase of extracellular and intracellular PRL after 3–7 days of treatment, while decreasing GH production (Tashjian and Hoyt, 1972; Haug and Gautvik, 1976; Tixier-Vidal *et al.*, 1978). This was observed in normal medium supplemented with 17β-estra- diol as well as in medium prepared from charcoal-dextran extracted serum, supplemented or not with 17β-estradiol. This effect seems specific for 17β- estradiol, since progesterone was found to exert a slight decreasing action and testosterone a very weak stimulating action on PRL secretion (Haug and Gautvik, 1976). The biological effect of 17β-estradiol is consistent with a selective uptake of that steroid by GH3 cells (Sonnenschein *et al.*, 1973) although no attempt has been made to correlate that uptake with the expression of a biological effect on PRL secretion.

In contrast, the mitogenic action of 17β-estradiol in PRL cells *in vivo* was not observed *in vitro* in GH3 cells, where it has been repeatedly found that this steroid does not affect cell growth (Sorrentino *et al.*, 1976; Clausen *et al.*, 1978; Tixier-Vidal *et al.*, 1978). It nevertheless acts on the DNA/protein ratio, which is decreased in medium supplemented with charcoal-dextran extracted serum and restored to a normal level in the presence of added 17β-estradiol (Brunet *et al.*, 1977). The absence of mitogenic action of estradiol on GH3 cells in culture contrasts with the fact that their ability to form tumors after *in vivo* injection is strictly dependent on the circulating level of estrogens (Sonnenschein *et al.*, 1973; Sorrentino *et al.*, 1976). The possibility that estrogen might act through the induction *in vivo* of polypeptide growth factors has been recently proposed (Sirbasku and Benson, in press).

Very few attempts have been made to look for a direct mitogenic effect of 17β-estradiol on normal pituitary cells in culture. In organ cultures, no effect was found on the induction of thymidine kinase after 24 or 48 h of treatment with 17β-estradiol (Le Guellec *et al.*, 1977).

### Dopamine and dopamine agonists

A large body of information suggests that dopamine (DA) may be the main inhibitory substance involved in the hypothalamic control of PRL secretion. Moreover, a direct inhibitory action of DA and of DA agonists on PRL secretion has been demonstrated in incubated rat hemi-pituitaries (MacLeod, 1969; MacLeod and Lamberts, 1978).

In primary cultures of dispersed rat anterior pituitary cells, DA and several dopaminergic agents, including ergot alkaloids, have been found to be potent inhibitors of PRL release. This effect is dose-dependent, stereospecific and can be closely correlated with the characteristics of the binding of [3]H-dihydroergocryptine to bovine anterior pituitary membranes (Labrie *et al.*, 1978). In addition, the inhibitory effect of DA agonists can be almost completely reversed by previous incubation with 17β-estradiol for 120 h (Labrie *et al.*, 1978; Raymond *et al.*, 1978). DA agonists also inhibited the TRH-induced stimulation of PRL release, an effect which is also prevented by previous incubation with 17β-estradiol (Raymond *et al.*, 1978). It appears therefore that the complex interaction between TRH, estradiol and DA in the *in vivo* regulation of PRL release is completely retained in primary cultures of normal rat anterior pituitary cells.

The situation is less clear in the GH3 cells. It has been shown that DA failed to inhibit PRL secretion by GH3 cells, when used under the same conditions and at the same concentrations that cause potent inhibition of PRL release in primary cultures. It was concluded that GH3 cells have a dopaminergic defect related to their tumoral origin (Malarkey *et al.*, 1977). Nevertheless, the ergot derivative CB154, a potent dopaminergic agonist, was found to be able to partially inhibit the spontaneous release of PRL when used at a rather high concentration, either

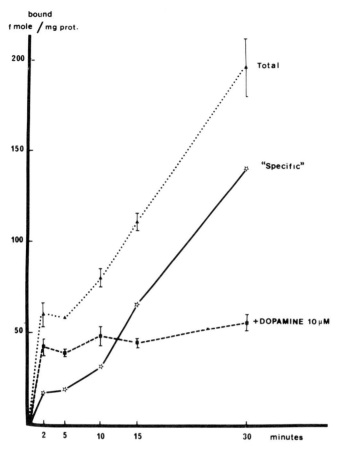

*Fig. 7.* Time course of ³H-dopamine binding by GH3/B6 cells previously grown for 5 days prior to the experiment, as described in the legend of Fig. 6. Before the experiment the medium was withdrawn and cells were rinsed with Ham F 10 solution containing 20 mM HEPES (pH 7.2). Fresh Ham F 10 solution supplemented with HEPES was thereafter used for incubation at 37°C in the absence or in the presence of ³H-DA (16 nM - 6 Ci/mM - NEN) (▲- - -▲) supplemented, or not, with 10 μM DA (■- - -■). Cell radioactivity was measured after washing the cells 4 times at 4°C with the same solution. Experiments were performed in triplicate. The curve for "specific" (x—x) binding was obtained by subtracting binding observed in the presence of excess unlabeled DA from the binding observed in absence of this excess of DA.

$3 \times 10^{-6}$ M for 3 h (Gautvik *et al.*, 1973) or $0.6 \times 10^{-6}$ M for 1-3 days (Gourdji *et al.*, 1973). Under the latter conditions CB154 inhibited the TRH-induced stimulation of PRL production by 80% (Gourdji *et al.*, 1973).

The GH3/B6 cell capacities to bind ³H-DA and to give a biological response was investigated. As illustrated on Fig. 7, intact cells bound ³H-DA. The curve representing the kinetics of binding displayed two components: a plateau at 2-5 min followed by a linear increase up to 30 min. In presence of an excess of unlabeled DA (10 μM), the first component was decreased by 30%, whereas the second component was decreased by 70%. The half-life of DA, as measured under the same experimental conditions, using specific radioenzymatic technique, was 30 min (Dr. J. P. Tassin, INSERM, U. 114). The second component of the curve therefore could be partially ascribed to tritiated DA metabolites. Nevertheless, a significant partial inhibition (31%) of PRL secretion was observed after 5 min as well as after 30 min of exposure. It seems therefore that GH3/B6 cells are not completely deprived of functional DA receptors. The latter might be partially masked, due to either tumoral transformation or to the presence or absence of some peripheric hormones.

In concluding this brief review, it appears that, concerning the mechanisms involved in the regulation of PRL secretion, the GH tumor-derived cell lines retain many of the receptors and the responsiveness of normal PRL cells. It must nevertheless be pointed out that these properties may be lost, simultaneously or separately, depending on the clones and/or the culture conditions. For example, GH3 cells grown for months in charcoal-dextran extracted serum lose most of their TRH receptors and their ability for hormone secretion (Brunet *et al.*, 1977). It has also been reported that GH3 cells which displayed estradiol responsiveness prior to 1974 have thereafter "spontaneously" lost this property (Dannies *et al.*, 1977). The occurrence of similar events *in vivo*, which might explain the variations in PRL-responsiveness among patients with pituitary adenomas cannot be excluded.

## REFERENCES

Bácsy, E., Tougard, C., Tixier-Vidal, A., Marton, J. and Stark, E. (1976). *Histochemistry* **50**, 161–174.

Baker, B. L., Reel, J. R., Van Dewark, S. D. and Yu, Y. Y. (1974). *Anat. Rec.* **179**, 93–106.

Bancroft, F. C., Levine, L. and Tashjian, A. H. (1969). *J. Cell Biol.* **43**, 432–441.

Brunet, N., Gourdji, D., Moreau, M. F., Grouselle, D., Bournaud, F. and Tixier-Vidal, A. (1977). *Ann. Biol. Anim. Biochem. Biophys.* **17** (3B), 413–424.

Buonassisi, V., Sato, G. and Cohen, A. I. (1962). *Proc. Nat. Acad. Sci., USA* **48**, 1184–1190.

Clausen, O. P. F., Gautvik, K. M. and Haug, E. (1978). *J. Cell Physiol.* **94**, 205–214.

Dannies, P., Yen, P. M. and Tashjian, A. H., Jr. (1977). *Endocrinology* **101**, 1151–1156.

De Léan, A., Ferland, L., Drouin, J., Kelly, P. A. and Labrie, F. (1977). *Endocrinology* **100**, 1496–1504.

Faivre-Bauman, A., Gourdji, D., Grouselle, D. and Tixier-Vidal, A. (1975). *Biochem. Biophys. Res. Commun.* **67**, 50–57.

Faivre-Bauman, A., Gourdji, D., Grouselle, D. et Tixier-Vidal, A. (1976). *J. Microsc. Biol. Cell.* **27**, p. 9a.

Furth, J. (1973). *In* "Human Prolactin" (J. L. Pasteels and C. Robyn, eds) 233–238. Elsevier, Amsterdam.

Furth, J. and Clifton, K. H. (1958). *Endocrinology* **12**, 3–18.

Gautvik, K. M., Hoyt, R. F. Jr. and Tashjian, A. H., Jr. (1973). *J. Cell Physiol.* **82**, 401–410.

Gourdji, D., Kerdelhué, B. and Tixier-Vidal, A. (1972). *C. R. Acad. Sci. Ser. D.* **274**, 437–440.

Gourdji, D., Morin, A. and Tixier-Vidal, A. (1973). International Congress Series No. 308. Proceedings of the International Symposium on Human Prolactin, Brussels, June 12–14, 1973, Excerpta Medica, Amsterdam.

Haug, E. and Gautvik, K. (1976). *Endocrinology* **99**, 1482–1489.

Hinkle, P., Woroch, E. L. and Tashjian, A. H., Jr. (1974). *J. Biol. Chem.* **249**, 3085–3090.

Labrie, F., Beaulieu, M., Caron, M. G. and Raymond, V. (1978). *In* "Progress in Prolactin Physiology and Pathology" (C. Robyn and M. Harter, eds) 121–136. Elsevier, Amsterdam.

Le Geullec, R., Kercret, H., Geullaen, G., Valotaire, Y. et Duval, J. (1977). *Biochimie* **59**, 853–855.

MacLeod, R. M. (1969). *Endocrinology* **85**, 916–923.

MacLeod, R. M. and Lamberts, S. W. J. (1978). *In* "Progress in Prolactin Physiology and Pathology" (C. Robyn and M. Harter, eds) 111–119. Elsevier, Amsterdam.

Malarkey, W. B., Groshong, J. C. and Milo, G. E. (1977). *Nature* **266**, 640–641.

Martin-Comin, J. and Robyn, C. (1976). *J. Histochem. Cytochem.* **24**, 1012–1016.

Masur, S. K., Holtzman, E. and Bancroft, F. C. (1974). *J. Histochem. Cytochem.* **22**, 385–394.

Meites, J. and Nicoll, C. S. (1965). *In* "Proceedings of the first International Congress on Hormonal Steroid," Vol. II, 307–316. Academic Press, New York and London.

Olivier, L., Vila-Porcile, E., Racadot, O., Peillon, F. and Racadot, J. (1975). *In* "The Anterior Pituitary Gland" (M. G. Farquhar and A. Tixier-Vidal, eds) 231–276. Academic Press, New York and London.

Pasteels, J. L. (1963). *Arch. Biol.* **74**, 439–553.

Perrone, M. H. and Hinkle, P. M. (1978). *J. Biol. Chem.* **253**, 5168–5173.

Raymond, V., Beaulieu, M., Labrie, F. and Boissier, J. (1978). *Science* **200**, 1173–1175.

Sirbasku, D. A. and Benzon, R. H. (in press).

Sonnenschein, C., Posner, M., Saududdin, S. and Krasnay, M. (1973). *Exp. Cell Res.* **78**, 41–46.

Sorrentino, J. M., Kirkland, W. L. and Sirbasku, D. A. (1976). *J. National Cancer Inst.* **56**, 1149–1154.

Tashjian, A. H., Jr. and Hoyt, R. F. Jr. (1972). *In* "Molecular Genetics and Developmental Biology" (M. Sussman, ed) 353–387, Prentice-Hall, New Jersey.

Tashjian, A. H., Jr., Yasumura, Y., Levine, R., Sato, G. H. and Parker, M. L. (1968). *Endocrinology* **82**, 342–352.

Tashjian, A. H., Jr., Bancroft, F. C. and Levine, L. (1970). *J. Cell Biol.* **47**, 61–71.

Tashjian, A. H., Jr., Barowsky, N. J. and Jensen, D. K. (1971). *Biochem. Biophys. Res. Commun.* **43**, 516–523.

Tixier-Vidal, A. (1975). *In* "The Anterior Pituitary Gland" (M. G. Farquhar and A. Tixier-Vidal, eds) 181–229. Academic Press.

Tixier-Vidal, A., Gourdji, D. and Tougard, C. (1975a). *Intern. Rev. Cytol.* **41**, 173–239.

Tixier-Vidal, A., Gourdji, D., Pradelles, P., Morgat, J. L., Fromageot, P. and Kerdelhué, B. (1975b). *In* "Hypothalamic Hormones" (M. Motta, P. G. Crosignani and L. Martini, eds) 89–107. Academic Press, London and New York.

Tixier-Vidal, A., Tougard, C. and Picart, R. (1976). *In* "First International Symposium on Immunoenzymatic Techniques" (Feldmann *et al.* eds) 307–321. North-Holland, Amsterdam.

Tixier-Vidal, A., Brunet, N. and Gourdji, D. (1978). *In* "Progress in Prolactin Physiology and Pathology" (C. Robyn and M. Harter, ed) 29–43. Elsevier, Amsterdam.

Tougard, C., Tixier-Vidal, A., Kerdelbué, B. and Jutisz, M. (1977). *Biologie Cellulaire* **28**, 251–260.

Ueda, G., Moy, P. and Furth, J. (1973). *Int. J. Cancer* **12**, 100.

Vale, W., Blackwell, R., Grant, G. and Guillemin, R. (1973). *Endocrinology* **93**, 26–33.

Vale, W., Rivier, C. and Brown, M. (1977). *Ann. Rev. Physiol.* **39**, 473–527.

Waelbroeck-Van Gaver, C. and Potvliège, P. (1969). *Eur. J. Cancer* **5**, 99–117.

Yasumura, Y., Tashjian, A. H. Jr. and Sato, G. H. (1966). *Science* **154**, 1186–1189.

# MICROADENOMAS, STRUCTURE AND FUNCTION*

F. Peillon, J. Racadot, L. Olivier and E. Vila-Porcile

*Laboratory Histology and Embryology, (CNRS ERA 484), Faculté de Médicine Pitié-Salpêtrière, 75013 Paris, France*

Among the large series of secreting and non-secreting pituitary adenomas collected in our laboratory over fourteen years (more than a thousand cases) three main categories of hormone-secreting microadenomas may be described, classified on the basis of clinical criteria: microadenomas producing Cushing's disease, acromegaly and the amenorrhea-galactorrhea syndrome.

In this series, we encountered no example of adenomas secreting gonadotropic hormones, and very few examples (only five) of microadenomas secreting thyrotropic hormone, these last cases being discovered at post-mortem examinations in patients with primary hypothyroidism.

The microadenomas producing Cushing's disease and the amenorrhea-galactorrhea syndrome will be described separately, because of their different characteristics.

## MICROADENOMAS PRODUCING CUSHING'S DISEASE

### General considerations

In the history of these adenomas, the pioneer work of Harvey Cushing (1932) must be emphasized. It is well known that in eight of ten cases of adrenocortical hyperactivity, Cushing found at autopsy "minute" adenomas, six composed of

*This work was supported by grants from the CNRS (ERA 484) and the INSERM (CRAT No. 77-81).
We would like to thank Professors Caron, Comoy, Derome, Fohanno, Guiot, Pertuiset, Philippon and Sachs for their authorization to use their cases. We gratefully acknowledge Mrs Brandi and Drouet for their excellent technical assistance and Mrs Combrier for help in the preparation of the manuscript.

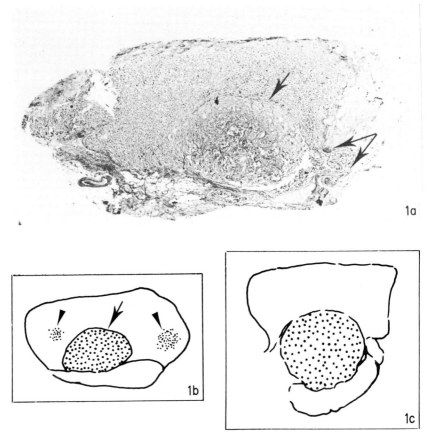

*Fig. 1.* (a)  Basophilic microadenoma located near the posterior lobe of the pituitary in a case of Cushing's disease (transverse arrow). An invasive extension is observed on the right part of the microadenoma (double arrow) × 10.

(b)  Drawing of the pituitary at the level of the basophil microadenoma (transverse arrow). Two hyperplastic areas (one poorly granulated, the other composed of somatotrophic cells) are present in the normal anterior lobe (arrowheads).

(c)  Drawing of the basophilic microadenoma shown by Harvey Cushing himself in his original manuscript × 4.

basophilic elements, two "undifferentiated". The pituitary glands appeared to be of normal size. The definition of microadenomas was thus established: a normal-sized pituitary gland containing a minute adenoma related to hormonal hyper-secretion disease.

Since then the frequency and nature of the hypophyseal adenomas in Cushing's disease became the matter of discussion (Racadot *et al.*, 1967). However, the surgical technique of transsphenoidal selective adenomectomy (Guiot and Thibaut, 1959) has permitted repeated verification of this pioneer work, with the discovery of basophilic microadenomas in Cushing's disease and the possibility to cure the patients in this way (Wilson and Dempsy, 1978).

Our experience is based upon 19 cases of microadenomas of a total of 48 cases of adenomas in Cushing's disease (including Nelson's syndrome). In only one case

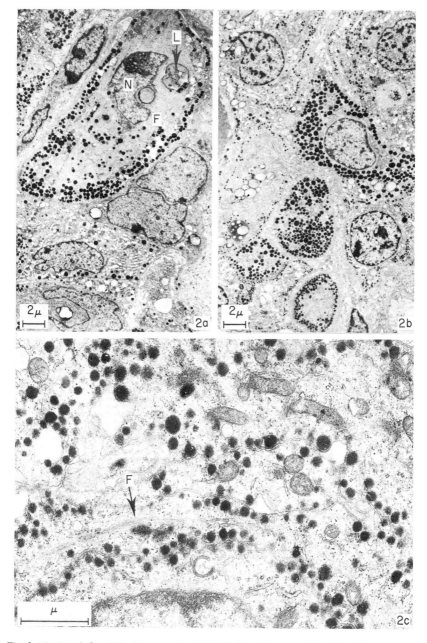

*Fig. 2.* (a) Crooke's cell in the normal residual pituitary in a case of Cushing's disease. Perinuclear ring of filaments (F), enclosing secretory granules and large lysosomes (L). Nucleus (N). Small marginal granules along the cell periphery.

(b) Normal anterior cells from the non-adenomatous pituitary in a case of Cushing's disease.

(c) Variable diameters of secretory granules in a microadenoma producing Cushing's disease. Bundle of filaments (F).

was no microadenoma discovered, although the patient was operated on twice.

Most of these microadenomas were small in size (3 to 5 mm) (Fig. 1a, b) while one of 10 mm occupied nearly all the anterior lobe, in transition between micro- and macroadenoma. The majority were located in the central part of the gland, while some of them were near the posterior part of the pituitary, as in one Cushing's case (Fig. 1c).

## Structure in the light microscope

Although the architecture of most of these microadenomas was of the trabecular type, in some of them the cell cords were regular, with palisaded cells, and in other cases the adenomas were partly papillary. No difference was observed in this between micro- and macroadenomas. The cells, whose average size was 15 to 20 $\mu$m, had a large nucleus and a clearly defined nucleolus. In all cases secretory granules were present. They were blue with Herlant's tetrachrome (1960) and positive to PAS and lead hematoxylin. They corresponded to the basophilia of the granules, as indicated by Cushing (1932). Their number varied from one microadenoma to another, but they were always present in the cells, in contrast with macroadenomas in the same disease or in Nelson's syndrome, which sometimes appeared chromophobic.

Some cells of the microadenomas showed a cytoplasmic hyalinization, similar to that of Crooke's hyaline cells observed in the residual hypophysis (Fig. 2a) (Porcile and Racadot, 1966; Olivier et al., 1975). When it was possible (in nine of these cases) examine the non-adenomatous parts of the anterior pituitary, these Crooke's cells were one of the main abnormal features found. In one of three cases where the whole pituitary was examined at autopsy, a second poorly granulated microadenoma was found at some distance from the basophilic one (Fig. 1b). In the other cases no hyperplasia of the ACTH-MSH cells, as described by Saeger (1977), was found, but only small fragments of the non-adenomatous pituitary were studied (Fig. 2b). However, as no well-defined capsule surrounded the microadenomas, "normal" cords of pituitary cells were observed together with cords of basophilic cells. Moreover, in nearly half of the cases, although the microadenoma was small, there was an invasive tendency towards the adjacent "normal" pituitary or the overlying dura and periosteum of the sella (Fig. 1a).

## Ultrastructure of the microadenomas

The granular heterogeneity was a dominant feature of these cases, with secretory granules of several sizes (Fig. 2c). Their calibre varied from cell to cell, as it did in individual cells from one adenoma to another. Three groups of granules could be distinguished according to their size (from 400 to 500 nm to 100 to 200 nm diam.).

A distinctive feature of these granulated cells was the frequent occurrence of intracytoplasmic filaments associated with secondary lysosomes (Olivier et al., 1975). Among the other features observed in these adenomas, we noticed important variations in the cell size in the same adenoma and alterations in the blood vessels probably related to diabetes.

**Physio-pathological problems**

*Comparison between the structures of the micro-
and macroadenomas in Cushing's disease*
   No important structural differences were observed between these two categories of adenomas. One minor difference concerned basophilic granules which
were always found in microadenomas while larger tumors sometimes appeared
chromophobic. Another point was the more frequent cytological abnormalities
in the biggest tumors, which appeared to be more undifferentiated than the
smaller ones (Racadot *et al.*, 1967, 1975). However, most of the structural
findings were identical in micro- and macroadenomas. This favored a similar
pathological process being observed at different steps of its evolution.

*Hormonal content*
   Two types of data allowed us to consider these granular cells to be secreting
ACTH and MSH. Hormonal assays of some tumors led to the conclusion that
they contained ACTH and MSH (Bahn *et al.*, 1960; Nelson and Sprunt, 1965;
Abe *et al.*, 1967) and the granular cells corresponded to the cortico-melanotrophic
cells described in the normal human pituitary (Phifer *et al.*, 1970; Dubois, 1973).
Cytoimmunological explorations of our personal cases (8 microadenomas, 14
macroadenomas) favored the notion that they contained not only ACTH and $\alpha$
or $\beta$ MSH but also $\alpha$ and $\beta$ endorphins (Dubois, personal communication 1978,
unpublished data). These findings, observed in the two categories of adenomas,
enhanced the argument that they were identical pathological processes. Moreover,
these cytoimmunological findings have been encountered in two cases of basophilic macroadenomas discovered only as tumors, without any endocrine disease.
This underlines the fact that basophilic adenomas exist without adrenal hyperfunction, i.e. "non-functional adenomas" with the occurrence of the abnormal
hormonal secretions found in Cushing's disease only detected by the immunofluorescence technique.
   The existence of these non-functional basophilic macroadenomas must be
related to the discovery at post mortem examination of non-functional basophilic microadenomas in a normal-sized pituitary. According to the authors, the
frequency of these basophilic macroadenomas varies from 3 to 7%. Susman
(1935) found 8 of these processes in 260 examined pituitaries while Costello
(1935) found 72 basophilic microadenomas in 1000 pituitaries. But Costello
underlined that the incidence of these basophilic microadenomas increased with
age. This remark must be taken into account since many authors have repeated the
observation of Lucien (1929) for hyperplastic tendency of the basophilic cells in
old people.
   It may be possible that these non-functional basophilic microadenomas (like
the non-functional basophilic macroadenomas we quoted above) are secreting
hormones in the blood but in such small amounts that they are not causing endocrine disease. Abnormality of the secretion is less likely, since the immunofluorescence technique was able to detect, in these non-functional basophil adenomas,
the same hormones as in Cushing's disease.

## MICROADENOMAS PRODUCING THE AMENORRHEA-GALACTORRHEA SYNDROME*

### General considerations

The scientific study of these microadenomas most probably begins with Erdheim and Stumme (1909). Studying the pituitaries of 118 pregnant women, these authors focused their attention on the numerous pregnancy cells of the anterior pituitary and found 14 intrapituitary microadenomas, 6 of them being composed of pregnancy cells. Later, the relation between these pregnancy cells and the occurrence of amenorrhea and galactorrhea was evoked by Cushing (1933). Describing a case of transitory acromegaly in a woman with post-partum amenorrhea and continuing lactation, he wrote: "it is not inconceivable that it may have been an adenoma arising from the pregnancy cells" and wondered "whether the cells of the patient's tumor secreted a lactogenic hormone corresponding to the "prolactin" of Riddle (1931)". However, until the clinical description of the amenorrhea-galactorrhea syndrome by Forbes *et al.* (1954), the histological characterization of the adenomas by Herlant *et al.* (1965) and the development of the immunoassay for human prolactin (Friesen *et al.*, 1972a), these adenomas were considered to be chromophobic.

At present, the PRL-secreting adenomas represent the most important category among secreting and non-secreting pituitary adenomas (Hardy *et al.*, 1978; Landolt, 1978). This is also our experience, as demonstrated by the percentages of the different types of pituitary adenomas collected in our laboratory from 1964 to 1976 (Peillon *et al.*, 1978). From 1964 to 1968, chromophobe adenomas represented 45% of the cases, against 6% of PRL-secreting adenomas and 49% of other types (Cushing's disease and acromegaly). From 1972 to 1976, chromophobe adenomas represented only 20%, against 39% of PRL-secreting adenomas. This clearly shows the "relative" increase in the last few years of correctly identified PRL-secreting adenomas, thanks to the progress in the different histological methods and the systematic evaluation of plasma PRL levels.

Fifty-three cases of microadenomas have been collected, 49 of them during the last three years. In nine cases, a fluid or hemorrhagic cystic lesion was found, with no possibility of histological identification. In four other cases (three women with amenorrhea and galactorrhea, one in a man with gynecomastia and galactorrhea) no circumscribed microadenoma was found and the whole pituitary was infiltrated by cords of PRL-secreting cells (Fig. 3a, b).

In most of the cases, the consistency of the microadenomas was compared with ACTH or GH microadenomas. They were soft and appeared grey, whitish or milky, as already reported by Hardy *et al.* (1978). The lesion was found in the basal lateral wing of the pituitary, sometimes on the left side (20 of the 35 cases where the localization has been mentioned) or in the right basal wing (12 cases). Two were observed in the central part of the gland and one near the posterior pituitary.

No microadenomas were found in 50 male cases of PRL-secreting adenomas.

---

*It seems to be better to use the denomination of PRL-secreting adenomas or prolactinomas, since these adenomas may also be responsible for amenorrhea without galactorrhea and for gynecomastia, with or without galactorrhea, and impotence in males.

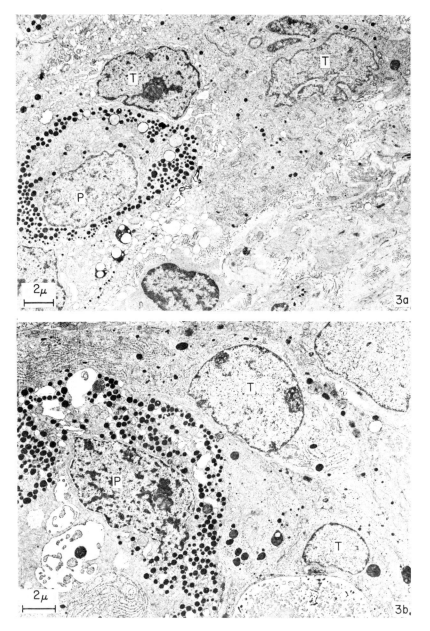

*Fig. 3.* (a) Cords of tumoral PRL-secreting cells infiltrating the normal residual pituitary (P).
(b) Another area of the same pituitary.

## Structure in the light microscope

The architecture was sometimes of the parenchymatous type with cells arranged in a diffuse pattern. In other cases, although less frequent, there were well-defined cords. In many cases the parenchyma was disrupted by hemorraghic areas with extravasated blood cells. Small colloid follicles were frequently observed and microcalcospherites were seen in 20% of the cases. The cells were often small (10-15 $\mu$m) and packed tight. They had a clear nucleus and a prominent nucleolus. The cytoplasm showed a true basophilia due to a well-developed ergastoplasm (Racadot *et al.*, 1972). Erythrosinophilic secretory granules were frequently found (2/3 of the cases), in contrast with macroadenomas, where they were more rarely observed. The granules, often very small, were dispersed throughout the cytoplasm or located along the cell membrane (Fig. 4a). Mitotic figures were seen in 6 cases. In 9 of 18 cases where the paraadenomatous pituitary tissue was examined, many cords of PRL-secreting cells were observed inside the remnant pituitary. As in Cushing's disease, there was no defined capsule surrounding the microadenoma.*

## Ultrastructure

In some parts of the adenomas, the cells were closely associated. In other parts of the tumor, a lack or a fragmentation of the parenchymal basal laminae was observed and the cells were loosely arranged. Several features related to high secretory activity of the cells were always present: secretory granules, large Golgi area and prominence of a rough endoplasmic reticulum, and nucleolar hypertrophy (Pasteels, 1963; Racadot *et al.*, 1972; Pasteels *et al.*, 1972) (Fig. 4b and 5a).

Two main categories of secretory granules were observed: large granules (400-500 nm diam.) and more often, smaller ones (100-150 nm). The large granules were usually irregular and crescent shaped, as described in the literature. They could be associated with smaller ones. These small granules were spheroidal and enclosed in a vesicle limited by a well-defined membrane. They might represent the only granular type. Histochemical reactions showed aspects rather similar to the reaction pattern observed in normal prolactin cells (Vila-Porcile *et al.*, 1973).

## Physiopathological problems

*Comparison of micro- and macroprolactinomas*
As in Cushing's disease, no major structural differences were observed between these two kinds of adenomas. Secretory granules were more often found in the microadenomas than in bigger tumors, which frequently appeared chromophobic. This may be one of the reasons why these PRL-secreting tumors were not discovered earlier. Another difference consisted in the number of mitoses, which

---

*In 5 cases where Bromocriptine treatment was administered for several months, no major differences were found compared to untreated cases.

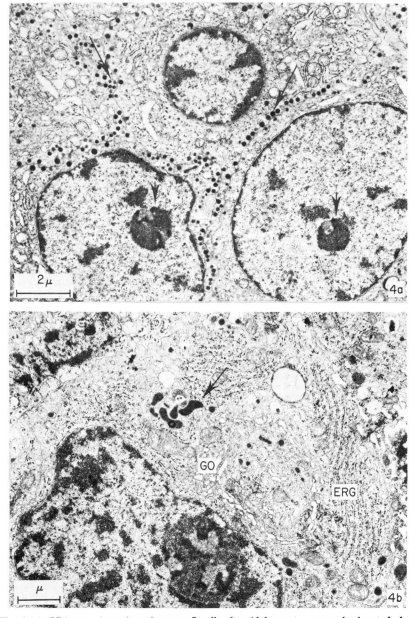

*Fig. 4.* (a) PRL-secreting microadenoma. Small spheroidal secretory granules located along the cell membrane (transverse arrows). Nucleolar hypertrophy (arrowheads).

(b) PRL-secreting cell from another microadenoma. Large and irregular granules (transverse arrows). Nucleolar hypertrophy; well-developed endoplasmic reticulum (ERG). Large Golgi area (GO).

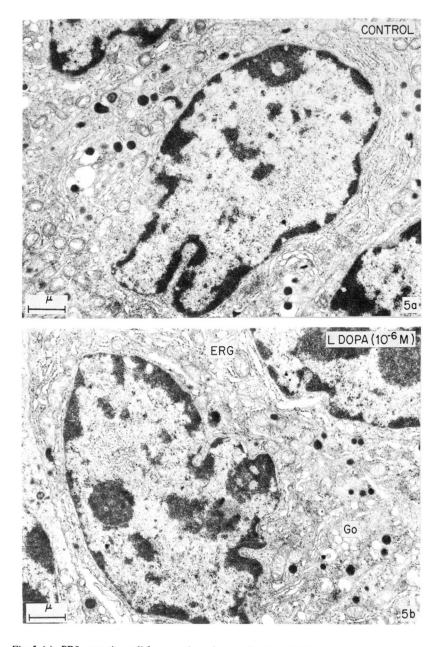

*Fig. 5.* (a)  PRL-secreting cell from a microadenoma incubated 4 h.

    (b)  PR L-secreting cell from the same adenoma incubated 4 h with L Dopa ($10^{-6}$ M). Enlargement of the rough endoplasmic reticulum (ERG). Secretory granules in the Golgi apparatus (GO).

were more frequent in macroadenomas, in particular in those with extra-sellar extensions. Indeed, they were present in more than 21% of these cases (66% of "giant" tumors) while they were present in only 7% of microadenomas. This shows that the bigger tumors have a greater proliferative potentiality than the microadenomas and explains in part the greater volume of the tumor. Another explanation is suggested by comparison of the mean durations of the disease in micro- and macroadenomas. When it has been possible to evaluate this (taking into account the first clinical symptom), the duration of the disease in microadenomas was 6 y (range 1-18 y) while it was 9 y (range 2-31 y) in macroadenomas with large supra-sellar extensions and even 12 y (range 2-16 y) in "giant" tumors. However the experience of everyone and the ranges cited above also demonstrate that a microadenoma may have a long duration, while a giant tumor may be explosive. So at least two factors may contribute to the size of the tumor: a longer or shorter duration of the disease and a particular proliferative potentiality of the tumor.

*Nature of the secretion*

These differences observed between micro- and macroadenomas do not indicate that they are of different natures. Both of them induce the same clinical disorders. Both of them secrete prolactin, as shown by radioimmunoassay (RIA), and no other hormone in excess. When PRL was studied in 35 cases of microadenomas, compared to an identical number of macroadenomas, the average plasma levels were respectively, 203 ng (range 33-530 ng/ml; normal < 30 ng/ml) and 565 ng/ml (range 29-13035 ng/ml). Though a lower mean level was observed in microadenomas, large tumors might be accompanied by low PRL levels and small microadenomas might secrete high amounts of PRL.

Since these two sorts of prolactinoma give the same clinical syndrome, have the same histological structure and secrete the same hormone in excess, PRL, we can consider that they are identical processes observed at different steps of their evolution.

In vitro *experiments*

Few *in vitro* experiments have been performed with microadenomas because of the lesser amounts of tumor compared to macroadenomas. When experimentation was possible, the behavior of these microadenomas in culture was identical to that observed with bigger tumors. Six PRL-secreting adenomas (3 microadenomas, 3 macroadenomas) were incubated for 4 h with dopaminergic drugs. The same amounts of Dopamine ($5.2 \times 10^{-7} - 5.2 \times 10^{-5}$ M), L Dopa ($10^{-6} - 10^{-4}$ M), and bromocriptine ($6.5 \times 10^{-6} - 6.5 \times 10^{-4}$ M) were introduced into the medium. All experiments were done in triplicate and PRL assayed by RIA. As no dose-related reponse was observed, pooled data for the same treatment were compared to those of the controls (Table I). In all the cases a decrease in PRL secretion was observed, which was significant most of the time. This correlated well with the *in vivo* results. Electron microscopy of two cases (1 micro-, 1 macroadenoma) showed an enlargement of the rough endoplasmic reticulum (Fig. 5b). as already observed by MacLeod and Lehmeyer (1972) with rat pituitary gland incubated with catecholamines. There was no modification of the Golgi apparatus

Table I.  *In vitro* and *in vivo* effects of dopaminergic drugs upon PRL secretion from human prolactinomas.

| Treatments | Prolactinomas | | | | | |
| --- | --- | --- | --- | --- | --- | --- |
| | A | B | C | D | E | F |
| | PRL : ng/µg protein | | | | ng/mg tissue | |
| *In vitro* | | | | | | |
| None | $61 \pm 16$ | $16.4 \pm 5$ | $425 \pm 54$ | $596 \pm 220$ | $3227 \pm 924$ | $734 \pm 311$ |
| L Dopa | $34 \pm 7^c$ | $1.9 \pm 2.9^c$ | $287 \pm 37^a$ | $254 \pm 94^b$ | $1571 \pm 639^c$ | $444 \pm 264$ |
| Dopamine | $32 \pm 5^c$ | | | $286 \pm 123$ | | $265 \pm 141^c$ |
| CB 154 | $37 \pm 7^c$ | | | | | $428 \pm 376$ |
| *In vivo* | PRL : ng/ml | | | | | |
| None | 200 | 150 | 5000 | 35 | 325 | 500 |
| L Dopa | 76 | 14 | 1000 | 7 | 126 | 235 |
| CB 154 | 45 | | | | | 196 |

$^a P < 0.05$
$^b P < 0.025$
$^c P < 0.01$.
Tumors A, B, E are microprolactinomas.
Tumors C, D, F are macroprolactinomas.

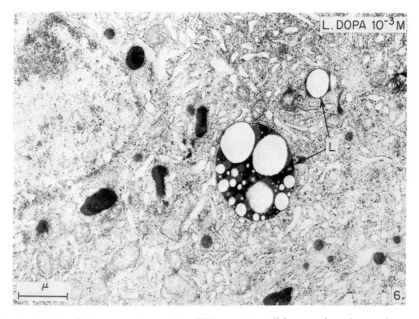

*Fig. 6.*  Autophagic lysosomes (arrows) in a PRL secreting-cell from a microadenoma incubated 4 h with L Dopa ($5 \times 10^{-3}$ M).

nor of the organelles. Higher doses of L Dopa ($5 \times 10^{-3}$ M) induced autophagic lysosomes (Fig. 6) identical to those observed after long-term bromocriptine treatment (Beauvillain *et al.*, 1976; Racadot, unpublished data). PRL-secreting micro- and macroadenomas have also been incubated with TRH ($2.7 \times 10^{-7}$ M) for 1 h (Cesselin and Peillon, unpublished data). In only 2 out of 6 tumors, TRH increased PRL *in vitro*. One of the 2 cases was a microadenoma, with a good correlation between *in vivo* and *in vitro* results. The other case was a macroadenoma, with no PRL increase after TRH *in vivo*, as is frequently observed when the plasma PRL level is above 100 ng/ml (Derome *et al.*, 1978, to be published).

The different agents used above have direct effects upon the PRL secretion and the morphology of PRL-secreting adenomas. This effect, nearly identical for micro- and macroadenomas, favors the argument of an identical process in the two cases. This process appears to be partly independent of the hypothalamus, since PRL-secreting adenomas are able to secrete large amounts of prolactin when cultured for several hours or days. In long-term organ culture of tumors from acromegalic patients, it has been shown that the secretion and synthesis of GH and PRL occurred for 15 days after the beginning of the culture. Though these results were in favour of an autonomous secretion by the pituitary adenomas, however, they did not rule out a possible hypothalamic control. It has been shown, indeed, that somatostatin, TRH or dopaminergic drugs may have an effect on PRL and/or GH secretion from these adenomas *in vivo* as well as *in vitro*. Moreover, in long-term organ culture of somatotropic tumors, it has been shown that PRL secretion and synthesis increased with time, in contrast to a decrease in GH during the same culture time (Peillon *et al.*, 1978). These findings suggest that pituitary tumors may function *in vivo* similar to normal pituitary tissue and under partial hypothalamic control even if they are able to have an autonomous secretion.

*Role of estrogens*

Our attention was focused some years ago on the role played by estrogens upon pituitary adenomas. We were impressed indeed by the aggravation observed in different kinds of pituitary adenomas (chromophobe, somatotrope or prolactin-secreting) in women and even in a man submitted to estrogen therapy. There were clinical symptoms of intracranial hypertension and visual disturbances like those observed in some cases of pituitary adenomas stimulated during pregnancy. The morphology of the tumors demonstrated proliferative signs, such as mitoses and interstitial hemorrhages (Peillon *et al.*, 1970). Later, some correlations were established between the frequency of hematoma or pituitary apoplexy in PRL-secreting adenomas and the estrogen therapy given to reinstitute normal cycle in women.

It has not been proved, up to now, that estrogen-progesterone therapy given to patients with spanomenorrhea or pills given as contraceptives are able to provoke PRL-secreting adenomas. However some careful attention must be focused upon this possibility.

It is well known that in rats, estrogens given at high doses lead to experimental PRL-secreting adenomas (Furth and Clifton, 1966). It has been shown that after diethylstilbestrol treatment the number of lactotrophs stimulated to mitoses were as many as 30% of the total number of the mitotic cells in the rat's pituitary, with an increase in the serum PRL levels followed by an increase in the pituitary PRL (Jacobi et al., 1977).

In women, during pregnancy prolactin cells undergo extensive hypertrophy with a rise in serum PRL which parallels that of estrogens (Friesen et al., 1972b). In these particular situations, the amounts of estrogens delivered are very high. Besides these conditions, however, it has been shown that the PRL serum levels parallel those of estrogens. In adult women, there is a progressive decline in serum PRL levels with age while in men the serum PRL levels remain unchanged between 15 and 65 y (Vekemans and Robyn, 1975). As also reported, doses of estrogens contained in sequential oral contraceptives are high enough to increase significantly the basal and TRH-induced prolactin secretion in women (Reymond and Leamrchand-Béraud, 1976). In 15 patients taking oral contraceptives or submitted to estrogen-progesterone therapy for abnormal menstrual cycles, we found after withdrawal of the therapy, symptoms such as amenorrhea or spanomenorrhea, galactorrhea and/or infertility. These patients had a normal basal level of prolactin but a highly enhanced response of PRL to TRH. The basal plasma PRL level was indeed multiplied by 10 or more after TRH. The plasma level of progesterone, studied in the luteal phase when present, was very low ($< 0.50$ ng/ml), while estradiol was more often in the low normal range (60–100 pg/ml). An exaggerated response of LH to LHRH was found, while FSH exhibited a normal response (Peillon, Vincens and Doumith unpublished data). We wonder whether, in these cases, an excess of pituitary PRL reserve due to estrogen therapy might be the reason for the abnormal symptoms. It may be one of the explanations of the post-pill amenorrhea, with or without galactorrhea, and of the more frequent impaired fertility observed in nulliparous women after discontinuing oral contraception, when compared to other forms of contraception (Vessey et al., 1978). Some of the patients described above received bromocriptine therapy (2.5 mg per day), which led to ovulatory cycles in some of them and pregnancy in two cases. One may ask whether in such cases, a continued estrogen therapy would have changed a functional disease into an organic one, such as a PRL-secreting micro- or macroadenoma. In 4 cases of the 57 cases described above, the entire pituitary was infiltrated by cords of PRL-secreting cells, as is observed in pregnancy or the post-partum pituitary, and no microadenoma was found. It may sometimes be difficult to differentiate, even at the structural level, a functional amenorrhea-galactorrhea syndrome from an organic one.

Some questions arise in view of the unusual frequency of the discovery of prolactinomas during these last years. The attention focused upon slight modifications of the sella turcica in women with abnormal cycles, galactorrhea or infertility, combined with PRL determination is certainly one of the reasons. We may ask also whether the discovery of such microadenomas will lead to the disappearance in the next years of large tumors such as the so-called ancient chromophobe. The answer will be obtained in the future, if a decrease in the number of macroadenomas is observed as compared to some years ago. However, we must not exclude the possibility that there is a true increase in prolactinomas as well as the development of functional disease in relation to estrogen and/or neuroleptic therapy.

In conclusion, the discovery of secreting microadenomas represents undoubtedly one of the major progresses in pituitary tumoral pathology in these last few years. If we consider micro- and macroadenomas to be identical in their structure, their secretion and their physiopathological behavior, we may hope that the discovery and removal of the former will lead to the disappearance of the latter. However, though no functional syndrome has been observed in Cushing's disease and in acromegaly, this is not the case in hyperprolactinemia. The sometimes difficult differentiation between a functional disease and a tumoral one in the amenor-rhea-galactorrhea syndrome must lead to assertion of the occurrence of a micro-adenoma only on the basis of carefully chosen criteria.

## REFERENCES

Abe, K., Island, D. P., Liddle, G. W., Fleischer, N. and Nicholson, W. E. (1967). *J. Clin. Endocr. Metab.* **35**, 635.

Bahn, R., Ross, G. T. and MacCarty, C. S. (1960). *Proc. Staff. Meet. Mayo Clin.* **35**, 635.

Beauvillain, J. C., Tramu, G., Mazzucca, M., Christiaens, J. L., L'Hermite, M., Asfour, M., Fossati, P. and Linquette, M. (1976). *Ann. Endocrinol. (Paris)* **37**, 117.

Costello, R. T. (1935). *Proc. Staff. Meet. Mayo Clin.* **10**, 449.

Cushing, H. (1932). *In* "Papers Related to the Pituitary Body, Hypothalamus and Parasympathetic Nervous System" (Ch. C. Tomas) 113-174. Springfield, Illinois.

Cushing, H. (1933). *Arch. Intern. Med.* **51**, 487.

Dubois, M. P. (1973). *Bull. Ass. Anat. (Nancy)* **156**, 63.

Erdheim, J. and Stumme, E. (1909). *Beitr. Path. Anat.* **46**, 1-132.

Forbes, A. P., Henneman, P. H., Grinwald, G. C. and Albright, F. (1954). *J. Clin. Endocr. Metab.* **14**, 265.

Friesen, H., Guyda, H., Hwang, P., Tyson, J. E. and Barbeau, A. (1972a). *J. Clin. Invest.* **51**, 706.

Friesen, H., Kwang, P., Guyda, H., Tolis, G., Tyson, J. and Myers, R. (1972b). *In* "Prolactin and Carcinogenesis" (A. R. Boyns and K. Griffiths, eds) 64-97. Alpha Omega Alpha Publishing, Cardiff.

Furth, J. and Clifton, K. H. (1966). *In* "The Pituitary Gland" (G. W. Harris and B. T. Donovan, eds) Vol. II, 460-497. Butterworths, London.

Guiot, G. and Thibaut, B. (1959). *Neurochirurgia* (Stuttgart) **1**, 133.

Hardy, J., Beauregard, H. and Robert, F. (1978). *In* "Progress in Prolactin Physiology and Pathology" (C. Robyn and M. Harter, eds) 361-370. Elsevier, Amsterdam.

Herlant, M. (1960). *Bull Micr. Appl.* **10**, 37.

Herlant, M., Laine, E., Fossati, P. and Linquette, M. (1965). *Ann. Endocrinol. (Paris)* **26**, 65.

Jacobi, J., Lloyd, H. M. and Mears, J. D. (1977). *J. Endocr.* **72**, 35.

Landolt, A. M. (1978). *In* "Advances and Technical Standards in Neurosurgery" (H. Krayenbühl, ed) Vol. V, 4-49. Springer Verlag, Wien.

Lucien, M. (1929). *R. Fr. Endocrinologie* **7**, 441.

MacLeod, R. M. and Lehmeyer, J. E. (1972). *In* "Lactogenic Hormones" (G. E. W. Wolstenholme and J. Knight, eds) 53-82. Churchill, Livingstone, London.

*F. Peillon et al.*

Nelson, D. H. and Sprunt, J. G. (1965). *Proc. Int. Congr. Endocrinol.* 2nd International Congress Series No. 83, 1053–1057.

Olivier, L., Vila-Porcile, E., Peillon, F. and Racadot, J. (1972). *C. R. Soc. Biol.* **166**, 1591.

Olivier, L., Vila-Porcile, E., Racadot, O., Peillon, F. and Racadot, J. (1975). *In* "The Anterior Pituitary" (A. Tixier-Vidal and M. G. Farquhar, eds) 231–276. Academic Press, New York and London.

Pasteels, J. L. (1963). *Arch. Biol.* **74**, 439.

Pasteels, J. L., Gausset, P., Dangy, A., Ectors, F., Nicoll, C. S. and Varavudhi, P. (1972). *J. Clin. Endocr. Metab.* **34**, 359.

Peillon, F., Vila-Porcile, E., Olivier, L. and Racadot, J. (1970). *Ann. Endocrinol. (Paris)* **31**, 259.

Peillon, F., Cesselin, F., Garnier, P. E., Brandi, A. M., Donnadieu, M., L'Hermite, M. and Dubois, M. P. (1978). *Acta Endocrinol.* **87**, 701.

Peillon, F., Racadot, J., Moussy, D., Vila-Porcile, E., Olivier, L. and Racadot, O. (1978). *In* "Treatment of Pituitary Adenomas" (R. Falhbusch and V. K. Werder, eds) 114–122. Thieme Verlag, Stuttgart.

Phifer, R. F., Spicer, S. S. and Orth, D. N. (1970). *J. Clin. Endocr. Metab.* **31**, 347.

Porcile, E. and Racadot, J. (1966). *C. R. Acad. Sci. (Paris)* **263**, 948.

Racadot, J., Girard, F., Peillon, F. and Binoux, M. (1967). "Le syndrome de Cushing", 1–59. Masson, Paris.

Racadot, J., Vila-Porcile, E., Peillon, F. and Olivier, L. (1972). *Ann. Endocrinol. (Paris)* **32**, 298.

Racadot, J., Vila-Porcile, E., Olivier, L. and Peillon, F. (1975). *In* "Progress in Neurological Surgery" (H. Krayenbühl, ed) Vol. VI, 95–141. Karger, Basel.

Reymond, M. and Lemarchand-Béraud, Th. (1976). *Clin. Endocr.* **5**, 429.

Riddle, O. and Braucher, P. F. (1931). *Am. J. Physiol.* **97**, 617.

Saeger, W. (1977). *Virchow's Arch. A. Path. Anat. Histol.* **372**, 299.

Susman, W. (1935). *Brit. J. Surg.* **22**, 539.

Vekemans, M. and Robyn, C. (1975). *Brit. Med. J.* **4**, 738.

Vessey, M. P., Wright, N. H., McPherson, K. and Wiggins, P. (1978). *Brit. Med. J.* **1**, 265.

Vila-Porcile, E., Olivier, L. and Racadot, O. (1973). *In* "Human Prolactin" (J. L. Pasteels and C. Robyn, eds) 56–59. Excerpta Medica American Elsevier, New York.

Wilson, C. B. and Dempsey, L. C. (1978). *J. Neurosurg.* **48**, 13.

# BIOLOGY OF PITUITARY MICROADENOMAS

A. M. Landolt*

*Department of Neurosurgery, Universitätsspital, 8091 Zürich, Switzerland*

> With all this stress upon the tumor and its local manifestations we
> must not overlook the fact that the constitutional indications of
> pituitary disease may bear little relation to the size of the lesion...
>
> Harvey Cushing (1914)

## INTRODUCTION

Four different types of space-occupying lesions of the pituitary have been described in the last 155 years. The first was the endocrine-inactive macroadenoma. Rayer (1823) described four men who suffered from pituitary tumors and showed bilateral amaurosis and apathy and a 20-year-old woman who had in addition to that amenorrhea. Verga (1864) observed the presence of an endocrine-active pituitary macroadenoma in a patient with acromegaly. The first endocrine-active microadenoma causing acromegaly which was situated entirely within the pituitary was found by Erdheim (1910). Erdheim (1903) also described the first incidental subclinical microadenoma.

The functions of these different adenoma types were elucidated only during this century. Gubler (1900) and Benda (1901) (Fraenkel *et al.*, 1901) suggested the endocrine activity of the pituitary adenomas in acromegaly. They thought that the adenoma was directly responsible for the abnormal growth. Cushing (1914) found that the degree of the endocrine activity was not necessarily related

---

*The author thanks Dr. R. Smith, Phoenix, Arizona for his help in translation of the manuscript, Miss Cécile Elsener for her typing and Mrs. Verena Links and Miss Sabine Huber for their technical assistance.

to the size of adenoma. This was illustrated by his description of pituitary baso-
philism (Cushing, 1932). Details concerning the pathology of the pituitary lesions
in 6 of Cushing's 16 patients were available. All 6 adenomas had diameters of less
than 7 mm. They belonged therefore to the class of endocrine-active microadenomas.

The pathogenesis and function of the incidental, subclinical microadenomas
remained unclear. Erdheim and Stumme (1909), as well as Cushing (1912), were
not able to decide whether these lesions were true adenomas or focal hyperplasias.
They noted, however, that these lesions were not separated from the normal
glandular tissue by a collagenous capsule. They were inclined therefore to classify
the lesions as non-neoplastic. Löwenstein (1907) favored a neoplastic nature. He
suggested that the subclinical microadenomas consist of pluripotent, embryonal
cells and that all types of larger pituitary adenomas originate from them. Costello
(1936), who had examined 1000 subclinical microadenomas, also thought that
they represented neoplasms, which might under the influence of an unknown
stimulus, start to secrete hormones and produce clinical symptoms. Intensive
research has not yet been able to solve the problems of pathogenesis, development
and function of the different types of pituitary adenomas. Our current knowledge
about the natural history of the different proliferative processes of the human
adenohypophysis will here be presented.

## DEFINITIONS

The different terms used in pituitary pathology are not clearly defined and are
used simultaneously for different items. This leads to misunderstanding. Therefore
we will define the terms used in this article. Some of the definitions need additional explanations which will be given in the following paragraphs.

All disturbances of pituitary growth leading to occupation of space are called
proliferative processes. They are subdivided into hyperplasias and neoplasms. A
diffuse increase in the number of a certain cell type is called diffuse hyperplasia.
Focal hyperplasia is morphologically similar to a microadenoma but does not
cause clinical symptoms. It is equivalent to the terms minute adenoma, incidental
microadenoma, subclinical adenoma and glandular hyperplasia.

A pituitary adenoma is a benign neoplasm with either autonomous growth,
autonomous function or both. Autonomy need not be absolute. A certain degree
of hypothalamic dependence may exist. The dependence may be lost gradually
during the evolution of the adenoma. Endocrine-active adenomas produce increased
amounts of one or several pituitary hormones which cause clinical symptoms and
can be detected in the patients' blood. These adenomas are named according to
the hormone produced (Landolt, 1978). Microadenomas cause signs of endocrine
hyperfunction. According to the definition of Hardy (Hardy, 1969; Hardy *et al.*,
1973), they have diameters of 10 mm or less and are usually located within the
sella. Endocrine-inactive adenomas show in neither clinical examination nor
endocrine testing signs of hormone secretion. They manifest their presence by
local pressure symptoms. They lack evidence of hormone production because:
(1) the adenoma cells have lost the ability to produce hormones as a result of
degeneration (oncocytomas); (2) the adenoma cells produce normal hormones

in such small amounts that the resulting blood concentrations are not elevated above normal; (3) the adenoma cells secrete abnormal substances that are recognized neither by the biological receptor nor by the antibodies used in the radio immunoassay.

## INCIDENCE OF PROLIFERATIVE PROCESSES IN THE PITUITARY

Focal hyperplasia is rather frequent but a great variety of incidences has been reported: Hardy (1969) 2.7%, McCormick and Halmi (1971) 9%, Erdheim and Stumme (1909) 10%, Saeger (1977a) 12%, Haugen (1973) 19%, Costello (1936) 22.5%. The incidence depends on the method of preparation of the material. Costello (1936) cut the hypophysis in multiple 1 to 1.5 mm thick slices and examined each one histologically. He would have overlooked only lesions with diameters of less than 1 mm. We found an incidence of 13% when we examined two random sections per gland.

Both sexes are equally affected (Costello, 1936). The age incidence was examined by the same author. His youngest subject was 2, the oldest 86 years old. The greatest incidence was present in the sixth decade of life. We have calculated the relative distribution of the total focal hyperplasias (=100%) in the different age groups in the living population from Costello's data (Fig. 1). The highest frequency (23.3%) shifts to the fourth decade, with an average age of 39.4 years. This calculation allows comparison with the data obtained from symptomatic adenomas.

The annual incidence of symptomatic adenomas is 1.5 per 100 000 population (95% confidence interval: 0.5-3.9%) (Kurland, 1958). This is 1.5 × $10^4$ times fewer than the incidence of focal hyperplasias. Only 1 in 15 000 people with focal hyperplasias will develop symptoms of a pituitary adenoma per year. Hypophysial adenomas are somewhat more frequent in men than in women. The relation used

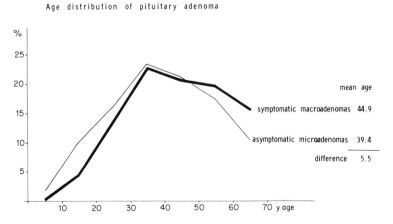

*Fig. 1.* Age distribution of asymptomatic pituitary microadenomas, corresponding to our focal hyperplasias, and symptomatic pituitary macroadenomas (data from Costello 1936; Earle and Dillard 1973).

to be 53:47 (Saeger, 1977a). But this and other statistical data may change since we now detect frequent microprolactinomas in young women.

The age distribution of symptomatic adenomas (Earle and Dillard, 1973) is similar to the curve found in focal hyperplasias but is shifted towards older ages (Fig. 1). The mean age of symptomatic adenomas is 5.5 years greater than in focal hyperplasias. This time difference may indicate that symptomatic adenomas originate from focal hyperplasias, as proposed by Löwenstein (1907). The mean duration of preoperative symptoms and signs in a group of 306 symptomatic adenomas was 2–6 years (Earle and Dillard, 1973). This is only half of the time shift obtained from the statistical analysis. But the tumor growth may have started in many adenomas a longer time before the first symptoms were noticed since compression symptoms appear late and since the onset of symptoms is often insidious, so that the duration of the preoperative history may have been under-estimated.

## MORPHOLOGY OF PITUITARY PROLIFERATIVE LESIONS

### Focal hyperplasia

We found in our own series of 100 routine autopsies (material obtained by courtesy of Th. Hardmeier, Dept. of Pathology, Kantonsspital Münsterlingen) 14 examples of focal hyperplasia in 13 pituitaries. They had diameters between 0.3 and 8.0 mm (mean 1.7 mm, median 1.2 mm). Their shapes were usually spherical. Their architecture was different from the normal gland. This was seen best in reticulum-stained tissue sections (Fig. 2) (Velasco et al., 1977). They usually contained much less connective tissue than the normal gland. The lobules of the immediately surrounding hypophysis were oriented tangentially to the surface of the lesion. They were smaller than usual and seemed to be compressed. The connective tissue fibers of the normal lobules could be seen to extend into the nodule. No capsule of the nodule was present.

Staining with Herlant's tetrachrome (Herlant, 1960) revealed that the majority contained several cell types. We have disregarded chromophobe cells in the following enumeration, since they are either interpreted as degranulated chromophile cells (Romeis, 1940) or fixation artefacts (McCormick and Halmi, 1971). We found 1 chromophile cell type in 2 nodules, 2 cell types in 5, 3 cell types in 4, and 4 cell types in another 2 nodules. Thirteen nodules contained cells which belong to the serous group and 11 nodules contained cells which belong to the mucoid group. The predominant cell type was serous in 2 cases, mucoid in 6 cases and ungranulated in 5 cases. One nodule could not be evaluated because of bad fixation. This distribution does not correspond to the situation in either the normal gland or in adenomas. Light microscopy results are confirmed and extended by immunohistologic findings (Heitz, 1978). Only 8 of 44 clinically silent nodules contained a single hormone. The remaining 36 were multihormonal. Ten specimens contained 2, 10 contained 3, 12 contained 4, 3 contained 5, and 1 contained 6 hormones. The most frequent hormones were luteinizing hormone/follicle stimulating hormone (LH/FSH) (35 cases of 44) followed by growth hormone (GH) (30 cases of 44), β-lipotropin (β-LPH) (9 cases of 17), adrenocordicotropic hormone (ACTH) (20 cases of 44), prolactin (PRL) (15 cases of 34) and thyrotropic hormone (TSH) (18 cases of 44 examined).

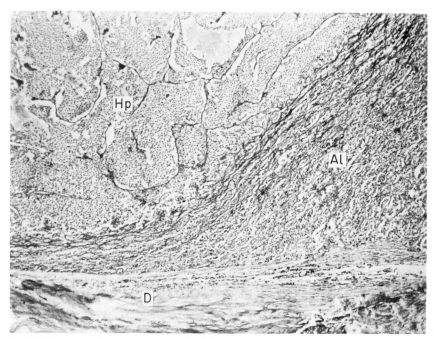

*Fig. 2.* Periphery of an asymptomatic focal hyperplasia with a diameter of 8 mm seen in low power light microscopy. The hyperplastic area (Hp) contains less connective tissue than the adjacent normal anterior lobe (Al). There is no interposed fibrous capsule. The immediately surrounding lobules of the normal gland are compressed and orientated tangentially to the surface of the space-occupying process. D: dura. –60-year-old man, formalin fixation, reticulum stain, × 36.

### Symptomatic adenomas

The sizes of hypophysial adenomas can vary from a few millimeters to that of a man's fist (Zülch, 1956). Adenomas with diameters of less than 10 mm are defined as microadenomas. Three architectural types have been described on the basis of the distribution of blood vessels and connective tissue observed in histologic sections of the tumors (Nurnberger and Korey, 1953; Kernohan and Sayre, 1956): the diffuse, sinusoidal and papillary types.

Hypophysial adenomas consist usually of one cell type but exceptions to this rule are known. The transitional cell adenoma (Kraus, 1914) contains chromophile, granulated cells, various grades of degranulated cells and chromophobe cells. This chromophilic variation is interpreted as an expression of the secretory cycle of the adenoma cells. The true mixed adenoma contains different cell types involved in secretion of different hormones. In acromegaly 11–33% of the patients show a concomitant elevation of the blood growth hormone and blood prolactin (Franks *et al.*, 1975; Halmi and Duello, 1976; Landolt, 1978). A concomitant elevation of prolactin has also been observed in corticotropic, gonadotropic and thyrotropic adenomas (for review see Landolt, 1978; Duello and Halmi, 1977). Corticotropic adenomas in Cushing's disease often simultaneously secrete β-LPH and ACTH (Heitz, 1978). It is not clear from morphologic studies whether one or two cell types are involved in the secretion of two hormones and further studies will be necessary to solve this problem. Rare inclusions of groups of granulated cells displaying a different staining character have been described (Kernohan and Sayre, 1956; Saeger, 1977a). It is not known if these groups are of neoplastic origin or if they are remnants of the destroyed, adjacent adenohypophysis.

In electron microscopy the measurement of secretory granules diameters has often been used for cell type identification in normal and adenomatous hypophysis (for review see Landolt, 1975). But a comparison of the morphological findings with the hormone secretions of adenomas showed that the diamater of the hormone granules depends on their rate of formation and exocytosis rather than on the nature of the hormone produced. The granules grow during their intracellular storage. Adenomas with fast granule release contain, therefore, few

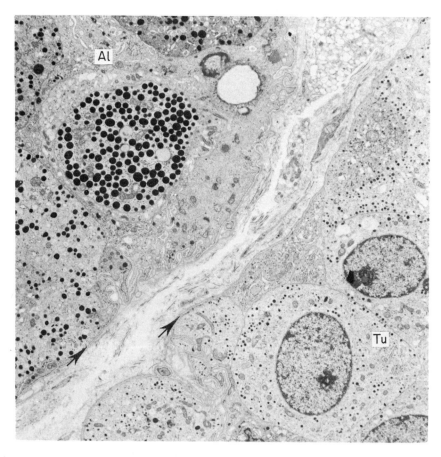

*Fig. 3.* Electron micrograph of the periphery of a prolactinoma (Tu) separated from the adjacent normal pituitary by two basement membranes (arrows) and some interposed collagen fibrils. Note the large osmiophilic secretory granules in the normal PRL cell in comparison with the small granules in the prolactinoma cells. 49-year-old woman, glutaraldehyde-osmium fixation, epon embedding, × 4400.

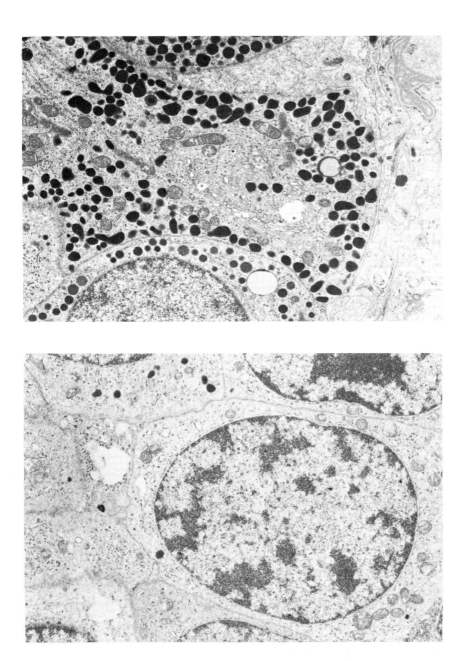

*Fig. 4.* (a) Prolactin cells with accumulation of large, deformed PRL granules in the normal hypophysis adjacent to a prolactinoma. (b) Prolactinoma cell of the same patient containing only a few and smaller granules than the normal PRL-cell, suggesting faster hormone release. 22-year-old woman, glutaraldehyde-osmium fixation, epon embedding, × 8200.

and small granules whereas adenomas with long storage periods contain numerous large granules (Landolt, 1975; Landolt and Rothenbühler 1977a). However, certain other morphological features of the adenoma, when present, may provide insight into the nature of the secreted hormone (for review see Landolt 1975, 1978).

The demarcation between adenoma and normal gland is usually sharp in acromegaly and in prolactinomas (see Fig. 27 of Landolt, 1978). No capsule can be seen. Even the electron microscope shows only an interposition of two basement membranes and few collagen fibrils between the neoplasm and the normal tissue (Fig. 3). A deposit of a larger amount of connective tissue, which usually has the width of less than one adenoma cell layer, is quite rare. Invasive growth of the adenoma into the normal hypophysis can be observed in patients with Cushing's disease and even more often in Nelson's syndrome. Indeed, malignant changes and true metastatic spreading are seen relatively more often in association with corticotropic adenomas than with any other cell type (Landolt, 1975). However, recently we have also observed invasion of the adenoma into the underlying dura and periosteum of the sella floor in half of our patients with prolactinomas (Landolt, unpublished results).

Saeger (1977b) has examined the normal gland adjacent to pituitary adenomas. He described increased numbers of ACTH-cells in 10 and 12 cases with Cushing's syndrome, forming nodular hyperplasias in 7. The para-adenomatous acidophils were hyperplastic in 3 out of 6 patients with prolactinomas. He suggested that the adenomas originated from the hyperplasias, which had been caused by a hypothalamic disturbance. No similar hyperplasias were seen in acromegaly and endocrine inactive adenomas.

We have compared the ultrastructure of the prolactin cells in the adenoma and the gland in 5 women suffering from prolactinomas (Fig. 4a, b). The prolactin cells in the adenoma and in the normal gland were identified by immuno-histologic staining of semi-thin sections. The ultrastructures of the two types of prolactin cells differed markedly. The adenoma cells were usually smaller, had larger nuclei, less cytoplasm and fewer and smaller secretory granules. The prolactin cells of the normal gland were densely filled with bigger and deformed granules. This indicates that their secretory activity was low or at least lower than in the adjacent adenoma (Landolt, 1975). Secretion was blocked either directly by the hormone secreted by the adenoma or indirectly via an interaction with the hypothalamus. Similar pictures of blocked prolactin cells have been seen in prolactinomas which were transplanted into "nude" mice and treated with bromocriptine (Landolt, 1978). These human prolactinomas demonstrated an increased number and size of the stored secretory granules when compared with fragments of the same transplanted adenoma which had not been treated with the secretion-inhibiting substance (Fig. 5a, b).

Bergland (1975) has claimed that in acromegaly small adenomas are usually eosinophilic whereas the majority of larger adenomas are chromophobic. This means that small adenomas store more secretory granules than larger ones. We have reinvestigated the problem of morphological differences between micro- and macroadenomas in 49 prolactinomas (Landolt, unpublished results). The ultrastructures of the 10 smallest, range 3–6 mm (average diameter 5.1 mm), and of the 10 largest tumors, range 33–50 mm (average diameter 40.3 mm) were com-

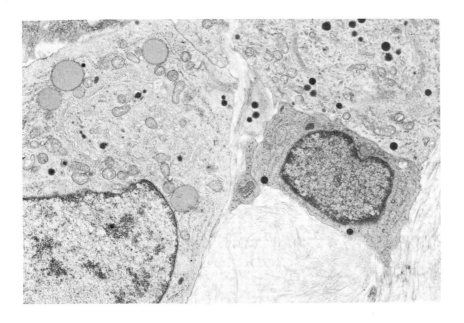

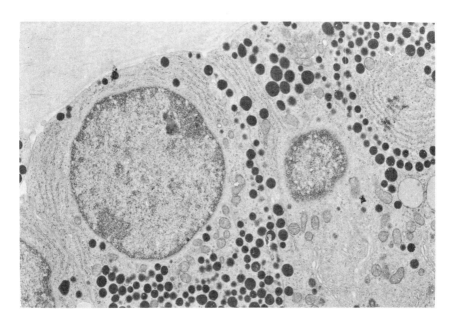

*Fig. 5.* (a) Electron micrograph of a human prolactinoma one week after transplantation into the cutis of an immunoincompetent "nude" mouse. The cells contain only few small secretory granules. (b) Same prolactinoma as in (a) kept in another "nude" mouse for one week and treated with bromocriptine. Note the increased content of larger secretory granules in this pharmacologically blocked specimen. Glutaraldehyde-osmium fixation, epon embedding × 8200.

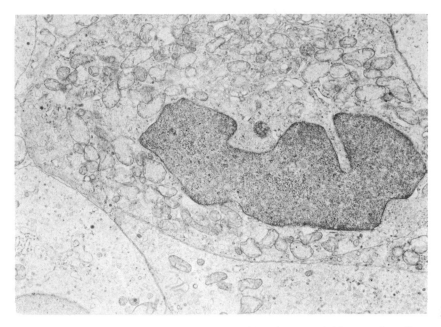

*Fig. 6.*   Oncocyte in a large prolactinoma (diameter 40 mm) surrounded by secreting cells containing normal mitochondria. 56-year-old man. Osmium fixation, epon embedding, × 11 000.

pared. There was no difference in the cell size, nuclear shape, extension of the cisterns of the rough surfaced endoplasmic reticulum, dimension of the Golgi cisterns, presence of annulate lamellae, storage of secretory granules, content of lipids, presence of intracytoplasmic filaments, formation of follicles, or occurrence of intra-adenomatous calcifications. Only one morphological finding was significantly different ($P < 0.001$): nine of ten large adenomas contained dispersed oncocytes (Fig. 6) and accumulation of oncocytic mitochondria whereas such cells could only be observed in one of ten microadenomas. We interpret the presence of oncocytes as a sign of secondary degeneration, which occurs in the interior of larger adenomas.

## NATURAL HISTORY OF PITUITARY ADENOMAS

Our knowledge of the natural history of the different proliferative processes of the pituitary is still rudimentary and several of the connections presented in our tentative scheme (Fig. 7) remain hypothetical and will need experimental and/or clinical confirmation. But it is clear that the normal hypophysis can undergo a number of structural changes.

Diffuse hyperplasia of a particular pituitary cell type can be caused by direct or indirect (via hypothalamus) action of a hormonal alteration as, e.g. in pregnancy, estrogen application, or hypothyroidism. The change is fully reversible after elimination of the basic cause (Erdheim and Stumme, 1909).

Focal hyperplasia may be due to age (Costello, 1936), parietal destruction of

Natural history of pituitary proliferative lesions

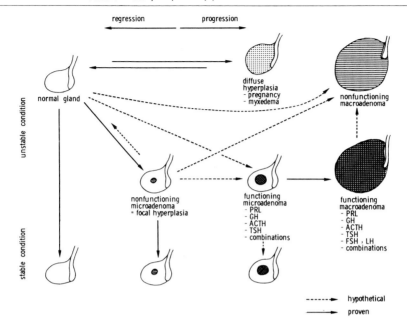

*Fig. 7.* Tentative relationships between the different proliferative processes of the hypophysis.

the normal hypophysis (Landolt, 1973) and possibly also to alteration of the hormonal equilibrium. It is neither autonomous in function nor in growth and therefore does not deserve the name "adenoma" in spite of its structural similarities. The majority of these lesions contain several hormonal cell types, as shown by light microscopy and immuno-histology. It is possible that the lesions are reversible. This might explain their decreasing incidence in the age groups over 40 years (Fig. 1).

The functioning microadenoma may be caused occasionally by peripheral hormone disturbances, as for example in prolonged high dosage estrogen treatment of laboratory animals (El Etreby and Günzel, 1973) or in the course of long lasting, severe thyroid insufficiency (Linquette *et al.*, 1973). They only gradually gain full independence from the hypothalamus and may even be reversible in an early stage of development (Guinet *et al.*, 1972). There are four criteria which must be fulfilled by adenomas resulting from peripheral gland disorders: (1) the original endocrine deficit must be of peripheral origin, and not secondary to the hypophysial lesion; (2) the blood level of the corresponding pituitary tropic hormone must be elevated; (3) the blood level of this hormone must return to normal after removal of the adenoma or hypophysectomy; (4) the pituitary adenoma must be composed of cells that produce the tropic hormone involved (Linquette *et al.*, 1973). But no cause can be found in the majority of the microadenomas. We do not think that focal hyperplasia is the precursor of symptomatic microadenomas, as suggested by statistical analysis, because of the different cellular compositions of the two types of lesions. The majority of hyperplasias contain a multitude of endocrine cell types whereas adenomas usually show the production of only one or two hormones. Gonadotropic adenomas are extremely rare but the same cell type is present in more than two thirds of the hyperplasias. Prolactin production is seen in less than half of the hyperplasias but is present in the largest group of the symptomatic adenomas.

Symptomatic microadenomas do not necessarily secrete lesser amounts of hormones than endocrine-active macroadenomas. No relation exists in the majority of prolactinomas between the observed prolactin level and the adenoma diameter. The computed linear least square regression line obtained from 46 cases of our own series had the following characteristics: $y = 116.59 \times -1262, r^2 = 0.17$. The low coefficient of determination means that only 17% of the total variation observed can be explained by the alteration of $x$ by linear regression. This is not surprising, since the ultrastructure examination of different adenomas shows signs of different degrees of secretory activity (Landolt, 1975). The secretory activity per unit volume therefore varies considerably from biopsy to biopsy. In addition to that, the secretory activity can be altered by external and internal factors.

The endocrine-active microadenomas may grow and become endocrine macroadenomas, they may remain stable over longer periods of time, or they may very rarely regress spontaneously. Spontaneous regression may occur because of a hemorrhage in the microadenoma, as first observed by Erdheim and Stumme (1909). Such intraadenomatous bleedings can be produced by estrogens (Peillon *et al.*, 1970) and are not necessarily related to incarceration of a large adenoma in the opening of the diaphragma sellae (Rovit and Fein, 1972). A number of microadenomas probably remain unchanged and do not grow over long intervals of time. This is suggested by the large number of microprolactinomas which are now detected in young women and which will ultimately alter our "well-established" statistics. Probably not all of these lesions will progress to the stage of a macroadenoma, because this would have resulted in a different sex distribution of the adenomas than was actually observed in earlier statistics. Sheline (1973) observed two patients in a group of 16 who did not show radiological or clinical evidence of tumor progression over observation periods of 4 and 20 years.

The majority of endocrine-active microadenomas grow and reach the stage of macroadenoma. This growth may be stimulated by endocrine factors, such as estrogen administration and pregnancy for prolactinomas or adrenalectomy for corticotropic adenomas (Nelson's syndrome). Simultaneously, some adenoma cells degenerate and become oncocytes. Intraadenomatous calcifications are not a sign of degeneration because they are present in micro- and macroadenomas with equal frequency; they are signs of prolactin production (Landolt and Rothenbühler, 1977b). It is possible that an endocrine-active adenoma may lose a smaller or larger part of its secretory activity by oncocytic transformation, but the larger majority of the endocrine-inactive macroadenomas probably originate directly from the normal hypophysis. There are no data available which allow a further description of the processes involved.

Pituitary adenomas usually grow expansively and only a few have invasive growth tendencies. Invasive growth occurs in every hormonal type but it is relatively more frequent in stimulated corticotropic adenomas. Invasive growth can be microscopic or macroscopic. Macroscopic invasion of the structures surround-

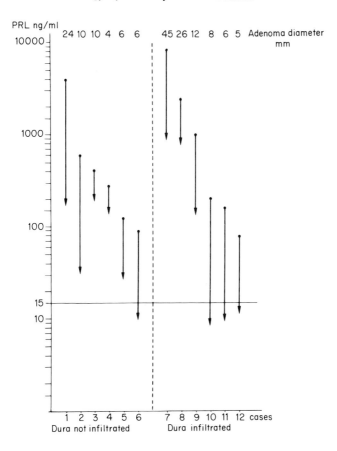

*Fig. 8.* Preoperative (●) and postoperative (▾) PRL blood levels and diameters in six prolactinomas without and six prolactinomas with invasion of the basal dura of the sella turcica.

ing the pituitary by extension beyond the dural capsule into the cavernous sinus, middle cranial fossa, temporal lobe, diencephalon, clivus, sphenoid sinus, and epipharynx is usually considered as a sign of malignancy (Jefferson, 1954). But an invasion can be of only microscopic dimensions. This is not related to the size of the tumor. Even microadenomas may show this type of invasion. These adenomas infiltrate the adjacent normal pituitary and the overlying dura and periosteum of the sella. Such microinvasion seems to be rather frequent, contrary to the above described macroinvasion. We have examined the histology of the basal dura in a series of 12 prolactinomas. Six biopsies showed infiltrative growth. In some cases it affected only the innermost collagen layers, whereas it extended through the whole thickness of the collagen tissue in others. We were surprised to find that this growth pattern did not seem to affect the immediate postoperative PRL levels (Fig. 8). This may be due to the fact that we routinely treat the adenoma cavity at the end of the surgical procedure with absolute alcohol which may destroy some of the infiltrating cells. But only a long term follow-up of our patients will tell us more about the significance of the microinvasion.

The surgical results in terms of normalization of the hypersecretion of pituitary adenoma hormones do not necessarily depend only on the tumor size and growth pattern but indicate that other factors may be involved. In prolactinomas one of the most important seems to be the preoperative PRL blood level. We have collected 162 prolactinomas operated on by the transsphenoidal approach from the literature and from our own material (Antunes *et al.*, 1977; Chang *et al.*, 1977; Tindall *et al.*, 1978; von Werder *et al.*, 1978). Only 6 out of 81 patients with a preoperative PRL level above 200 ng/ml (upper level of normal 15–25 ng/ml) showed normal postoperative PRL values whereas 56 of 81 with a preoperative level below 200 ng/ml were normalized after surgery. This difference in outcome is highly significant ($P < 0.0001$). Additional irradiation did not improve the

*Table I.*   Surgical prognosis of prolactinomas (results of transsphenoidal operation of 38 patients). Percentage of patients with postoperative normal PRL levels in relation to preoperative PRL and to adenoma size.

|  | Preoperative prolactin | | |
|---|---|---|---|
|  | > 200 ng/ml %  | < 200 ng/ml %  |  |
| Adenoma diameter |  |  |  |
| > 10 mm | 0 | 66 | 22 |
| ≤ 10 mm | 29 | 75 | 45 |
|  | 8 | 69 |  |

The four framed values present the combined effect of both parameters, whereas the four marginal values indicate their individual effects.

results in our material. The comparison of the influences of the preoperative PRL level and the adenoma diameter (Table I) in our own material demonstrated that the size of the adenoma in terms of micro- or macroadenoma was not as important in prediction of the surgical results as the preoperative PRL. The most reliable prognosis was obtained when the two parameters were combined. We believe that the hyperplasia of the PRL-cells in the normal gland adjacent to the adenoma may be responsible for the remaining hyperprolactinemia in some cases. A postoperative elevation of the PRL level would in this situation not indicate in every case an incomplete removal of the adenoma. The situation might then be handled more adequately with antisecretory drugs and not with reoperation or additional X-ray treatment. The situation is different in acromegaly. There surgical results depend mainly on size and extension of the tumor (Hardy, 1973). No hyperplasia of somatotropic cells is observed in the adjacent adenohypophysis (Saeger, 1977b). A postoperative elevation of the GH level therefore indicates the presence of a remaining tumor fragment.

## REFERENCES

Antunes, J. L., Housepian, E. M., Frantz, A. G., Holub, D. A. Hui, R. M., Carmel, P. W. and Quest, D. O. (1977). *Ann. Neurol.* **2**, 148–153.

Bergland, R. M. (1975). *Progr. Neurol. Surg.* **6**, 62–94.

Chang, R. J., Keye, W. R., Young, J. R., Wilson, C. B., Jaffe, R. B. (1977). *Am. J. Obstet. Gynecol.* **128**, 356–363.

Costello, R. J. (1936). *Amer. J. Path.* **12**, 205–215.

Cushing, H. (1912). "The Pituitary Body and its Disorders". J. B. Lippincott, Philadelphia and London.

Cushing, H. (1914). *J.A.M.A.* **63**, 1515–1525.

Cushing, H. (1932). "Papers Relating to the Pituitary Body, Hypothalamus and Parasympathetic Nervous System" pp. 113–174. Springfield.

Duello, T. M. and Halmi, N. S. (1977). *Virchow's Arch. A Path. Anat. Histol.* **376**, 255–265.

Earle, K. M. and Dillard, S. H. (1973). *In* "Diagnosis and Treatment of Pituitary Tumors" (P. O. Kohler and G. T. Ross, eds) 3–16. Excerpta Medica, Amsterdam, American Elsevier, New York.

El Etreby, M. F. and Günzel, P. (1973). *Arneim.-Forsch.* **23**, 1768–1790.

Erdheim, J. (1903). *Beitr. path. Anat.* **33**, 158–236.

Erdheim, J. (1910). *Frankf. Z. Path.* **4**, 70–86.

Erdheim, J., Stumme, E. (1909). *Beitr. path. Anat.* **46**, 1–132.

Fraenkel, A., Stadelmann, E. and Benda, C. (1901). *Dtsch. Med. Wschr.* **27**, 513–517, 536–539, 564–566.

Franks, S., Jacobs, H. S. and Nabarro, J. D. N. (1975). *J. Endocrinol.* **65**, 25P–26P.

Gubler, R. (1900). *Corresp.-Bl. Schweiz. Aerz.* **30**, 761–771.

Guinet, G., Tournaire, J., Orgiazzi, J. and Robert, M. (1972). *Ann. Endocr. (Paris)* **33**, 376–389.

Halmi, N. S. and Duello, T. (1976). *Arch. Pathol. Lab. Med.* **100**, 346–351.

Hardy, J. (1969). *Clin. Neurosurg.* **16**, 185–216.

Hardy, J. (1973). *In* "Diagnosis and Treatment of Pituitary Tumors" (P. O. Kohler and G. T. Ross, eds) 179–194. Excerpta Medica, Amsterdam.

Hardy, J., Robert, F., Somma, M. and Vezina, J. L. (1973). *Neurochirurgie* **19** suppl. 2, 1–184.

Haugen, O. A. (1973). *Acta Path. Microbiol. Scand. Sect. A Path.* **81**, 425–431.

Heitz, Ph. U. (1978). *Hormone Res.* (in press).

Herlant, M. (1960). *Bull. Micr. Appl.* **10**, 37–44.

Jefferson, G. (1954). "The Invasive Adenomas of the Anterior Pituitary". University Press of Liverpool, Liverpool.

Kernohan, J. W. and Sayre, G. P. (1956). "Tumors of the Pituitary Gland and Infundibulum". Atlas of Tumor Pathology, section X, fascicle 36, Armed Forces Institute of Pathology, Washington.

Kraus, E. J. (1914). *Beitr. path. Anat.* **58**, 159–210.

Kurland, L. T. (1958). *J. Neurosurg.* **15**, 627–641.

Landolt, A. M. (1973). *J. Neurosurg.* **39**, 35–41.

Landolt, A. M. (1975). *Acta Neurochir. (Wien)* Suppl. 22.

Landolt, A. M. (1978). *In* "Advances and Technical Standards in Neurosurgery" (H. Krayenbühl, ed) Vol. V, 4–49. Springer Verlag, Wien.

Landolt, A. M. and Rothenbühler, V. (1977a). *Acta Endocr. (Kbh)* **84**, 461–469.

Landolt, A. M. and Rothenbühler, V. (1977b). *Arch. Pathol. Lab. Med.* **101**, 22–27.

Linquette, M., Fossati, P. and Derrien, G. (1973). *Actual. Endocrinol.* **13**, 247–256.

Löwenstein, D. (1907). *Virchow's Arch.* **188**, 44–65.

McCormick, W. F. and Halmi, N. S. (1971). *Arch. Pathol. (Chicago)* **92**, 231–238.

Nurnberger, J. L. and Korey, S. R. (1953). "Pituitary Chromophobe Adenomas. A Clinical Study of the Sellar Syndrome: Neurology, Metabolism, Therapy". Springer Publishing Comp., New York.

Peillon, F., Vila-Porcile, E., Olivier, L. and Racadot, J. (1970). *Ann. Endocr. (Paris)* **31**, 259–270.

Rayer, P. (1823). *Arch. Gén. de Méd.* **3**, 350–367.

Romeis, B. (1940). *In* "Handbuch der mikroskopischen Anatomie des Menschen" (W. v. Möllendorff, ed) Vol. VI, part 3. Springer, Berlin.

Rovit, R. L. and Fein, J. M. (1972). *J. Neurosurg.* **37**, 280–288.

Saeger, W. (1977a). *In* "Veröffentlichungen aus der Pathologie" (W. Büngeler, M. Eder, K. Lennert, G. Peters, W. Sandritter and G. Seifert, eds) Heft 107. G. Fischer Verlag, Stuttgart.

Saeger, W. (1977b). *Virchow's Arch. A Path. Anat. Histol.* **372**, 299–314.

Sheline, G. E. (1973). *In* "Diagnosis and Treatment of Pituitary Tumors" (P. O. Kohler and G. T. Ross, eds) 201–216. Excerpta Medica, Amsterdam, American Elsevier, New York.

Tindall, G. T., McLanahan, C. S. and Christy, J. H. (1978). *J. Neurosurg.* **48**, 849–860.

Velasco, M. E., Sindley, S. D. and Roessmann, U. (1977). *J. Neurosurg.* **46**, 548–550.

Verga, A., (1864). *Reale Istituto Lombardo di Scienze e lettere. Rendiconti. Classe di Scienze Matematiche e Natruali.* **1**, 111–117. Republished (1964). *Atti Accad. Med. Lombard.* **19**, 1363–1379.

von Werder, K., Fahlbusch, R. Landgraf, R., Pickardt, C. R., Rjosk, H. K. and Scriba, P. C. (1978). *J. Endocrinol. Invest.* **1**, 47–58.

Zülch, K. J. (1956). *In* "Handbuch der Neurochirurgie" (H. Olivecrona and W. Tönnis, eds) Vol. III, 1–702. Springer, Berlin.

# PITUITARY ADENOMAS ASSOCIATED WITH HYPERPROLACTINEMIA: MORPHOLOGICAL AND IMMUNOCYTOLOGICAL ASPECTS*

K. Kovacs and E. Horvath

*Department of Pathology, St. Michael's Hospital, University of Toronto, Toronto, Ontario, Canada*

With the introduction of radioimmunoassay, endocrinolgy attained scientific respectability. Sensitive and reliable measurements of various hormones in blood and tissues provided a deeper insight into endocrine function and hormone metabolism and unraveled correlations which had been unknown so far. One of the significant advances was the discovery of human prolactin (Frantz and Kleinberg, 1970; Hwang *et al.*, 1971). Further progress was achieved by the finding that diverse endocrine conditions and various drugs can affect prolactin production and/or release (Horrobin 1976; Frantz, 1977; Martin *et al.*, 1977; Frantz, 1978). The existence of prolactin-secreting pituitary adenomas also became firmly established (Forbes *et al.*, 1954; Herlant *et al.*, 1965; Peake *et al.*, 1969; Racadot *et al.*, 1971; Friesen *et al.*, 1972; Guinet *et al.*, 1973; Antunes *et al.*, 1977; Kleinberg *et al.*, 1977; Frantz, 1978). These tumors are clinically often associated with galactorrhea, amenorrhea, infertility, decrease of libido and impotence. In some cases, however, no pronounced clinical symptoms are apparent.

In order to shed light on the structural features of pituitary tumors accompanied by enhanced prolactin secretion, a detailed morphologic study was undertaken, including immunocytology and electron microscopy, on pituitary adenomas

---

*This work was supported in part by the Medical Research Council of Canada (Grant MA-6349). We wish to thank Mrs. G. Ilse, Miss D. McComb and Mrs. N. Ryan for excellent technical assistance, and Mrs. W. Wlodarski for invaluable secretarial help.

removed by surgery from patients with hyperprolactinemia. Some of the results have been reported elsewhere (Horvath and Kovacs, 1974; Kovacs *et al.*, 1975; Corenblum *et al.*, 1976; Horvath and Kovacs, 1976; Sirek *et al.*, 1976; Horvath *et al.*, 1977b; Kovacs, 1977; Kovacs *et al.*, 1977a). The present work was focused on seeking answers to the following two questions: (1) Is it possible to diagnose prolactin-producing pituitary adenomas by morphology and to distinguish them from other adenoma types? (2) Are cytologic techniques valuable in revealing the cellular origin of pituitary tumors?

## MATERIAL AND METHODS

The material consists of 67 pituitary adenomas removed by surgery from 29 male and 38 female patients of various ages. Surgery was indicated because of local symptoms (visual disturbances, severe headaches, signs of increased intra-cranial pressure) or endocrine abnormalities unaffected by medical treatment. All the patients had hyperprolactinemia. Plasma prolactin levels were measured by radioimmunoassay. The upper limit of normal was considered to be 30 ng/ml; hence, plasma levels higher than this value were regarded as indicating hyper-prolactinemia.

For light microscopy, tumor tissue was fixed in 10% buffered formalin, de-hydrated in graded ethanol and embedded in paraffin. Sections of 4-6 μm thick-ness were cut and stained with hematoxylin-phloxine-saffron, the PAS technique, and in many cases with lead hematoxylin, aldehyde fuchsin, aldehyde thionin, orange G, Goldberg-Chaikoff's trichrome, Herlant's erythrosin and Brookes' carmoisine methods.

For immunocytologic localization of prolactin, growth hormone and, in some cases, other adenohypophysial hormones, the immunoperoxidase technique (Sternberger *et al.*, 1970) was used as described in detail elsewhere (Kovacs *et al.*, 1976). Paraffin sections of 4-6 μm thickness were cut and immunostained, using antibodies raised in rabbits against prolactin (donated by Dr. H. Friesen, Depart-ment of Physiology, University of Manitoba, Winnipeg, Canada), growth hormone (Imperial Cancer Research Foundation, London, England), [1-24] ACTH (Organon, Oss, Holland; donated by Dr. S. Hane and Dr. P. H. Forsham, Metabolic Unit, University of California Medical Center, San Francisco, California, USA), FSH and LH (β-subunit, donated by the National Pituitary Agency, University of Maryland School of Medicine and National Institute of Arthritis, Metabolic and Digestive Diseases, Bethesda, Maryland, USA), and TSH (Imperial Cancer Research Foundation, London, England). Duration of exposure to the primary antibody varied from 30 minutes to 3 hours; dilution of the primary antibody from 1:100 to 1:1000.

Binding sites of the immunologic reaction were demonstrated by using the horseradish peroxidase-antihorseradish peroxidase complex (Cappel Labora-tories, Inc., Downingtown, Pennsylvania, USA), and 3,3'-diaminobenzidine. The specificity of immunostaining was verified by serial dilution of the antibodies and by replacing the antibodies with normal rabbit serum as well as with phosphate buffered saline. For control purposes, several non-tumorous pituitary glands, obtained at surgery (hypophysectomy was performed because of disseminated breast cancer, carcinoma of prostate, severe diabetes mellitus) or from unselected autopsies, were also immunostained, using the same primary antibodies and staining procedure.

For electron microscopy, small pieces of tumor tissue were fixed in 2.5% glutaraldehyde in Sorensen's buffer, postfixed in 1% osmium tetroxide in Millonig's buffer, dehydrated in graded ethanol, processed through propylene oxide and embedded in Epon 812 or in an Epon–Araldite mixture. Semithin sections were stained with toluidine blue and appropriate areas selected for fine structure study. Thin sections were cut with a Porter-Blum MT-2 ultramicrotome, stained with uranyl acetate and lead citrate and investigated with a Philips 300 electron microscope.

## RESULTS

Based on their morphologic features, it was possible to divide pituitary adenomas associated with hyperprolactinemia into five distinct entities: (1) densely granulated prolactin cell adenoma; (2) sparsely granulated prolactin cell adenoma; (3) mixed adenoma composed of growth hormone cells and prolactin cells; (4) acidophil stem cell adenoma; (5) undifferentiated cell adenoma not consisting of prolactin cells.

These five adenoma types will be separately described.

### (1)  Densely granulated prolactin cell adenoma

Only one adenoma appeared to belong to this type, thus this entity seems to be rather rare. The patient was a 19-year-old woman with galactorrhea, amenorrhea and enlarged sella turcica.

By light microscopy, the tumor cells showed intense cytoplasmic staining with phloxine or orange G, and also with Herlant's erythrosin or Brookes' carmoisine techniques, claimed to specifically detect secretory granules of prolactin cells (Herlant and Pasteels, 1967; Peak *et al.*, 1969; Pasteels *et al.*, 1972; Guyda *et al.*, 1973; Zimmerman *et al.*, 1974). No positive staining was obtained with PAS, lead hematoxylin, aldehyde fuchsin, aldehyde thionin or aniline blue. The immunoperoxidase technique revealed the presence of immunoreactive prolactin in the form of brown deposits in the cytoplasm of adenoma cells.

By electron microscopy, the adenoma cells resembled those seen in the nontumorous pituitaries (Fig. 1). They were oval or oblong and contained an oval, not uncommonly pleomorphic nucleus. The rough-surfaced endoplasmic reticulum was well developed and was composed of long parallel rows of ribosome-studded membranes, usually located at the periphery of the fairly large cytoplasm. The Golgi complex was moderately prominent and usually contained dense, immature, pleomorphic secretory granules. The secretory granules were numerous, spherical, oval or pleomorphic, exhibited high electron density and measured up to 1200 nm in diameter, averaging about 600 nm in diameter. The large size and oval or pleomorphic shape of the secretory granules distinguished this tumor type from growth hormone cell adenomas in which the secretory granules were smaller and always spherical (Horvath and Kovacs, 1976; Kovacs *et al.*, 1977a).

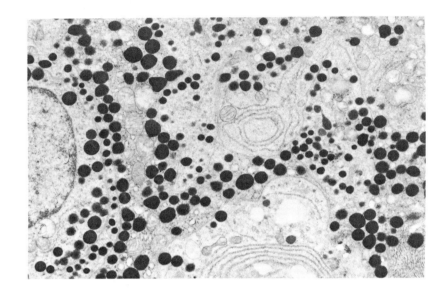

*Fig. 1.* Densely granulated prolactin cell adenoma showing well-developed rough-surfaced endoplasmic reticulum membranes and large, partly pleomorphic secretory granules. × 8000.

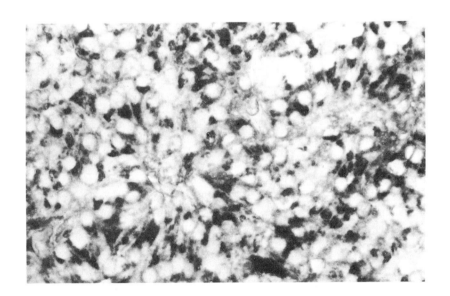

*Fig. 2.* Immunoreactive prolactin is evident in the cytoplasm of sparsely granulated adenomatous prolactin cells. Immunoperoxidase technique. Original magnification × 300.

## (2) Sparsely granulated prolactin cell adenoma

Fifty-five tumors were classified as sparsely granulated prolactin cell adenomas, indicating that this tumor type represents the most frequently occurring entity among pituitary neoplasms associated with hyperprolactinemia. Clinically, some of the patients showed galactorrhea, amenorrhea, infertility, decrease of libido and impotence, while others appeared to be symptomless.

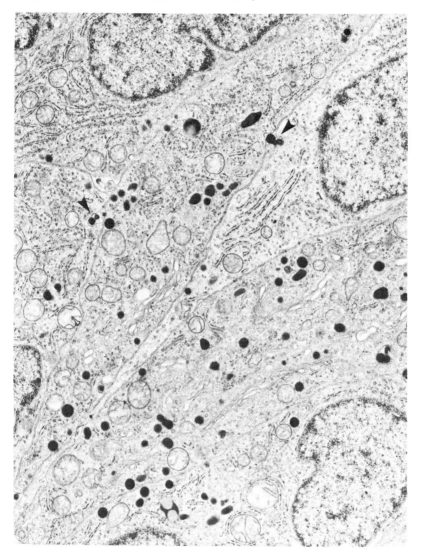

*Fig. 3.* Sparsely granulated prolactin cell adenoma exhibiting abundance of rough-surfaced endoplasmic reticulum membranes, prominence of Golgi complexes and misplaced exocytosis (arrowheads). × 10 000.

By light microscopy, the tumors showed the characteristic features of those of chromophobic adenomas, exhibiting no cytoplasmic staining with PAS, lead hematoxylin, aldehyde fuchsin, aldehyde thionin, aniline blue or with acid dyes, except for a few acidophilic granules in some adenoma cells. By Herlant's erythrosin or Brookes' carmoisine techniques, small positively staining secretory granules were disclosed in the cytoplasm. By the immunoperoxidase technique, brown deposits were apparent in the cytoplasm, usually arranged in streaks, frequently adjacent to the nucleus or to the plasma membranes (Fig. 2).

By electron microscopy, the adenoma cells were closely apposed and polyhedral with large oval, or pleomorphic nuclei (Fig. 3). The rough-surfaced endoplasmic reticulum was extensively developed and was composed of numerous parallel rows of ribosome-studded cisternae, occupying large portions of the cytoplasm. Nebenkern formations, composed of concentric whorls of rough-surfaced endoplasmic reticulum membranes, were frequent. Free ribosomes and polysomes were numerous. The Golgi apparatus was prominent and occupied, in some cells, as much as one-third of the cytoplasm. The Golgi sacculi were slightly or moderately dilated and regularly contained a variable number of dense, immature secretory granules. The secretory granules in the cytoplasm were dense, spherical or pleomorphic, but not numerous and, in general, were much smaller than those seen in nontumorous prolactin cells or in the densely granulated prolactin cell adenoma. Their largest diameter was only 130–350 nm, averaging about 250 nm.

A characteristic fine structural feature of this tumor type was the extrusion of secretory granules on the lateral cell membranes, into the intercellular space, distance both from the perivascular spaces and also from the intercellular extensions of the basement membrane. This phenomenon has been termed "misplaced exocytosis" (Horvath and Kovacs, 1974) to emphasize that granule extrusions occur on the far side and not on the capillary side of the cell where exocytosis usually occurs.

The cells of the sparsely granulated prolactin cell adenomas differed considerably from resting nontumorous prolactin cells or from densely granulated prolactin adenoma cells or from other pituitary cell types. They most resembled the estrogen-stimulated prolactin cells in the animal pituitaries (Hymer et al., 1961; Lundin and Schelin, 1962). Similar adenoma cells were seen in the rat pituitary in cases of estrogen-induced tumors (Schelin et al., 1964; Tiboldi et al., 1967; Schelin and Lundin, 1971) or in some spontaneously occurring adenomas noted with advancing age (Kovacs et al., 1977b).

### (3) Mixed adenomas composed of growth hormone cells and prolactin cells

Six tumors were classified into this group. Clinically, these patients had various degrees of acromegaly, elevated blood growth hormone levels and hyperprolactinemia. Symptoms related to enhanced prolactin production were frequently overshadowed by acromegaly.

By light microscopy, these tumors were composed mainly of chromophobic or slightly acidophilic cells. Some cells showed orangeophilia, while others seemed to contain erythrosinophil or carmoisinophil granules in their cytoplasm. The immunoperoxidase technique revealed the presence of growth hormone and prolactin in the cytoplasm of some adenoma cells. Growth hormone and prolactin seemed to be located in separate cells. Thus, this tumor type appears to represent a real mixed adenoma consisting of two distinct cell types.

By electron microscopy, the tumor cells corresponded either to growth hormone cells or to prolactin cells (Fig. 4), and their ultrastructural details were identical to those seen in pure growth hormone cell adenomas or prolactin cell adenomas. Groups of densely or sparsely granulated growth hormone cells were mixed with densely or sparsely granulated prolactin cells and transitional forms between the two cell types were not observed.

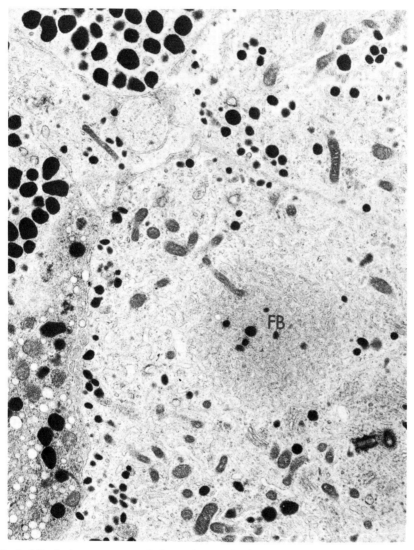

*Fig. 4.* Mixed adenoma composed of sparsely granulated growth hormone cells and densely granulated prolactin cells. Note the fibrous body (FB) in a growth hormone cell and the large pleomorphic secretory granules in the prolactin cells. × 10 500.

## (4)  Acidophil stem cell adenoma

Three pituitary adenomas were classified as acidophil stem cell adenomas.
Clinically, neither acromegaly nor galactorrhea were evident and hyperprolactinemia was the only sign which indicated active secretion by the tumor.

By light microscopy, the tumors corresponded to chromophobic or sparsely
granulated acidophilic adenomas with the predominance of chromophobic cells.
In a few cells, small cytoplasmic granules were disclosed which stained with
orange G. Herlant's erythrosin and Brookes' carmoisine techniques revealed the
presence of a few small secretory granules in the cytoplasm. By the immunoperoxidase technique, a varying number of adenoma cells stained positively for
growth hormone. In the same parts of the adenomas, the majority of the cells
showed a strong cytoplasmic positivity when antihuman prolactin was used as the
primary antibody. The reaction product exhibited the same intracytoplasmic
localization and microscopic appearance as seen in sparsely granulated prolactin
cell adenomas. Growth hormone and prolactin seemed to be present in the cytoplasm of the same cells, suggesting that the adenoma cells produced two separate
hormones. This is, however, a very difficult question, since even if consecutive
sections were immunostained, not the same cells are compared.

By electron microscopy, the adenoma cells were closely apposed, elongated
and sometimes quite attenuated with oval or markedly irregular nuclei and dense,
oval nucleoli (Fig. 5). The rough-surfaced endoplasmic reticulum was well developed in most cells and formed parallel stacks, densely studded with ribosomes
or widely scattered dilated profiles. Free ribosomes were usually numerous. The
Golgi apparatus was only moderately developed, even inconspicuous and contained only a few small, immature secretory granules. The number and volume

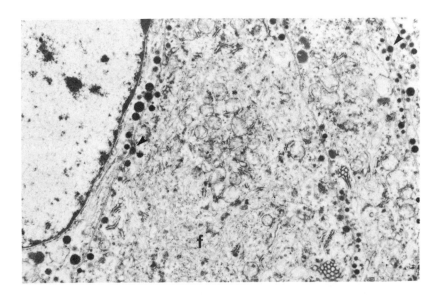

*Fig. 5.*  Acidophil stem cell adenoma showing accumulation of type II microfilaments (f), as
well as misplaced exocytosis (arrowheads). × 9000.

density of the mitochondria were increased in several cells. The mitochondria showed marked alterations, such as loss of cristae, enlargement, slight swelling in some cells and extreme ballooning in others. Centrioles were conspicuous in the Golgi region. Multiple or immature centrioles and procentriolar bodies were also apparent. Secretory granules were spherical or pleomorphic, not numerous and measured 150–300 nm in diameter. In a few cells, larger secretory granules with a diameter of up to 600 nm were also observed. Misplaced exocytosis, type II

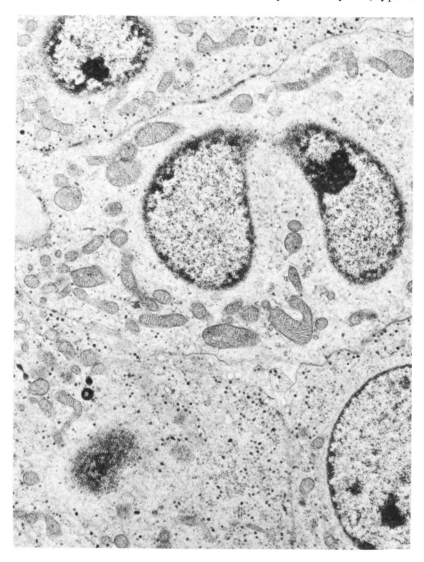

*Fig. 6.* Undifferentiated cell adenoma. The cytoplasm contains only a few rough-surfaced endoplasmic reticulum profiles. The secretory granules are small and dense. Note the abundance of cytoplasmic microtubules. × 8000.

microfilaments and fibrous bodies were noted occasionally within the same cell.

Thus, although these tumors showed some resemblance to those of undifferentiated cell adenomas, the adenoma cells exhibited distinctive fine structural features of both sparsely granulated adenomatous growth hormone cells and prolactin cells. The fibrous bodies, the multiple centrioles which are characteristic markers of sparsely granulated growth hormone cell adenomas (Kovacs *et al.*, 1974; Horvath and Kovacs, 1976; Horvath *et al.*, 1976; Kovacs *et al.*, 1977a) and the presence of misplaced exocytosis, typical of sparsely granulated prolactin cell adenomas (Horvath and Kovacs, 1974; Horvath and Kovacs, 1976; Kovacs *et al.*, 1977a) were accompanied by mitochondrial abnormalities, endowing this tumor type with its own characteristic appearance. These electron microscopic findings, as well as the results of immunostaining, suggested that these tumors derived from the common committed precursor of the two acidophil cell lines and the term acidophil stem cell adenoma seemed to be appropriate to designate this entity.

### (5)   Adenomas not composed of prolactin cells

In 2 cases, the pituitary adenomas did not consist of prolactin cells. Clinically, in these patients there were no signs suggesting endocrine overactivity, and local symptoms necessitated the surgical removal of the tumors.

By light microscopy, these tumors corresponded to chromophobic adenomas, exhibiting no PAS, lead hematoxylin, aldehyde fuchsin, aldehyde thionin or aniline blue positivity. Stainings with acid dyes, with Herlant's erythrosin or Brookes' carmoisine techniques gave negative results, and the immunoperoxidase technique revealed no prolactin in the cytoplasm of the tumor cells. Immunostainings for growth hormone, ACTH, FSH, LH and TSH were also negative.

By electron microscopy, the tumors were not composed of prolactin cells but of undifferentiated cells (Fig. 6). They were classified as undifferentiated cell adenomas (Horvath and Kovacs, 1976; Kovacs *et al.*, 1977a) and elevated blood prolactin levels were interpreted as representing examples of "stalk section effect" (Turkington *et al.*, 1971; Frantz *et al.*, 1972).

### DISCUSSION

The present results clearly indicate that morphologic study of pituitary adenomas can provide important information to the clinical endocrinologist. Histology combined with immunocytology and electron microscopy can disclose which hormones are stored in the adenoma cells and can reveal the cellular origin as well as the composition of the tumors. Thus, in patients with hyperprolactinemia, morphologic investigation can separate tumors capable of producing prolactin from those which are not composed of prolactin cells and are unassociated with prolactin secretion. In the latter cases, it is apparent that elevation of blood prolactin level is due to an enhanced discharge of prolactin from the nontumorous portion of the pituitary.

Prolactin-producing adenomas exhibit different fine structural features and can be divided into four distinct entities. Although details related to the clinical course and functional activity of these tumor types have yet to be established, unpublished studies, using ultrastructural morphometry, seem to indicate that there is an inverse correlation between volume density of secretory granules and hormonal overactivity.

The incidence of prolactin-producing adenomas remains to be established. By using radioimmunoassay, elevated blood prolactin levels were found in 25-79% of all patients with hypophysial neoplasms (Franks *et al.*, 1975; Jacobs *et al.*, 1976; Antunes *et al.*, 1977; Horvath *et al.*, 1977a; Kleinberg *et al.*, 1977; Frantz, 1978). It is known, however, that rises in blood prolactin level occur in a variety of conditions (Turkington *et al.*, 1971; Frantz *et al.*, 1972; Friesen and Hwang, 1973; Tolis *et al.*, 1973; Boyar *et al.*, 1974; Tolis *et al.*, 1974) and that hyperprolactinemia itself does not prove that the hormone is secreted by a prolactin-producing adenoma, since different neoplasms may compress the hypophysial stalk and hypothalamus and interference with the production and release of various hypothalamic regulatory substances or with their flow to the anterior lobe can cause increased discharge of prolactin from the nontumorous pituitary. Morphologic studies represent a valuable approach to distinguish between these alternatives and to assess the incidence of prolactin-producing adenomas, since these tumors can be recognized by morphology and can be differentiated from those not consisting of prolactin cells. In our laboratory, during the last 8 years, among 181 surgically-removed pituitary adenomas that have been studied by conventional histology, immunocytology and electron microscopy, 76 were composed of or contained prolactin cells, indicating that prolactin-producing adenomas constitute one of the most frequently occurring pituitary tumor types. Hence, problems related to their pathogenesis, diagnosis and treatment are regarded as representing a major challenge to endocrinologists.

Since immunocytology and electron microscopy are valuable procedures in the diagnosis of prolactin-producing adenomas and of other pituitary adenoma types, we wish to recommend that these techniques be widely introduced and routinely used in the assessment of pituitary tumors. More work is required, however to elucidate whether or not the morphologic features of pituitary adenomas can be correlated with secretory activity, biological behavior, growth rate, recurrence, and furthermore, to clarify the role of the hypothalamus in their pathogenesis.

## REFERENCES

Antunes, J. L., Housepian, E. M., Frantz, A. G., Holub, D. A., Hui, R. M., Carmel, P. W. and Quest, D. O. (1977). *Ann. Neurol.* **2**, 148–153.

Boyar, R. M., Kapen, S., Finkelstein, J. W., Perlow, M., Sassin, J. F., Fukushima, D. K., Weitzman, E. D. and Hellman, L. (1974). *J. Clin. Invest.* **53**, 1588–1598.

Corenblum, B., Sirek, A. M. T., Horvath, E., Kovacs, K. and Ezrin, C. (1976). *J. Clin. Endocrinol. Metab.* **42**, 857–863.

Forbes, A. P., Henneman, P. H., Griswald, G. C. and Albright, F. (1954). *J. Clin. Endocrinol. Metab.* **14**, 265–271.

Franks, S., Murray, M. A. F., Jequier, A. M., Steel, S. J., Nabarro, J. D. N. and Jacobs, H. S. (1975). *Clin. Endocrinol.* **4**, 597–607.

Frantz, A. G. (1977). *Adv. Exp. Med. Biol.* **80**, 95–133.

Frantz, A. G. (1978). *New Engl. J. Med.* **298**, 201–207.

Frantz, A. G. and Kleinberg, D. L. (1970). *Science* **170**, 745–747.

Frantz, A. G., Kleinberg, D. L. and Noel, G. L. (1972). *Rec. Progr. Hormone Res.* **28**, 527-573.

Friesen, H. and Hwang, P. (1973). *Ann. Rev. Med.* **24**, 251-270.

Friesen, H., Webster, R., Hwang, P., Guyda, H., Munro, R. E. and Read, L. (1972). *J. Clin. Endocrinol. Metab.* **34**, 192-199.

Guinet, P., Girod, C., Pousset, G., Trouillas, J. and L'Hermite, M. (1973). *Ann. Endocrinol.* **34**, 407-417.

Guyda, H., Robert, F., Colle, E. and Hardy, J. (1973). *J. Clin. Endocrinol. Metab.* **36**, 531-547.

Herlant, M. and Pasteels, J. L. (1967). *Meth. Achievm. exp. Path.* **3**, 250-305.

Herlant, M., Laine, E., Fossati, P. and Linquette, M. (1965). *Ann. Endocrinol.* **26**, 65-71.

Horrobin, D. F. (1976). "Prolactin", 1-208. Eden Press, Montreal.

Horvath, E. and Kovacs, K. (1974). *Arch. Path.* **97**, 221-224.

Horvath, E. and Kovacs, K. (1976). *Can. J. Neurol. Sci.* **3**, 9-21.

Horvath, E., Kovacs, K. and Ezrin, C. (1976). *Path. Europ.* **11**, 81-86.

Horvath, E., Kovacs, K., Ryan, N., Singer, W. and Ezrin, C. (1977a). *IRCS Med. Sci.* **5**, 447.

Horvath, E., Kovacs, K., Singer, W., Ezrin, C. and Kerenyi, N. A. (1977b). *Arch. Pathol. Lab. Med.* **101**, 594-599.

Hymer, W. C., McShan, W. H. and Christiansen, R. G. (1961). *Endocrinology* **69**, 81-90.

Hwang, P., Guyda, H. and Friesen, H. (1971). *Proc. Natl. Acad. Sci. USA* **68**, 866-869.

Jacobs, H. S., Franks, S., Murray, M. A. F., Hull, M. G. R., Steele, S. J. and Nabarro, J. D. N. (1976). *Clin. Endocrinol.* **5**, 439-454.

Kleinberg, D. L., Noel, G. L. and Frantz, A. G. (1977). *New Engl. J. Med.* **296**, 589-600.

Kovacs, K. (1977). *Clin. Endocrinol.* **6** (Suppl.) 71s-79s.

Kovacs, K., Horvath, E., Stratmann, I. E. and Ezrin, C. (1974). *Acta anat.* **87**, 414-426.

Kovacs, K., Horvath, E., Corenblum, B., Sirek, A. M. T., Penz, G. and Ezrin, C. (1975). *Virchows, Arch. A Path. Anat. Histol.* **366**, 113-123.

Kovacs, K., Corenblum, B., Sirek, A. M. T., Penz, G. and Ezrin, C. (1976). *J. Clin. Path.* **29**, 250-258.

Kovacs, K., Horvath, E. and Ezrin, C. (1977a). *Path. Annu.* **12** (part 2) 341-382.

Kovacs, K., Horvath, E., Ilse, R. G., Ezrin, C. and Ilse, D. (1977b). *Beitr. Path.* **161**, 1-16.

Lundin, M. and Schelin, U. (1962). *Acta path. microbiol. Scand.* **54**, 66-74.

Martin, J. B., Reichlin, S. and Brown, G. M. (1977). "Clinical Neuroendocrinology", 129-145. Davis Co., Philadelphia.

Pasteels, J. L., Gausset, P., Danguy, A., Ectors, F., Nicoll, C. S. and Varavudhi, P. (1972). *J. Clin. Endocrinol. Metab.* **34**, 959-967.

Peake, G. T., McKeel, D. W., Jarett, L. and Daughaday, W. H. (1969). *J. Clin. Endocrinol. Metab.* **29**, 1383-1393.

Racadot, J., Vila-Porcile, E., Peillon, F. and Olivier, L. (1971). *Ann. Endocrinol.* **32**, 298-305.

Schelin, U. and Lundin, P. M. (1971). *Acta endocrinol.* **67**, 29-39.

Schelin, U., Lundin, P. M. and Bartholdson, L. (1964). *Endocrinology* **75**, 893-900.

Sirek, A. M. T., Corenblum, B., Horvath, E., Rewcastle, B., Ezrin, C. and Kovacs, K. (1976). *Can. Med. Ass. J.* **114**, 225-229.

Sternberger, L. A., Hardy, P. H. Jr., Cuculis, J. J. and Meyer, H. G. (1970). *J. Histochem. Cytochem.* **18**, 315–333.

Tiboldi, T., Viragh, S., Kovacs, K., Hodi, M. and Julesz, M. (1967). *J. Microscopie* **6**, 677–689.

Tolis, G., Goldstein, M. and Friesen, H. (1973). *J. Clin. Invest.* **52**, 783–788.

Tolis, G., Somma, M., Van Campenhout, J. and Friesen, H. (1974). *Am. J. Obst. Gynec.* **118**, 91–101.

Turkington, R. W., Underwood, L. E. and Van Wyk, J. J. (1971). *New Engl. J. Med.* **285**, 707–710.

Zimmerman, E. H., Defendini, R. and Frantz, A. G. (1974). *J. Clin. Endocrinol. Metab.* **38**, 577–585.

# PITUITARY ADENOMAS: SURGICAL VERSUS POST MORTEM FINDINGS TODAY

L. Mosca, E. Solcia, C. Capella and R. Buffa

*Department of Morbid Anatomy and Histopathology, The State University of Pavia, 27100 Pavia and Histopathology, Histochemistry and Ultrastructure Center, The University of Pavia at Varese, 21100 Varese, Italy*

The relationship between clinically apparent and clinically silent pituitary adenomas has been investigated in 66 tumors removed surgically, mainly by transphenoidal hypophysectomy (mean age 42 years; 47% intrasellar; 62% in women) and 24 microadenomas found in adults by careful sections of 100 pituitaries removed at autopsy.

## METHODS

An indirect *immunofluorescence procedure* (Coons *et al.*, 1955) has been applied to paraformaldehyde-, Bouin-, or Zamboni-fixed sections using rabbit anti-human TSH serum (from Dr. A. Parlow, through the National Institute of Arthritis, Metabolism and Digestive Disease, Bethesda), rabbit anti-human ACTH serum (Wellcome), rabbit anti-human chorionic gonadotrophin (HCG) serum known to react with human pituitary LH in radioimmunoassay tests (Wellcome, England), rabbit anti-human growth hormone (GH) serum (Sorin, Saluggia, Italy) or a rabbit anti-human placental lactogen (HPL) serum detecting human prolactin in radioimmunoassay tests (Behringwerke, Marburg, West Germany), at dilutions 1:250 to 1:1000, followed by goat (Hyland, England) or pig (Dagopatts, Denmark) anti-rabbit $\alpha$-globulin serum. The anti-TSH serum was applied directly or after addition of excess HCG (Serono, Roma) to remove $\alpha$ chain antibodies cross-reacting with gonadotrophins (Moriarty, 1973). The anti-HCG serum was also combined, in some tests, with excess human TSH (Organon, Holland). Controls were performed: (a) by adsorbing the specific antihormone serum with excess purified pituitary hormone, (b) by substituting non-immune serum for the specific serum and (c) by omitting the first step of the indirect test. Other sections, after incubation with the immune serum, were first treated with swine anti-rabbit serum IgG, then with peroxidase–antiperoxidase (P.A.P.) immune complex (Dakopatts) and finally with a 3,3′-diaminobenzidine-$H_2O_2$ mixture (Sternberger, 1974). Controls were carried out as for immunofluorescence. Parallel immunohistochemical tests were performed on sections of human non-tumor pituitaries; some of these sections, showing GH, ACTH, TSH or HCG immunofluorescent cells, were photographed and then restained with Grimelius's silver. Immunofluorescent staining survived these procedures and allowed us to compare each immunofluorescent cell with argyrophilic cells in the same section.

For electron microscopy small specimens of surgically removed tumor tissue and normal hypophysis were fixed in a mixture of 2% paraformaldehyde and 2.5% glutaraldehyde in 0.1M phosphate buffer at pH 7.3. Specimens of all cases were post-fixed in 1% osmium tetroxide, dehydrated in ethanol and embedded in Epon. Sections were stained with uranyl acetate and lead citrate and viewed in a Zeiss EM10 electron microscope. Specimens of several cases and normal hypophysis were cut with a Smith Farquhar tissue sectioner (Sorvall), and 100–150 $\mu$m sections were stained with Grimelius's silver technique. They were then dehydrated and embedded in Epon. Sections of silver-impregnated blocks were observed in the electron microscope with and without uranyl acetate counter-staining.


# RESULTS

On the basis of histological, immunohistochemical and electron microscopic findings (Mosca and Vassallo, 1970; Solcia *et al.*, 1977), as well as on the basis of the correlation between endocrine symptoms and hormone assays, 24 of 66 surgical tumors are classified as prolactin cell adenomas (36.5%), 14 as GH cell adenomas (21.2%), 10 as mixed GH and prolactin cell adenomas (15%), 13 as argyrophil adenomas (19.7%) and 5 as ACTH cell adenomas (7.6%).

*GH cell adenomas* (57% extrasellar; 71% in females; mean age 46.1 y) were all associated with acromegaly; a large majority of these tumors are highly differentiated diffuse acidophil adenomas and show immunohistochemical and ultrastructural patterns corresponding to those of normal GH cells.

*Mixed GH and prolactin cell adenomas* (30% extrasellar; 50% in females, mean age 38.6 y) are found in acromegalic patients. In some cases the hypersecretion of GH was accompanied by hyperprolactinemia; only in two cases was galactorrhea present. Histologically, the adenomas are not distinguishable from pure GH cell acidophil tumor; but immunohistochemical and electron microscopic methods reveal a prolactin cell component consisting of well-differentiated densely granulated cells.

*Prolactin cell adenomas* (41% extrasellar; 71% in females; mean age: in males 44.1 y, in females 32.2 y). Constant endocrine symptoms were amenorrhea in females and loss of libido in males, while galactorrhea was present in 45% of cases. Under the light microscope, the majority of these tumors can easily be confused

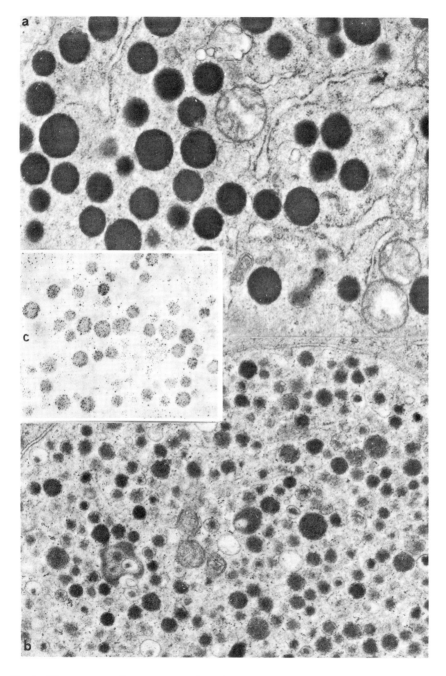

*Fig. 1.* Ultrastructure of secretory granules in immunohistochemically proven ACTH cell tumor (a) and TSH cell tumor (b). *c* = silver deposits on secretory granules of the same tumor of *b*, stained with Grimelius's silver. All × 25 000.

with diffuse chromophobe adenomas. Electron microscopical study of these tumors revealed in 23 cases sparsely granulated prolactin cells with prominent endoplasmic reticulum, large Golgi area and frequent granule exocytosis on the lateral cell surface.

Of the five *ACTH cell tumors* (two extrasellar; all in females; mean age 41.2 y) three tumors were clinically and biochemically silent, one was associated with Nelson's syndrome and one with Cushing's syndrome. All these tumors were composed of solid nests and sheets of PAS- and lead-haematoxylin positive cells that under the electron microscope always showed abundant, large round secretory granules (250–450 nm in diameter) closely similar to those of the ACTH cell of the normal human pituitary (Fig. 1a).

*Argyrophil adenomas* are chromophobic trabecular tumors showing numerous positive cells when stained with Grimelius's silver method. Among these adenomas two tumors consisted of densely granulated and intensely immunoreactive TSH cells which, ultrastructurally, showed osmiophilic, small, round granules (140–150 nm in diameter), quite comparable to those of the normal human TSH cell (Figs 1b, c and 2). Both cases of *TSH cell adenomas* were extrasellar, in males and associated with hypothyroidism. The other 11 cases of argyrophil cell adenomas (73% extrasellar; 37% in females; mean age 51.2 y), except for one case in which a few cells reacted with anti-human glycoprotein α subunit antibodies, did not reveal the presence of GH, ACTH, LH-FSH or PRL cells. Ultrastructurally, all these adenomas were composed of closely packed small cells with irregular contours, abundant mitochondria and variable amounts of small, round, cored or vesicular granules of mean diameter varying from case to case (from 150 to 90 nm). These

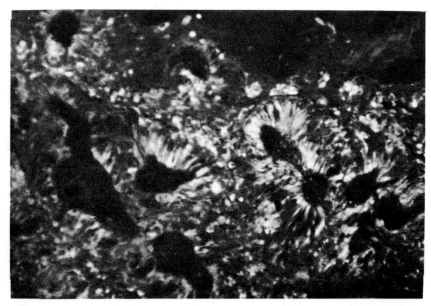

*Fig. 2.* Same tumor as in Fig. 1b and c, stained with immunofluorescence using anti-TSH antiserum absorbed with HCG. Note sinusoidal pattern of growth with tumor cells palisading around fibrovascular structures. × 100.

tumor cells seem to correspond to the small argyrophil cells we have found in non-tumor human pituitary, which differ from TSH cells and from all other types of functionally identified adenohypophyseal cells (Capella *et al.*, 1978).

Of the 24 *autoptic microadenomas* (all intrasellar, ranging from 0.2 to 5 mm in diameter, lacking any clinical sign of local growth; 45.8% in women; age range from 28 to 98 y; mean age 61.2 of tumor bearing subjects and 72.6 of 100 autopsied cases) only two were coupled with signs of endocrine hyperfunction, one showing overt Cushing's syndrome, the other bilateral hyperplasia of adrenal cortex. They were histochemically identified as ACTH cell tumors. Of the remaining 22 clinically silent microadenomas, three were identified as GH cell tumors, two as PRL tumors, one as mixed GH and PRL cell tumor, five as ACTH cell nodular hyperplasias invading the neurohypophysis, one as argyrophil cell tumor (Fig. 3) and one as a chromophobe tumor showing small, apparently agranular cells (so-called fetal adenoma). Of the remaining nine cases, poor preservation or inappropriate fixation of tumor tissue prevented a precise and reliable identification of tumor cells, although some reactivity with conventional granule stains was detectable (Mosca *et.*, 1975).

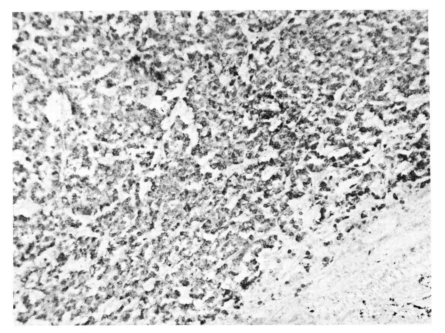

*Fig. 3.* Argyrophil, asymptomatic microadenoma of the pituitary found at autopsy. Grimelius's silver. × 120.

## CONCLUSIONS

A cytological and functional classification of surgically removed pituitary adenomas is easily achieved by combining histochemical, ultrastructural and histopathologic studies. Using the same procedures (with the exception of electron microscopy) an exact classification of autoptic adenomas is less easily obtained. However, a number of such tumors have been identified histochemically and histologically. As a rule, the same types of tumor cells seem to occur in both surgical and in p.m. material. Thus, in principle, it might be accepted that at least part of the silent microadenomas found incidentally at autopsy represent a preclinical stage of pituitary adenomas.

The evidence that, in spite of the abundance of microadenomas in "normal" adult people, not very many reach conspicuous bulk probably points to either a late onset and very slow enlargement of most adenomas or to spontaneous regression (hemorrhages, necrosis) of some of them with advancing age.

## REFERENCES

Capella, C., Usellini, L., Frigerio, B., Buffa, R., Fontana, P. and Solcia, E. (1978). Submitted to *Virchow Archiv A*.

Coons, A. H., Leduc, E. H. and Connolly, J. M. (1955). *J. exp. Med.* **102**, 49–63.

Moriarty, G. C. (1973). *J. Histochem. Cytochem.* **21**, 855–894.

Mosca, L. and Vassallo, G. (1970). *Atti. Soc. It. Endocrinol.* **13**, 339–401.

Mosca, L., Buffa, R., Castello, A. and Gaspa, L. (1975). *Rev. Franc. Endocr. Clin.* **16**, 433–443.

Solcia, E., Capella, C., Buffa, R., Frigerio, B., Fontana, P. and Usellini, L. (1977). *Pathologica* **69**, 333–346.

Sternberger, L. A. (1974). "Immunocytochemistry". Prentice-Hall, Englewood Cliffs, New Jersey.

# HUMAN PITUITARY MICROADENOMAS IN ORGAN CULTURE*

Structural organization, function and physiological reactivity; and
cellular and subcellular effects of ionizing radiation: viability,
sublethal and lethal damage.

M. Anniko[1], P. Eneroth[2], S. Werner[3] and J. Wersäll[1]

[1] *Department of Otolaryngology, Karolinska sjukhuset, and King Gustaf V
Research Institute, Karolinska Institutet, S-104 01 Stockholm 60;*
[2] *Hormone Research Laboratory, Karolinska sjukhuset;*
[3] *Department of Endocrinology and Metabolism, Karolinska sjukhuset, Sweden*

## INTRODUCTION

The anterior lobe of the pituitary gland is less available for study than many
other glands, particularly from human material. Until the early 1970s, most
studies were performed in animals *in vivo*. Recently, interest has been shown in
developing an *in vitro* system for a combined morphological and physiological/
biochemical study of human anterior pituitary cells. These investigations have
been focused on adenoma/microadenoma tissue obtained at surgical removal of
the tumor.

The present paper correlates structure and function of growth hormone and
prolactin producing adenoma tissue in organ culture.

A well characterized and controlled *in vitro* system constitutes a suitable
experimental model for the morphologic elucidation of the sequential development
of radiation-induced damage, which in the present investigation was analysed
following a single dose of 7000 rad.

*Supported by grants from Karolinska Institutet, The Swedish Medical Research Council
(grant No. 12X-720) and The Swedish Society of Medical Sciences.

## MATERIAL AND METHODS

### Material

Pituitary adenoma tissue was obtained after transanthrosphenoidal removal of seven growth hormones and three prolactin producing neoplasms.

### Organ culture technique

Immediately after excision, the tumor was sectioned into small fragments under sterile conditions and explanted to the *in vitro* system. The nutrient solution consisted of Neuman and Tytell's serumless medium supplemented with 10% FCS (fetal calf serum) and 1% 1-glutamine. The culture medium was changed every 2-3 days (dishes) or after one week (culture flasks) and analysed for hormone content. Probes of 0.2-0.3 ml of medium were drawn from the culture flasks every 2-3 days. Antibiotics/antimycotics were not used. For details see Anniko *et al.* (1978a).

### Testing of physiological reactivity *in vitro*

The influence of thyrotropin releasing hormone (TRH) and LH releasing hormone (LHRH) on growth hormone producing specimens was analysed after incubation with (physiological)concentrations of $10^{-6}$ to $10^{-8}$ $\mu g/ml$ for 10 min to 24 h.

### Irradiation of organ cultures

This technique was originally described by Rähn and Anniko (1978). After explantation of the tumor, the specimens were kept *in vitro* for at least 3-4 days prior to further handling. The irradiation was performed with $^{60}$Co gamma rays with a dose of 7000 rad, given as a single dose. During irradiation cultures were kept outside the incubator but within a water bath of the same temperature as inside the incubator (+ 37°C ± 0.2°C). Controls were treated the same way except for the irradiation.

## RESULTS

### Structural and functional considerations

Specimens were analysed at the ultrastructural level after 1-32 days in culture. The nutrient solution was assayed for both growth hormone (GH) and prolactin (PRL) content to allow a correlation of morphology and physiological hormone production.

A high degree of stability was obtained during the first two weeks of culture. If structural alterations occurred, these were observed after only 1-2 days following explantation and showed a central necrosis of the specimens if they had been too large for the *in vitro* conditions. In very dense cell-rich tissue, single cells in

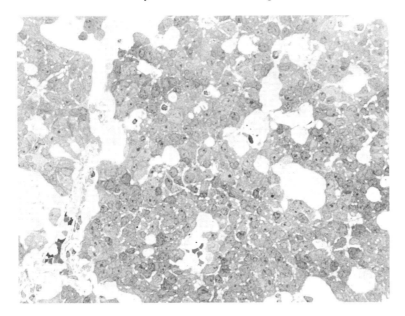

*Fig. 1.* Light microscopy (LM). Prolactin-producing adenoma tissue cultured *in vitro* for 14 days. Well-preserved cells.

groups of cells sometimes degenerated giving a glandular structure as a whole. Thereafter, the *in vitro* system showed stable conditions for at least two weeks, often 2–3 weeks. Many specimens were preserved morphologically for an even longer time with an unchanged *in vitro* hormone production. There was no divergence in structural preservation between GH and PRL producing microadenomas *in vitro* (Figs 1 and 2).

The assays of GH and PRL contents in the culture medium revealed that the pituitary cells of the specimens produced only one of the two hormones, as had also been documented preoperatively *in vivo*. The organ culture system could therefore be correlated to morphologic structure and physiologic hormone production. *In vivo* endocrinologically very active tissue retained this characteristic also *in vitro* (Fig. 3).

If the culture medium was changed more often than every third day, e.g. every day or even every hour, an increased growth hormone release occurred. However, repeated changes after an interval of only 10 min rapidly decreased the hormone content in the medium after a few changes.

### (2) Influence of TRH and LHRH on growth hormone secretion *in vitro*

A stimulatory effect was obtained after incubation of the specimens with concentrations of $10^{-6}$ to $10^{-8}$ $\mu$g/ml of TRH and $10^{-6}$ to $10^{-7}$ $\mu$g/ml of LHRH.

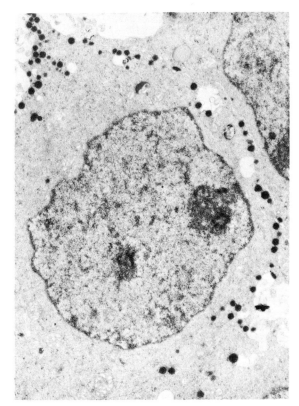

*Fig. 2.* Electron microscopy (EM). Ultrastructurally well-preserved morphology in a growth hormone producing cell cultured *in vitro* for 19 days.

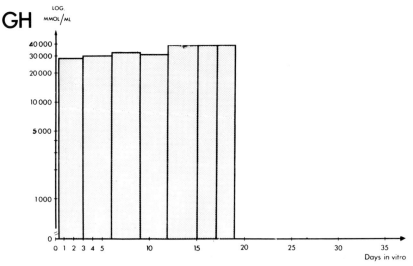

*Fig. 3.* Diagram illustrating the growth hormone production *in vitro* for 19 days, thereafter the specimen was prepared for morphological analysis (compare Fig. 2).

When the incubation period was extended from 10 min to 24 h (the same specimen as a control after an interval of several days) no considerable increase in hormone extrusion occurred.

### (3) Early irradiation-induced morphological changes (Fig. 4)

Following a single dose of 7000 rad, the first cytological alterations, observed at the ultrastructural level after 2-4 h, were cytoplasmic vesiculations. Thereafter this vacuolization increased and reached a maximum at 24-36 h post-

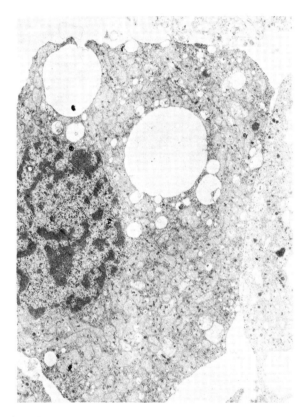

*Fig. 4.* EM. Growth hormone-producing cell cultured *in vitro* for 4 days, thereafter it was irradiated with 7000 rad ($^{60}$Co) and investigated 24 h post irradiation. The structure is altered as compared with controls, showing vacuolization of cytoplasm and swelling of the cell.

irradiation. At this stage, many pituitary cells were swollen and blebs occurred from the outer cell membrane. Only occasionally were pyknotic pituitary cells found in the specimens. In cultures, normal morphology was now gradually restored. In investigation of specimens six days post-irradiation, no difference in cell shape or ultrastructural morphology could be found between the irradiated cells and the controls.

## DISCUSSION

A good correlation occurs between ultrastructural preservation and hormonal secretory capacity of human pituitary microadenomas in this type of organ culture. Differentiation of growth hormone and prolactin cell types was maintained, as was also the regulation/stimulation of secretory activity in growth hormone producing cells. The hormonal content of the medium was concluded to be mainly due to physiological hormone release by living cells (Anniko *et al.*, 1978a, 1978a, b).

Morphological research on the adenohypophysis—both in animals and man—is often restricted by the identification problem both in light and electron microscopy. During *in vitro* conditions, this can be supported by the analysis of hormonal activities and the hormonal spectrum in the medium. In the present study, the organ culture system was working with "pure" neoplasms, at least with regard to growth hormone and prolactin production, thereby correlating the functional and the structural state of the specimens.

The potential capacity of the pituitary tissue in organ culture to produce hormone may in the *in vitro* system be depressed when the hormone concentration reaches a certain level (feedback control *in vitro*)—as it is *in vivo* conditions. Thus, Schofield (1967) reported an increased growth hormone release when the culture medium was changed frequently, e.g. every hour. However, these observations may also be influenced by the half-life of the hormone *in vitro*.

The organ culture system establishes a suitable experimental model for early changes following irradiation. In general, a clear difference occurs in dose-survival response of rapidly dividing cells as compared with cells in a static phase of growth. It is nowadays agreed that there is no difference between sensitivity to radiation *in vivo* and *in vitro* (Trowell, 1966).

The first morphological changes were observed after a few hours, reaching a maximum 1–2 days later, but 6 days after irradiation few morphological alterations could be detected in the surviving cells, indicating a restoration of cell morphology (Rähn and Anniko, 1978). These morphologic events are in agreement with the clinical observations on the hormone response in patients given the same dose stereotactically to the microadenoma (Rähn, 1978, personal communication). Initially, a high serum level of the hormone was obtained. We have interpreted this as an effect on the cell membrane with release of granules. On the second and third days post-irradiation, hormone concentrations were depressed, probably due to a swelling of the pituitary cell and an initially reversible metabolic dysfunction. After approximately one week, the serum levels in blood returned to pre-irradiation values, showing the reversible effects of irradiation on pituitary cells in the early stages of post-irradiation damage. Following these (acute) changes the cells must have sustained damage to the nucleus and the genetic code, but this is not recognized until later when the cell metabolism requires further information to replace consumed material. This process may take weeks or months before it is detected and the cell subsequently degenerates. It is supported by the clinical observations that show a late decrease in serum hormone concentration and an X-ray visualized regression of the tumor, a few to several months after irradiation.

Studies are now in progress to correlate structural and functional data following irradiation with various doses in different human pituitary cell types *in vitro*.

## REFERENCES

Anniko, M., Eneroth, P., Werner, S. and Wersäll, J. (1978a). To be published.
Anniko, M., Eneroth, P., Werner, S. and Wersäll, J. (1978b). To be published.
Rähn, T. and Anniko, M. (1978). To be published.
Schofield, J. G. (1967). *Biochem. J.* **103**, 331–341.
Trowell, O. A. (1966). *In* "Cells and Tissues in Culture" (E. N. Willmer, ed) Vol. III, 53–149. Academic Press, London and New York.

# STUDIES OF HORMONE SECRETION BY TRYPSIN ISOLATED
# PITUITARY TUMOR CELLS *IN VITRO*\*

S. W. J. Lamberts[1†], R. M. MacLeod[1] and D. T. Krieger[2]

[1]*Departments of Medicine, University of Virginia School of Medicine,
Charlottesville, Virginia, 22908 and* [2] *Mount Sinai School of Medicine,
New York, 10028, USA*

## INTRODUCTION

In the past several years the therapeutic use of several neuroactive drugs in patients with pituitary tumors has become widely accepted. The mechanism of action by which these drugs lower the circulating hormone levels in patients with prolactinomas, acromegaly and Cushing's disease is not clear.

Experimental studies which supported the clinical usefulness of these drugs in man were derived partially from research in which transplantable hormone-secreting pituitary tumors of the rat were used (MacLeod and Lehmeyer, 1973). However these studies were not always directly applicable to human pathology (Lamberts and MacLeod, 1979). In the present report we describe *in vitro* studies of prolactin (PRL), growth hormone (GH), and adrenocorticotropin (ACTH) secretion from trypsin dispersed pituitary tumor cells prepared from the mixed PRL/GH-secreting tumor MtTW15 and from the mixed PRL/ACTH-secreting tumor 7315a. Hormone suppressive (cyproheptadine, ergocryptine, GABA, clonidine, methysergide) substances were studied.

---

\*This work was supported by USPHS Research Grants CA–07535 and CA–166694–3 from the National Cancer Institute.
†On leave from the Department of Internal Medicine III and Clinical Endocrinology, University Hospital Dijkzigt, Erasmus University, Rotterdam, The Netherlands.

## METHODS

Female rats of 100–220 g were used for tumor implantation (Wistar-Furth in the case of the MtTW15 tumor and Buffalo rats for the 7315a tumor). Tumor homogenate was injected into the scapular region 6–8 weeks before the animals were studied, as described previously (MacLeod et al., 1969).

Isolated tumor cells were prepared by mincing 5 g of the tumor in 10 ml Medium 199 containing 1.5 mg/ml trypsin (Worthington) and 100 μg/ml bovine serum albumin. Tissue fragments were incubated for 20 min at 37°C under an atmosphere of 95% $O_2$, 5% $CO_2$.

Following this incubation, the tissue fragments were allowed to return to room temperature, and then were drawn up and expelled 25 times through a plastic Pasteur pipette. The debris and large fragments were allowed to settle 5 min and the supernatant containing the isolated cells was aspirated. Trypsin inhibitor (Worthington) was added to this suspension (1.5 mg/ml) and the acutely dispersed cells were pipetted into plastic vials (final volume 1 ml) and incubated for different time periods up to 5 h in a Dubnoff shaker at 37°C in an atmosphere of 95% $O_2$, 5% $CO_2$, followed by centrifugation at 3500 $g$ for 10 min. After centrifugation the medium and cell pellet were separated and stored.

The tumor cell content of the incubation medium was counted in a hematological counting chamber. The percentage of viable cells, as determined by the exclusion of trypan blue, was 95% prior to the incubation and 85% after a 5 h incubation.

The PRL and GH content of the incubation medium were measured by a double antibody radioimmunoassay using the materials and protocols supplied by the NIAMDD Rat Pituitary Hormone Distribution program. The reference hormones used were PRL RP-1 prolactin and GH-RP-1 growth hormone. ACTH was measured by a slight modification of the method described in Krieger et al. (1977). The results are expressed as mean ± s.e.m. and statistical analysis was performed by analysis of variance.

## RESULTS

A linear release of PRL was observed from trypsin-dispersed pituitary tumor cells during a 4 h incubation (Fig. 1). The addition of 5 mM dbcAMP significantly increased PRL release from dispersed pituitary tumor cells prepared from both the MtTW15 (Fig. 2a) and the 7315a tumor (Table I).

A direct in vitro effect of cyproheptadine on hormone secretion was detected: both 6 and 12 μM cyproheptadine inhibited the release of PRL significantly ($P < 0.01$; Fig. 2a). The addition of dbcAMP to incubation medium containing cyproheptadine was only partially stimulatory for PRL secretion during the first 2.5 h and was without effect during the subsequent 2.5 h (data not shown). During a 5 h incubation of trypsin-dispersed MtTW15 tumor cells a linear release of GH was observed (Fig. 2b). The stimulatory effects of dbcAMP and the inhibitory effects of cyproheptadine of PRL secretion were observed in a way parallel to GH secretion (Fig. 2b).

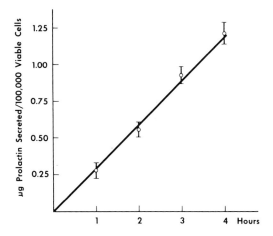

*Fig. 1.* Basal PRL secretion by trypsin dispersed pituitary tumor cells incubated for 4 h.

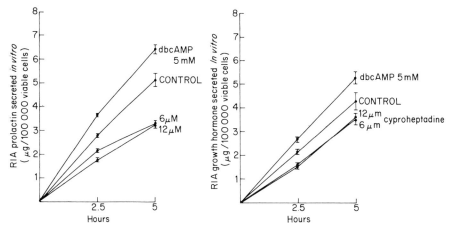

*Fig. 2.* The effect of dbcAMP and cyproheptadine on PRL and GH secretion by trypsin dispersed pituitary tumor cells prepared from the mixed PRL/GH secreting tumor MtTW15.

In two experiments the effect of the ergot alkaloid ergocryptine was investigated in trypsin-dispersed cells from the experimental pituitary tumor 7315a. Ergocryptine 0.1 μM suppressed PRL release from these cells during the first 2.5 h of incubation ($P < 0.05$), but this effect was not significant after a 5 h incubation. At higher concentration ergocryptine (1 μM) suppressed PRL secretion significantly after 5 h in both experiments (Table I; $P < 0.01$). This suppression was overcome by coincubation with the specific dopamine receptor antagonist haloperidol (50 nM). Clonidine (10 μg/ml), methysergide (5 μg/ml) and GABA (5 μg/ml) did not affect PRL secretion by dispersed pituitary tumor cells.

*Table I.* The effect of dbcAMP, ergocryptine, cyproheptadine and clonidine on prolactin secretion by trypsin-dispersed pituitary tumor cells.

| | Radioimmunoassayable prolactin in medium ($\mu$g PRL/100 000 viable cells) | |
| | 0–2.5 h | 0–5 h |
| --- | --- | --- |
| *Experiment I* | | |
| Control | $1.38 \pm 0.10$ | $3.80 \pm 0.32$ |
| dbcAMP 5mM | $2.35 \pm 0.08^{b}$ | $7.39 \pm 1.12^{a}$ |
| Ergocryptine 0.1 $\mu$M | $0.99 \pm 0.09^{a}$ | $3.07 \pm 0.20$ |
| Ergocryptine 1 $\mu$M | $0.90 \pm 0.12^{a}$ | $2.43 \pm 0.08^{b}$ |
| Cyproheptadine 6 $\mu$M | $0.70 \pm 0.10^{b}$ | $1.71 \pm 0.12^{b}$ |
| *Experiment II* | | |
| Control | $1.70 \pm 0.09$ | $3.81 \pm 0.18$ |
| dbcAMP 5mM | $3.15 \pm 0.18^{b}$ | $6.11 \pm 0.46^{b}$ |
| Ergocryptine 1 $\mu$M | $1.46 \pm 0.09$ | $2.89 \pm 0.02^{b}$ |
| Ergocryptine 1 $\mu$M + Haloperidol 50 nM | $1.55 \pm 0.04$ | $3.24 \pm 0.14$ |
| Clonidine 10 $\mu$g/ml | $1.66 \pm 0.06$ | $3.86 \pm 0.22$ |

Five flasks per group, mean ± s.e.m.
[a]$P < 0.05$ *vs* control.
[b]$P < 0.01$ *vs* control.

*Table II.* The effect of ergocryptine and cyproheptadine on ACTH and prolactin secretion by trypsin-dispersed pituitary tumor cells.

| | RIA ACTH in medium (ng/100 000 viable cells) | RIA prolactin in medium ($\mu$g PRL/100 000 viable cells) |
| --- | --- | --- |
| Control | $0.24 \pm 0.22$ | $1.22 \pm 0.15$ |
| Ergocryptine 1 $\mu$M | $0.08 \pm 0.04^{a}$ | $0.73 \pm 0.08^{a}$ |
| Cyproheptadine 10 $\mu$M | $0.09 \pm 0.07^{a}$ | $0.51 \pm 0.09^{a}$ |

Duration of incubation 3 h.
Three flasks per group, mean ± s.e.m.
[a]$P < 0.01$ *vs* control.

In another experiment (Table II) the secretion of radioimmunoassayable ACTH by dispersed tumor cells prepared from the 7315a tumor was investigated. ACTH secretion was suppressed parallel to PRL secretion, either in response to cyproheptadine (10 $\mu$M) or ergocryptine (1 $\mu$M).

## DISCUSSION

In this study the characteristics of hormone secretion by dispersed pituitary tumor cells *in vitro* were analyzed. After a 5 h incubation at least 85% of the cells were considered to be viable as measured by trypan blue exclusion. PRL was released during incubation in a linear fashion and hormone secretion was stimulated significantly by the addition of dbcAMP to the incubation medium.

Cyproheptadine directly inhibits PRL secretion by dispersed pituitary tumor cells. We showed previously that *in vitro* application of the drug $IC_{50}$ 100 nM inhibits PRL release by normal whole pituitary glands (Lamberts and MacLeod, 1978b). The cyproheptadine effect was not blocked by coincubation with low concentrations of the specific dopamine receptor antagonists perphenazine, pimozide and haloperidol, which suggests that this direct *in vitro* effect is not mediated via dopamine receptors. In addition, the observation that serotonin has no direct effect on PRL secretion by the pituitary *in vitro* (Lamberts and MacLeod, 1978a) precludes the possibility that the cyproheptadine effect is a specific antagonistic action on a serotonin receptor. Cyproheptadine was shown to have a selective effect on PRL secretion without exerting an influence on the synthesis or release of growth hormone in the same normal whole pituitary glands. This suggests that these findings are not the result of a toxic effect of the drug (Lamberts and MacLeod, 1978c). PRL secretion by dispersed pituitary tumor cells was also directly inhibited by cyproheptadine, while a parallel inhibition of the secretion of GH was observed in cells prepared from the mixed PRL/GH secreting tumor MtTW15. Since GH release by normal pituitary glands was shown not to be affected by cyproheptadine, it is concluded that GH secretion by this mixed pituitary tumor has acquired properties of the normal PRL secreting cell.

In man contradictory effects of cyproheptadine administration on GH secretion in acromegaly have been described. Feldman *et al.* (1976) reported a suppressive effect of cyproheptadine (16 mg daily for 2 days) on plasma GH concentrations during oral glucose tolerance tests in four of six patients with active acromegaly. Chiodini *et al.* (1976), however, did not observe a change in plasma GH in response to the administration of a single dose of 8 mg cyproheptadine, or during chronic treatment of four acromegalic patients for 2 weeks with 12 mg cyproheptadine per day.

PRL secretion by dispersed pituitary tumor cells *in vitro* was significantly inhibited by ergocryptine in a concentration of 0.1 $\mu$M. This effect is probably mediated via a dopamine agonistic action because it was prevented by coincubation with low concentrations of the specific dopamine receptor antagonist haloperidol. The suppressive effect of ergocryptine on PRL secretion by these dispersed tumor cells, however, was relatively poor, compared to the strong inhibitory effect of the drug on normal PRL secretion. 10 nM ergocryptine decreased PRL release by normal dispersed pituitary cells by 65% (Lamberts *et al.*, 1978).

Interestingly, ACTH secretion by the dispersed pituitary tumor cells prepared from the mixed PRL/ACTH-secreting pituitary tumor 7315a was inhibited in a manner similar to PRL secretion by both cyproheptadine and ergocryptine. It was shown previously that ACTH secretion was suppressed both by the administration of cyproheptadine and the ergot alkaloid bromocriptine in patients with Cushing's disease (Krieger *et al.*, 1975; Lamberts and Birkenhäger, 1976a). Treatment with these drugs, however, did not produce a long-term remission of Cushing's disease in all patients (Krieger and Luria, 1976; Lamberts *et al.*, 1977). The greatest ACTH-lowering effect of bromocriptine administration was observed in a patient with Nelson's syndrome, who also had raised plasma PRL concentrations and galactorrhea (Lamberts and Birkenhäger, 1976b).

We suggest that in pateints with GH or ACTH secreting pituitary tumors, chronic treatment with cyproheptadine and/or bromocriptine may be expected to be more successful when a certain degree of undifferentiation of these tumors has occurred toward the direction of normal PRL secretion.

## REFERENCES

Chiodini, P. G., Liuzzi, A., Müller, E. E., Botalla, L., Cremascoli, G., Oppizzi, G., Verde, G. and Silvestrini, F. (1976). *J. Clin. Endocr. Metab.* **43**, 356–363.
Feldman, J. M., Plonk, J. W. and Bivens, C. H. (1976). *Clin. Endocrinol. (Oxf).* **5**, 71–78.
Krieger, D. T. and Luria, M. (1976). *J. Clin. Endocr. Metab.* **43**, 1179–1182.
Krieger, D. T., Amorsa, L. and Linick, F. (1975). *N. Engl. J. Med.* **293**, 893–896.
Krieger, D. T., Liotta, A. and Brownstein, M. J. (1977). *Proc. Natl. Acad. Sci.* **74**, 648–652.
Lamberts, S. W. J. and Birkenhäger, J. C. (1976a). *J. Endocr.* **70**, 315–316.
Lamberts, S. W. J. and Birkenhäger, J. C. (1976b). *Lancet* **II**, 811.
Lamberts, S. W. J. and MacLeod, R. M. (1978a). *Endocrinology* **103**, 287–295.
Lamberts, S. W. J. and MacLeod, R. M. (1978b). *Endocrinology* **103**, 1710–1717.
Lamberts, S. W. J. and MacLeod, R. M. (1978c). Submitted for publication.
Lamberts, S. W. J. and MacLeod, R. M. (1979). *Endocrinology* **104**, 65–70.
Lamberts, S. W. J., Timmermans, H. A. T., de Jong, F. H. and Birkenhäger, J. C. (1977). *Clin. Endocrinol. (Oxf.)* **7**, 185–193.
Lamberts, S. W. J., Thorner, M. O. and MacLeod, R. M. (1978). Abstr. No. 556, 60th Annual Meeting, Endocrine Society, Endocrinolgy 353 A.
MacLeod, R. M. and Lehmeyer, J. E. (1973). *Cancer Res.* **33**, 849–854.
MacLeod, R. M., Abad, A. and Eidson, L. L. (1969). *Endocrinology* **84**, 1475–1482.

# PROLACTIN AND GROWTH HORMONE SECRETION BY DISPERSED CELL CULTURES OF SOMATOTROPHIC, LACTOTROPHIC AND MIXED PITUITARY ADENOMAS*

K. Mashiter and E. F. Adams

*Endocrine Unit, Department of Medicine, Royal Postgraduate Medical School, Hammersmith Hospital, Du Cane Road, London W12 OHS, UK*

## INTRODUCTION

The control of pituitary hormone secretion has been extensively studied *in vitro* using rat hemi-pituitaries, dispersed cells, isolated rat somatotrophs, mammotrophs and thyrotrophs (Tixier-Vidal, 1975; Vale *et al.*, 1972; Snyder *et al.*, 1977; Hymer *et al.*, 1974). In addition, cell-lines of rat pituitary tumors secreting one or more hormones have been produced (Tashjian and Hoyt 1972; Gautvik and Fossum, 1976). Despite the greatly increased knowledge derived from these studies it is clear that many hormonal responses observed in patients with pituitary adenomas are "inappropriate", possibly due to altered pituitary membrane receptors, and this situation is not adequately represented by any of the animal models. It has become increasingly important, therefore, that studies of the cellular mechanisms controlling hormone secretion by pituitary adenomas be carried out directly on human tissue. This paper summarizes the results of experiments designed to develop such an *in vitro* system and its use for the examination of basal and modulated hormone secretion by human somatotrophic, lactotrophic and mixed pituitary adenomas.

---

*This work was generously supported by grants from the University of London Central Research Fund, The Humane Trust, The Smith Kline and French Foundation, The Medical Research Council and Cancer Research Campaign. Reagents for TSH and PRL assays were generously donated by the N.I.A.M.D.D., USA.

We are greatly indebted to a number of our colleagues who include Susan Van Noorden, Dr. G. F. Joplin, Dr. I. Brajkovich, Dr. M. White, Dr. L. De Marco and technical staff of the laboratories.

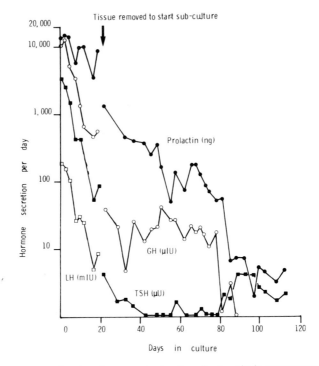

*Fig. 1a.* Hormone secretion in primary explant culture from a pituitary tumor removed by the transsphenoidal route from a woman with hyperprolactinemic-amenorrhea. Culture medium was changed every 3 or 4 days. Radioimmunoassayable PRL, GH, LH and TSH secretion are represented as the mean outputs per 24 h. FSH secretion (not shown) was very similar to that of LH. Normal and neoplastic tissue were demonstrated by immunocytochemistry. (Mashiter *et al.*, 1977).

## RESULTS AND DISCUSSION

### Source of adenoma tissue

Previous studies have shown that somatotrophic, lactotrophic, adrencortico-trophic and non-functioning adenomas removed by the transsphenoidal or trans-frontal route secrete in culture not only the tumor hormone but also other pituitary hormones (Kohler *et al.*, 1969; Lipson *et al.*, 1978). The presence of multiple hormones suggested that the specimens were heterogeneous and contained both adenoma and adjacent normal pituitary tissue. To test this we obtained specimens via the transsphenoidal route as well as biopsies during the procedure of [90]Yttrium implant for therapeutic ablation. Since the objective of the implant is to place a radioactive seed into the centre of the adenoma, needle aspiration biopsies obtained at this time should not be contaminated with normal tissue.

Specimens were sectioned into cubes of approximately 1mm$^3$ and placed in primary explant culture for two consecutive periods of three days. Hormone

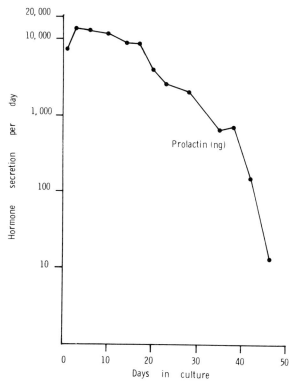

*(b)* PRL secretion by a biopsy of a lactotrophic adenoma in primary explant culture. Conditions as for Fig. 1a. No other pituitary hormones were secreted and the tissue gave positive immunostaining solely with antisera to PRL. (Mashiter *et al.*, 1977).

secretion into the medium (Minimum Essential Medium, HEPES buffered) was measured by specific radioimmunoassays and compared with tumor immuno-cytochemistry and clinical presentation. Specimens obtained by transsphenoidal hypophysectomy from two acromegalics and a woman with hyperprolactinemic-amenorrhea secreted prolactin (PRL), growth hormone (GH), luteinizing hor-mone (LH), follicle stimulating hormone (FSH) and thyroid stimulating hormone (TSH) in culture (Fig. 1a), and were shown to contain both neoplastic and normal pituitary tissue by immunocytochemistry. In contrast, for the needle aspiration biopsies obtained from five patients there was a high degree of correlation between the hormone secretion in culture (Fig. 1b), the immunocytochemical and the clinical findings. Two adenomas secreted solely PRL, one solely GH, two were mixed adenomas, one with a preponderance of GH over PRL and the other with a preponderance of PRL over GH cells (Mashiter *et al.*, 1979).

It follows that in any studies of human pituitary adenoma in culture considera-tion must be given to the nature of the specimen, since use of heterogeneous preparations may lead to difficulties of interpretation when responses are attri-buted to adenoma cells but actually belong to those of adjacent normal cells.

Whereas this does not exclude the use of material obtained by transsphenoidal or transfrontal adenomectomy, confirmation of the nature of the tissue should be sought by immunocytochemistry and the clinical presentation of the patient, as well as hormone secretion in culture.

### Hormone secretion in explant culture

The results in Fig. 1a show that secretion of GH, LH, FSH and TSH declines rapidly whether from adenomatous or normal tissue, confirming the earlier work of Kohler et al. (1969). There have been few studies of PRL secretion in short or long-term explant culture of human pituitary adenomas. Whereas a rise in PRL secretion would be predicted on the basis of removal from the tonic inhibitory influence of the hypothalamus, this has not been a consistent finding. In the present experiments only two of seven cultures demonstrated increased PRL secretion over the six days and in long-term culture PRL secretion from a lacto-trophic adenoma remained relatively stable for twenty days but then declined (Fig. 1b). Peillon et al. (1978) obtained convincing increases in PRL secretion in only one of four somatotrophic adenomas in explant culture and there was considerable variability in the results obtained with explants from the same adenoma. We believe this variability arises from inconstant degrees of cell differentiation or tissue necrosis over the longer term as well as the problems associated with initial distribution of the tissue. Explant culture is unlikely therefore to provide a reproducible experimental system in which to examine cellular control of hormone secretion by human pituitary adenomas.

### Dispersed cell culture of human pituitary adenomas

Although the advantages of using dispersed cell cultures are now well established there have been few applications to the study of human pituitary adenomas. Our procedure (Adams et al., submitted for publication) is to obtain pituitary tissue from selective transsphenoidal hypophysectomies and to establish the nature of the tissue by immunocytochemistry and, subsequently, hormone secretion in culture. The tissue is minced and the adenoma cells dissociated by incubation with 40 ml 0.1% trypsin in phosphate-buffered saline, pH 7.3 (PBS) for 1 h at 37°C with stirring by a Teflon®-coated magnet. The resulting suspension is centrifuged at 700 $g$ for 4 min at 4°C and the cell pellet thoroughly washed with more PBS. The cells are re-suspended in Minimum Essential Medium (MEM), HEPES buffered, containing 10% foetal calf serum and antibiotics. Cell number is determined by haemocytometer and viability, which is never less than 95%, by trypan blue exclusion; 2-4 × $10^5$ cells are distributed into tubes containing 2 ml medium.

### Basal secretion

Figure 2 shows the 24 h secretion of PRL and GH by 4 × $10^5$ cells of a mixed somatotrophic-lactotrophic adenoma in various culture media over a period of 36 days. PRL secretion increased in all but one medium (MEM, HEPES buffered)

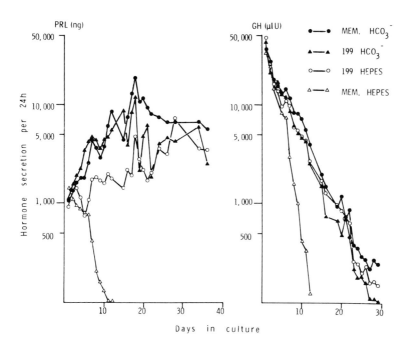

*Fig. 2.* Long-term secretion of PRL and GH by $4 \times 10^5$ dispersed cells of a mixed somatotrophic-lactotrophic adenoma in various culture media. Results represent the means of duplicate determinations. Culture medium was changed every 24 h. MEM, Minimum Essential Medium; 199, Medium 199, $HCO_3^-$, 26.2 mm bicarbonate buffered; HEPES, $N$-2-hydroxyethylpiperazine-$N'$-ethane sulphonic acid buffered.

reaching concentrations 18- and 16-fold those attained initially in bicarbonate-buffered MEM and Medium 199 respectively. GH secretion declined in all media but did so more rapidly in the HEPES buffered MEM. The inability of this medium to support increased PRL output was not confirmed in subsequent experiments with lactotrophic adenomas, where secretion of PRL increased at very much the same rates in the different media although the bicarbonate buffered media still tended to maintain the highest output.

Secretion of PRL from a normal pituitary (removed from a woman with breast cancer) similarly increased with time in culture whilst GH secretion declined rapidly (data not shown).

## MODULATED SECRETION

Various factors are known to affect hormone secretion from human pituitary adenoma *in vivo* and animal pituitaries *in vitro*. We report on the effects of some of those which have been used to test the integrity of our dispersed cell culture system, particularly in regard to GH and PRL secretion. Figures 3 and 4 summarize these data.

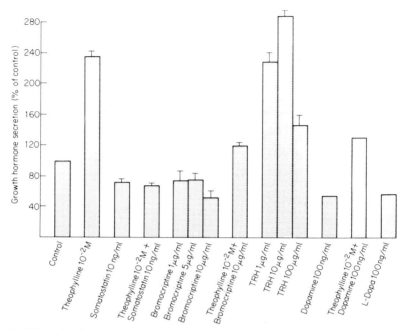

**Fig. 3.** Effect of various agents on GH secretion by dispersed cell cultures of somatotrophic and mixed somatotrophic-lactotrophic adenomas in dispersed cell culture. The results represent cumulative data from a series of experiments and have been normalized with respect to the control in each experiment to allow comparison on a percentage change basis. Incubations were for 4 h and at least duplicate cultures were used for each variable.

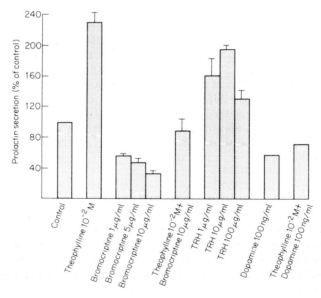

**Fig. 4.** Effect of various agents on PRL secretion by dispersed cell cultures of lactotrophic and lactotrophic-somatotrophic adenomas in dispersed cell culture. Conditions as for Fig. 3.

### Theophylline

Theophylline consistently stimulated GH and PRL secretion from a mixed somatotrophic-lactotrophic adenoma and GH secretion from somatotrophic adenomas during 4 h experiments. These effects were dependent on the time the adenoma cells had been in culture. GH secretion could be stimulated at 4 or 28 days but not at 49 days whereas PRL secretion was unaffected after 4 days but manifested significant stimulation after 28 days culture.

### Somatostatin

Although somatostatin inhibits GH secretion in patients with active acromegaly (Besser *et al.*, 1974), we have been unable to demonstrate a consistent inhibitory effect on GH secretion from somatotrophic cells in culture during 4 h experiments at doses from 1–10 ng/ml somatostatin. However, under the same conditions somatostatin (10 ng/ml) completely blocked the effect of theophylline, in agreement with a similar action on dibutyryl-cyclic-AMP-induced GH release from rat pituitary somatotrophs (Borgeat *et al.*, 1974), suggesting its effect to be at a stage beyond the generation of cyclic AMP (Snyder *et al.*, 1977).

### Bromocriptine

Bromocriptine inhibited GH and PRL secretion by mixed somatotrophic-lactotrophic adenomas and GH secretion by somatotrophic adenomas in a dose responsive manner with increasing effects up to the maximal used (10 µg/ml). Furthermore, bromocriptine (10 µg/ml) inhibited the theophylline-induced increase in both GH and PRL secretion. This effect of bromocriptine on GH secretion, first reported by Mashiter *et al.* (1977) using explant culture, was not a consistent finding with every adenoma, in a manner similar to the variability encountered with the clinical results in patients with GH-secreting adenomas (Cessar *et al.*, 1977). Although we have only examined *in vivo*, with subsequent *in vitro* testing, a single acromegalic patient who came to surgery, bromocriptine produced very similar responses under these different circumstances, these being 37% suppression *in vitro* and 57% *in vivo*.

### Thyrotrophin releasing hormone (TRH)

GH and PRL secretion from a mixed pituitary adenoma were stimulated in a dose-dependent manner by TRH during a 4 h incubation. Maximal effects were achieved with a dose of 10 ng/ml TRH. Removal of the TRH during a subsequent 4 h incubation resulted in a decline in hormone secretion to basal levels. Again there was variability from tumor to tumor and in the one acromegalic patient where *in vivo* and *in vitro* GH responses to TRH were compared, results were negative in each case.

### Dopaminergic compounds

Dopamine (100 ng/ml) inhibited both basal PRL and GH and theophylline-stimulated PRL and GH secretion by a mixed pituitary adenoma that had been cultured for six days. L-Dopa (100 ng/ml) had a similar effect after 1 day's culture. No significant changes were observed in similar experiments with the adenomas that had been cultured for longer periods. In one acromegalic patient no significant change in GH secretion occurred following administration of L-dopa (500 mg) *in vivo* and no change *in vitro* with either L-dopa (100 ng/ml) or dopamine (100 ng/ml) after 3 days' culture of the adenoma.

## CONCLUSIONS

The results of these studies show that dispersed cell cultures of human pituitary adenomas provide a useful system for the investigation of the cellular control of tumor hormone secretion and have significant advantages over explant techniques. Basal secretion of PRL continues at increased rates for periods up to 36 days and responds to stimulation by theophylline and TRH. Both basal and theophylline-stimulated PRL secretion are suppressed by bromocriptine, L-dopa and dopamine. Basal GH secretion declines with time in culture but is stimulated by theophylline and sometimes TRH. Bromocriptine inhibits basal and bromocriptine, somatostatin, L-dopa and dopamine block theophylline-induced GH secretion. In the single acromegalic patient who came to survery, *in vivo* and *in vitro* responses to a number of these compounds were in complete agreement, providing further evidence for the integrity of the system as a model for the human pituitary tumor.

## REFERENCES

Adams, F., Brajkovich, I. and Mashiter, K. (submitted for publication).

Besser, G. M., Mortimer, C. H., Carr, D., Schally, A. V., Coy, D. H., Evered, D., Kastin, A. J., Tunbridge, W. M. G., Thorner, M. O. and Hall, R. (1974). *Br. Med. J.* 1, 352–355.

Borgeat, P., Labrie, F., Drouin, J. and Belanger, A. (1974). *Biochem. Biophys. Res. Commun.* 56, 1052–1059.

Cassar, J., Mashiter. and Joplin, G. F. (1977). *Metabolism* 26, 539–545.

Gautvik, M. and Fossum, S. (1976). *Biochem. J.* 159, 119–125.

Hymer, W. C., Snyder, J., Wilfinger, W., Swanson, N. and Davis, J. A. (1974). *Endocrinology* 95, 107–122.

Kohler, P. O., Bridson, W. E., Rayford, P. L. and Kohler, S. E. (1969). *Metabolism* 18, 782–788.

Leuschen, M. P., Tobin, R. B. and Moriarty, C. M. (1977). *Endocrinology* 102, 509–518.

Lipson, L. G., Beitins, I. Z., Kornblith, P. D., McArthur, J. W., Friesen, H. G., Kliman, B. and Kjellberg, R. N. (1978). *Acta. Endocronologica* 88, 239–249.

Mashiter, K., Adams, E., Beard, M. and Holley, A. (1977). *Lancet* 2, 197–198.

Mashiter, K., Van Noorden, S., De Marco, L., Adams, E. and Joplin, G. F. (1979). *J. Clin. Endocrinol. Metab.* 48, 108–113.

Peillon, F., Cesselin, F., Garnier, P. E., Brandi, A. M., Donnadien, M., L'Hermite, M. and Dubois, M. P. (1978). *Acta. Endocrinologia.* 87, 701–715.

Snyder, G., Hymer, W. C. and Snyder, J. (1977). *Endocrinology* 101, 788–799.

Tixier-Vidal, A. (1975). *In* "The Anterior Pituitary" (A. Tixier-Vidal and M. Farquhar, eds) 181–229. Academic Press, New York and London.

Tashjian, A. H. Jr. and Hoyte, R. F. Jr. (1972). *In* "Molecular Genetics and Developmental Biology" (M. Sussman, ed) 353–387. Prentice-Hall, New Jersey.

Vale, W., Grant, G., Amoss, M., Blackwell, R. and Guillemin, R. (1972). *Endocrinology* 91, 567–572.

Yen, S., Siler, T. and De Vane, G. (1974). *N. Engl. J. Med.* 290, 935–938.

# PRESENCE OF A DOPAMINE-SENSITIVE ADENYLATE-CYCLASE IN FUNCTIONING HUMAN PITUITARY ADENOMAS*

P. De Camilli[1] **, A. Spade[2], P. Beck-Peccoz[2], P. Moriondo[2],
M. Giovanelli[3] and G. Faglia[2]

[1] *CNR Center of Cytopharmacology, Department of Pharmacology,
University of Milan, Italy.* [2] *Endocrine Unit, II Medical Clinic, University
of Milan, Italy.* [3] *Department of Neurosurgery, University of Milan, Italy*

## INTRODUCTION

Dopamine (DA) is known to be a potent activator of adenylate-cyclase (AC) in various regions of the brain (Kebabian *et al.*, 1972; Clement-Cormier and Robinson, 1977). In contrast, in the normal anterior pituitary (AP), where the presence of DA receptors that modulate prolactin (PRL) secretion is now well established (MacLeod and Lehmeyer, 1974; Brown *et al.*, 1976; Calabro and MacLeod, 1978), an effect of DA on AC has never been demonstrated. Furthermore, an activation of AC in cells of the AP by DA would be puzzling, since strong evidence indicates that cAMP is stimulatory for AP hormone secretion (Hill *et al.*, 1976; Labrie *et al.*, 1976) while the action of DA at the pituitary level is primarily inhibitory (MacLeod and Lehmeyer, 1974; Camanni *et al.*,

*Acknowledgements: The authors thank G. Tonon and Dr. S. Nicosia for helpful suggestions and Dr. J. Meldolesi for critical discussion. Data shown in Fig. 2B are courtesy of Dr. P. G. Crosignani.

**Dr. De Camilli's present address is: Dept of Pharmacology, Yale University School of Medicine, New Haven, Connecticut 06510, USA.

This work has been partially supported by CNR contribution No. 78.02121.04.115.3936

1977). Since the existence of a DA-mediated modification of AC in normal AP might have been obscured by the very marked heterogeneity of the cell population, we decided to reinvestigate the problem of possible coupling of DA and AC at the pituitary level by studying the effects of dopaminergic and antidopaminergic agents on AC in tissues composed of cell populations meeting the following criteria: (a) homogeneity, and (b) responsiveness to DA. Human PRL- or growth hormone (GH)-secreting adenomas are good experimental models that fulfil these criteria. In fact, PRL adenomas, at variance with some pituitary tumour cell lines for which a defective dopaminergic regulation has recently been reported (Malarkey *et al.*, 1977), are in the large majority of cases sensitive to both DA and dopaminergic drugs (Kleinberg *et al.*, 1977; Friesen *et al.*, 1973; De Camilli *et al.*, this volume). In GH adenomas some evidence indicates that the paradoxical dopaminergic inhibition that can be observed in a good proportion of acromegalic patients (Liuzzi *et al.*, 1972) is due to a direct action of the drug on DA receptors of adenomatous somatotrophs (Camanni *et al.*, 1977; Mashiter *et al.*, 1977).

## MATERIALS AND METHODS

DA, norepinephrine and phosphocreatine were purchased from Sigma Chemical Company, ATP and cAMP from Boehringer, apomorphine from Merck, Sharpe and Dohme, and Creatinephosphokinase from Worthington Biochemical Corporation.

The following drugs were obtained as gifts: trifluoperazine from Maggioni, fluphenazine from Squibb, sulpiride from Ravizza, and CH 29-717 from Sandoz Pharmaceuticals.

Pituitary adenomas were removed by selective adenomectomy through the transnasosphenoidal route. In all cases endocrinological tests were carried out *in vivo* before surgery to establish the responsiveness to dopaminergic drugs. Small aliquots of the tissue fragments obtained at operation were immediately fixed for morphological examination by light and electron microscopy, to assess the actual adenomatous nature of the tissue. The remaining portions of the fragments were frozen at $-20°C$ until used for AC assay.

AC assay was carried out by a procedure based on the method of Salomon *et al.* (1974), with some modifications. Tissue was homogenized with a Teflon® pestle in 2mM EGTA, 2mM Tris-maleate pH 7.4. The final incubation mixture contained: 80 mM Tris-maleate, pH 7.4, 10 mM theophylline, variable concentrations of ATP (0.5 mM in cases 1, 2 and 1'; 0.15 mM in all other cases), 1 mM cAMP, 0.2 mM EGTA, variable concentrations of $MgSO_4$ (2 mM in cases 1, 2 and 1'; 0.6 mM in cases 3 and 3'; 1.5 mM in all other cases), phosphocreatine (1.8 mg/ml) creatinephosphokinase (0.2 mg/ml; 35U/mg) and about 100 µg of tissue protein. The incubation time was 8 min at 30°C; the reaction was started by the addition of the tissue homogenate. Values reported in the figures and tables are means ± s.e.m. for at least three replicate determinations.

*Table 1.* Effects of DA on AC *in vitro* and on hormonal secretion *in vivo* in PRL- and GH-secreting adenomas.

| Cases | Adenylate-cyclase activity | | | Effect of dopaminergic drugs on | |
|---|---|---|---|---|---|
| | cAMP formed (pmole/mg prot/8 min) | | Variation induced by Dopamine 10 μM (%) | PRL secretion *in vivo* | GH secretion *in vivo* |
| | Control | Dopamine 10 μM | | | |
| PRL-secreting adenomas 1 | 165.52 ± 13.76 | 111.76 ± 8.31[a] | −32.48 | → | |
| PRL-secreting adenomas 2 | 204.56 ± 17.14 | 144.40 ± 4.76[a] | −29.41 | → | |
| PRL-secreting adenomas 3 | 193.60 ± 1.60 | 118.08 ± 1.16[c] | −39.01 | → | |
| PRL-secreting adenomas 4 | 53.44 ± 0.78 | 45.84 ± 2.00[b] | −14.22 | → | |
| PRL-secreting adenomas 5 | 112.48 ± 2.37 | 89.11 ± 7.68[a] | −20.77 | → | |
| PRL-secreting adenomas 6 | 50.79 ± 1.59 | 44.21 ± 0.66[a] | −12.95 | → | |
| PRL-secreting adenomas 7 | 55.69 ± 1.30 | 56.98 ± 1.67 | – | ↑ | |
| GH-secreting adenomas 1' | 45.84 ± 7.12 | 25.36 ± 2.18[a] | −44.67 | | → |
| GH-secreting adenomas 2' | 324.88 ± 7.12 | 320.56 ± 5.36 | – | | → |
| GH-secreting adenomas 3' | 57.68 ± 2.82 | 87.76 ± 0.32[b] | +52.15 | | ↑ |
| GH-secreting adenomas 4' | 139.76 ± 8.08 | 242.40 ± 1.88[b] | +73.44 | | → |
| GH-secreting adenomas 5' | 35.06 ± 0.62 | 35.12 ± 1.92 | – | | ↑ |
| GH-secreting adenomas 6' | 563.54 ± 3.30 | 755.88 ± 6.29 | +34.13 | | ↑ |

[a] = $P < 0.05$
[b] = $P < 0.005$
[c] = $P < 0.001$

Downwards arrows indicate a decrease of the circulating PRL or GH of more than 50%.

## RESULTS

### PRL adenomas

Table I shows the effects of DA on basal AC in the homogenates of seven different pituitary adenomas, as well as the action of dopaminergic drugs on secretion *in vivo* before adenomectomy. AC activity in six of the seven cases was significantly inhibited by 10μM DA. As can be seen in the same table, a good correlation was found between the effects of DA on AC *in vitro* and the action of dopaminergic agents *in vivo* on PRL secretion before surgery.

Figures 1A and 1B show that the inhibitory effect of DA was clearly dose-dependent. Low doses of antidopaminergic agents such as trifluoperazine (Fig. 1A) and fluphenazine (data not shown) strongly counteracted the DA action in a competitive way, L-NA was also inhibitory to the cyclase, but higher doses of L-NA than of DA were required to inhibit the enzyme activity to the same amount (Fig. 1B), thus suggesting that the action of DA is not due to occupance by DA of α-adrenergic receptors. The action of DA could be mimicked by apomorphine (data not shown) and by the dopaminergic ergot CH 29-717* (Fig. 1C). This compound had even greater affinity for the DA binding site that mediates the inhibition of AC, since it was effective at doses at which DA was still inactive (Fig. 1C; compare with Fig. 1B, same case).

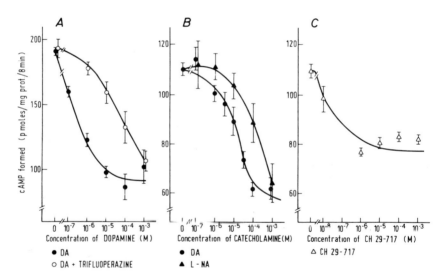

*Fig. 1.* Effects of drugs on basal AC activity in homogenates of PRL-secreting adenomas. A: effect of various doses of DA in the absence and presence of trifluoperazine 0.1μM (case 3). B: effects of DA and L-NA (case 5). C: effects of various doses of the dopaminergic ergot CH 29-717 (case 5).

---

\* The dopaminergic ergot CH 29-717 (8 α-amino-ergoline) is even more potent than CB 154 in inhibiting PRL secretion and much more soluble in water (Flückiger *et al.*, in press). Therefore it is more suitable than CB 154 for *in vitro* studies.

Sulpiride, at a dose which *per se* is inactive on AC, fully reversed the inhibitory effect of 10 $\mu$M DA (Fig. 2A). This figure also shows (Fig. 2B) that this effect paralleled the *in vivo* antagonism of sulpiride of the DA-mediated inhibition of PRL secretion in the same case. That this *in vivo* effect of sulpiride occurred through a specific blockade of dopaminergic receptors is indicated by the finding that, as is often the case in hyperprolactinemic patients (Kleinberg *et al*., 1977; Friesen *et al*., 1973), sulpiride alone did not induce any increase in the circulating PRL.

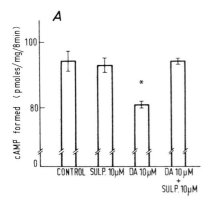 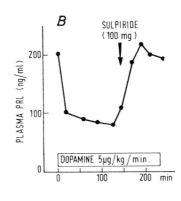

*Fig. 2.* A: effects of sulpiride alone or in combination with DA on cAMP formation in a PRL-secreting adenoma (case 5). B: effects of sulpiride administration during DA infusion *in vivo* (same case). * = $P < 0.05$ relative to control and $< 0.02$ relative to DA + sulp.

### GH adenomas

The effects of 10 $\mu$M DA on basal AC in homogenates of six different GH-secreting adenomas are shown in Table I. The table also shows the effects of dopaminergic drugs *in vivo* on GH secretion before adenomectomy. At variance with the situation observed in PRL adenomas, the effects of DA on AC in homogenates of GH adenomas were found to be variable. Either inhibitory, stimulatory effects or no effect at all were observed. Furthermore, as it appears from Table I, except for case 1'*, no correlation was found between the effect of DA on AC and the effect of DA and dopaminergic drugs on GH secretion. In particular, stimulation of the enzyme by DA was found in cases in which dopaminergic agents had either no effect or were even inhibitory for GH secretion *in vivo* (case 3', 4' and 6').

Figure 3A shows the effects of various doses of DA on AC in case 4'. The effect of DA was dose-dependent and specific, because: (a) it could be competitively inhibited by low doses of fluphenazine (Fig. 3A); (b) it was not due to

---

* Case 1' is the only case in which, in addition to high GH plasma level (100 ng/ml), a very high PRL plasma level (180 ng/ml) was also detected before adenomectomy. It is therefore not surprising that this tumour displays characteristics similar to those of PRL adenomas.

occupance by DA of alpha-adrenergic receptors (Fig. 3A); and (c) it could be at least partially mimicked by the dopaminergic agonist apomorphine (Fig. 3B). However, at variance with what was found for PRL adenomas, the dopaminergic agent CH 29-717 was almost ineffective in mimicking the action of DA (data not shown) and L-sulphiride (Fig. 3C) was totally ineffective as an antagonist.

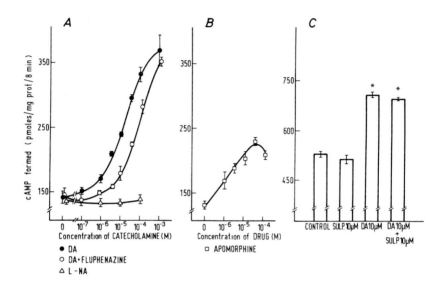

Fig. 3. Effects of drugs on basal AC activity in homogenates of GH-secreting adenomas. A: effects of various doses of DA (in the absence or presence of fluphenazine 1µM) and of L-NA (case 4'). B: effects of various doses of Apomorphine (case 4'). C: effects of sulpiride alone or in combination with DA (case 6'). * = $P < 0.001$ relative to control.

## DISCUSSION

The results of the present study clearly indicate that in pituitary tissue also, at least in particular cases (such as in adenomatous tissue), a coupling between DA receptors and AC can be demonstrated.

The different results obtained in PRL adenomas and in GH adenomas are rather surprising. They point to the existence of differing DA receptors on mammotrophs and somatotrophs and do not support the concept that there is a common mechanism of action of DA in inhibiting PRL and GH secretion.

The DA receptor on adenomatous mammotrophs displays unique characteristics as compared to DA receptors known so far: (a) it is coupled with AC, but DA binding to the receptor produces an inhibition rather than a stimulation of the enzyme; and (b) the DA effect on the cyclase is mimicked by dopaminergic ergots and antagonized by sulpiride, drugs which are ineffective in mimicking or antagonizing the DA-mediated AC stimulation which occurs in various regions of the brain (Fuxe *et al.*, 1978; Trabucchi *et al.*, 1975). Both these properties are in agreement with the properties of the DA receptor on mammotrophs, expected from the secretion studies. Point (a) is in agreement with the line of evidence which attributes a stimulatory role for cAMP on PRL secretion (Hill *et al.*, 1976; Labrie *et al.*, 1976; Dannies *et al.*, 1976); point (b) gives further support to the hypothesis that the DA receptor on mammotrophs has different pharmacological properties than the AC-coupled DA receptor of the CNS in its ability to bind agonists and antagonists (Calabro and MacLeod, 1978; Kebabian, 1978). Our study indicates that this receptor is also able to induce an opposite effect on AC and suggests that DA might inhibit PRL secretion through a decrease in the intracellular concentration of cAMP.

Further studies are needed to establish whether DA is able to inhibit AC in normal mammotrophs also. However, there is excellent correlation between the ability of DA to inhibit PRL secretion and to inhibit AC in the seven tumors. We have examined points on the existence of a causal relationship between the two phenomena peculiar to the physiology of the PRL cell. In the normal pituitary, the effect of DA on AC might be masked by the background of AC in cells unresponsive to DA. It is also possible that for some reason tumoral growth amplifies the coupling between DA receptor and AC. Crosignani *et al.* (1977) recently reported data supporting the hypothesis of lowered dopaminergic activity in hyperprolactinemic patients. If this were actually the case, the AC inhibition might be more clearly detectable because DA receptors might be in a supersensitive state (Cheung and Weiner, 1976).

The data obtained in GH adenomas (with the exception of case 1') are puzzling. In particular, it is nard to interpret a stimulation of AC by DA in cases in which DA is inhibitory for secretion (case 4'). A similar finding has been reported in a study of four cases of acromegaly by Matsukura *et al.* (1977), who however did not further characterize the DA receptors responsible for this effect. Moreover, dopaminergic ergots which are agonists of DA in its inhibitory effect on secretion are not agonists of DA in its stimulatory effect on the cyclase. The DA receptor which is responsible for the effect on AC in GH adenomas seems to have little to do with GH secretion.

The similarity between the AC-coupled DA receptors in brain and in these GH adenomas is remarkable. They seem to have the same characteristics both in relation to the effects of DA on AC and to the binding properties for agonists and antagonists. In fact, at both sites dopaminergic ergots are ineffective as agonists and sulpiride as antagonist. As has been recently proposed (Kebabian, 1978), a definite type of specificity for agonists and antagonists might be a general property of those DA receptors which exhibit an excitatory coupling with AC. It will be interesting to investigate in the future whether DA is also able to inhibit AC at other sites, in which pharmacological studies have suggested that there are DA receptors with a type of specificity different from that of the classical AC-coupled DA receptors as in pituitary mammotrophs. It is worth noting that at one such site, i.e. the DA autoreceptors of DA neurons (Di Chiara *et al.*, 1977; Fuxe *et al.*, 1977), DA and cAMP induce opposite effects, DA being inhibitory (Bunney and Aghajanian, 1975), and cAMP excitatory for the function of the DA neurons (Anagnoste *et al.*, 1974; Goldstein *et al.*, 1975).

## REFERENCES

Anagnoste, B., Shirron, C., Friedman, E. and Goldstein, M. (1974). *J. Pharmac. Exp. Ther.* **191**, 370.

Brown, G. M., Seeman P. and Lee, T. (1976). *Endocrinology* **99**, 1407.

Bunney, B. S. and Aghajanian, G. K. (1975). *In* "Pre- and Post- Synaptic Receptors" (E. Usdin and W. E. Bunney Jr, eds) pp. 89–122. Dekker, New York.

Camanni, F., Massara, F., Belforte, L., Rosatello, A. and Molinatti, G. M. (1977). *J. Clin Endocr. Metab.* **44**, 465.

Calabro, M. A. and MacLeod, R. M. (1978). *Neuroendocrinology* **25**, 32.

Cheung, C. Y. and Weiner, R. I. (1976). *Endocrinology* **99**, 914.

Clement-Cormier, Y. C. and Robinson, G. A. (1977). *Biochem. Pharmac.* **26**, 1719.

Crosignani, P. G., Reschini, E., Peracchi, M., Lombroso, G. C., Mattei, A. and Caccano, A. (1977). *J. Clin. Endocr. Metab.* **45**, 841.

Dannies, P. S., Gautvik, K. M. and Tashjian A. H. Jr. (1976). *Endocrinology* **98**, 1147.

Di Chiara, G., Vargiu, L., Porceddu, M. L. and Gessa, G. L. (1977). *In* "Advances in Biochemical Psychopharmacology" (E. Costa and G. L. Gessa, eds) Vol. XVI, 443–446. Raven Press, New York.

Flückiger, E., Briner, U., Doenfner, W., Kowacs, E., Marbach, P. and Wagner, H. R. (in press). *Experientia.*

Friesen, H., Tolis, G., Shin, R. and Hwang, P. (1973). *In* "Human Prolactin" (J. L. Pasteels and C. Robyn, eds) p. 11. Excerpta Medica. Amsterdam.

Fuxe, K., Agnati, L., Everitt, B. J., Hökfelt, T., Ljungdahl, A. and Perez De La Mora, M. (1977). *In* "Advances in Biochemical Psychopharmacology" (E. Costa and G. L. Gessa, eds) Vol. XVI, 489–494. Raven Press, New York.

Fuxe, K., Fredholm, B. B., Agnati, L. F., Ogren, S. O., Everitt, B. J., Jonsson, G. and Gustafsson, J. A. (1978). *Pharmacology* **16** (suppl 1).

Goldstein, M., Ebstein, B., Bronaugh, R. L. and Roberge, C. (1975). *In* "Chemical Tools in Catecholamine Research" (G. Jonsson, T. Malmohors, C. Sachs, O. Almgen, A. Carlsson and J. Engel, eds) pp 257–264. North Holland, Amsterdam.

Hill, M. K., MacLeod, R. M. and Orcutt, P. (1976). *Endocrinology* **99**, 1612.

Kebabian, J. W., Petzold, G. L. and Greengard, P. (1972). *Proc. Natl. Acad. Sci. USA* **69**, 2145.

Kebabian, J. W. (1978). Abstracts of the Symposium on "Receptors of Dopamine Antagonists: New Biochemical Approaches". Janssen Pharmaceutica, Belgium.

Kleinberg, D. L., Noel, G. I. and Frantz, A. G. (1977). *New Engl. J. Med.* **296**, 589.

Labrie, F. G., Pelletier, G., Borgeat, P., Drouin, J., Ferland, L. and Belanger, A. (1976). *In* "Frontiers in Neuroendocrinology" (L. Martini and W. F. Ganong, eds) Vol. IV, 63. Raven Press, New York.

Liuzzi, A., Chiodini, P. G., Botalla, L., Cremascoli, G. and Silvestrini, F. (1972). *J. Clin, Endocr. Metab.* **35**, 941.

MacLeod, R. M. and Lehmeyer, J. E. (1974). *Endocrinology* **94**, 1077.

Malarkey, W. B., Groshong, J. C. and Milo, G. E. (1977). *Nature* **266**, 640.

Mashiter, K., Adams, E., Beard, M. and Holley, A. (1977). *Lancet* **2**, 197.

Matsukura, S., Kakita, T., Hirata, J., Yoshimi, H., Fukase, M., Iwasaki, Y., Kato, Y. and Imura, H. (1977). *J. Clin. Endocr. Metab.* **44**, 392.

Salomon, Y., Londos, C. and Rodbell, M. (1974). *Anal. Biochem.* **58**, 451.

Trabucchi, M., Longoni, R., Fresna, P. and Shano, P. F. (1975). *Life Sci.* **17**, 1551.

# CHARACTERIZATION OF CORTICOLIPOTROPIC PEPTIDES
# IN A PITUITARY ADENOMA OF CUSHING'S DISEASE*

J. C. Lissitzky, M. Guibout, P. Jaquet, C. Lucas, J. Hassoun,
C. Charpin, P. Martin, F. Grisoli and C. Oliver

*Laboratoire des Hormones Protéiques, Faculté de Médecine,
27 Bd. Jean-Moulin, 13385 Marseille Cédex 4, France*

Adrenocorticotropic hormone (ACTH) and β-lipotropin (βLPH) are two closely related peptides originating from the same prolipocortin precursor molecule. Although this has been demonstrated in a mouse tumoral cell line (Mains *et al.*, 1977; Roberts and Herbert, 1977), indirect evidence has been obtained that this also applies to human ACTH-secreting tissues (Yalow and Berson, 1971, 1973) ACTH and βLPH have been demonstrated in the anterior pituitary (Rubinstein *et al.*, 1977; Lissitzky *et al.*, 1978) and their identical control, including corticosteroid negative feedback, stress, circadian rhythm, CRF stimulation and α-adrenergic inputs (Gilkes *et al.*, 1975; Bachelot *et al.*, 1977; Krieger *et al.*, 1977; Jeffcoate *et al.*, 1978; Raymond *et al.*, 1978) suggested secretion of both compounds in parallel. On the contrary, in the intermediate pituitary lobe, as proposed by Lowry and Scott (1975), ACTH and βLPH seem to be further processed into α melanocyte stimulating hormone (αMSH) and corticotropin-like intermediate lobe peptide (CLIP) (Scott *et al.*, 1974) and γ-lipotropin (γLPH) and β-endorplin (βEND), (Lissitzky *et al.*, 1978), respectively. Furthermore, the control of secretion, best documented for ACTH and αMSH (Kraicer *et al.*, 1973; Greer *et al.*, 1975; Kraicer and Morris, 1976) seems to be very different here than in the anterior hypophysis. The human pituitary, which lacks the intermediate lobe,

---

* We are indebted to the National Pituitary Agency, NIH (Bethesda, USA) for providing hβMSH and hACTH$_{1-39}$, to Dr. P. J. Lowry (London) for hβLPH and anti hβLPH antiserum, to Dr. F. Girard (Paris) for anti hβMSH antiserum, to Dr. F. Labrie (Quebec) for anti hACTH antiserum and to Dr. Rittel (CIBA Geigy) for the supply of the ACTH fragments. This work was supported by INSERM grants No. 78.5.034.4 and 46 7778.

appears to be differentiated like the pars distalis of other species in so far as it contains mainly ACTH and βLPH (Liotta *et al.*, 1978; Abe *et al.*, 1967; Scott and Lowry, 1974). In this study, the nature of the corticolipotropic peptides contained in an adenoma of Cushing's disease and in the patient's blood has been investigated.

## CLINICAL HISTORY

Melanoderma restricted to the trunk and the face and headache were the only clinical symptoms shown by the 36-year-old male patient from whom the plasma samples and tumor fragments were obtained. Other signs of Cushing's syndrome were absent. The basal 24-hour 17-hydroxysteroid urinary excretion was elevated (28 mg/24 h). It was insensitive to either the dexamethasone test or the metyrapone indirect stimulation test. Plasma cortisol was elevated and did not fluctuate during the day. Tomograms of the sella turcica and pneumoencephalography revealed a state II grade B pituitary adenoma, which was removed surgically through successive transsphenoidal and transfrontal routes. The tumoral tissue investigated was a fragment of the suprasellar expansion.

## RADIOIMMUNOASSAYS

The specific radioimmunoassays used for the detection of βLPH, γLPH, βEND, αMSH, βMSH and ACTH are summarized in Table I. As indicated, the βLPH N-terminal assay (N-βLPH) was able to detect βLPH and γLPH, the βLPH C-terminal assay (C-βLPH) to detect βEND, $\beta LPH_{61-87}$ and βLPH. Since βLPH crossreacted in the two assays (50 % and 25 % on a weight basis, respectively), purification of biological material was required for accurate measurement of βLPH, γLPH and βEND. Peptides were extracted from plasma with silicic acid to avoid non-specific serum interference in the assays. High extraction yields were observed with all the peptides investigated (90 %), whatever labeled or unlabeled molecules were used as controls.

## βLPH AND ACTH PLASMA LEVELS

Basal N-βLPH and C-βLPH immunoreactive-like materials in the plasma were elevated, 1358 ± 111 pg/ml γLPH equivalent (m ± s.e.; *n* = 10) and 571 ± 34 pg/ml βEND equivalent, respectively. ACTH was increased to a lesser extent, 130 ± 20 pg/ml. The levels of the ACTH, N- and C- βLPH immunoreactive materials were not sensitive to bromocriptine (5 mg, p.o.), TRH (200 μg, i.v.), L-DOPA (100 μg, i.v.) or insulin hypoglycemia, and the nyctohemeral rhythms of these peptides were suppressed. During the metyrapone test, N- and C-βLPH increased (1450 – 2270 pg/ml and 465 – 1025 pg/ml respectively), whereas ACTH and the 17-hydroxysteroids did not increase, revealing a dissociation in the regulation of the ACTH and βLPH immunoreactive-like materials. Removal of the intrasellar tumor did not lower the blood levels of the assayed peptides, which did drop after the ablation of the suprasellar expansion. Remission was not

Table 1. Description of the radioimmunoassays.

| Assay | Antibody | Immunogen | Labeled antigen and standard | Titer | Sensitivity (pg) | Cross-reacting peptides[a] | No Cross reaction[b] with |
|---|---|---|---|---|---|---|---|
| hβLPH N-term | HA58 | purified hβLPH | hγLPH | $20000^{-1}$ | 10 | hβLPH (50) | hβEnd<br>hβMSH<br>hACTH<br>hβMSH |
| hβLPH C-term | 334 | synthetic hβEnd | hβEND | $10000^{-1}$ | 20 | hβLPH (25)<br>hβLPH 61–87(100) | MetEnk<br>αEND<br>γEND<br>$ACTH_{1-39}$ |
| ACTH N-term | 105 | synthetic $hACTH_{1-24}$ | $hACTH_{1-39}$ | $70000^{-1}$ | 10 | $hACTH_{1-24}$ (100)<br>$hACTH_{11-24}$ (0.25)<br>$hACTH_{1-13}$ (0.1) | $hACTH_{1-10}$<br>$hACTH_{17-39}$<br>αMSH<br>hβMSH<br>hβEND |
| αMSH | 3 | synthetic αMSH | αMSH | $40000^{-1}$ | 5 | $ACTH_{1-13}$ (100)<br>$ACTH_{1-16}$ (1) | $hACTH_{1-39}$<br>1–24<br>4–10<br>hβMSH<br>γLPH |
| hβMSH | 3315 | ACTH powder | hβMSH | $40000^{-1}$ | 5 | hγLPH (20)<br>hβLPH (10) | $hACTH_{1-39}$<br>$hACTH_{1-24}$<br>hβEND<br>αMSH |

[a] Cross reaction ratios (figures in parentheses) were calculated as $100\ x/y$ where $x$ and $y$ are the mass of standard and cross-reacting peptide, respectively, which produced a 50% decrease of antibody bound tracer.

[b] Cross reaction inferior to 0.1%.

only quantitative, since N- and C- βLPH and ACTH dropped to 300, 130, 20 pg/ml, respectively, but was also functional, since 17-hydroxysteroids fell from 2.4 to 0.4 mg/24 h under dexamethasone and increased to 19.6 mg/24 h with metyrapone.

Histological examination of the tumor revealed a PAS +, hematoxylin +, basophilic adenoma which stained specifically for ACTH and βLPH by immuno-histochemical methods (case I, Hassoun *et al.*, this symposium).

## TUMOR ANALYSIS

A tumoral fragment was extracted with 2M boiling acetic acid and the extract was filtered on a G-50 Sephadex column (2.5 × 200 cm). Fractions (8 ml) were collected and freeze-dried. Each of them was assayed for immunoreactive material. The column was calibrated with unlabeled βLPH (elution fraction F.48), βEND (F.67) and ACTH$_{1-39}$ (F.74) which despite having a larger size than βEND eluted reproducibly in a larger elution volume. In control runs no reactive material appeared in the void volume (F.38) indicating that there was no aggregation.

The immunoreactive peptides in the tumoral extract were resolved by gel filtration into five peaks (Fig. 1). Some information on the nature of the peptides contained in these peaks was inferred from their antigenic characteristics and elution volumes relative to markers. Peak I which was eluted in the void volume

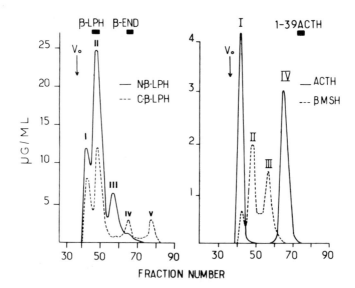

*Fig. 1.* Gel filtration profile on an ACTH-secreting pituitary adenoma extract. Sephadex G-50 (2.5 × 200 cm) equilibrated with 1M acetic acid. After freeze-drying, fractions (8 ml) were assayed in various radioimmunoassay systems. Right panel : N-βLPH RIA (full line), C-βLPH RIA (dotted line). Left panel : N-terminal ACTH RIA (full line), βMSH RIA (dotted line). Position of markers is indicated by closed rectangles.

(F. 38–40), contained material cross-reacting in the ACTH, βMSH, N- and C-βLPH assays, thus showing the immunological features of the prolipocortin precursor molecule. Peak II (F. 48) contained material co-eluting with the βLPH marker and cross-reacting in the βMSH, N- and C- terminal assays, thus resembling βLPH in all respects. Peak III (F. 56) migrated at an intermediate position between βLPH and βEND and disclosed the immunological characteristics of γLPH (competition in the βMSH and N-βLPH assays only). Peak IV (F. 66–67) included material showing ACTH and C-βLPH determinants and co-migrating with the βEND marker. The ACTH-like material eluting in this volume could not be immunoprecipitated by an excess of C-βLPH serum and therefore was not related to the C-βLPH immunoreactivity, which had the same chromatographic behavior as βEND. The ACTH-immunoreactive-like material migrating faster than native ACTH may either have a larger mol.wt and thus resemble one of the various "intermediate ACTH" already described (Eipper and Mains, 1976; Orth and Nicholson, 1977) or have slight structural modifications which would reduce its interaction with the gel matrix. Peak V (F. 77) contained only C-βLPH immunoreactivity. Because of its molecular size and antigenicity, this material should belong to the 77–91 part of βLPH, from the fact that γ endorphin (γEND) did not cross-react in the C-βLPH assay. Trace amounts of αMSH like material were found in the expected elution volume (F. 80) for a peptide of this size. No other slower migrating immunoreactive material could be detected in the column eluate, which was assayed completely. In all the assays, both the tumoral peptides and standards produced parallel dose-response curves (Fig. 2). It appeared therefore that the concentration of βLPH (taking into account cross-reaction ratios) was roughly 8 times greater than γLPH and 40 times greater than βEND.

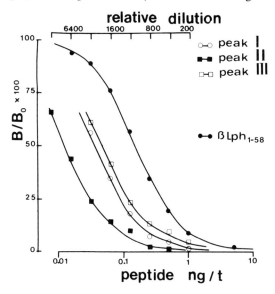

*Fig. 2.* Competitive inhibition of $^{125}$-I-labeled γLPH binding to the anti-hβLPH antiserum by unlabeled hγLPH and serial dilutions of the various N-βLPH immunoreactive peaks from gel filtration of an ACTH secreting pituitary tumor extract (Fig. 1).

The prolipocortin cross-reaction ratio was not tested. However, assuming a most favorable full cross-reaction, it would give a concentration of about two thirds that of $\beta$LPH. Similarly, the peak IV ACTH amount was one-tenth that of $\beta$LPH.


## DISCUSSION

Since the $\gamma$LPH and $\beta$END contents of the tumor were much lower than its $\beta$LPH content, it appears that the processing pathway of $\beta$LPH in this tumor was in this respect very similar to that of normal pituitary tissue and did not shift to an intermediate lobe-like differentiation pattern, in which almost all the $\beta$LPH appears to be processed. The finding of small amounts of $\alpha$MSH-like immuno-reactive material strengthens this interpretation. The presence of $\gamma$LPH and $\beta$END is probably related to artefactual proteolysis which has been shown to be enhanced by tissue freezing and to be only partially inhibited by extraction with boiling acetic acid. Similarly, the small amount of $\alpha$MSH-like material detected was most probably an ACTH degradation product (possibly $ACTH_{1-13}$, which cannot be distinguished from $\alpha$MSH in the assay used). No chromato-graphic analyses were performed on the plasma samples and extrapolation of its hormonal content from the knowledge of data obtained in the tumor could be hazardous, although parallelism between peptidic cell content and secretion has often been demonstrated. Nevertheless, estimation of plasma N- and C-$\beta$LPH, and ACTH activities yielded figures very different from those obtained in normal human plasma as well as in Cushing's disease (Krieger *et al.*, 1977; Jeffcoate *et al.*, 1978), and which demonstrated a good correlation between ACTH and $\beta$LPH in the basal state (ACTH/$\beta$LPH ratio fluctuating from 1.2 to 1.6), and after stimulation. These results correlated well with the concept that $\beta$LPH and ACTH arise from a common precursor molecule. On the contrary, in the case studied concentrations of N-$\beta$LPH and C-$\beta$LPH were 10 times and 5 times greater than that of ACTH-like material. Furthermore N- and C-$\beta$LPH regulation appeared to be dissociated from that of ACTH. Defects in the biosynthesis and/or the secretion mechanisms of ACTH could be suggested to be a workable explanation for this discrepancy.

The tumoral tissue differed from normal pituitary tissue, which was shown to contain mainly native ACTH (Yalow and Berson, 1971, 1973), in so far as it contains very large amounts of ACTH-like material in the form of precursor molecules (previously named big ACTH). Big ACTH has already been described as the major synthesis and secretion product of ectopic ACTH-producing tumors (Yalow and Berson, 1971). It has been shown in the medium of cultured human adenomatous cells (Krieger *et al.*, 1973) as well as in the plasma of a normal human tested with metyrapone (Yalow and Berson, 1971). The abnormal precursor content found in Cushing's disease could arise from a defect of the precursor-processing pathways and/or could be the reflection of highly stimulated state leading to the secretion of immature molecular forms. Further *in vivo* and *in vitro* studies are in progress to test this possibility. If validated, a search for precursor molecules in the plasma could be a valuable aid in the diagnosis of Cushing's disease.

## REFERENCES

Abe, K. D., Island, D., Liddle, G. W., Fleischer, N. and Nicholson, W. E. (1967). *J. Clin. Endocrinol. Metab.* **27**, 46–52.

Bachelot, I., Wolfen, A. R. and Odell, W. D. (1977) *J. Clin. Endocrinol. Metab.* **44**, 939–956.

Eipper, R. E. and Mains, B. A. (1976). *J. Biol. Chem.* **251**, 4115–4120.

Gilkes, J. J. H., Bloomfield, G. A., Scott, A. P., Lowry, P. J., Ratcliffe, J. G., Landon, J. and Rees, L. H. (1975). *J. Clin. Endocrinol. Metab.* **40**, 450–457.

Greer, M. A., Allen, C. F., Panton, P. and Allen, J. P. (1975). *Endocrinology* **96**, 718–724.

Jeffcoate, W. J., Rees, L. H., Lowry, P. J. and Besser, G. M. (1978). *J. Clin. Endocrinol. Metab.* **47**, 160–167.

Kraicer, J. and Morris, A. R. (1976). *Neuroendocrinology* **20**, 79–96.

Kraicer, J., Gosbee, J. L. and Bencosme, S. A. (1973). *Neuroendocrinology* **11**, 156–176.

Krieger, D. T., Choi, H. S. H. and Anderson, B. (1973). *Clin. Endocrinol.* **5**, 455–459.

Krieger, D. T., Liotta, A. and Li, C. H. (1977). *Life Science* **21**, 1971–1978

Liotta, A. S., Suda, T. and Krieger, D. (1978). *Proc. Natl. Acad. Sci., USA* **75**, 2950–2957.

Lissitzky, J. C., Morin, O., Dupont, A., Labrie, F., Seidah, N. G., Chretien, M., Lis, M. and Coy, D. H. (1978). *Life Science* **22**, 1715–1722.

Lowry, P. J. and Scott, A. P. (1975). *Gen. Comp. Endocrinol.* **26**, 16–23.

Mains, R. E., Eipper, B. A. and Ling, N. (1977). *Proc. Natl. Acad. Sci., USA* **74**, 3014–3018.

Orth, D. N. and Nicholson, W. E. (1977). *J. Clin. Endocrinol. Metab.* **44**, 214–217.

Raymond, V., Lepine, J., Lissitzky, J. C., Ferland, L. and Labrie, F. (1978) International Narcotic Research Conference, Noordwikerhout.

Roberts, J. L. and Herbert, E. (1977). *Proc. Natl. Acad. Sci., USA* **74**, 4826–4830.

Rubinstein, M., Stein, S., Gerber, L. D. and Udenfriend, S. (1977). *Proc. Natl. Acad. Sci., USA* **74**, 3052–3055.

Scott, A. P. and Lowry, P. J. (1974). *Biochem. J.* **139**, 593–602.

Scott, A. P., Lowry, P. J., Bennet, H. P. J., McMartin, C. and Ratcliffe, J. G. (1974). *J. Endocrinol.* **61**, 355–367.

Yalow, R. S. and Berson, S. A. (1971). *Biochem. Biophys. Res. Commun.* **44**, 439–445.

Yalow, R. S. and Berson, S. A. (1973). *J. Clin. Endocrinol. Metab.* **36**, 415–423.

# HYPOTHALAMIC CRF-ACTIVITY IN DOGS WITH PITUITARY-DEPENDENT HYPERADRENOCORTICISM: RELATION TO PATHOGENESIS

J. C. Meijer[1], G. H. Mulder[2], A. Rijnberk[1] and R. J. M. Croughs[3]

[1] *Small Animal Clinic, Veterinary Faculty, State University of Utrecht, The Netherlands.* [2] *Department of Pharmacology, Medical Faculty, Free University of Amsterdam, The Netherlands.* [3] *Third Department of Internal Medicine, University Hospital Dijkzigt, Rotterdam, The Netherlands*

## INTRODUCTION

Evidence for the pathogenesis of pituitary-dependent Cushing's syndrome in man is still controversial. The central question is whether the excessive secretion of adrenocorticotrophic hormone (ACTH) by the pituitary gland is due to a derangement at the hypothalamic or at the pituitary level.

An animal model for this disease, permitting more basic research, would be helpful in solving this controversy. In the dog, spontaneous hyperadrenocorticism is known to occur rather frequently (Rijnberk *et al.*, 1968). Canine Cushing's syndrome is most frequently associated with bilateral adrenocortical hyperplasia, but may also result from an adrenocortical tumour (Siegel *et al.*, 1967; Kelly *et al.*, 1971; Lubberink, 1977).

The pituitary-dependent form of this syndrome is characterized by an excessive and non-rhythmic secretion of cortisol and by the relative resistance of the elevated plasma cortisol levels to dexamethasone suppression (Meijer *et al.*, 1978).

These characteristics of canine pituitary-dependent hyperadrenocorticism, being identical with the hallmarks of pituitary-dependent Cushing's syndrome in man, were the reason to propose the canine disease as a model for the study of the pathogenesis of its human counterpart (Meijer *et al.*, 1978). Using this model, we have approached the study of the pathogenesis of pituitary-dependent hyperadrenocorticism by measuring corticotrophin-releasing factor (CRF) activity in extracts of hypothalamic tissue.

## METHODS

In five dogs with spontaneous hyperadrenocorticism the diagnosis was made from the results of a low dose dexamethasone suppression test. Relative resistance of the elevated plasma cortisol levels to suppression with dexamethasone was found in four dogs and led to the diagnosis of pituitary-dependent hyper-adrenocorticism, whereas absolute resistance to dexamethasone in the remaining dog was found to be concurrent with adrenocortical adenoma. For these dogs we obtained permission for further post-mortem examination and hypothalamic tissue was removed for measurement of CRF activity. In addition, CRF activity was measured in hypothalamic tissue from normal dogs, either untreated or treated with cortisone or corticotrophin for a period of two months in amounts sufficient to produce signs of hyperadrenocorticism.

Within 15 min of euthanasia, achieved by i.v. administration of pentobarbitone (100 mg/kg), a block of hypothalamic tissue was removed. The pituitary stalk was cut and a block of the hypothalamus including the median eminence was excised by cutting through the optic chiasm, along the lateral borders of the hypothalamus, and just posterior to the mammillary bodies, a final horizontal cut was made at a depth of 3 mm. The tissue was placed in ice cold 0.1 M-HCL and stored frozen at $-20°C$ until processed in the CRF-assay.

Extracts of hypothalamic tissue were used to stimulate isolated rat pituitary cells in a superfusion column. The amount of ACTH released into the superfusate was determined by an adrenal cortex cell bioassay. Details and evaluation of this procedure as an assay for CRF have been described by Mulder *et al.* (1976) and Mulder and Smelik (1977). The CRF activity in canine samples was expressed in terms of the resulting ACTH release, relative to the release of ACTH caused by a standard rat HME preparation. The doses of dog preparations used were equivalent to 1/25 of the hypothalamus, while the standard rat preparation (HME) was equivalent to 1 rat hypothalamus.

## RESULTS

The CRF activities of hypothalamic extracts of the eight dogs studied have been summarized in Table I.

Hypothalamic CRF content of normal dogs was not influenced by treatment with cortisone or corticotrophin. In all dogs with spontaneous hyperadrenocorticism, irrespective of its etiology, hypothalamic CRF content was low, and in two cases even undetectable.

*Table I.* CRF activity in hypothalamic extracts of control dogs and of dogs with spontaneous hyperadrenocorticism.

| Dog | Sex (M/F) | Age (y) | Diagnosis/treatment | Duration of the disease or treatment (Months) | Relative hypothalamic CRF activity (%) |
|---|---|---|---|---|---|
| 1 | M | 5 | control, none | – | 100 |
| 2 | M | 6 | control, cortisone | 2 | 99 |
| 3 | F | 6 | control, corticotrophin | 2 | 92 |
| 4 | F | 5 | p.d. HAC[a] | 6 | 0 |
| 5 | F | 7 | p.d. HAC | 8 | 40 |
| 6 | F | 11 | p.d. HAC, pituitary tumor | 4 | 47 |
| 7 | M | 9 | p.d. HAC, pituitary tumor | 7 | 0 |
| 8 | M | 12 | adrenocortical adenoma | 10 | 57 |

[a] Pituitary-dependent hyperadrenocorticism.

## DISCUSSION

Several theories postulating a defect at the hypothalamic or central level in pituitary-dependent Cushing's syndrome are subject to criticism.

The lack of responsiveness of plasma corticosteroids to insulin-induced hypoglycaemia in subjects with pituitary-dependent Cushing's syndrome was interpreted as indicating a fundamental defect at the hypothalamic or cerebral level (James *et al.*, 1968). The possibility that this phenomenon might be secondary to hypercorticism *per se* was ruled out by the authors because of the observation that administration of corticosteroids or ACTH to normal subjects was less effective in reducing the plasma corticosteroid response to insulin-induced hypoglycaemia than a similar degree of hypercorticism in patients with pituitary-dependent Cushing's syndrome. However, their arguments are invalidated by the observation of a recurrence of responsiveness of plasma ACTH to insulin-induced hypoglycaemia after correction of hypercortisolism by bilateral adrenalectomy (Croughs *et al.*, 1977).

The lack of responsiveness of plasma growth hormone to insulin-induced hypoglycaemia in subjects with pituitary-dependent Cushing's syndrome was interpreted as indicating a central origin of the disease (Krieger and Glick, 1972). These observations were made both in untreated patients and in patients treated by irradiation of the pituitary, in some of them combined with partial adrenalectomy (Krieger and Glick, 1972). However, recently Tyrrell *et al.* (1977) convincingly demonstrated the return of normal growth hormone responsiveness to insulin-induced hypoglycaemia in subjects with pituitary-dependent Cushing's syndrome after correction of hypercortisolism by bilateral adrenalectomy.

Partial restoration of growth hormone responsiveness to insulin-induced hypoglycaemia in pituitary-dependent Cushing's syndrome after pre-treatment with the dopamine agonist bromocriptine was the main argument underlying the postulation of a localized dopaminergic depletion in this disease (Lamberts *et al.*, 1977). However, no control studies were performed. The observations can also be explained by the significant decrease in the plasma cortisol levels following pre-treatment with bromocriptine.

In summary, it appears that the above mentioned theories are based on a specific phenomena related to hypercorticism *per se*.

The cyproheptadine-induced remission in three patients with pituitary-dependent Cushing's syndrome (Krieger *et al.*, 1975) was interpreted as indicating a disturbance in serotoninergic control of hypothalamic CRF secretion in this disease. However, no restoration of normal regulation of pituitary-adrenocortical function was found. Cortisol secretion remained non-rhythmic and a paradoxical response of urinary steroid excretion was found after administration of high doses of dexamethasone. Recently, return of normal circadian periodicity of plasma ACTH concentration has been observed in a patient with Nelson's syndrome after longterm therapy with cypropheptadine (Krieger and Condon, 1978). This observation is very interesting, but direct evidence for an exclusively central action of the drug is still lacking. In fact, high concentrations of serotonin have also been found in the anterior pituitary gland (Piezzi *et al.*, 1970), which may be another site of action of cyproheptadine.

The therapeutic value of cyproheptadine appears to be limited. Remissions of pituitary-dependent Cushing's syndrome have been demonstrated in some studies, but temporary improvement or negative results have been found more frequently.

In dogs with pituitary-dependent hyperadrenocorticism we could not demonstrate any effect of cyproheptadine therapy (Meijer *et al.*, unpublished observations).

In contrast to the above-mentioned theory, the results of sophisticated pituitary surgery involving selective removal of pituitary adenomas (Lagerquist *et al.*, 1974; Bigos *et al.*, 1977; Salassa *et al.*, 1978; Tyrrell *et al.*, 1978) point to a primary pituitary origin of pituitary-dependent Cushing's syndrome. Following removal of pituitary adenomas these authors found complete restoration of the pituitary-adrenal system and normal cortisol production rates.

In the present study we have demonstrated evidence for a considerably reduced hypothalamic CRF content in dogs with spontaneous hyper-adrenocroticism.

Decreased hypothalamic CRF content has also been found in rats after treatment with corticosteroids *in vivo* (Buckingham and Hodges, 1977). Jones *et al.* (1976) found that corticosterone *in vitro* had inhibitory effects on synthesis as well as on release of CRF, resulting in either unchanged or increased CRF contents, depending on the moment of observation after treatment with steroid. Thus, hypothalamic CRF content may not be directly related to CRF secretion.

Nevertheless it is likely that the rate of secretion of CRF is low in the presence of persistently high concentrations of cortisol in the plasma, regardless of whether this hypercortisolaemia is produced by the administration of cortisone or ACTH or by an adrenocortical tumour. Under the latter circumstances, there may eventually be a secondary inhibition of CRF production. The absence of any difference in hypothalamic CRF activity between normal dog 1 and dogs 2 and 3 with iatrogenic Cushing's syndrome may be explained by the short period of treatment and by the intermittent character of hypercortisolaemia in dogs 2 and 3. In contrast, hypothalamic CRF activity was low in dog 8, which had long-standing permanent cortisol excess due to an adrenocortical adenoma.

In the four dogs with pituitary-dependent hyperadrenocorticism, the low or even undetectable hypothalamic CRF contents can either be explained by longstanding persistent hypercortisolaemia, fitting with a primary pituitary etiology, or by assuming an abnormal CRF secretion which continues at a rate which does not permit storage of CRF within the hypothalamus. In the latter case the occurrence of pituitary adenomas then can be thought to result from excessive stimulation of ACTH-producing cells by CRF. Differentiation between these two possible etiologies can only be made after measurement of CRF dynamics, involving CRF secretion into the hypothalamo-hypophysial portal blood in various disease states. Therefore, at present the etiologies of both canine pituitary-dependent hyper-adrenocorticism and pituitary-dependent Cushing's syndrome remain uncertain. Furthermore it is unclear whether this disease is a homogenous entity or whether several subgroups do exist.

## REFERENCES

Bigos, S. T., Robert, F., Pelletier, G. and Hardy, J. (1977). *J. clin. Endocr. Metab.* **45**, 1251-1260.

Buckingham, J. C. and Hodges, J. R. (1977). *J. Endocr.* **74**, 297-302.

Croughs, R. J. M., Timmermans, H., Vingerhoeds, A. C. M., Vermeulen, A., Smals, A., Kloppenborg, P. W. C. and Meyer, J. C. (1977). *Acta Endocr.* **86**, 578-582.

James, V. H. T., Landon, J., Wynn, V. and Greenwood, F. C. (1968). *J. Endocr.* **40**, 15-28.

Jones, M. T., Hillhouse, E. and Burden, J. (1976). *In* "Frontiers in Neuro-endocrinology" (L. Martini and W. Ganong, eds.) vol. 4, 195-226. Raven Press, New York.

Kelly, D. F., Siegel, E. T. and Berg, P. (1971). *Vet. Path.* **8**, 385-400.

Krieger, D. T. and Glick, S. M. (1972). *Am. J. Med.* **52**, 25-40.

Krieger, D. T. and Condon, E. M. (1978). *J. clin. Endocr. Metab.* **46**, 349-352.

Krieger, D. T., Amoroso, L. and Linick, F. (1975). *New Engl. J. Med.* **293**, 893-896.

Lagerquist, L. G., Meikle, A. W., West, C. D. and Tyler, F. H. (1974). *Am. J. Med.* **57**, 826-830.

Lamberts, S. W. J., Timmermans, H. A. T., de Jong, F. H. and Birkenhäger, J. C. (1977). *Clin. Endocr.* **7**, 185-193.

Lubberink, A. A. M. E. (1977). Diagnosis and Treatment of Canine Cushing's Syndrome. Ph. D. Thesis, University of Utrecht, Drukkerij Elinkwijk, Utrecht.

Meijer, J. C., de Bruijne, J. J., Rijnberk, A. and Croughs, R. J. M. (1978). *J. Endocr.* **77**, 111-118.

Mulder, G. H. and Smelik, P. G. (1977). *Endocrinology* **100**, 1143-1152.

Mulder, G. H., Vermes, I. and Smelik, P. G. (1976). *Neuroscience Letters* **2**, 73-78.

Piezzi, R. S., Larin, F. and Wurtman, R. J. (1970). *Endocrinology* **86**, 1460-1462.

Rijnberk, A., der Kinderen, P. J. and Thijssen, J. H. H. (1968). *J. Endocr.* 41, 397–406.

Salassa, R. M., Laws, E. R., Carpenter, P. C. and Northcutt, R. C. (1978). *Mayo Clin. Proc.* 53, 24–28.

Siegel, E. T., O'Brien, J. B., Pyle, L. and Schryver, H. F. (1967). *J. Am. vet. med. Ass.* 150, 760–766.

Tyrrell, J. B., Wiener-Kronish, J., Lorenzi, M., Brooks, R. M. and Forsham, P. H. (1977). *J. clin. Endocr. Metab.* 44, 218–221.

Tyrrell, J. B., Brooks, R. M., Fitzgerald, P. A., Cofoid, P. B., Forsham, P. H. and Wilson, C. B. (1978). *New Engl. J. Med.* 298, 753–758.

# DIFFERENT CORTICOID FEEDBACK EFFECTS ON ADENOMATOUS AND ANTERIOR LOBE TISSUE IN CUSHING'S DISEASE * †

D. K. Lüdecke[1], J. Bansemer[1], J. Resetić[2] and M. Westphal[1]

[1] *Department of Neurosurgery, University of Hamburg, West Germany*
[2] *Department of Endocrinology, University of Zagreb, Yugoslavia*

## INTRODUCTION

The good results in Cushing's disease (C.D.) of selective adenomectomy reported by several investigators (i.e. Hardy, 1973; Müller and Fahlbusch, 1978; Wilson and Dempsey, 1978; Salassa *et al.*, 1978) and ourselves supply the most practical argument for the concept that the essential defect of C.D. lies within the ACTH-cell adenoma. On the other hand, the assumption of a primary hypothalamic disturbance is supported by the absence of adenomas in several cases (Saeger, 1974) which could be cured by hypophysectomy (Lüdecke *et al.*, 1976). Several abnormalities of ACTH regulation (Fehm *et al.*, 1978) and therapeutic effects e.g. of antiserotonergic drugs (Krieger *et al.*, 1975), led to the discussion that a heterogeneous group of disorders might be causes of C.D. (Liddle, 1977).

Nevertheless a decrease in the negative glucocorticoid feedback is characteristic for all cases of C.D. Therefore, we employed different *in vitro* methods to study the direct actions of cortisol on human ACTH cell adenomas as well as on para-adenomatous pituitary tissue. Our knowledge about the mechanism in the human pituitary tissue, especially in C.D., is still limited (Bansemer *et al.*, 1976) whereas the direct negative corticoid feedback has been well established in

*Supported by Deutsche Forschungsgemeinschaft, SFB 34 – D1 –
† This paper is dedicated to Prof. Dr. R. Kautzky on his 65th birthday.

pituitary tissues of animals, e.g. by Fleischer and Vale (1968), Portanova and Sayers (1973) and Mulder and Smelik (1977).

A summary of our results, which will be the subject of more detailed publications elsewhere, will be given here.

## MATERIALS AND METHODS

### General methods

Tissue for *in vitro* studies was obtained by transnasal operations*, from patients with Cushing's disease, with or without pituitary adenomas and from cases of palliative hypophysectomy for cancer. In the last six cases of C.D., a selective adenomectomy was performed but a small specimen of anterior lobe was also removed. The extent of the studies had to be adapted to the material available. Portions of the tissues were always taken for parallel microscopic evaluation†. Immediately after removal, all suspensions were prepared as described by Portanova *et al.* (1970) by mild trypsination and mechanical agitation. The cells were resuspended in KRBG buffer with trypsin inhibitor (LBI, Sigma).

### Static incubation

Aliquots of 900 $\mu$l of all suspensions were transferred to Teflon® beakers. Parallel incubations of at least triplicates were carried out in a Dubnoff metabolic shaker for 15, 30, 60 and 75 min. The following substances were used: hydrocortisone (Hoechst), lysin-vasopressin (LVP, Ferring or Sandoz), Dexamethasone (Merck) and pressinoic acid (Ferring). Medium and cells were separated by high speed centrifugation and deep frozen for later ACTH assay.

### Superfusion system

Aliquots of 1 ml of the cell medium were transferred to 6 superfusion chambers which were constructed according to Mulder and Smelik (1977). The various substances were added to the continuous flow of the medium (Fig. 4), 1.2 ml of which was collected over 3 min intervals. ACTH was measured by RIA, using the method of Berson and Yalow (1968), and most samples were also measured by the bioassay of Sayers *et al.* (1971).

### Perioperatively

Perioperatively serial ACTH and cortisol plasma levels were measured by RIA. Substitution therapy was administered according to clinical needs (Lüdecke *et al.*, 1978).

---

*Operations performed by either R. Kautzky or D. K. Lüdecke.
†Microscopic work done by W. Saeger, Institute of Pathology, UKE.

### Statistical analyses

These were performed by the Student's *t*-test (static incubation), Bartlett's test for nonhomogenous variances and Anova for uneven subclasses (superfusion system).

## RESULTS

### Perioperative ACTH and cortisol plasma levels

In five cases of selective adenomectomy, the perioperative ACTH and cortisol levels measured can be seen in Fig. 1. ACTH and cortisol decreased to a subnormal range in four of five cases. Clinical and laboratory evidence of ACTH deficiency persisted for different time intervals up to six months. The patient who did not demonstrate this defect, but had normal plasma ACTH levels, developed a recurrence after a short remission of about six months.

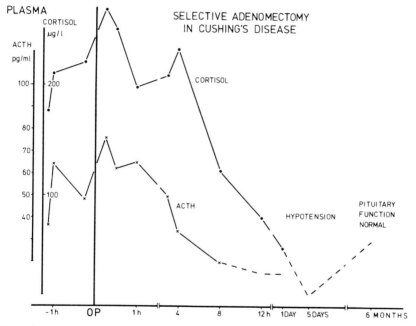

*Fig. 1.* Plasma ACTH (RIA) and cortisol levels during and after selective adenomectomy in Cushing's disease.

### Static incubation

*Basal ACTH secretion*

As shown in Fig. 2, basal ACTH release by anterior lobe (a.l.) tissue in C.D. varies widely as compared with that of normal a.l. tissue obtained by

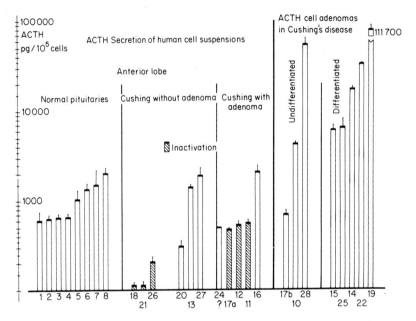

**Fig. 2.** Spontaneous ACTH release (bioassay) by isolated human pituitary cells of various origin. Inactivation: predominant Crooke's hyaline changes

hypophysectomy from cases with carcinomas. In three cases without adenomas, which microscopically showed merely inactivation signs (Crooke's hyaline changes), ACTH secretion was nearly abolished. These were special cases which were not cured by hypophysectomy. Ectopic ACTH secretion must be assumed.

In most of the cases with ACTH-cell adenomas, the ACTH release from a.l. tissue was significantly lower than in cases of palliative hypophysectomy.

ACTH secretion by undifferentiated adenomas was relatively low. These adenomas were larger in size than the others.

*Corticoid feedback*

(a) In the case of normal hypophyseal cells, the basal ACTH secretion could be suppressed by cortisol or dexamethasone. The stimulatory effect of LVP was decreased but not completely suppressed in most cases. One case showed a paradoxical response to the addition of corticoids. Microscopically, ACTH-cell hyperplasias were detected in this case.

(b) Pituitary cells without concomitant adenoma in Cushing's disease were studied in six cases. Three cases have to be excluded (Fig. 2, cases 18, 21, 26) for the reasons explained. Of the remaining three cases, two did not respond to corticoids. Only one showed an inhibitory effect of cortisol on LVP stimulation.

(c) Para-adenomatous tissue in C.D. showed a "paradoxical" rise in ACTH secretion after incubation with corticoids in two of five cases. This effect was significant in one case after a 15 min incubation. Higher doses produced an adverse effect. LVP stimulation was enhanced once. In general, the effects were equivalent to those on normal pituitary tissue.

(d) In the case of adenomatous tissue six of seven cases exhibited a "paradoxical" rise in ACTH in response to corticoids, as shown in Fig. 3. However, the effects were heterogeneous with respect to incubation time and doses applied. In two cases the stimulation was present only at 15 min and later no significant changes were seen. In all these cases, incubation of cortisol together with LVP or pressinoic acid enhanced the ACTH release.

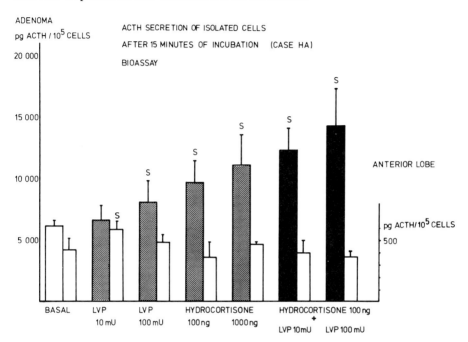

*Fig. 3.* ACTH secretion by isolated cells from Cushing's disease in a static incubation system. Significant (S) enhancement by cortisol of basal and LVP stimulated ACTH secretion in adenoma cells. Significant suppression of LVP stimulation by cortisol in para-adenomatous cells.

(e) Feedback action of cortisol and LVP were studied twice in the adenomatous and para-adenomatous tissues of the same patient.

Figure 3 summarizes the results of various incubations after 15 min. While the basal secretion of the anterior lobe cells was not significantly influenced by the presence of cortisol in the medium, the adenoma cells exhibited a marked increase in ACTH secretion.

LVP induced a release of ACTH in both tissue types. The effect of LVP was diminished by cortisol co-incubation in the case of anterior lobe cells. The adenoma cells, on the other hand, showed a paradoxical additional ACTH release.

These results were reproduced in an additional case. The divergent effects of cortisol and, in this case of dexamethasone as well, were most marked after 30 min of incubation. Dexamethasone had a stimulatory effect on adenoma cells and an inhibitory effect on anterior lobe cells.

Basal ACTH secretion by anterior lobe cells was significantly suppressed by cortisol, whereas no influence on adenoma cells was seen. Pressinoic acid, which as an inconstant CRF-like activity (Jones *et al.*, 1976) was without effect alone but caused a significant ACTH release in combination with cortisol.

### Superfusion system

In three additional patients, the reactivities of adenoma and pituitary cells to LVP and cortisol were compared using a superfusion technique. By this method, kinetic studies can be better adapted to the *in vivo* situation. In one case the para-adenomatous tissue exhibited an initial "paradoxical" rise in response to cortisol, identical to that of the adenoma. In another case a suppressive effect of cortisol on adenomatous and nonadenomatous cells was found, as can be seen in Fig. 4. Whereas LVP stimulation was completely abolished in the a.l. tissue, it was still present in the adenoma cells.

After cessation of cortisol addition, ACTH release from the a.l. cells increased significantly. In the third case similar results were reproduced.

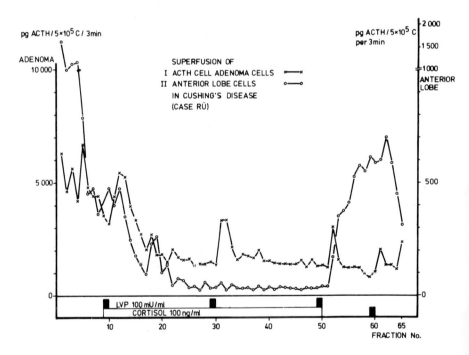

*Fig. 4.* ACTH secretion (RIA) by isolated cells from Cushing's disease in a superfusion system. In adenomatous tissue (upper curve, left scale), all LVP stimulations were significant. They were not seen in para-adenomatous cells (lower curve, right scale) after cortisol addition. Suppression of basal ACTH release by cortisol was evident in both tissue types.

## DISCUSSION

The transient subnormal ACTH secretion in cases of successful selective adenomectomy supports the concept of an inhibition of the para-adenomatous ACTH cells. This mechanism was found by other authors as well (Liddle, 1977; Salassa *et al.*, 1978; Kageyama, 1978, personal communication). Though longer follow-ups are still limited, these findings are best explained by the presence of an autonomous adenoma rather than a primary CRF hypersecretion. Most of our results from *in vitro* studies are concordant with the theory of an intact corticoid feedback on the para-adenomatous tissue in C.D. On the other hand, throughout all our experiments with C.D., corticoids did not adequately suppress LVP-induced ACTH secretion in ACTH cell adenomas. A paradoxical positive feedback of cortisol could be demonstrated. Because of the fast response, a mechanism different from nuclear steroid actions must be considered. Kummer *et al.* (1978), who found the equivalent in sophisticated *in vivo* studies, came to the conclusion that C.D. is characterized by a conversion of the negative rate-sensitive steroid feedback mechanism into a positive one, while the delayed dose-sensitive feedback mechanism remains undisturbed. We found this type of reaction in the superfusion system as well. These findings indicate a pathological differentiation of receptor sites in adenoma cells, whereas the ACTH cells of the adjacent anterior lobe usually seem to be intact. However, it must be taken into consideration that microscopic and *in vitro* findings in some exceptional cases have given evidence of a disturbance of ACTH cells in the para-adenomatous tissue as well. The clinical significance of these results is still unclear.

From our new results and the results of the authors quoted in the introduction, we would now come to the conclusion that for case of circumscribed adenomas in Cushing's disease, selective adenomectomy should be the first step in therapy.

## REFERENCES

Bansemer, J., Lüdecke, D., Neuss, M., Resetic, J. and Saeger, W. (1976). $V^{th}$ *Internat. Congr. Endocrinology, Abstract* **497**, 203.

Berson, A. and Yalow, S. (1968). *Clin. Invest.* **47**, 2725.

Fehm, H. L., Voigt, K. H. and Pfeiffer, E. F. (1978). *In* "Treatment of Pituitary Adenomas" (R. Fahlbusch and K. V. Werder, eds) pp. 77–86. Thieme Verlag, Stuttgart.

Fleischer, N. and Vale, W. (1968). *Endocrinology* **83**, 1232.

Hardy, J. (1973). *In* "Diagnosis and Treatment of Pituitary Tumors" (P. O. Kohler and G. T. Ross, eds) pp. 197–198. Exerpta Medica, Amsterdam.

Jones, M. T., Hillhouse, E. and Burden J. (1976). *In* "Frontiers in Neuroendocrinology" (L. Martini and W. F. Ganong, eds) Vol. 4, 195–226. Raven Press, New York.

Krieger, D. T., Amorosa, L. and Linick, F. (1975). *N. Engl. J. Med.* **293**, 893.

Kummer, G., Beinart, K. E. and Lang, R. (1978). *Acta endocr. (Kbh) (Suppl.* 215) **21**, 13.

Liddle, G. W. (1977). *In* "ACTH and Related Peptides: Structure, Regulation and Action" (D. T. Krieger and W. F. Ganong, eds) Vol. 297, 594–601, Annals of the New York Academy of Science, New York.

Lüdecke, D., Kautzky, R., Saeger, W. and Schrader, D. (1976). *Acta Neurochirurgica* **35**, 27.

Lüdecke, D., Kautzky, R., Bansemer, J. and Montz, H. R. (1978). *In* "Treatment of Pituitary Adenomas" (R. Fahlbusch and K. v. Werder, eds). Thieme Verlag, Stuttgart.

Mulder, G. H. and Smelik, P. G. (1977). *Endocrinology* **100**, 1143–1152.

Muller, O. A. and Fahlbusch, R. (1978). *Acta endocr. (Kbh.) (Suppl.* 215) **21**, 23–24.

Portanova, R. and Sayers, G. (1973). *Neuroendocrinology* **12**, 236–248.

Portanova, R., Smith, D. K. and Sayers, G. (1970). *Exp. Biol. Med.* **133**, 573–576.

Saeger, W. (1974). *Virchows Arch. Path. Anat. Histol.* **362**, 73–88.

Salassa, R. M., Laws, E. R., Carpenter, P. C. and Northcutt, R. C. (1978). *Majo Clinic Proc.* **53**, 24–28.

Sayers, G., Swallow, R. L. and Giordano, N. D. (1971). *Endocrinology* **88**, 1063.

Wilson, C. B. and Dempsey, L. C. (1978). *J. Neurosurg.* **48**, 13–22.

# PITUITARY BASOPHILIC ADENOMA. OPTIC, ELECTRON MICROSCOPIC AND IMMUNOCYTOCHEMICAL STUDY OF FOUR CASES*

J. Hassoun[1], C. Charpin[1], J. C. Lissitsky[2], C. Oliver[2], P. Jaquet[3] and M. Toga[1]

[1] *Laboratoire de Neuropathologie, Faculté de Médecine, 27, Bd Jean Moulin, 13385 Marseille Cedex IV, France*
[2] *Laboratoire de Médecine expérimentale, Faculté de Médecine Nord, Bd Pierre Dramard, 13015 Marseille, France*
[3] *Laboratoire des Hormones protéiques, Faculté de Médecine, 27 Bd Jean Moulin, 13385 Marseille Cédex IV, France*

Pituitary basophilic adenomas are classically found in patients with Cushing's disease. From a morphological point of view, ACTH and MSH production have been correlated with tumor cells on the basis of their histochemical and ultrastructural similarities with normal cortico-melanotrophic cells (Olivier *et al.*, 1975). However, only very few studies using immunocytochemical methods were performed on these tumors (Bigos *et al.*, 1977). It seemed interesting to investigate our own cases with such methods which possess a greater specificity and to look for the presence of ACTH, βLPH derived from the same molecule, "31 K" (Mains *et al.*, 1977) or "big ACTH" (Lazarus *et al.*, 1976) and correlated hormonal peptides such as MSH, endorphin and enkephalins. Four basophilic adenomas were investigated in patients with Cushing's disease proved on a clinical and biological basis. Case 1 is extensively described elsewhere in this symposium (Lissitzky *et al.*).

---

*We are grateful to Dr. P. J. Lowry for his gift of anti-hβLPH serum and purified hβLPH. We thank Mrs. M. N. Lavaut for her helpful technical assistance.

## MATERIAL AND METHODS

Fragments from the four tumors were fixed in Bouin Hollande and embedded in paraffin for optic microscopy. Five micron thick sections were stained with Herlant's tetrachrome, PAS, and Lead-hematoxylin. Other tumor fragments were fixed in 2.5% or 3.7% glutaraldehyde in cacodylate buffer, post-fixed in 1% osmic acid in the same buffer, dehydrated and embedded in araldite for electron microscopy. Ultrathin sections were stained with lead citrate uranyl acetate and photographed with an electron microscope Philips EM 300. Immunoperoxidase reactions were studied by optic microscopy in the four cases and by electron microscopy in cases 1, 2 and 4. using an unlabeled peroxidase-anti-peroxidase complex according to Sternberger (1974) and rabbit sera prepared against porcine purified ACTH (dilution : 1/500), synthetic $\alpha$MSH (1/250), purified h$\beta$LPH (1/500), synthetic $\beta$ endorphin (1/500), synthetic Leucine-enkaphalin (1/500) and synthetic methionine-enkephalin (1/100). Anti-$\alpha$MSH serum (Usategui et al., 1976) cross-reacted with ACTH 1–13 (100 % on a molar basis) but not with ACTH 1–39, 1–24, 4–10, 11–24, 25–39. Anti-Leucine-enkephalin serum cross-reacted only with methionine-enkephalin (3 % on a molar basis) and anti-methionine-enkephalin serum only with Leucine-enkephalin (5 %). Anti-$\beta$ endorphin (anti-$\beta$LPH-COOH terminal determinant) serum cross-reacted only with h$\beta$LPH (50 % on a molar basis). Anti-$\beta$LPH and anti-ACTH sera were heterogeneous and were partially immunoabsorbed with various peptides (anti-$\beta$LPH serum with ACTH 1–39, $\beta$ endorphin, $\alpha$ MSH, met- and Leu-enkephalin; anti-ACTH serum with h$\beta$LPH, h$_\beta$endorphin, $\alpha$ MSH, $\beta$ MSH, met- and Leu-enkephalin). Anti-$\beta$ LPH serum, so prepared, cross-reacted only with h$\beta$ LPH and not with ACTH, h $\beta$ endorphin, or $\alpha$ MSH. Partially immunoabsorbed anti-ACTH serum cross-reacted with ACTH 1–24 and 1–39 but not with ACTH 17–39, 4–10, 11–24, 1–10 and 34–39, $\alpha$ MSH, $\beta$ LPH, or h$\beta$ endorphin. For all anti-sera, negative controls were obtained by substituting totally immunoabsorbed sera and/or normal rabbit serum.

## RESULTS

### Optic microscopy

The histological features of the four adenomas were very similar (Fig. 1). The tumors displayed a massive architecture with some papillary pattern in cases 1 and 3. The tumors cells were ovoid or angular in shape. The nuclei were often bizarre and showed obvious nucleoli. Mitoses were rare. With Herlant's tetrachrome, tumor cells showed basophilic cytoplasm and secretory granules in all cases. Moreover, in case 3, erythrosinophilic granules were observed in some cells. PAS and Lead-hematoxylin were positive in the four cases, especially in case 1.

### Electron microscopy

In the three cases investigated by electron microscopy (cases 1, 2 and 4), the nuclei of the tumor cells were irregularly outlined, showing deep invaginations of the nuclear membrane, a densely packed chromatin and one or

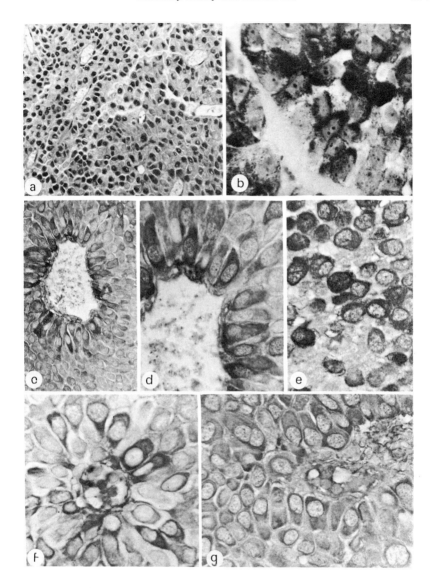

*Fig. 1.* Basophilic adenoma: optic microscopy.
a, General view of a massive pituitary tumor (Herlant's tetrachrome. × 190). b, Lead-hematoxylin staining ( × 500). c, Immunocytochemical staining with anti-ACTH serum ( × 190). d, Detail of "c" ( × 500). e, Staining with anti-βLPH serum ( × 500).
f, Staining with anti-leucine enkephalin serum ( × 500). g, Staining with anti-methionine enkephalin serum ( × 500).

two nucleoli. The granule content of the cytoplasm varied from one case to another. In cases 1 and 4, secretory granules were located beneath the plasma membrane or gathered in clumps in the juxta-nuclear area. Some aspects of exocytosis were seen as well as granules free in the extra-cellular space. The

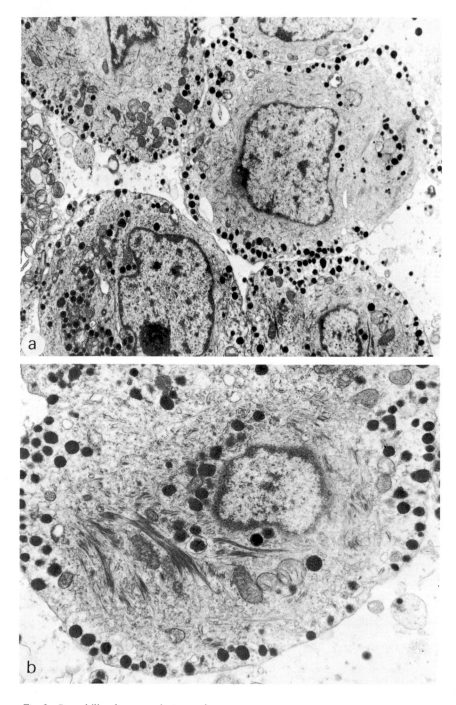

*Fig. 2.* Basophilic adenoma: electron microscopy.
a, Tumor cells dissociated by edema ( × 5140). b, Crooke cell with characteristic
filamentous bundles and marginal secretory granules ( × 9000).

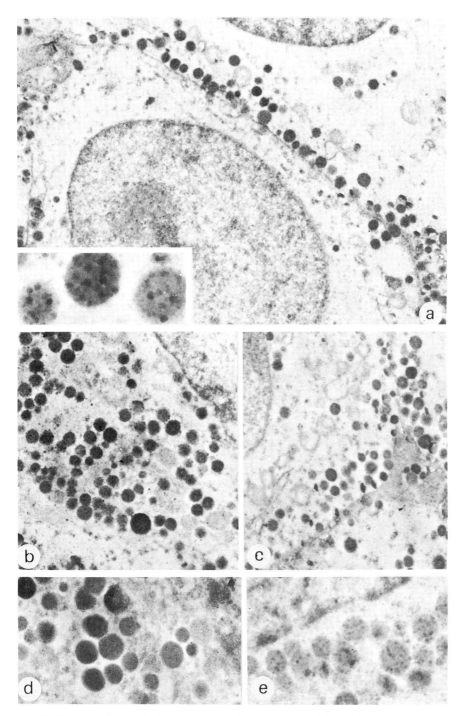

*Fig. 3.* Electron microscopic immunocytochemistry. Immunostaining of the secretory granules of the tumor cells with anti-ACTH serum (a, × 12 600; insert, × 40 000), anti-αMSH serum (b, × 16 000), anti-βendorphin serum (c, × 12 600), anti-Leu-enkephalin (d, × 24 500) and anti-met-enkephalin (e, × 24 500) sera.

granules were 180 $\mu$m in diameter (ranging from 120 to 200 $\mu$m). Numerous 70 A$^\circ$ cytoplasmic filaments formed thick and waved fibrils, especially in case 1 where they filled the major part of some cells (Fig. 2). In case 2, secretory granules were more regularly spread throughout the cytoplasma. Their average diameter was 320 $\mu$m. Mitochondria were increased in number and pleiomorphic. Filaments were not obvious in this case. In all cases, blood capillaries showed fenestrated endothelial cells with numerous pinocytotic vesicules and Weibel-Palade tubular bodies.

### Immunoperoxidase study

Immunoperoxidase reactions were studied in the four cases, by optic microscopy only in case 3, by optic and electron microscopy in the other cases. The same anti-sera were applied to 5 $\mu$m paraffin sections, 1 $\mu$m and ultrathin araldite sections. Electron microscopic immunocytochemical reactions appeared to be more discriminative and revealed some positive granules in cells which seemed to be negative by optic microscopy. Cells and granules were considered positive only when control immuno-absorbed anti-sera or normal rabbit serum gave negative results on serial sections. Only anti-ACTH and anti-methionine-enkephalin sera gave positive reactions with the four adenomas. The other anti-sera gave various reactions from one case to another (Fig. 3). The intensity of

*Table I.*   Immunoperoxidase reactions of the four basophilic adenomas with anti-ACTH, anti-$\alpha$MSH, anti-$\beta$LPH, anti-$\beta$endorphin, anti-leucine-enkephalin, anti-methionine-enkephalin sera.

| Patient | Antiserum | ACTH 1/500 | $\alpha$MSH 1/250 | $\beta$LPH 1/500 | $\beta$Endor. 1/500 | Leu - Enk. 1/500 | Met - Enk. 1/1000 |
|---|---|---|---|---|---|---|---|
| 1. Ben. . . | | + | + | + | + | + | + |
| 2. Per . . . | | + | – | + | + | – | + |
| 3. Art . . . | | + | + | + | + | + | + |
| 4. Gui. . . | | + | – | – | – | + | + |

The dilution is indicated for each antiserum. This table summarizes optic and/or electron microscopy data.

positiveness varied according to the anti-serum and to the case; but in each case, the positive cells were always the same in serial sections whatever the antiserum. Moreover, they were always prominent around the vessels. In all positive cases, only a few cells or granules appeared negative. Table 1 summarizes the results of the immuno-cytochemical reactions in the four cases.

## COMMENTS

From a clinical point of view, all cases showed typical signs of Cushing's disease. However, case 1 presented only slight facial dysmorphism but a striking brown pigmentation of the skin. In all patients plasma ACTH concentrations were increased or at the upper limit of normal level but with loss of circadian periodicity; plasma cortisol and urinary 17-OHCS leves were increased and sensitive to suppression by dexamethasone. These results agreed with the diagnosis of Cushing's disease by ACTH-secreting pituitary adenoma.

Histologically, all the tumors were basophilic with Herlant's tetrachrome. No chromophobe adenoma was found, as has been described (Racadot *et al.*, 1973). Case 3 showed fine erythrosinophilic intra-cytoplasmic granules as noted also by Herlant and Decourt (1964) in Cushing adenomas. As expected, PAS and Lead hematoxylin were positive in the four cases. All these aspects are classically found in ACTH-MSH pituitary adenomas (Racadot *et al.*, 1973).

The fine structure of these tumors corresponded to previous descriptions (Olivier *et al.*, 1975). The two categories of secretory granules (180–320 µm) were also reported by Landolt (1975). Tumor cells loaded with filamentous bundles were similar to Crooke's cells as described by electron microscopy by Porcile and Racadot (1966) in non-tumoral Cushing pituitary and by Landolt (1975) in ACTH adenoma secondary to Addison's disease.

Immunocytochemical data deserve more extensive comments. Specific ACTH immunoreactivity was demonstrated in the four tumors by optic and electron microscopy. However such expected results were only reported by Bigos *et al.* (1977) in a Cushing microadenoma, using immunocytochemical staining. Likewise, Tramu *et al.* (1978) could demonstrate ACTH 17–39 in a basophilic adenoma without clinical or biological hypercorticism. On the other hand, Kovacks *et al.* (1978) in a similar case proved the presence of ACTH 1–24. In our cases, with the anti-serum cross-reacting with both ACTH 1–24 and ACTH 1–39, it was not possible to rule out the presence of the C-terminal fragment of corticotropin. With radioimmunoassay coupled with gel filtration of Cushing adenoma extracts and culture medium, Krieger *et al.* (1976) found an ACTH of large molecular size which could correspond to a tumoral pro-hormone. This possibility has been confirmed in our case 1 by similar methods (see Lissitzky *et al.* in this symposium).

The presence of βMSH in Cushing adenoma or in the plasma of the patients had been demonstrated by radioimmunoassay (Bahn *et al.*, 1960) but had never been investigated by immunocytochemical methods. However, this peptide is now considered to be a probable artefact of extraction produced by cleavage from βLPH during the technical procedure (Scott and Lowry, 1974). Thus, we preferred to test for h βLPH. In three cases (1, 2 and 3), anti-hβLPH serum stained the same tumor cells as contained immunoreactive ACTH. Similar co-existence has been demonstrated with the same methods in normal human anterior pituitary for ACTH and βMSH (Phifer *et al.*, 1970), for ACTH and βLPH (Pelletier *et al.*, 1977), and in various species for ACTH, βMSH and βLPH (Dubois, 1972). In Cushing's disease and Nelson's syndrome, high concentrations of β or γLPH in plasma and tumor extracts were found concomitantly with ACTH increase (Bertagna *et al.*, 1977; Tanaka *et al.*, 1978). So it seems that LPH normally present in ACTH cells follows the same pathological fluctuation as corticotropin. However, the exact physiological role of LPH is still obscure since it seems not to present any true remarkable lipolytic, steroidogenic or morphino-mimetic activity (Lazarus *et al.*, 1976; Tanaka *et al.*, 1978).

The quantity of αMSH in the normal human pituitary does not exceed 2 % of the total MSH as estimated by bio-assay (Abe *et al.*, 1967). Nevertheless, in the same tissue, Phifer *et al.* (1974) proved the presence of strongly stained immunoreactive αMSH cells possessing also ACTH and βMSH (i.e. βLPH) activity. Our findings in Cushing adenomas can be related to these results since in two cases, anti-αMSH serum immunostained the same tumors cells as anti-ACTH and anti-hβLPH sera. Cases 2 and 4 did not react with anti-αMSH serum. No relationship could be established between these results and the skin pigmentation of the patients. Anti-αMSH serum did not cross-react with ACTH 1-39, 1-24 or several fragments (ACTH 4-10, 11-24, 25-39), but cross-reacted with ACTH 1-13. This cross-reaction would tend to make the immunostaining doubtful. Thus it is not definitely possible to exclude the presence of this ACTH fragment any more than to rule out the presence of immunoreactive αMSH.

β Endorphin (βLPH 61-91) was demonstrated by immunofluorescence methods in the pars intermedia and pars distalis of the rat pituitary (Bloom *et al.*, 1977). However according to Liotta *et al.* (1978) β endorphin-like immuno-reactivity in man might represent the COOH terminal determinant of βLPH only. β Endorphin immunoreactivity was found in three of our cases and was absent in case 4 which lacked βLPH. Thus it is possible that here also, the immunoreactivity corresponds in fact to βLPH. But a double secretion of βLPH and β endorphin was found in ACTH-secreting mouse pituitary tumor (Giagnoni *et al.*, 1977; Scherrer *et al.*, 1978) and in a human pancreatic islet cell carcinoma causing an ectopic ACTH syndrome (Orth *et al.*, 1978).

In the rat pituitary, enkephalins are restricted to pars intermedia and to the nervous lobe (Rossier *et al.*, 1977). For some other authors, enkephalins are only found in rat brain tissue (Miller *et al.*, 1978). As far as we are aware, the exact distribution of enkephalins has not yet been studied in human hypophysis. This peptide was only demonstrated in human adrenal pheochromocytoma and ganglioneuroma secreting adrenaline and nor-adrenaline (Sullivan *et al.*, 1978). Immunoreactive leucine and methionine-enkephalins were present in the four Cushing adenomas, with a more intense staining for methionine-enkephalin. So the main endogenous opioid peptides known to date were found in these ACTH tumors on an immunocytochemical basis.

Two complementary hypotheses can be argued to explain these results:

(1) ACTH, αMSH, βLPH, β endorphin and enkephalins are secreted separately by the same tumor cells, with some quantitative variations from one case to another. They are all probably present in the normal pituitary. In Cushing's disease, the constant ACTH hypersecretion by itself could explain the entire clinical expression of these tumors, including skin pigmentation (Tanaka *et al.*, 1978). But there is still little information concerning physiological activity or pathological involvement of human αMSH, LPH, endorphins and enkephalins. Regarding the two latter opiate peptides, their basic plasma concentrations and their response to various stimulations remain to be evaluated.

(2) ACTH, αMSH, βLPH, β endorphin and enkephalins detected in Cushing's adenomas could be the cleavage products of a larger molecule. Mains *et al.* (1977) in a clonal ACTH-secreting pituitary tumor cell line (ALT 20/D 16V) demonstrated a 31000 dalton molecule from which ACTH, LPH and endorphins could originate. In normal human pituitary and in pathological conditions, Orth and Nicholson (1977) and Orth *et al.* (1978) showed that ACTH, βLPH, α and β endorphins are derived from a "big" ACTH glycopeptide. Moreover hypophyseal

βLPH could be a precursor of endorphins and methionine-enkephalin (Lazarus *et al.*, 1976; Rubinstein *et al.*, 1978). Though cleavage enzymes for these precursors have not yet been identified and though the exact origin of immunoreactive leucine-enkephalin has not been proved, it is possible that all the ACTH-related peptides including opioid peptides demonstrated in the normal pituitary, in experimental tumors, in ectopic ACTH secreting tumors and, as here, in Cushing pituitary adenomas, derive from the same precursor, present with them in the same ACTH cells or even in the same secretory granules. The tumoral transformation of hypophyseal cells could account for metabolic changes which would explain the disappearance of one or several peptidic products in some adenomas.

## REFERENCES

Abe, K., Island, D. P., Liddle, G. W., Fleisher, N. and Nicholson, W. E. (1967). *J. Clin Endocrinol. Metab.* **27**, 46–52.

Bahn, R., Ross, G. T. and MacCarthy, C. S. (1960). *Proc. Staff Meet. Mayo Clin.* **35**, 623–652.

Bertagna, X., Luton, J. P., Donnadieu, M., Binoux, M., Girard, F. and Bricaire, H. (1977). *Nouv. Presse med.* **6**, 3299–3303.

Bigos, S. T., Robert, F., Pelletier, G. and Hardy, J. (1977). *J. Clin. Endocrinol. Metab.* **45**, 1251–1260.

Bloom, F., Battenberg, E., Rossier, J., Ling, N., Leppaluoto, J., Vargo, T. and Guillemin, R. (1977). *Life Sciences* **20**, 43–48.

Dubois, M. P. (1972). *Lille Med.* **27**, 1391–1394.

Giagnoni, G., Sabol, S. L. and Nirenberg, M. (1977). *Proc. Natl. Acad. Sci., USA.* **74**, 2259–2263.

Herlant, M. and Decourt, J. (1964). *Sem. Hôp. Paris.* **40**, 1426.

Kovacks, K., Horvath, E., Bayley, T. A., Hassaram, S. T. and Ezrim, C. (1978). *Amer. J. Med.* **64**, 492–499.

Krieger, D. T., Choi, H. S. H. and Anderson, P. J. (1976). *Clin. Endoc.* **5**. 455–472.

Landolt, A. M. (1975). Ultrastructure of human sella tumors. *Acta neurochir. Suppl. 22*, Springer Verlag, Wien and New York.

Lazarus, L. H., Ling, N. and Guillemin, R. (1976). *Proc. Natl. Acad. Sci., USA.* **73**, 2156–2159.

Liotta, A. S., Suda, T. and Krieger, D. T. (1978). *Proc. Natl. Acad, Sci., USA.* **75**, 2950–2954.

Mains, R. E., Eipper, B. A. and Ling, N. (1977). *Proc. Natl. Acad. Sci., USA.* **74**, 3014–3018.

Miller, R. J., Chang, K. J., Cooper, B. and Cuatrecasas, P. (1978) *J. Biol. Chem.* **253**, 531–538.

Olivier, L., Vila-Porcile, E., Racadot, O., Peillon, F. and Racadot, J. (1975). *In* "The Anterior Pituitary" (A. Tixier-Vidal and M. G. Farquhar, eds) Vol. 7, 231–276. Academic Press, New York and London.

Orth, D. N. and Nicholson W. E. (1977). *J. Clin. Endocrinol. Metab.* **44**, 214–217.

Orth, D. N., Guillemin, R., Ling, N. and Nicholson, W. E. (1978). *J. Clin. Endocrinol. Metab.* **46**, 849–852.

Pelletier, G., Leclerc, R., Labrie, F., Cote, J., Chretien, M. and Lis, M. (1977). *Endocrinology* **100**, 770–775.

Phifer, R. F., Spicer, S. S. and Orth, D. N. (1970). *J. Clin. Endocr.* **31**, 347–361.
Phifer, R. F., Orth, D. N. and Spicer S. S. (1974). *J. Clin. Endocrinol. Metab.* **39**, 684–692.
Porcile, E. and Racadot, J. (1966). *C. R. Acad. Sc. Paris.* **263**, 948–951.
Racadot, J., Peillon, F., Vila-Porcile, E. and Olivier, L. (1973). *Ann. Endocrinol. (Paris)* **34**, 753–754.
Rossier, J., Vargo, T. M., Minick, S., Ling, N., Bloom, F. E. and Guillemin, R. (1977). *Proc. Natl. Acad. Sci., USA* **74**, 5162–5165.
Rubinstein, M., Stein, S. and Udenfriend, S. (1978). *Proc. Natl. Acad. Sci., USA* **75**, 669–671.
Scherrer, H., Benjannet, S., Pezalla, P. D., Bourassa, M., Seidah, N. G., Lis, M. and Chretien, M. (1978). *Febs Letters* **90**, 353–356.
Scott, A. P. and Lowry, P. J. (1974). *Biochem. J.* **139**, 593–602.
Sternberger, L. A. (1974). "Immunocytochemistry". Prentice-Hall, Englewood Cliffs, New Jersey.
Sullivan, S. N., Bloom, J. R. and Polak, J. M. (1978). *Lancet* **8071**, 986–987.
Tanaka, K., Nicholson, W. E. and Orth, D. N. (1978). *J. Clin. Invest.* **62**, 94–104.
Tramu, G., Beauvillain, J. C., Mazzuca, M., Linquette, M., Lefebvre, J., Fossati, P. and Christiaens, J. L. (1978). *Ann. Endocrinol. (Paris)* **39**, 51–52.
Usategui, R., Oliver, C., Vaudry, H., Lombardi, G., Rozenberg, I. and Mourre, A. M. (1976). *Endocrinology* **98**, 189–196.

# IMMUNOENZYMATIC STUDY OF PITUITARY
# ADENOMAS IN ACROMEGALIC PATIENTS

T. Fukaya[1], N. Kageyama[1], A. Kuwayama[1], M. Takanohashi[1],
J. Yoshida[1] and Y. Osamura[2]

[1] *Department of Neurosurgery, Nagoya University School
of Medicine, Nagoya, Japan*
[2] *Department of Pathology, Tokai University School
of Medicine, Kanagawa, Japan*

It has been postulated that the usual light- and electronmicroscopical
findings of pituitary adenomas do not always correspond with their clinical
features. For example, the adenoma cells in acromegaly are usually eosinophilic,
but in some cases are chromophobe. The electronmicroscopical findings of the
adenomas show that the amount or size of the granules and development of cytoplasmic organellae are not so constant as those of normal pituitary glands. Because
of these variations, the functional character or ability of the adenoma may not be
properly evaluated by the morphological findings alone.

Recently several papers reported that more than two hormones can be secreted
from a single adenoma. This phenomenon cannot be confirmed by usual light- and
electronmicroscopical studies.

In order to establish a functional classification of such tumors, indirect
methods of immunoperoxidase stains developed by P. Nakane were applied to
tumors removed from acromegalic patients and these findings were compared with
various pituitary hormone levels in blood.

## PATIENTS AND METHODS

As shown in Table I, 24 patients with active acromegaly were studied. The
plasma GH levels ranged from 27 to 279 ng/ml with an average of 97 ng/ml. In
9 patients hyperprolactinemia was associated with elevated GH. Galactorrhea was

220

*Table I.* Serum hormone level and immunostain of cells.

| Case | Age | Sex | HE stain | sGH ng/ml | Immuno-stain | sPRL ng/ml | Immuno stain | sLH ng/ml | Immuno-stain | Galactorrhea |
|---|---|---|---|---|---|---|---|---|---|---|
| 1.T.Y. | 28 | F | eosino | 279 | +++ | 21 | ++ | 10 | + | + |
| 2.M.S. | 49 | F | eosino | 271 | +++ | 400 | - | 11 | ++ | + |
| 3.J.M. | 45 | F | eosino | 269 | ++ | 93 | ++ | 12 | ++ | |
| 4.M.S. | 29 | F | mixed | 157 | + | 203 | + | 10 | + | + |
| 5.M.T. | 38 | M | mixed | 125 | +++ | 96 | + | 12 | - | + |
| 6.K.T. | 31 | M | eosino | 121 | ++ | 45 | + | 11 | + | |
| 7.E.N. | 50 | M | eosino | 115 | +++ | 189 | + | 7 | + | |
| 8.S.K. | 49 | F | eosino | 102 | + | 14.2 | not done | 12 | + | |
| 9.M.W. | 51 | M | eosino | 86.5 | + | 508 | + | 17 | - | + |
| 10.T.T. | 41 | M | eosino | 82 | +++ | 16 | - | 8 | - | |
| 11.F.K. | 23 | M | eosino | 79 | +++ | 8 | + | 7 | - | |
| 12.Y.K. | 39 | M | mixed | 77 | + | 20 | + | 5 | - | |
| 13.T.Y. | 39 | M | eosino | 77 | + | 2.6 | + | 6 | not done | |
| 14.S.K. | 27 | F | eosino | 70 | ++ | 27 | - | 42 | + | |
| 15.S.C. | 32 | M | eosino | 58 | + | 46 | - | 17 | - | |
| 16.K.S. | 39 | F | eosino | 54 | +++ | 17.3 | - | ? | + | + |
| 17.H.I. | 38 | F | mixed | 52 | + | 234 | + | 12 | + | |
| 18.T.F. | 43 | M | eosino | 50 | + | 24 | - | 17 | - | |
| 19.M.S. | 52 | M | mixed | 46 | + | ? | + | 3 | - | |
| 20.T.A. | 27 | M | mixed | 41 | +++ | 2.9 | + | 1 | + | + |
| 21.T.T. | 50 | M | mixed | 40 | +++ | 16 | - | 8 | - | |
| 22.S.A. | 41 | M | eosino | 33 | ++ | 11.8 | - | 15 | + | |
| 23.M.S. | 49 | F | mixed | 30.5 | + | 5 | not done | 4 | - | |
| 24.T.K. | 47 | M | mixed | 27 | ++ | 9.5 | + | 6 | + | |

found in 3 female and 3 male hyperprolactinemic patients and amenorrhea in all 4 hyperprolactinemic female patients. Galactorrhea was also found in 1 patient with normal serum prolactin levels.

All patients showed detectable plasma LH levels, which ranged from 1 to 42 mIU/ml. No abnormally high levels of plasma FSH and TSH were found.

The adenoma tissues were all collected by transsphenoidal approach and fixed in 4% paraformaldehyde or 10% formalin, below 4°C, and embedded in paraffin. The tissue was cut in 3 to 6 $\mu$n slices. After confirming the existence of adenoma tissue by H. E. stain, the other slices were subjected to the enzyme-labelled antibody method.

The deparaffinized tissue sections were bathed in phosphate buffer saline (PBS 0.01 M, pH 7.2) 3 times for 15 min each. The slices were soaked in PBS for 15 min to wash out antiserum from the tissues after each step. The slices were reacted with the first antiserum (anti-hGH, anti-prolactin and so on) in the moist chamber for 15 min. After soaking in PBS, the second antiserum (horseraddish peroxidase conjugated with anti-rabbit-gamma-globulin) was layered on these slices for 15 min. Cytoplasmic sites of immunological reaction were demonstrated by 3,3'-diaminobenzidine with 0.005% $H_2O_2$ for 10 min. The cells were counter-stained with methyl green. Anti-GH and anti-LH serums were kindly supplied by Calbiochemical Co., Ltd and anti-PRL serum by the National Institute of Arthritis, Metabolism and Digestive Diseases (NIAMDD).

## RESULTS

GH-positive adenoma cells were observed in all 24 patients with acromegaly, although the amount of GH-positive adenoma cells was different in each case. According to the amount of GH-positive adenoma cells, they were classified into 3 groups (Fig. 1): (+++) - - most adenoma cells were GH positive: (+) - - few cells were positive; and (++) - - number of GH positive cells was in between the above 2 types. Nine of 24 cases were classified as (+++), 5 as (++) and the other 10 were (+), as shown in Table I.

The plasma GH levels ranged from 40 to 279 ng/ml (average, 121 ng/ml) in Group (+++), from 27 to 269 ng/ml (average, 103 ng/ml) in Group (++) and from 30.5 to 157 ng/ml (average, 73.6 ng/ml) in Group (+) (Table I). The plasma GH levels and the amounts of GH-positive adenoma cells are not always parallel if compared individually. However, cases with more GH positive cells as a whole demonstrate higher GH levels in the serum.

The enzyme-labelled antibody method with anti-human PRL serum was applied to 22 cases of acromegaly. As shown in Table I, immunoreactive prolactin was revealed in the cytoplasm of the tumor cells in 13 cases. In some cases a moderate amount of cells reacted positively (++), but in others only some cells reacted positively (+) (Fig. 2). PRL-positive adenoma cells were counted in only 7 of 10 cases with hyperprolactinemia. On the other hand, among 12 cases with normal serum prolactin level, 5 cases had PRL-positive adenoma cells. No significant correlation was found between the plasma PRL levels and the results of enzyme-labelled anti-PRL stains. By careful observation with this anti-body method, it was found that PRL-positive adenoma cells have coarse granules

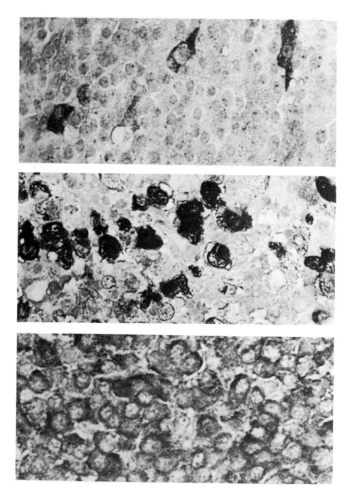

*Fig. 1.* Immunoenzymatic stains show three types of adenoma as regards GH-positive cells, as shown in this figure, a: a small number of cells are GH-positive (+), c: most adenoma cells are GH-positive (+++), b: the number of GH-positive cells is in between those of the above two types (++). × 350.

aggregated in a certain part of the cytoplasm. This phenomenon seems to be characteristic of PRL-positive cells, since GH-positive and LH-positive cells have uniform granules diffusely distributed in the cytoplasma.

LH-positive adenoma cells were found in 13 of 23 cases. In these cases sparse PAS positive cells were found in the adenoma tissues by the PAS stain.

The same histochemical technique using anti-FSH, anti-TSH and anti-ACTH serum was applied to 6 cases. A few cells reacted positively to anti-FSH serum only in one case, but tumor cells reacted negatively to the antisera to FSH, TSH

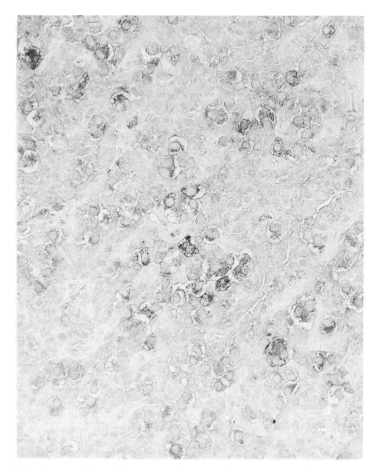

*Fig. 2.* This photograph shows immunoreactive LH cells in an acromegalic patient. LH cells are distributed in the adenoma. × 300.

and ACTH in the other cases.

Electronmicroscopical observations were performed in 14 out of 24 cases. Each adenoma cell had a different amount of secreting granules of different sizes. The development of intracellular organelles also differed from case to case. No correlations were established between the electronmicroscopical findings and the results of enzyme-labelled antibody method.

Mirror sections of the adenomas with 3 μm thickness were made in 4 cases, one for anti-GH and the other for anti-PRL stains to verify if these two hormones could be secreted concomitantly from the same cells or from different cells. In view of the results so far examined, these two hormones seem to be secreted from different adenoma cells.

## DISCUSSION

Our results with the immunoenzymatic method clearly show that in all cases with acromegaly GH-positive cells can be confirmed and in more than half of total cases PRL-positive and LH-positive cells also coexist. From the fact that there are few FSH-, TSH- and ACTH- positive cells, it would be inferred that PRL- and LH- positive cells in the adenoma tissues are not an admixture of normal pituitary cells, but are one of the constituents of the adenomas.

The question why the plasma PRL and LH levels were in the normal ranges in cases with clearly positive cells to these hormones arises. Possible answers would be as follows:

(1)   Only a minimal part of the adenomas can be analysed by the histological studies and the hormonal activities of the adenomas in total can not be assessed by this technique.

(2)   The immunoenzymatic method can only reflect the amount of each hormone stored in the cells, and does not reflect the ability of the adenoma cells to synthesize and secrete the hormones.


## CONCLUSION

(1)   Immunoenzymatic histochemical studies were made in 24 cases with active acromegaly. GH-positive cells were confirmed in all cases and in 13 cases PRL-positive and LH-positive cells were found. In 8 of these 24 cases, 3 kinds of these hormones were positive. In 5 cases GH-positive and PRL-positive cells were found. In another 5 cases GH-positive and LH-positive cells were present. In the other 5 cases only GH-positive cells were found. LH activity was not tested for in 1 case. These results suggest that more than two hormones can be secreted from the pituitary adenomas.

(2)   GH-positive cells and PRL-positive cells seem to be different cells, in view of the study by the mirror section method performed in 4 cases.


## REFERENCES

Corenblum, B., Sirek, A. M. T., Horvath, E., Kovacs, K. and Ezrin, C. (1976). *J. Clin. Endocrinol. Metab.* **42**, 857–863.

Guyda, H., Robert, F., Colle, E. and Hardy, J. (1973). *J. Clin. Endocrinol. Metab.* **36**, 531–547.

Kovacs, K., Horvath, E., Colenblum, B., Sirek, A. M. T., Peuz, G. and Ezrin, C. (1975). *Virchows Arch. A. Path. Anat. Histol.* **366**, 113–123.

Kovacs, K., Corenblum, B., Sirek, A. M. T., Peuz, G. and Ezrin, C. (1976). *J. Clin. Path.* **29**, 250–258.

Nakane, P. K. and Pierce, G. B. (1966). *J. Histochem. Cytochem.* **14**, 929–931.

Nieuwenhuyzen, K. A. C., Bots, G. T. A. M. and Lindeman, J. (1976). *Cancer* **38**, 1163–1170.

Zimmerman, E. A., Defendini, R. and Frantz, A. G. (1974). *J. Clin. Endocrinol. Metab.* **38**, 577–585.

# THE ROLE OF CONTRACEPTIVE STEROIDS IN THE
# PATHOGENESIS OF PITUITARY TUMOURS IN
# VARIOUS EXPERIMENTAL ANIMALS AND IN MAN

M. F. El Etreby*

*Research Laboratories of Schering AG, Berlin/Bergkamen,
Federal Republic of Germany*

The author is indebted to Mrs R. Biermann, B. Schilk and U. Tüshaus-Bussmann for their highly qualified assistance and Dr. P. Günzel for his advice and encouragement.

## INTRODUCTION

The hypothalamic-pituitary system has a multitude of functional units that control different hormonal effector systems such as reproductive activity, thyroid function, adrenal function and growth as well as metabolism in general. The target secretions of these different effector systems may, in turn influence hypothalamic-pituitary function via a feedback mechanism. Therefore an imbalance at the level of the target organs may involve a complementary imbalance at the level of the pituitary gland (for reviews, see Ganong and Martini, 1978; Reichlin *et al.*, 1978).

Steroid hormones are important factors in the control of the function of the different centres for hormone synthesis and release at the hypothalamic and/or pituitary level. A disturbance in the serum levels of sex or adrenal steroids may lead to multiple functional and structural deviations of the hypothalamic pituitary system itself (e.g. atrophy, hyperplasia, tumours etc.) as well as to

---

*Author's address: Dr. M. F. El Etreby, Department of Experimental Toxicology, Schering AG, Müllerstr. 170/178, D-1000 Berlin 65, Federal Republic of Germany.

changes in the structure and function of the different specific effector systems controlled by the trophic hormones of the pituitary gland (cf. El Etreby *et al.*, 1979).

Pituitary tumours mostly occur in the form of an adaptive hyperplasia of certain cell types in the pituitary gland. These biologically benign tissue proliferations are controlled growth processes, which are caused by protracted disturbance of the hypothalamic-pituitary system. Therefore, it seems probable that some pharmacological agents which are able to stimulate trophic hormone synthesis and secretion may also, under certain circumstances, cause pituitary tumours. This holds true especially in the case of long-term treatment with high doses of biologically active steroid hormones (e.g. oestrogens) (for reviews, see El Etreby and Günzel, 1973; Saeger, 1977).

The object of the present paper is to evaluate and summarize knowledge of the role of contraceptive steroids in the pathogenesis of pituitary tumours in various experimental animals and in man.

## MICE AND RATS

Spontaneously-occurring pituitary tumours (chromophobe cell adenomas) in both mice and rats are commonly observed in older animals. The frequency rate is subject to considerable variation in the various strains (genetic disposition). The majority of these pituitary adenomas consist of highly active and partly degranulated prolactin (PRL) cells. Growth hormone (GH) and adrenocorticotrophin (ACTH) cells are occasionally observed in them. In contrast, undifferentiated adenomas are found less frequently (for further details see Kwa, 1961; Furth and Clifton, 1966; El Etreby and Günzel, 1973, 1975).

Triggering of pituitary tumours by hormonal disturbance in the gonadal-pituitary-hypothalamic system (e.g. by continuous endogenously enhanced production or exogenous administration of oestrogens) has been known for many years to occur in both mice and rats (cf. Kwa, 1961; Furth and Clifton, 1966; El Etreby and Günzel, 1973). The Committee on Safety of Medicines, CSM (1972) evaluated the carcinogenic activities of different contraceptive steroids by incorporating them into the diets of mice and rats for 80 and 104 weeks respectively, the doses being identified only as low (2 - 5 times the human contraceptive dose); medium (50 - 150 times) and high (200 -400 times). The amounts were not further specified. These long-term systemic tolerance and carcinogenicity studies suggest that high doses of certain sex steroids (oestrogens, certain progestogens and progestogen–oestrogen combinations) may stimulate the development of pituitary tumours in mice and rats (see Tables I and II). Mice were particularly susceptible to the effects of different steroids, there being a clear difference in incidence of pituitary tumours in comparison with the corresponding controls. The higher incidences were found mainly in the medium and high dose groups. However, in other studies using the same or different strains of mice some oestrogens, progestogens or oestrogen–progestogen combinations were shown not to promote this reaction. In rats it was uncertain whether contraceptive steroids had such an effect, owing to large differences in incidence between different groups in several studies. In

*Table I.*

| Contraceptive steroids which have caused increased incidence of pituitary tumours in mice |
|---|
| ethinyloestradiol |
| mestranol |
| norethynodrel |
| norethisterone |
| norethynodrel + mestranol (25 + 1) |
| (66 + 1) |
| norethisterone + mestranol (20 + 1) |
| norethisterone acetate + ethinyloestradiol (50 + 1) |
| ethynodiol diacetate + ethinyloestradiol ( 2 + 1) |
| (20 + 1) |
| ethynodiol diacetate + mestranol ( 1 + 1) |
| (10 + 1) |
| (20 + 1) |
| dl- norgestrel + ethinyloestradiol (10 + 1) |
| chlormadinone acetate + mestranol (25 + 1) |

*Table II.*

| Contraceptive steroids which have caused a slight increased incidence of pituitary tumours in rats |
|---|
| ethinyloestradiol |
| mestranol |
| oestrone |
| norethynodrel |
| norethisterone oenanthate |
| norethynodrel + mestranol (25 + 1) |
| (66 + 1) |
| norethisterone acetate + ethinyloestradiol (50 + 1) |
| ethynodiol diacetate + ethinyloestradiol (2 + 1) |

some of these studies, an unexplained inhibitory effect of certain sex steroids on the development of pituitary tumours in rats could even be assumed. However, this may also reflect a variation in the spontaneous incidence of pituitary tumours (for further details see CSM report, 1972; El Etreby and Günzel, 1973; Leonard, 1974; IARC Monograph, 1974; El Etreby *et al.*, 1979).

The steroid-related pituitary tumours are closely similar to those observed spontaneously in old mice and rats. They consist mainly of PRL cells (PRL cell adenomas or prolactinomas). However, single or small groups of GH and ACTH cells are also observed. This may explain their predominantly mammotrophic and to some extent somatotrophic and/or corticotrophic activity (for further details see Kwa, 1961; Furth and Clifton, 1966; Waelbroeck-van Gaver and Potvliege, 1969; El Etreby and Günzel, 1973, 1974; El Etreby *et al.*, 1979).

In general, the development of these PRL cell tumours in mice and rats seems to be dependent on the strain, age and sex of the animals, housing conditions and especially on the quality of the biological effect (e.g. oestrogenic effect) of the substance administered, dosage, mode of administration, continuity and duration of treatment. The other sex steroids (apart from oestrogens) which stimulate the development of these pituitary tumours (Tables I and II) are either progestogens with inherent oestrogenic activity in these species or progestogen-oestrogen combinations in ratios in which only the oestrogen component would be expected to exert an effect in mice and rats — in total contrast to the situation in primates (cf. Neumann and Gräf, 1978). The role of the oestrogenic activity may be explained by the fact that oestrogens were shown to stimulate PRL synthesis and secretion in a dose-dependent manner, both directly and indirectly (via the hypothalamus, see Fig. 1). The stimulatory effect of oestrogens on PRL

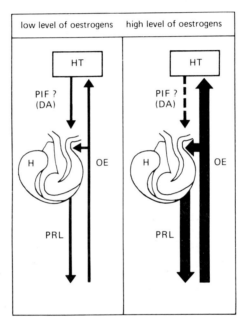

*Fig. 1.* The stimulatory effect of oestrogens (Oe) on PRL secretion at both the pituitary (H) and hypothalamus (HT) levels.

DA = dopamine
PIF = PRL-inhibiting factor

secretion at the pituitary level holds true for both baseline secretion and dopamine-induced inhibition. Simultaneous administration of other steroid hormones in addition to oestrogens can result in a synergistic or antagonistic effect on the development of these pituitary tumours, which is the same as the situation with regard to the effect on PRL secretion. Synergism or antagonism depends on the factors listed above, on the absolute dose of the individual components and on the dose ratio (cf. El Etreby and Günzel, (1973).

## RABBITS, HAMSTERS AND GUINEA PIGS

Spontaneous pituitary tumours have rarely been described in rabbits, hamsters and guinea pigs (cf. Dobberstein and Tamaschke, 1958). Furthermore, information regarding the influence of contraceptive steroids on the development of pituitary tumours in these species is lacking as they are not usually used in the long-term tolerance and carcinogenicity studies of such steroid hormones. However, general hyperplasia of presumptive PRL cells with no evidence of the development of adenomas was described in rabbits and hamsters with suspected endocrine hyperfunction of the gonads and following oestrogen treatment (cf. El Etreby and Günzel, 1973). On the other hand, in the hamster, long-term treatment with oestrogens results in hyperplastic and neoplastic changes in the melanocyte stimulating hormone (MSH) cells of the pars intermedia of the pituitary gland and elevated serum MSH concentrations. These oestrogen-dependent pituitary changes persist for at least nine months after cessation of treatment (Saluja *et al.*, 1978).

## DOGS

The spontaneous pituitary tumours of aged dogs, originate in both the pars distalis and pars intermedia of the pituitary gland. The relative frequency of the two types seems to depend on the breed of dogs involved. The basophil and chromophobe adenomas are the most predominant types of the pituitary tumours of the pars distalis (for reviews, see Capen *et al.*, 1967; Dämmrich, 1967; Potel, 1968; Michaelson, 1970; Jubb and Kennedy, 1970). Capen *et al.* (1967) have shown that the majority of the chromophobe adenomas in the canine pituitary gland in their series were associated with the clinical syndromes of hyperadrenocorticism. They were further able to find ultrastructural evidence of secretory activity and similarity between the tumour cells and those thought to produce ACTH in other laboratory animals (Capen and Koestner, 1967). Using the immunoperoxidase technique, it has been recently shown that the frequent pituitary tumours in old dogs arise from the ACTH/MSH cells of both the pars distalis and pars intermedia of the canine pituitary gland (Fig. 2). On the contrary, GH and PRL cell adenomas seem to be rare in the dog (El Etreby *et al.*, 1978).

In contrast to the effect of progestogens, which stimulate GH rather than PRL cells, long-term treatment of the beagle bitch with oestrogens (17β-oestradiol) causes marked stimulation of PRL cells in the pituitary gland Consequently, marked diffuse hyperplasia and/or hypertrophy of PRL and/or GH cells was usually observed as a result of the treatment with oestrogens and/or progestogens (cf. El Etreby *et al.*, 1977; El Etreby and Fath El Bab, 1977, 1978). In spite of these findings, steroid-related pituitary tumours were not observed in systemic tolerance and carcinogenicity studies of oestrogens, progestogens and their combinations in the beagle dog (Wazeter *et al.*, 1973, 1976; Geil and Lamar, 1977).

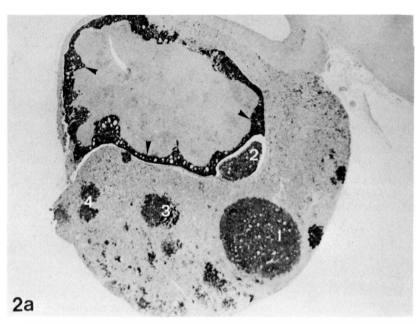

2a

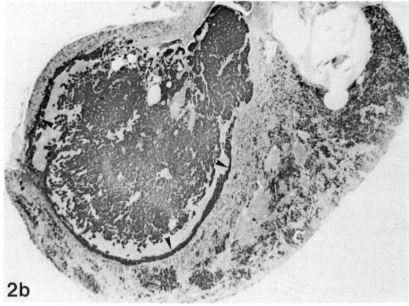

2b

*Fig. 2.* Immunoperoxidase staining of ACTH/MSH cells in the pituitary glands of two old dogs using anti-porcine ACTH serum and 3,3'-diaminobenzidine-hydrogen peroxide as substrate. The nuclei were lightly counterstained with hematoxylin. $\times$ 16.

    a : Multiple microadenomas and nodular hyperplasia of the pars distalis. They are labelled (1–4). These nodules are of different sizes and may cause pressure atrophy of the surrounding parenchyma. The pars intermedia (see arrows) shows positive staining (ACTH/MSH cells).

    (Beagle bitch, seven years old, benign mammary tumour, progressive transformation of adrenal cortex.)

    b : Pituitary ACTH/MSH cell adenoma of the pars intermedia which infiltrates the pars nervosa. The ACTH/MSH cells of the pars distalis and pars intermedia (see arrows) are also shown.

    (Alsatian bitch, > ten years old, adenocarcinoma of mammary gland, adenoma of adrenal cortex.)

## MONKEYS

Pituitary tumours have rarely been described as spontaneous or induced neoplasms in monkeys and other non-human primates (Ruch, 1967; O'Gara and Adamson, 1972; Spies and Clegg, 1972).

In the rhesus monkey, long-term (ten years) studies with high doses of oestrogens, progestogens and their combinations are in progress. Monkeys dying during the test have not had any pituitary tumours, but a definite conclusion cannot be made until the experiments are completed (Wazeter *et al.*, 1973, 1976; Geil and Lamar, 1977). However, this species may, as is the case with the dog, be resistant to development of pituitary tumours (prolactinomas) in spite of long-term treatment with high doses of these biologically active steroids. On the other hand, based on morphological (diffuse PRL cell hyperplasia and hypertrophy) and radioimmunoassay data, it can be concluded that PRL synthesis and secretion were enhanced by oestrogens (El Etreby and Günzel, 1974; Herbert and Hayashida, 1974) and progestogens (e.g. cyproterone acetate, chlormadinone acetate and progesterone (Herbert *et al.*, 1977 and unpublished results) in the rhesus monkey.

## MAN

According to a recent study, the human pituitary adenomas could be classified into acidophil GH cell and PRL cell adenomas, mucoid ACTH cell and Thyrotropin (TSH) cell adenomas, oncocytic and undifferentiated adenomas (Saeger, 1977). The pathogenesis of the PRL cell tumours (prolactinomas) is of special interest with regard to the role of the sex steroids. This type of pituitary tumour appears in men with impotence, testicular atrophy, gynaecomastia and galactorrhoea, and in women as part of the known clinical picture of tumorigenic amenorrhoea-galactorrhoea without acromegaly (cf. El Etreby and Günzel, 1973; Saeger, 1977).

Both in the case of protracted endogenous oestrogen impregnation by oestrogen-producing tumours (chorio-epithelioma of the testis, adrenal cortical tumours) and after exogenous administration of oestrogens in very large dosages in long-term treatment of prostatic cancer or angina pectoris, PRL cell hyperplasia or adenomas, gynaecomastia and galactorrhoea may occur in men. Moreover, in women too, endogenous oestrogen impregnation (pregnancy) or exogenous administration of oestrogens or oestrogen–progestogen combinations can exert a stimulatory effect on existing prolactinomas in the sense of acceleration of tumoural processes or a worsening of clinical symptoms (cf. Schrader and Weber, 1958; Poujol *et al.*, 1964; Goluboff and Ezrin, 1969; Peillon *et al.*, 1970; Hachmeister, 1972; Hachmeister *et al.*, 1972; Pasteels *et al.*, 1972; El Etreby and Günzel, 1973, 1974; Saeger, 1977). However, it is obvious from the observations of Linquette *et al.* (1967) and Goluboff and Ezrin (1969) that differences exist in the sensitivity and responsiveness of certain individuals to this stimulatory effect of oestrogens. In a recent study of 191 women with secondary amenorrhoea, the cause was found to be pituitary tumours in 26 % of 69 former users of oral contraceptives but only in 13 % or 122 women whose amenorrhoea was not associated with oral contraception. The difference is statistically significant (Population Reports, 1977). This study may cause some concern that contra-ceptive steroids can in some cases affect the pituitary adversely i.e. they may stimulate the development of tumours. In another study, the difference between the incidence of prolactinomas in patients with postpill amenorrhoea-galactorrhoea (10/31 = 32 %) and the incidence of these tumours (16/39 = 41 %) in patients with amenorrhoea-galactorrhoea unrelated to oral contraceptives was not statistically significant (Campenhout *et al.*, 1977). Moreover, the cases described in the literature so far show that the stimulating effect of oestrogens and oestrogen–progestogen combinations on pituitary tumours of women was only noticed when endocrine regulation was already disturbed or pathological changes had taken place in the hypothalamic-pituitary system before the commencement of treatment (cf. El Etreby and Günzel, 1973). However, these findings would appear particularly interesting in the light of recent results showing that oestrogens, certain progestogens and oestrogen–progestogen-combinations may stimulate PRL synthesis and secretion in humans. Thus, it has been shown that oral contraceptives composed of oestrogens and progestogens (either the combination or the sequential type) evoked a significant increase in basal serum PRL levels in women (Robyn *et al.*, 1973; Schmidt-Gollwitzer and Saxena, 1975; Abu-Fadil *et al.*, 1976; Dericks-Tan and Taubert, 1976). A significantly increased release of PRL following either hypoglycaemia or TRH treatment in women using combined oral contraceptives for a long period of time was also observed (Mishell *et al.*, 1977). These findings are in agreement with those of Buckman and Peake (1973), who reported that phenothiazine stimulation of PRL secretion was significantly greater in women taking oral contraceptives than that in control women. It has also been reported that oestro-gens alone increase the PRL response to TRH. However, in a recently published (non-randomized) study, PRL levels after TRH stimulation were similar both in women taking oral contraceptives (d-norgestrel, cyproterone acetate) and in those receiving no hormonal medication (controls) (cf. Bellmann *et al.*, 1978). Since PRL secretion is enhanced by oestrogen (Yen *et al.*, 1974; Siler *et al.*, 1974; Schmidt-Gollwitzer and Saxena, 1975; Ehara *et al.*, 1976; Rutlin *et al.*, 1977), it is not known to what extent the progestogens contributed to hypersecretion of PRL in those women treated with a combination of oestrogens and progestogens. However, it has been recently reported that women taking the minipill composed of a synthetic progestogen had significantly elevated serum PRL values (Dericks-Tan and Taubert, 1976). Medroxyprogesterone acetate was also found to significantly raise PRL levels in treated women over those observed in control subjects. It was also observed that the same drug enhanced release of PRL in response to the suckling stimulus in lactating women (cf. Mishell *et al.*, 1977; Chaudhury *et al.*, 1977). Similarly, Fonzo *et al.* (1977) have reported the occurrence of hyperprolactinaemia in girls with idiopathic precocious puberty undergoing prolonged treatment with cyproterone acetate. Recently, Graf *et al.* (1978) substantiated the role of this synthetic progestogen in the stimulation of PRL secretion in human subjects. On the other hand, Robyn *et al.* (1973, 1976) have shown that some progestational agents were ineffective in stimulating PRL in women.

The above-mentioned findings suggest that women taking sex steroids should be watched for amenorrhoea or other indications of hypothalamic-pituitary dysfunction, which could be considered as occasional undesirable effects of contraceptive steroids and common symptoms of pituitary tumours (prolactinomas). Moreover, careful documentation, investigation and follow-up of the relationship between sex steroids and pituitary tumours in humans are still required and full prospective and retrospective studies should be undertaken. Until then, a possible association between long-term use of contraceptive steroids and a higher risk of pituitary tumours in humans should be borne in mind.

## REFERENCES

Abu-Fadil, S., DeVane, G., Siler, T. M. and Yen, S. S. C. (1976). *Contraception* **13**, 79–85.

Bellman, O., Bröschen-Zywietz, C. and Fichte, K. (1978). *Arch. Gynäk.* **225**, 31–42.

Buckman, M. T. and Peake, G. T. (1973). *J. clin. Endocr. Metab.* **37**, 977.

Campenhout van, J., Blanchet, P., Beauregard, H. and Papas, S. (1977). *Fertil. Steril.* **28**, 728–732.

Capen, C. C. and Koestner, A. (1967). *Path. vet.* **4**, 326–347.

Capen, C. C., Martin, S. L. and Koestner, A. (1967). *Path. vet.* **4**, 301–325.

Chaudhury, R., Chompootaweep, S., Dusitsin, N., Friesen, H. and Tankeyoon, M. (1977). *Brit. J. Pharmacol.* **59**, 433–434.

Committee on Safety of Medicines (1972). "Carcinogenicity Tests of Oral Contraceptives". H.M.S.O., London.

Dämmrich, K. (1967). *Zbl. Vet. Med.* **14A**, 137–154.

Dericks-Tan, J. S. E. and Taubert, H.-D. (1976). *Contraception* **14**, 1–8.

Dobberstein, J. and Tamaschke, C. (1958). *In* "Pathologie der Laboratorium-stiere" (P. Cohrs, R. Jaffe and H. Meessen, eds) pp. 470–586. Springer-Verlag, Berlin.

Ehara, Y., Siler, T. M. and Yen S. S. C. (1976). *Am. J. Obstet. Gynec.* **125**, 455–458.

El Etreby, M. F. and Fath El Bab, M. R. (1977). *Cell Tiss. Res.* **183**, 177–189.

El Etreby, M. F. and Fath El Bab, M. R. (1978). *Cell Tiss. Res.* **191**, 205–218.

El Etreby, M. F. and Günzel, P. (1973). *Arzneimittel-Forsch. (Drug. Res.)* **23**, 1768–1790.

El Etreby, M. F. and Günzel, P. (1974). *Acta endocr. (Copenh.) Suppl.* **189**, 1–15.

El Etreby, M. F. and Günzel, P. (1975). *Verh. Dtsch. Ges. Path.* **59**, 391–393.

El Etreby, M. F., Schilk, B., Soulioti, G., Tüshaus, U., Wiemann, H. and Günzel, P. (1977). *Endokrinologie* **69**, 202–216.

El Etreby, M. F., Fath El Bab, M. R., Müller-Peddinghaus, R. and Trautwein, G. (1978). Paper held at: 27. Tagung "Europ. Ges. Vet. Path.", May 15–16, Wien.

El Etreby, M. F., Fräf, K.-J., Günzel, P. and Neumann (1979). *Arch Toxicol.* (in press).

Fonzo, D., Angeli, A., Sivieri, R., Andriolo, S., Frajria, R. and Ceresa, F. (1977). *J. clin. Endocr. Metab.* **45**, 164–168.

Furth, J. and Clifton, K. H. (1966). *In* "The Pituitary Gland" (G. W. Harris and B. T. Donovan, eds) Vol. 2, 460–497. Butterworths, London.

Ganong, W. F. and Martini, L. (1978). "Frontiers in Neuroendocrinology". Raven Press, New York.

Geil, R. G. and Lamar, J. K. (1977). *J. Toxicol. Environ. Health* **3**, 179–193.

Goluboff, L. G. and Ezrin, C. (1969). *J. clin. Endocr. Metab.* **29**, 1533–1538.

Gräf, K.-J., Schmidt-Gollwitzer, M., Koch, U. J., Lorenz, F. and Hammerstein, J. (1978). *Acta endocr. (Copenh.) Suppl.* **215**, 96.

Hachmeister, U. (1972). *Verh. Dtsch. Ges. Path.* **56**, 535–539.

Hachmeister, U., Fahlbusch, R. and v. Werder, K. (1972). *Acta endocr. (Copenh.) Suppl.* **159**, 42.

Herbert, D. C. and Hayashida, T. (1974). *Gen. Comp. Endocrinol.* **24**, 381–397.

Herbert, D. C., Schuppler, J., Poggel, A., Günzel, P. and El Etreby, M. F. (1977). *Cell Tiss. Res.* **183**, 51–60.

IARC Monographs on the Evaluation of Carcinogenic Risk of Chemicals to Man (1974). "Sex Hormones" Vol. 6, International Agency for Research on Cancer, Lyon.

Jubb, K. V. F. and Kennedy, P. C. (1970). "Pathology of Domestic Animals". Academic Press, New York and London.

Kwa, H. G. (1961). "An Experimental Study of Pituitary Tumours". Springer Verlag, Berlin.

Leonard, B. J. (1974). *In* "Pharmacological Models in Contraceptive Development" (M. H. Briggs and E. Diczfalusy, eds) pp. 34–73. WHO Research and Training Centre on Human Reproduction, Karolinska Institutet, Stockholm.

Linquette, M., Herlant, M., Laine, E., Fossati, P. and Dupont-Lecompte, J. (1967). *Annls. Endocr. (Paris)* **28**, 773–780.

Michaelson, S. M. (1970). *In* "The Beagle as an Experimental Dog" (A. C. Anderson, ed) pp. 412–449. Iowa State University Press, Iowa.

Mishell, D. R. Jr., Kletzky, O. A., Brenner, P. F., Roy, S. and Nicoloff, J. (1977). *Am. J. Obstet. Gynecol.* **128**, 60–74.

Neumann, F. and Gräf, K.-J. (1978). *In* "Pharmacological Methods in Toxicology" (G. Zbinden and F. Gross, eds). Pergamon Press, Oxford.

O'Gara, R. W. and Adamson, R. H. (1972). *In* "Pathology of Simian Primates" (R. N. T-W-Fiennes, ed) Vol. 1, 190–238. Karger, Basel.

Pasteels, J. L., Gausset, P., Danguy, A. and Ectors, F. (1972). *In* "Prolactin and Carcinogenesis" (A. R. Boyns and K. Griffiths, eds) pp. 128–136. Alpha Omega Alpha, Cardiff.

Peillon, F., Vila-Porcile, D., Olivier, L. and Racadot, J. (1970). *Annls. Endocr. (Paris)* **31**, 259–270.

Population Reports (1977). Oral contraceptives, debate on oral contraceptives and neoplasia continues; answers remain elusive. Series A, No. 4. Department of Medical and Public Affairs. The George Washington University Medical Center, Washington.

Potel, K. (1968). *In* "Handbuch der speziellen pathologischen Anatomie der Haustiere" (J. Dobberstein, G. Pallaske and H. Stünzi, eds) pp. 150–163. Paul Parey Verlag, Berlin and Hamburg.

Poujol, J., Bacot, H., Darcourt, G. and Margat, C. (1964). *Rev. Franc. Endocrinol. Clin.* 5, 131–137.

Reichlin, S., Baldessarini, R. J. and Martin, J. B. (1978). "The Hypothalamus". Raven Press, New York.

Robyn, C., Delvoye, P., Nokin, J., Vekemans, M., Badawi, M., Perez-Lopez, F. R. and L'Hermite, M. (1973). *In* "Human Prolactin" (J. L. Pasteels and C. Robyn, eds) pp. 167–188. Excerpta Medica and American Elsevier Publishing Co., Inc., Amsterdam.

Robyn, C., Vekeman, M., Delvoye, P., Joosten-Defleur, V., Caufriez, A. and L'Hermite, M. (1976). *In* "Growth Hormone and Related Peptides (A. Pecile and E. E. Müller, eds) pp. 396–406. Excerpta Medica and American Elsevier Publishing Co., Inc., Amsterdam.

Ruch, T. C. (1967). "Diseases of Laboratory Primates". W. B. Saunders Company, Philadelphia.

Rutlin, E., Haug, E. and Torjesen, P. A. (1977). *Acta Endocr. (Copenh.)* 84, 23–35.

Saeger, W. (1977). "Die Hypophysentumoren", Gustav Fischer Verlag, Stuttgart and New York.

Saluja, P. G., Hamilton, J. M., Thody, A. J., Ismail, A. A. and Knowles, J. (1979). *Arch. Toxicol.* (in press).

Schmidt-Gollwitzer, M. and Saxena, B. B. (1975). *Acta Endocr. (Copenh.)* 80, 262–274.

Schrader, K. and Weber, W. (1958). *Ophthalmologica* 135, 44–50.

Siler, T. M., Ehara, Y. and Yen, S. S. C. (1974). *Gynec. Invest.* 5, 47–48.

Spies, H. G. and Clegg, M. T. (1972). *In* "Pathology of Simian Primates" (R. N. T-W-Fiennes, ed) Vol. 1, 399–413. Karger, Basel.

Waelbroeck-van Gaver, C. and Potvliege, P. (1969). *Europ. J. Cancer* 5, 99–117.

Wazeter, F. X., Geil, R. G., Berliner, V. R. and Lamar, J. K. (1973). *Toxicol. Appl. Pharmacol.* 25, 1 (Abstract No. 498).

Wazeter, F. X., Geil, R. G., Cookson, K. M., Berliner, V. R. and Lamar, J. K. (1976). *Toxicol. Appl. Pharmacol.* 37, 1 (Abstract No. 208).

Yen, S. S. C., Ehara, Y. and Siler, T. M. (1974). *J. Clin. Invest.* 53, 652–655.

# DEVELOPMENT OF PROLACTIN-SECRETING PITUITARY MICROADENOMAS IN THE RAT AFTER DMBA ADMINISTRATION

J. A. Heuson-Stiennon[1], A. Danguy[1], J. C. Heuson[2], and J. L. Pasteels[1]

[1] Laboratory of Histology, Free University of Brussels,
Medical School, Brussels, Belgium
[2] Laboratory of Mammary Oncology, Institut J. Bordet,
1000 Brussels, Belgium

Huggins *et al.* (1959) and Huggins and Yang (1962) were the first to observe that a single feeding of a chemical carcinogen such as dimethylbenz($\alpha$)anthracene (DMBA) induced hormone-dependent mammary carcinomas in the rat. Our purpose was to study the endocrine changes occurring at various intervals after carcinogen feeding.

## MATERIAL AND METHODS

Mammary tumors were induced in 42 Spragus-Dawley female rats by a single intragastric feeding of 20 mg DMBA at age 50 days. Estrous cycles were followed throughout the entire experience by daily vaginal smears. Groups of two experimental animals and one untreated control were killed by decapitation on days 0.5 (12 h), 1, 2, 3, 6, 10, 15, 20, 40, 60, 100, 150, 200, and 300 after DMBA feeding. Pituitary, mammary glands, adrenals, ovaries, uterus and vagina were prepared for light and electron microscopy. Histochemical identification of prolactin and ACTH cells was performed by immunoperoxidase methods (Furth *et al.*, 1976).

223

Prolactin cells were labelled with one antiserum to rat prolactin supplied by Dr. Parlow (NIAMDD) and corticotropes by immune serum to synthetic 17-39 ACTH prepared in our laboratory.


## RESULTS

The first morphological change observed was acute adrenocortical necrosis as previously reported by Huggins and Morii (1961). This phenomenon was apparent at 12 h after DMBA feeding and progressively disappeared within 2 - 3 weeks. Furthermore, profound changes occurred in the anterior pituitary.

Light microscopy and the immunoperoxidase method revealed hyperplasia of both prolactin and corticotropic cells, which was conspicuous on day two, reached a maximum on day 6 and then declined. After two or three weeks, the adenohypophysis of treated rats returned to a near normal state, as judged from the controls (Pasteels *et al.*, 1978). In electron microscopy the prolactin cells on day 6 displayed evidence of enhanced secretory activity and showed numerous images of exocytosis.

During the same period, the mammary gland showed enhanced secretory activity that gradually increased and became permanent for the entire life of the animal (Heuson-Stiennon *et al.*, 1974).

The first mammary tumors were detected on day 40 and, in agreement with Huggins and Morii (1961), we found a 100 % incidence of tumors in the experimental animals. In the animals that were allowed to survive for 150 - 300 days after DMBA feeding a 100 % incidence of pituitary adenomas were observed. A detailed description of the changes occurring in the mammary and adrenal glands will be reported elsewhere. This communication will describe the morphological changes appearing in the hypophysis.

The anterior lobe of the pituitary of every experimental animal contained at least one adenoma, but usually two or three tumors could be detected in the same section. In these tumors, the usually corded organization of the pituitary cells was replaced by a massive structure. This was due to extreme narrowing of the sinusoids. The tumor cells were poorly granulated and, in consequence they were only weakly labelled by the immunoperoxidase methods.

In electron microscopy (Fig. 1), the cell cytoplasm underwent a marked hypertrophy and we observed a disappearance of the plasma membranes in such a manner that the cytoplasm contained two or three nuclei. The rough endoplasmic reticulum was abundant but disrupted, and the different Golgi apparatuses were well-developed. The remaining secretory granules were irregular in shape, as are typical prolactin granules (Farquhar *et al.*, 1978). All these features are well known from now classical descriptions of mammotropic tumors (Olivier *et al.*, 1975; Furth *et al.*, 1976). In the surrounding non-tumoral tissue, the prolactin cells detected by the immunoperoxidase method (Fig. 2 b) were found to be more numerous than in comparable histological sections of control animals (Fig. 2 a).

Estrous cycles remained normal, as compared to the controls, despite the profound endocrine changes.

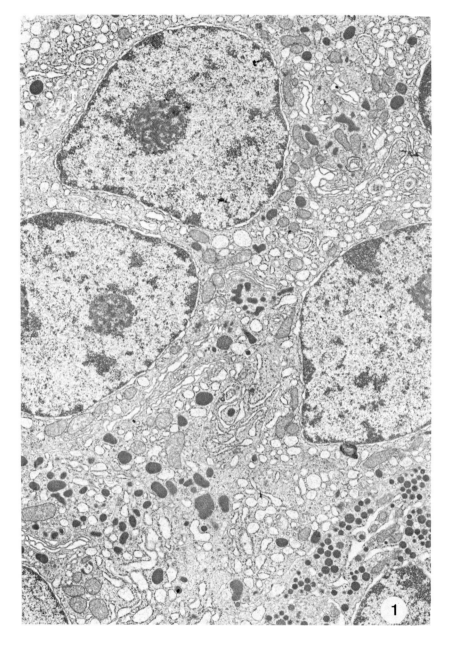

*Fig. 1.* Electron micrograph of a prolactin-secreting microadenoma cell, 160 days after DMBA. The cells are hypertrophied with well-developed rough endoplasmic reticulum and Golgi apparatus. Three nuclei are apparent in one cytoplasm.

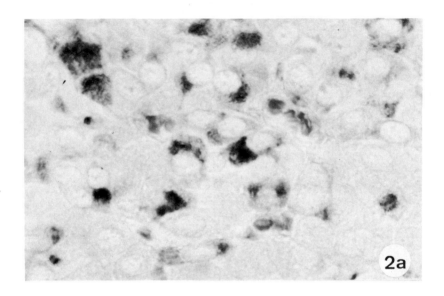

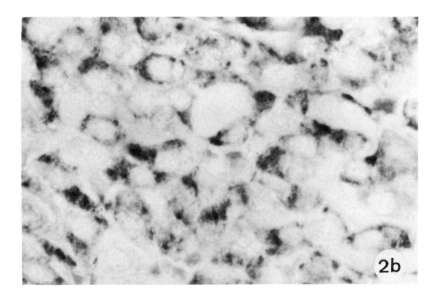

*Fig. 2.* Prolactin cells detected by the immunoperoxidase technique.
(a) Control animals.
(b) One hundred and sixty days after DMBA feeding. The prolactin cells are more numerous than in the controls.

## CONCLUSION

The first conclusion is that DMBA feeding induced early morphological changes suggesting stimulation of the prolactin cells. This probably resulted from the observed carcinogen-induced adrenal necrosis. Chen *et al.* (1976) reported that adrenalectomy increased prolactin release.

Later on, DMBA feeding induced pituitary and adrenal adenomas. It is well known that pituitary adenomas may develop in elderly rats and that their frequency of occurrence may be increased by carcinogenic treatment (Furth *et al.*, 1976). As reported here, most of these tumors were mammotropic. Moreover, hyperplasia of the prolactin cells was observed in the surrounding tissue.

These hormonal changes should be taken into account in studies of the endocrine control of growth of the DMBA-induced mammary tumors of the rat.

## REFERENCES

Chen, H. J., Bradley, C. J. and Meites, J. (1976). *Cancer Res.* **36**, 1414–1417.

Heuson-Stiennon, J. A. Gallez, G., Heimann, R. et Heuson, J. C. (1974). *J. Microscopie* **20**, 56a.

Huggins, C., Briziarelli, G. and Sutton, H. (1959). *J. exp. Med.* **109**, 25–53.

Huggins, C. and Morii, S. (1961). *J. exp. Med.* **114**, 741–759.

Huggins, C. and Yang, N. C. (1962). *Science* **137**, 257–262.

Farquhar, M. G., Reid, J. J. and Daniell, L. W. (1978). *Endocrinology* **102**, 296–311.

Furth, J., Nakane, P. and Pasteels, J. L. (1976). *In* "Pathology of Tumours in Laboratory Animals" (V. S. Turusov, ed) Vol. I, Part 2, 201–238. WHO International Agency for Research on Cancer, Lyon.

Olivier, L., Vila-Porcile, E., Racadot, O., Peillon, F. and Racadot, J. (1975). *In* "The Anterior Pituitary" (A. Tixier-Vidal and M. G. Farquhar, eds) Vol 7, 231–276. Academic Press, New York and London.

Pasteels, J. L., Heuson-Stiennon, J. A., Danguy, A., Legros, N. and Heuson, J. C. (1978). *In* "Progress in Prolactin Physiology and Pathology" (C. Robyn and M. Harter, eds) pp. 69–79. Elsevier North Holland Biomedical Press, Amsterdam.

# THE ENDOCRINOLOGY OF GROWTH HORMONE-SECRETING MICROADENOMAS

H.-J. Quabbe*

*Medical Clinic, Section of Endocrinology,
Klinikum Steglitz, Free University of Berlin,
Hindenburgdamm 30, D – 1000 Berlin 45, Federal Republic of Germany*

Growth hormone (GH)-secreting adenomas of the pituitary gland will produce
(1)   gigantism or acromegaly (depending on the age of manifestation),
(2)   a state of partial or total pituitary insufficiency if the adenoma causes compression and atrophy of the normal pituitary tissue, and
(3)   endocrine and metabolic derangements due to the excess of circulating GH.

This article will briefly review GH secretion and the peripheral effects of GH under physiological conditions and in acromegaly. It will then try to examine the question whether GH-secreting microadenomas differ from larger tumors and discuss the possible consequences of such differences.

## GH SECRETION AND ACTION IN NORMAL SUBJECTS

### Regulation of GH secretion

GH release from the pituitary gland occurs in episodic bursts. The temporal pattern of release is regulated by the CNS. The hypothalamus produces somatostatin, a GH-release-inhibiting hormone, and probably also GH-RH, a GH-release-stimulating hormone. Influences arising from extra-hypothalamic structures, especially in the limbic system, as well as sleep and possibly the

---

*The author gratefully acknowledges technical help from Ms. M. Mahlke, B. Mönnickes and M. Rösick and of secretarial help from Ms. J. Weirowski.

basic-rest-activity-cycle are important determinants of GH secretion in man. Several neurotransmitters are involved in the regulation, notably serotonin, dopamine and noradrenaline. Metabolic factors are important modulators of GH secretion. Glucose and free-fatty-acid excess inhibit, and a lack of these substrates as well as an excess of amino acids stimulates GH release. GH also seems to inhibit its own secretion, probably by a short loop feedback system (reviewed in Merimee and Rabin, 1973; Quabbe, 1977).

### Peripheral actions of GH*

GH has an important influence on the peripheral metabolism. It stimulates protein synthesis and does so in synergism with insulin. It stimulates lipolysis and inhibits glucose metabolism and in this respect is an antagonist of insulin. GH excess, experimental or in acromegaly, decreases glucose tolerance and eventually leads to diabetes mellitus. The hormone also stimulates the growth of practically all organs and tissues (with the possible exception of the brain) by its influence on cell replication and protein anabolism. However, many of these actions are not direct effects of GH. They are mediated by a heterogenous family of substances, the so-called somatomedins. The exact nature, origin and mode of action of the somatomedins is still a matter of investigation (see the section on "somatomedins").

## GH SECRETION AND ACTION IN ACROMEGALY AND GIGANTISM

### Pathology of GH secretion

In patients with GH-secreting pituitary adenomas, the plasma GH concentration is elevated to various degrees and cannot be suppressed adequately during a glucose-tolerance-test (GTT). In normal subjects, one or several GH values will usually be below 1 ng/ml during a 3-hour oral GTT. Patients with acromegaly may have a relatively low GH concentration with some decrease during a GTT, but they will not attain the normal range. In others, the GH concentration is not at all influenced by glucose. Some patients will even respond to glucose administration with a "paradoxical" increase of GH, rather than a decrease. The mechanism of this response is unknown. Speculatively, it could be explained by a direct stimulatory action of glucose on pituitary GH release and a lack of normal inhibitory influences. This would be in analogy with the suggested mechanism of TRH-stimulated GH release in acromegaly (Udeschini *et al.*, 1976). However, normal pituitary tissue *in vitro* does not respond with GH release to an increase of the glucose concentration (Schofield, 1967). Tissue from GH secreting adenomas has not been tested.

The "paradoxical response" of GH to glucose loading has been reported in a variety of other pathological conditions including renal failure, liver disease, Turner's syndrome, protein-losing enteropathy, malnutrition, diabetes mellitus

---

*Readers interested in a more thorough presentation of the actions of GH are referred to the appropriate chapters of the "Handbook of Physiology" (1974), (E. Knobil and W. H. Sawyer, eds) Section 7, Vol. IV, Part 2. Williams and Wilkins, Baltimore.

and endometrial carcinoma. Many of these patients did have one feature in common: decreased glucose tolerance. In several cases, improvement of glucose tolerance was associated with normalization of the GH response to glucose. The question may then be asked whether the paradoxical GH increase during glucose loading is a "normal" response in states of decreased glucose tolerance, possibly due to intracellular glucopenia relative to the extracellular glucose concentration. The reversibility of the paradoxical response which has been reported in some of these diseases may be taken to support such a view. However, in a group of 23 patients with acromegaly, we found no correlation between the presence of diabetes mellitus and the existence of a paradoxical GH response to oral glucose (Fig. 1). This makes it likely that at least in acromegaly the paradoxical response to glucose is independent of the metabolic situation. Another abnormality of GH

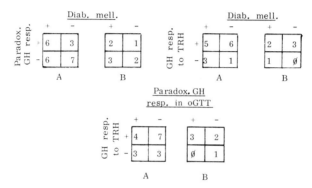

*Fig. 1.* Lack of correlation between existence of diabetes mellitus, paradoxical GH response to glucose and pathological GH response to TRH in a group of 23 acromegalic patients (A) and a subgroup of 8 patients with microadenomas (B).

secretion in acromegaly is a pathological response to LH-RH and/or TRH in approximately 20 and 60% of the patients, respectively (Faglia *et al.*, 1973a, 1973b; Quabbe, 1978). Normal subjects do not show this response. Again, this is not entirely specific for acromegaly, since it can also be seen in patients with other diseases (e.g. protein-calorie malnutrition and chronic renal failure). There is evidence that the pituitary somatotroph normally has receptors for at least TRH. It does not respond to TRH because of hypothalamic inhibition. In acromegalic patients, this inhibition may be lacking. This hypothesis is supported by a stimulation of GH secretion by small doses of TRH in rats bearing ectopic pituitary glands and by the GH response to TRH from the isolated perfused rat hypophysis (Udeschini *et al.*, 1976; Carlson *et al.*, 1974).

**Autonomous versus hypothalamus-dependent
GH secretion – the problem of the
"hypothalamic origin of acromegaly"**

In some patients with acromegaly, the plasma GH concentration responds to a certain degree to influences which are thought to be mediated via the hypothalamus (such as insulin-hypoglycemia or hyperglycemia). In view of these

and some other observations, the concept has been developed that GH
secretion in acromegaly remains under partial hypothalamic influence or
that at least in some patients acromegaly may be of "hypothalamic origin"
(Cryer and Daughaday, 1969; Lawrence et al., 1970; Sherman and Kolodny,
1971). This hypothesis is interesting not only from a pathophysiological point
of view, but also because it would open the way to treatment by centrally acting
drugs.

Two different possibilities could be envisaged:

(1)    Primary hypothalamic dysfunction causes chronic overstimulation of the
       pituitary somatotrophs. Some of them develop into a pituitary adenoma
       which later attains full or partial autonomy. In this case, more evidence
       of non-autonomous behavior would be expected in smaller than in large
       tumors.
(2)    A primary pituitary adenoma, possibly of monoclonal origin, evolves in the
       absence of increased hypothalamic stimulation. Its cells, however, attain
       only a limited degree of autonomy and respond to hypothalamic influences.
       In this case, the nature of the tumor, whether hypothalamus-dependent or
       autonomous, would be an "inborn characteristic" and would more probably
       be independent of its size and duration of existence.

How is it possible to differentiate between an autonomous and a hypothalamus-dependent GH-secreting adenoma? One approach would be the
determination of GH-RH and/or GH-RIH (somatostatin) in the hypophyseal stalk
or the jugular vein. In the case of an autonomous adenoma one would expect low
GH-releasing activity, since a feedback inhibition of GH on its own secretion
seems to exist. High releasing activity (or low GH-release-inhibiting activity)
would be expected in the case of hypothalamic overstimulation. Measurements of
the hypothalamic releasing and inhibiting hormones in the pituitary stalk or in
the jugular vein are not easily obtainable in man, but peripheral blood and CSF
have been examined.

Plasma from acromegalic patients has a higher stimulatory activity on GH
release from monkey pituitary glands than normal plasma (Hagen et al., 1971).
While this suggests that a circulating substance with GH-releasing activity is
increased in acromegaly, its nature is unknown and the finding needs confirmation. Normal somatostatin concentrations have been found in the CSF of
acromegalic patients (Patel et al., 1977), but it is not known whether CSF
somatostatin reflects hypothalamic somatostatin secretory activity or not. Thus,
there is at the present time no direct evidence for a hypothalamic overstimulation
of the pituitary gland in acromegaly.

Indirect evidence could come from histological examination of pituitary glands
of patients with acromegaly. It would be expected that hypothalamic overstimulation would lead to signs of increased activity in the tissue surrounding the
adenoma. This has been described for some but not all pituitaries harboring PRL-
and ACTH-producing adenomas and also for pituitaries which had developed TSH-
adenomas during long-standing primary hypothyroidism. There is so far no
evidence that the somatotrophs of the normal pituitary tissue are overstimulated
in patients with growth hormone-secreting tumors (Saeger, 1977).

One of the arguments for full or partial hypothalamic dependency of GH-secreting pituitary adenomas rests on their response to stimuli relayed via the hypothalamus, such as insulin-induced hypoglycemia or hyperglycemia. A response of the plasma GH concentration in acromegaly to stimulation by insulin-induced hypoglycemia and by arginin infusion and to suppression by hyperglycemia has been reported (Cryer and Daughaday, 1969; Lawrence *et al.*, 1970). The GH increase during exercise may also be observed in acromegaly (Johnson and Rennie, 1973). An important observation is the GH response to centrally acting drugs in some cases because of its implications for the possible conservative treatment of patients with acromegaly (Liuzzi and Chiodini, this volume).

What is the evidence that some or all of these GH responses in acromegaly are due to hypothalamic influences? The pattern of responses seems to represent part of the disease in a given patient. As long as the pituitary tumor is present, a patient usually continues to exhibit the same pattern when retested. After successful selective removal of an adenoma, the remaining pituitary tissue will respond in a normal manner (Lawrence *et al.*, 1970; Hoyte and Martin, 1975; Faglia *et al.*, 1978; Quabbe, 1978). This suggests that the pathological response of the tumor resides in the adenoma itself and not in the hypothalamus. However, by analogy to the TRH-induced GH response of the ectopic pituitary gland, another possibility may be considered. The pathological type of response may be potentially present in the normal pituitary but be inhibited under normal circumstances. Removal of the inhibition (due to feedback inhibition by elevated GH or due to a primary hypothalamic lack of inhibition?) would unmask the response. In this case, one would expect a certain homogeneity of pathological responses in a given patient, since they would be due to a common hypothalamic dysregulation. However, this is not the case. In our group of patients, no obvious correlation between the response to TRH and the paradoxical response to glucose was seen (Fig. 1). There is a lack of homogeneity of the response to TRH and the response to the dopamine agonist bromocriptine in 30% of the patients (Quabbe, 1978). No correlation between the response to TRH and that to other stimulatory or suppressive tests was found by Faglia *et al.* (1973b) in a group of 21 acromegalics. These results make it more likely that the pathological responses are an inherent characteristic of the adenoma than an expression of hypothalamic disregulation.

### Relation between the plasma GH concentration and the clinical activity of acromegaly

Plasma GH measurements have shown that there is only a poor relation between the plasma GH concentration and the apparent clinical activity of the disease. Patients with low GH concentrations may have marked acromegalic features and vice versa. While this may partly be due to different duration of GH excess, longer duration leading to a more severe expression of the disease, additional possibilities must also be considered. Difficulties in correlating tumor size, GH concentration in the plasma and clinical activity in a given patient arise from the heterogeneity of circulating GH molecules, the interposition of the

somatomedins between GH and many of the manifestations of acromegaly, and
from possible individual differences of the peripheral response to GH and the
somatomedins.

*Different molecular forms of growth hormone*

GH exists in different molecular forms in the plasma and in the pituitary of
normal subjects and of acromegalic patients. "Little" GH corresponds to the
monomeric GH molecule and "big" GH has a molecular weight about twice that
of the "little" form. Acromegalic plasma contains relatively more of the "little"
component than plasma from normals (Goodman *et al.*, 1972; Gorden *et al.*,
1976). The "little" GH has a higher reactivity in radioreceptor-assays (RRA)
and thus is probably biologically more active than "big" GH (Herington *et al.*,
1974; Gorden *et al.*, 1976). The "little" GH of acromegalics may be biologically
more active than the "little" GH from normals (Gorden *et al.*, 1976). The exact
relation of activity in the RRA's, which use receptor preparations from animals or
human lymphocytes, to the biological activity of the secreted GH *in vivo* in the
human body remains, however, to be established. These findings could explain
the presence of high concentrations of immunoreactive GH (which thus includes
biologically less active GH forms) in patients with a clinically mild form of
acromegaly. However, the difference in RIA- and RRA-measurable GH is not
important enough to account for all of the discrepancies between GH concentrations in the plasma and clinical severity of the disease. Other factors may be
more important.

*Somatomedins*

GH has no effect on the growth of cartilage or the epiphyseal growth zone
*in vitro*. Many of its *in vivo* effects depend on the generation of somatomedins
(SM), a heterogenous family of substances. One or several of them are probably
synthesized in the liver (McConaghey and Sledge, 1970). In addition to GH, other
hormones also have an influence on SM generation and action. Insulin participates
in the stimulation of SM release from the liver (Daughaday *et al.*, 1976), while
estrogens decrease the plasma SM concentration (Wiedemann and Schwartz, 1972;
Wiedemann *et al.*, 1976). Somatomedins may be bound specifically to a plasma
protein and this binding seems to be under the influence of GH (Moses *et al.*,
1976; Heinrich *et al.*, 1978). These interactions (Fig. 2) open the possibility
of secondary adjustments which could explain some discrepancies between GH
concentrations and the clinical expression of acromegaly.

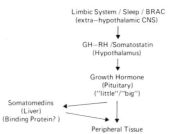

*Fig. 2.* Schematic presentation of the link between CNS – pituitary GH secretion – peripheral
GH action.

The mean concentrations of the somatomedins A and B are elevated in patients with acromegaly, but the correlation between the plasma concentration of GH and the SM concentration is only weak. There is also some overlap between normal and acromegalic values of somatomedin A and B (Yalow *et al.*, 1975; Takano *et al.*, 1976). Another somatomedin, NSILA-S (nonsuppressible-insulin-like-activity), has been reported to be either elevated (Schlumpf *et al.*, 1976; Heinrich *et al.*, 1978) or not to be different from normals in acromegalics (Megyesi *et al.*, 1977). The lack of a good correlation between the somatomedins and GH concentrations in acromegaly may be due in part to technical problems of the SM assays (presence of inhibitors?) and to the large variation of single GH values in the blood of patients with acromegaly. However, the details of interaction between GH, somatomedins and peripheral effects are still largely unknown. Other diseases with elevated SM activity have been described. Elevated SM levels in the presence of normal GH concentrations have been found in patients with hypopituitarism, associated with obesity and overgrowth (Finkelstein *et al.*, 1972; Hoffenberg *et al.*, 1977). In diabetes mellitus, elevated, but also low, SM values have been reported (Yde, 1969; Cohen *et al.*, 1977). Thus, more knowledge about the nature and regulation of SM activity is necessary before the exact role of these substances in acromegaly can be assessed.

### Difference in peripheral effects of growth hormone

A difference in the peripheral action of GH and/or the somatomedins between individual patients is another possibility for explaining discrepancies between the plasma concentration of these hormones and the clinical expression of the disease. For instance, estrogens antagonize the peripheral action of GH (Schwartz *et al.*, 1969). They decrease the plasma somatomedin activity in normals (Wiedemann *et al.*, 1976). The plasma concentration of estrogens, and possibly other hormones (testosterone, thyroid hormones, insulin?), may therefore modulate the peripheral effect of GH excess. For instance, it would thus be conceivable that the acromegalic manifestation becomes more pronounced when a large pituitary tumor induces gonadotrophin deficiency and thereby causes low estrogen concentrations in women. Longitudinal studies of untreated patients could reveal whether the clinical expression of acromegaly becomes more severe in women after the menopause, when estrogen concentrations decrease.

GH concentrations are elevated in patients with juvenile diabetes mellitus. Their mean 24-hour plasma concentration is often in a range which can also be found in some patients with active acromegaly (Johansen and Hansen, 1971; Table II). At the present time, it is unknown why these patients do not show acromegalic features, However, peripheral antagonism to the action of GH must be considered to be a possibility.

### Endocrine and metabolic response to GH excess

The endocrine and metabolic derangements associated with acromegaly have recently been reviewed (Quabbe, 1978). Here, only those which are due to the excess of GH and which have a certain clinical importance will be briefly discussed.

Overt diabetes mellitus is observed in about 20% of all patients and asymptomatic diabetes in another 12% (Wright *et al.*, 1970). In many other patients, glucose administration will reveal that normal carbohydrate tolerance is only achieved at the expense of elevated plasma insulin concentrations. GH excess causes an inhibition of glucose uptake by peripheral tissues in response to insulin. On the other hand, antagonism to the inhibitory action of insulin results in more hepatic glucose production (Bishop *et al.*, 1967). This increases the demand on insulin output. Additional consequences of GH excess, which may contribute to a deterioration of carbohydrate tolerance and yet promote high insulin secretion, are an increase in glucagon secretion (Goldfine *et al.*, 1972) as well as of secretin (Chisholm *et al.*, 1972). When even maximal insulin secretion can no longer balance carbohydrate tolerance, diabetes becomes manifest. Since the presence of diabetes mellitus is associated with increased mortality in acromegalic patients (Wright *et al.*, 1970), normalization of carbohydrate tolerance, including insulin secretion, should be one of the aims of treatment for any patient with acromegaly.

There is also a strong association between increased mortality in acromegaly and cardiovascular and cerebrovascular disease (Wright *et al.*, 1970). The pathogenesis of these conditions is, of course, complex. Could GH excess influence vascular disease by its action on lipid metabolism? Serum triglyceride concentrations increase during acute adminstration of GH to man (Friedman *et al.*, 1974), but this effect does not persist during chronic treatment (Aloia *et al.*, 1975). In acromegaly the mean serum triglyceride concentration is elevated (Nikkilä and Pelkonen, 1975), but this may be related to the presence of diabetes mellitus rather than being due to GH directly (Aloia *et al.*, 1972; Azizi *et al.*, 1973). On the other hand, GH depresses rather than elevates the plasma cholesterol concentration in animals and in human subjects during acute but not during chronic treatment (Friedman *et al.*, 1970, 1972, 1974; Aloia *et al.*, 1975). In acromegalic patients with otherwise normal pituitary function, the mean plasma cholesterol concentration is lower than in normals (Nikkilä and Pelkonen, 1975). In GH-deficient dwarfs with diabetes mellitus, serum triglyceride and cholesterol concentrations are elevated despite the absence of GH. Yet they do not have vascular disease (Merimee, 1978).

These observations support the conclusion that the influence of GH on vascular disease in acromegaly is not a direct consequence of its action on lipid metabolism. An effect of GH on the tissue of the vessel wall has been described (Brosnan *et al.*, 1973), but its possible role in the pathogenesis of vascular disease is unknown.

Hypertension may also play a role. It is found in approximately 23 - 45% of the patients (Wright *et al.*, 1970; McGuffin *et al.*, 1974). Probably it is more related to sodium and water retention caused by GH (Corvilain and Abramow, 1962) than to other endocrinological changes. An increased secretion rate of cortisol and corticosterone has been described (Roginsky *et al.*, 1966; Winkelmann *et al.*, 1968). Elevated urinary excretion of norepinephrine (Marek *et al.*, 1974) has also been reported, but the plasma concentration of both epinephrine and norepinephrine were normal in another group of acromegalic patients (Cryer, 1975). An effect of GH on aldosterone synthesis and secretion has also been described in rats (Venning and Lucis, 1962; Palkovits *et al.*, 1971), but its importance in man has been questioned (Birkhäuser *et al.*, 1975; McCaa *et al.*, 1978).

GH-secreting pituitary adenomas are associated with increased prolactin plasma concentrations in approximately 33% to 50% of the patients (Aubert, 1974; Von Werder *et al.*, 1976; Quabbe, 1978). In most cases this elevation is modest. Derangement of other pituitary hormones develops only as a consequence of pituitary compression due to the growth of the tumor, except for the very rare cases of tumors which secrete more than one hormone. Recently, a possible stimulatory influence of GH on parathyroid hormone secretion and on $1\alpha,25(OH)_2$-vitamin $D_3$ formation has received attention (Lancer *et al.*, 1976; Spanos *et al.*, 1978). At the present time, studies in patients with acromegaly are lacking, and the importance of these findings for the skeletal changes in this disease remains a matter of further investigation. However, in our own group of patients, the parathyroid hormone concentration in plasma samples taken in the morning after an overnight fast were within the normal limits ($n = 29$), except for borderline values in two patients and an excessive elevation in one patient with a coexistent parathyroid adenoma.*

## SPECIAL ASPECTS OF GH-SECRETING MICROADENOMAS

Growth hormone secreting microadenomas are being diagnosed more frequently during recent years due to the use of more refined roentgenological and endocrinological methods. By definition, a microadenoma is less than 10 mm in diameter; the sella turcica is normal in size on lateral roentgenograms, but there may be an asymmetry of the floor of the sella on tomograms (Vezina and Maltais, 1973; Hardy, 1973). Apart from their small size, are these microadenomas different from larger tumors? Some aspects of this question will be briefly discussed.

### Is there a relation between tumor size and plasma GH concentration?

Nests of proliferation or small adenomas are found in 25% of all pituitaries at routine autopsies (Daughaday, 1974). Patients with clinically manifest acromegaly usually do have signs of a pituitary tumor on roentgenological examination. These signs may be discrete, so that the tumor may be classified as a microadenoma. Such microadenomas may already produce markedly elevated plasma GH concentrations (Table I). On the other hand, some patients may have relatively large tumors with clinically indisputable acromegaly and yet have only a small elevation of GH concentrations (e.g. patients K.S. and W.W., Table II; Fig. 3). Moreover, there are even pituitary tumors without clinical evidence of hormonal activity, which histologically resemble GH-secreting adenomas and contain immunoreactive GH (Kirsch and Nakane, 1974).

Mims and Bethune (1974) observed five patients with acromegaly and low fasting GH concentrations, all of whom had 24-hour mean GH concentrations

---

*Determinations were kindly done by either Dr. Offermann, Berlin, using antiserum CH 12 M, which has a high affinity for the intact hormone (PTH 1 – 84 ($n = 7$) or by Dr. Hehrmann, Hannover, using antiserum S 469, which primarily recognizes C-regional fragments ($n = 30$).

*Table I.*  GH concentration in seven acromegalic patients with normal-sized sella turcica.

| | | X-Rays | | GH concentration during oGTT[a] (ng/ml) | Baseline GH concentration[b] (ng/ml) |
|---|---|---|---|---|---|
| Patient | Age (y) | Routine lateral and sagittal | Tomography | | |
| A.H. | 70 | borderline[c] | – | 20.2 | 16.4 |
| B.L. | 56 | normal | depression left floor | 8.3 | 4.5 |
| F.L. | 53 | borderline | depression midline floor | 27.8 | 25.0 |
| H.W. | 62 | normal | depression left floor | 30.7 | 46.0 |
| M.A.-F | 29 | normal | – | 21.1 | 21.8 |
| P.R. | 55 | normal | normal | 11.1 | 8.6 |
| W.F. | 66 | borderline | depression left floor | 35.0 | 43.7 |

[a]  Mean of six values during oral glucose tolerance test (100 g).
[b]  Mean of three different baseline concentrations.
[c]  Normal-sized sella but double contour of floor on routine lateral X-rays. of the skull and/or one-sided depression of floor on routine pa X-rays. No erosion of bone.

below 10 ng/ml. Three of them had an enlarged sella turcica. Sönksen *et al.* (1967) found a highly significant correlation between estimated volume of the pituitary fossa and plasma GH concentration in a group of 16 acromegalic patients. However, there was only moderate correlation of plasma GH concentrations with the sella area in a larger group of 84 acromegalic patients of Wright *et al.* (1969).

Thus, there is not necessarily a relation between the size of a GH-secreting tumor and the plasma GH concentration. The absence of a reliable relationship between these two is to be expected. Pituitary tumors may contain necrotic areas and cysts, so that sella or tumor size cannot necessarily be equated to secretory tumor tissue (Saeger, 1977). Furthermore, total GH secretion and not the number or size of GH-producing cells of an adenoma is responsible for the plasma GH concentration. A small adenoma with high secretory activity may cause higher plasma GH concentrations than a large adenoma with lower secretory activity. In general, there is good correlation between ultrastructural evidence of secretory activity and the plasma GH concentration (Landolt, 1975). The difficulties in relating plasma GH concentration to the clinical expression of acromegaly have been dealt with in the section on "Relation between the plasma GH concentration and the clinical activity of acromegaly".

Table II. Test results in five patients with GH concentrations below 10 ng/ml and mean GH concentrations in non-acromegalic patients with juvenile diabetes mellitus.[e]

| Patient | Sex | Age (y) | Size of sella[c] | Basal GH[a] (ng/ml) | Mean GH during oGTT[b] (ng/ml) | Paradoxical response to glucose[d] | Response to hypoglycemia[a] | Response to LH-RH/TRH[a] |
|---|---|---|---|---|---|---|---|---|
| G.K. | M | 47 | large | 7.3 | 18.3 | + | + | ∅ |
| K.S. | F | 38 | large | 6.6 | 4.2 | ∅ | ∅ | + |
| W.W. | M | 53 | large | 7.2 | 7.1 | ∅ | ∅ | ∅ |
| B.L. | F | 56 | small | 4.5 | 8.3 | + | + | + |
| P.R. | F | 55 | small | 8.6 | 11.1 | ∅ | + | + |
| | | | | | | | | |
| Juvenile diabetics[e] | | | | | | | | |
| good control | | | | 7.4[f] | | | | |
| poor control | | | | 8.3 | | | | |
| | | | | | | | | |
| Normal subjects[e] | | | | 2.0 | | | | |

[a] Mean of three different basal values.
[b] Mean of six values.
[c] Large sella: ballooning on routine lateral X-rays. Small sella: no definite pathology on routine lateral and pa X-rays.
[d] A response is defined as an increase of more than 50% above the baseline value.
[e] Data from Johansen and Hansen (1971).
[f] Half-hourly 24-hour profile.

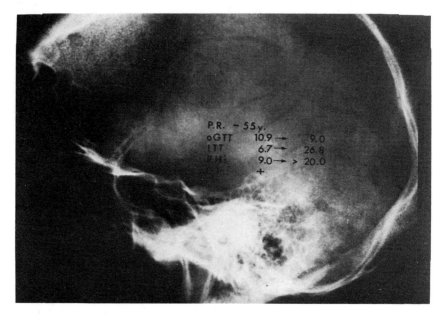

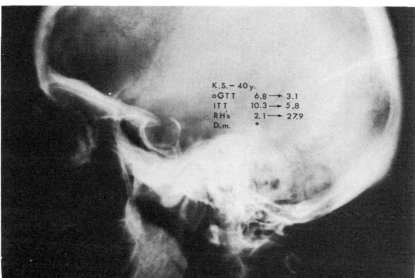

*Fig. 3.* Lateral skull X-rays of two acromegalic patients with normal-sized and enlarged sella respectively. Note that low basal GH concentrations and GH responses in oral GTT during insulin hypoglycemia and in the releasing hormone test (inset) are strikingly similar despite the difference in tumor size. Both patients have diabetes mellitus.

*Table III.* Comparison of patients with large and small sella turcica.

| Size of sella[a] | GH concentration[b] (ng/ml) | Paradoxical response to glucose[c] | Suppression by hyperglycemia[d] | Response to hypoglycemia[c] | Response to LH-RH/TRH[e] | All tests | Diabetes mellitus[f] |
|---|---|---|---|---|---|---|---|
| Large | 38.8 (17) | 7 (19) | 2 (19) | 12 (20) | 9 (12) | 30 (70) | 6 (18) |
| Small | 24.3 (7) | 2 (7) | 1 (7) | 5 (6) | 3 (3) | 11 (23) | 4 (6) |

In brackets: number of patients in whom the respective test was done.

[a] Large – larger than normal as judged by the roentgenologist, without actual measurement of the size. Includes one sella with obvious erosion of the bone, but no other evident enlargement.
Small – not increased on routine lateral X-rays.
[b] Mean of three different baseline concentrations.
[c] GH increase of more than 50% above the baseline concentration.
[d] GH decrease of more than 50% below the baseline concentration.
[e] LH-RH- and TRH-tests were done separately on most, but not all occasions. A response is defined as an increase of more than 50% at 30 min above the baseline concentration.
[f] Manifest or asymptomatic diabetes mellitus as judged from the oGTT.

### Are microadenomas more hypothalamus-dependent than larger tumors?

The answer to this question is of importance because of its implications for
the treatment of GH-secreting tumors. If microadenomas were often or usually
hypothalamus-dependent and would develop autonomy only in the later course of
their growth, conservative treatment (e.g. with modulators of neurotransmitter
action) might then possibly prevent them from becoming autonomous and could
cause them to regress into functional quiescence.

Unfortunately, microadenomas do not seem to be more often hypothalamus-
dependent than larger tumors, at least if the criterion of a response to various
stimulatory and suppressive tests is used (Fig. 1, Table III). Table III shows that
the relative incidence of GH responses in a group of 24 patients is not significantly
different in the subgroups with large and small adenomas respectively. Patients
with large tumor responded in 43% of all tests (30 times in 70 tests) and those
with small tumors in 48% of the tests (11 times in 23 tests). The group is too
small to be analyzed for group-relevant differences in single tests.

Together with the data discussed in the Section on "autonomous versus
hypothalamus-dependent GH secretion, the problem of the 'hypothalamic origin
of acromegaly' ", this suggests that the pattern of response to these different
tests is an inherent characteristic of a given adenoma and is not lost during growth
of the tumor. Thus, certain tumors may be more amenable to conservative
treatment independent of their size. On the other hand, others may not respond
from the beginning on. However, there are, at the present time, not enough
data available on the relationship between a GH response in the diverse
stimulatory and suppressive tests and a response to drug therapy. Our present
knowledge does not allow us to reliably predict the response to drug therapy of a
given adenoma from its behavior in these tests.

The problems related to pharmacological treatment of GH-secreting adenomas
will be examined in more detail in another contribution to this volume (Liuzzi
and Chiodini).

### Do all microadenomas evolve into macroadenomas?

The data cited in the section on "is there a relation between tumor size and
plasma GH concentration?" suggest that many pituitary adenomas never attain
a size that allows roentgenological recognition. Many also seem never to develop
excessive or uncontrolled secretory activity. If a considerable number of microadenomas never evolve into a macroadenoma, with the risk of visual impairment
and other complications due to para- or suprasellar expansion, one would feel
much safer to try long-term conservative treatment in these patients. There are
not many longitudinal observations of untreated patients with GH-secreting
microadenomas. In one report, five of seven untreated patients increased their GH
concentration within 12 - 48 months of the initial observation (Roth et al.,
1970). In another group, only one of nine untreated patients retested after more
than 12 months had an increase in his GH concentration, while the others
remained stable or had lower values (Hunter et al., 1974). These reports did not

differentiate between microadenomas and larger tumors, and no mention is made of changes in the tumor size. It is obvious, however, that all large tumors must have passed through the stage of a microadenoma. If the secretory potential of the cells of a given tumor is characteristic of that tumor, then it will also secrete more GH as it grows larger, notwithstanding the fact that among different tumors size is only poorly correlated with the plasma GH concentration. Consequently, unless a drug achieves normalization of GH concentration and of related endocrine and metabolic derangements and causes at least, arrest of growth of the adenoma if not regression, it cannot serve as an adequate mode of long-term treatment.

### Do we cure acromegaly by selectively removing a microadenoma?

If microadenomas are of "hypothalamic origin" i.e. if the cause of adenoma formation in the pituitary gland is a "hypothalamic overdrive", it cannot be expected that removal of the target gland adenoma cures the disease. On the contrary, one would expect recurrence of an adenoma after a certain time. On the other hand, if a GH-secreting adenoma develops autonomously, its complete selective removal would probably cure the patient, unless one assumes a generally increased potential of his pituitary somatotrophs to form adenomas. There are, at the present time, not enough long-term follow-up studies of patients with selectively removed GH-secreting microadenomas to answer this question. However, as more and more of such patients are successfully treated in this way, a preliminary answer will probably soon become available.

### REFERENCES

Aloia, J. F., Roginsky, M. S. and Field, R. A. (1972). *J. clin. Endocrin. Metab.* **35**, 921–923.

Aloia, J. F., Zanzi, I. and Cohn, S. H. (1975). *Metabolism* **24**, 795–798.

Aubert, M. L., Grumbach M. M. and Kaplan, S. L. (1974). *Acta Endocrinol. (Copenh.)* **77**, 460–476.

Azizi, F., Castelli, W. P., Raben, M. S. and Mitchell, M. L. (1973). *Proc. Soc. Exp. Biol. Med.* **143**, 1187–1190.

Birkhäuser, M., Gaillard, R., Riondel, A. M. and Zahnd, G. R. (1975). *Acta Endocrinol. (Copenh.)* **79**, 16–24.

Bishop, J. S., Steele, R., Altszuler, N., Rathgeb, I., Bjerknes, C. and de Bodo, R. C., (1967). *Amer. J. Physiol.* **212**, 272–278.

Brosnan, M. E., Sirek, O. V., Sirek, A. and Przybylska, K., (1973). *Diabetes* **22**, 243–250.

Carlson, H. E., Mariz, I. K. and Daughaday, W. H. (1974). *Endocrinology* **94**, 1709–1713.

Chisholm, D. J., Lazarus, L. and Young, J. D. (1972). *J. Clin. Endocrin. Metab.* **35**, 108–112.

Cohen, M. P., Jasti, K. and Rye, D. L. (1977). *J. Clin. Endocrin. Metab.* **45**, 236–239.

Corvilain, J. and Abramow, M. (1962). *J. clin. Invest.* **41**, 1230–1235.

Cryer, P. E. (1975). *J. Clin. Endocrin. Metab.* **41**, 542–545.

Cryer, P. E. and Daughaday, W. H. (1969). *J. Clin. Endocrin. Metab.* **29**, 386–393.

Daughaday, W. H. (1974). *In* "Textbook of Endocrinology", (5th Ed.) (R. H. Williams, ed) pp 31–79. W. B. Saunders, Philadelphia.

Daughaday, W. H., Phillips, L. S. and Mueller, M. C. (1976). *Endocrinology* **98**. 1214–1219.

Faglia, G., Beck-Peccoz, P., Travaglini, P., Paracchi, A., Spada, A. and Lewin, A. (1973a). *J. Clin. Endocrin. Metab.* **37**, 338–340.

Faglia, G., Beck-Peccoz, P., Ferrari, C., Travaglini, P., Ambrosi, B. and Spada, A. (1973b). *J. Clin. Endocrin. Metab.* **36**, 1259–1262.

Faglia, G., Paracchi, A., Ferrari, C. and Beck-Peccoz, P. (1978) *Clin. Endocrinol.* **8**, 373–380.

Finkelstein, J. W., Kream, J., Ludan, A. and Hellman, L. (1972). *J. Clin. Endocrin. Metab.* **35**, 13–17.

Friedman, M., Byers, S. O. and Elek, S. R. (1970). *Nature* **225**, 464–467.

Friedman, M., Byers, S. O., Rosenman, R. H. and Li, C. H. (1972). *Proc. Soc. Exp. Biol. Med.* **141**, 76–80.

Friedman, M., Byers, S. O., Rosenman, R. H., Li, C. H. and Neuman, R. (1974). *Metabolism* **23**, 905–912.

Goldfine, I. D., Kirsteins, L. and Lawrence, A. M. (1972). *Horm. Metab. Res.* **4**, 97–100.

Goodman, A. D., Tanenbaum, R. and Rabinowitz, D. (1972). *J. Clin. Endocrin. Metab.* **35**, 868–878.

Gorden, P., Lesniak, M. A., Eastman, R., Hendricks, C. M. and Roth, J. (1976). *J. Clin. Endocrin. Metab.* **43**, 364–373.

Hagen, T. C., Lawrence, A. M. and Kirsteins, L. (1971). *J. Clin. Endocr. Metab.* **33**, 448–451.

Hardy, J. (1973). *In* "Diagnosis and Treatment of Pituitary Tumors" (P. O. Kohler and G. T. Ross, eds) pp. 179–194. Elsevier, New York.

Heinrich, U. E., Schalch, D. S., Koch, J. G. and Johnson, C. J. (1978). *J. Clin. Endocrin. Metab.* **46**, 672–678.

Herington, A. C., Jacobs, L. S. and Daughaday, W. H. (1974). *J. Clin. Endocrin. Metab.* **39**, 257–262.

Hoffenberg, R., Howell, A., Epstein, S., Pimstone, B. L., Fryklund, L., Hall, K., Schwalbe, S. and Rudd, B. T. (1977). *Clin. Endocrinol.* **6**, 443–448.

Hoyte, K. M. and Martin, J. B. (1975). *J. Clin. Endocrin. Metab.* **41**, 656–659.

Hunter, W. M., Gillingham, F. J., Harris, P., Kanis, J. A., McGurk, F. M., McLelland, J. and Strong, J. A. (1974). *J. Endocr.* **63**, 21–34.

Johansen, K. and Hansen, Aa. P. (1971). *Diabetes* **20**, 239–245.

Johnson, R. H. and Rennie, M. J. (1973). *Clin. Sci.* **44**, 63–71.

Kirsch, W. M. and Nakane, P. K. (1974). *In* "5th International Congress of Neurological Surgery", 7 – 13 Oct. 1973, Tokyo, Japan. Excerpta Medica Int. Congr. Series No. 293, Amsterdam, p.35.

Lancer, S. R., Bowser, E. N., Hargis, G. K. and Williams, G. A. (1976). *Endocrinology* **98**, 1289–1293.

Landolt, A. M. (1975). "Ultrastructure of Human Sella Tumors", p.44. Springer Verlag, Wien and New York.

Lawrence, A. M., Goldfine, I. D. and Kirsteins, L. (1970). *J. Clin. Endocrin. Metab.* **31**, 239–247.

McCaa, R. E., Montalvo, J. M. and McCaa, C. S. (1978). *J. Clin. Endocrin. Metab.* **46**, 247–253.

McConaghey, P. and Sledge, C. B. (1970). *Nature* **225**, 1249–1250.

McGuffin, W. L., Jr., Sherman, B. M., Roth, J., Gorden, P., Kahn, C. R., Roberts, W. C. and Frommer, P. L. (1974). *Ann. Intern. Med.* 81, 11–18.
Marek, J., Horký, K., Kopecká, J., Mestan, J. and Srámková, J. (1974). *Endokrinologie* 63, 304–310.
Megyesi, K., Gorden, P. and Kahn, C. R. (1977). *J. Clin. Endocrin. Metab.* 45, 330–338.
Merimee, T. J. (1978). *New Engl. J. Med.* 298, 1217–1222.
Merimee, T. J. and Rabin, D. (1973). *Metabolism* 22, 1235–1251.
Mims, R. B. and Bethune, J. E. (1974). *Ann. Intern. Med.* 81, 781–784.
Moses, A. C., Nissley, S. P. and Cohen, K. L. (1976). *Nature* 263, 137–140.
Nikkilä E. A. and Pelkonen, R. (1975). *Metabolism* 24, 829–838.
Palkovits, M., de Jong, W., van der Wal, B. and de Wied, D. (1971). *J. Endocrinol.* 50, 407–411.
Patel, Y. C., Rao, K. and Reichlin, S. (1977). *New Engl. J. Med.* 296, 529–533.
Quabbe, H.-J. (1977). *Chronobiologia* 4, 217–246.
Quabbe, H.-J. (1978). *In* "Treatment of Pituitary Adenomas" (R. Fahlbusch and K. Von Werder, eds) pp. 47–60, Thieme Verlag, Stuttgart.
Roginsky, M. S., Shaver, J. C. and Christy, N. P. (1966). *J. Clin. Endocrin. Metab.* 26, 1101–1108.
Roth, J., Gorden, P. and Brace, K. (1970). *New Engl. J. Med.* 282, 1385–1391.
Saeger, W. (1977). "Die Hypophysentumoren". G. Fischer Verlag, Stuttgart and New York.
Schlumpf, U., Heimann, R., Zapf, J. and Froesch, E. R. (1976). *Acta Endocrinol. (Copenh.)* 81, 28–42.
Schofield, J. G. (1967). *Biochem. J.* 103, 331–341.
Schwartz, E., Wiedemann, E., Simon, S. and Schiffer, M. (1969). *J. Clin. Endocrin. Metab.* 29, 1176–1181.
Sherman, L. and Kolodny, H. D. (1971). *Lancet* 1, 682–685.
Sönksen, P. H., Greenwood, F. C., Ellis, J. P., Lowy, C., Rutherford, A. and Nabarro, J. D. N. (1967). *J. Clin. Endocrin. Metab.* 27, 1418–1430.
Spanos, E., Barrett, D., MacIntyre, I. Pike, J. W., Safilian, E. F. and Haussler, M. R. (1978). *Nature* 273, 246–247.
Takano, K., Hall, K., Ritzén, M., Iselius, L. and Sievertsson, H. (1976). *Acta Endocrinol. (Copenh.)* 82, 449–459.
Udeschini, G., Cocchi, D., Panerai, A. E., Gil-Ad, I., Rossi, G. L., Chiodini, P. G., Liuzzi, A. and Müller, E. E. (1976). *Endocrinology* 98, 807–814.
Venning, E. H. and Lucis, O. J. (1962). *Endocrinology* 70, 486–491.
Vezina, J. L. and Maltais, R. (1973). *Neurochirurgie* 19, Suppl. 2, 35–56.
Von Werder, K., Fahlbusch, R., Gay, R., Pickardt, C. R. and Schultz, B. (1976). *Klin. Wschr.* 54, 335–338.
Wiedemann, E. and Schwartz, E. (1972). *J. Clin. Endocrin. Metab.* 34, 51–58.
Wiedemann, E., Schwartz, E. and Frantz, A. G., (1976). *J. Clin. Endocrin. Metab.* 42, 942–952.
Winkelmann, W., Bethge, H., Schmitt, H., Solbach, H. G., Vorster, D. and Zimmermann, H. (1968). *Klin. Wschr.* 46, 1008–1010.
Wright, A. D., McLachlan, M. S. F., Doyle, F. H. and Fraser, T. R. (1969). *Brit. Med. J.* 4, 582–584.
Wright, A. D., Hill, D. M., Lowy, C. and Fraser, T. R. (1970). *Quart. J. Med.* 39, 1–16.
Yalow, R. S., Hall, K. and Luft, R. (1975). *J. Clin. Invest.* 55, 127–137.
Yde, H. (1969). *Acta med. scand.* 186, 293–297.

# PROLACTIN SECRETION IN ACROMEGALY

P. Moriondo, P. Travaglini, M. Rondena, P. Beck-Peccoz, F. Conti-Puglisi,
B. Ambrosi and G. Faglia

*2nd Medical Clinic, Endocrine Unit, University of Milan, Italy*

## INTRODUCTION

Hyperprolactinemia is frequently found in acromegalic patients. However, the interrelationships between prolactin (PRL) and growth hormone (GH) secretions have not as yet been clarified. Franks *et al.* (1976) did not find any overall correlation between GH and PRL secretions, though in 3 of 26 cases there was some evidence that both GH and PRL were hypersecreted by the tumor cells. Winkelmann *et al.* (1978) reported a PRL increase after TRH in 40% of hyperprolactinemic acromegalics, but the results were not compared with GH-responsiveness to the same stimulus.

The close concordance between GH-responsiveness to TRH and suppressibility by dopaminergic drugs (Liuzzi *et al.*, 1974) suggests that in responding patients GH secretion is similar to PRL secretion in normal subjects (Faglia *et al.*, 1975; Liuzzi *et al.*, 1975). However, PRL secretion is suppressed by dopaminergic drugs irrespective of GH-responsiveness to these agents. Furthermore, Camanni *et al.* (1977) and Schwinn *et al.* (1977) have reported that the regulation of GH and PRL in TRH-responsive patients is not exactly the same, since the administration of dopaminergic agents reduced the PRL but not the GH release after TRH. In the present study, the effects of TRH, anticatecholaminergic and dopaminergic drugs (administered separately or in combination) on serum PRL and GH were investigated in acromegalic patients, in order to clarify the extent to which and how PRL and GH secretions may be correlated.

## MATERIALS AND METHODS

Forty-two patients with active acromegaly (27 women and 15 men, aged between 18–73) volunteered for this study. All experiments were carried out in patients in bed after an overnight fast, blood specimens being taken through an indwelling needle kept permeable by slow saline infusion. Serum GH and PRL levels were measured in basal conditions on different occasions (at least 5 blood specimens), and after TRH (200 $\mu$g i.v.) or bromocriptine (2.5 mg. p.o.) administration. Blood was taken at $-30, 0, 30, 60$ and $120$ min after TRH and every 60 min for 6h during the bromocriptine test.

The serum GH response to TRH was considered positive when a net increase greater than 10 ng/ml and of at least 50% over basal values was observed. The serum PRL response to TRH was considered positive when an absolute increase greater than 25 ng/ml in women and 15 ng/ml in men and of at least 100% over basal values was observed. Patients were considered to be responders to bromocriptine when falls in serum GH and PRL values to at least 50% below the basal levels were obtained.

According to their basal serum PRL levels, patients were divided into two groups: normoprolactinemic (group A) and hyperprolactinemic (group B) and, on the basis of GH-responsiveness to TRH or to bromocriptine, they were subdivided into GH-responders and non-responders.

The modifications in serum PRL were also studied after sulpiride (100 mg i.m.) and chlorpromazine (0.7 mg/kg i.m.) administration; GH was evaluated only after sulpiride. The same criteria as those for TRH test were arbitrarily used for evaluating PRL and GH responses to these agents.

Dopamine (4 $\mu$g/kg/min) was infused over a 180 min period into 10 normo- and 5 hyperprolactinemic patients, 4 and 2 of whom, respectively, were GH responsive to TRH; blood was taken every 30 min.

In 10 patients (6 from group A and 4 from group B, 4 and 1 GH-responders to TRH, respectively) dopamine infusion was repeated and sulpiride injected (100 mg i.m.) at 120 min. In this experiment an additional blood sample was taken at 140 min. In the same patients the same procedure was repeated with injection of TRH (200 $\mu$g i.v.) instead of sulpiride.

Four normoprolactinemic (3 of them GH-responders to TRH) and 2 hyperprolactinemic patients received metergoline (4 mg p.o.), blood being taken every 30 min over a 4 h period; the experiment was repeated in the same subjects with sulpiride (100 mg i.m.) at 180 min., an additional blood sample being taken at 200 min. Serum PRL and GH were determined by specific RIA methods (hGH Kit, Dow-Lepetit, Milan, Italy; hPRL Kit, Biodata-Serono, Rome, Italy): no cross reaction between PRL and GH was observed.

## RESULTS

### Basal values

Serum GH concentrations ranged between 9 and 200 ng/ml. Serum PRL levels were normal in 29 patients (69%; PRL = 4-24 ng/ml) and elevated in 13 (31%; PRL = 33-256 ng/ml). No overall correlation between GH and PRL levels was found (Fig. 1).

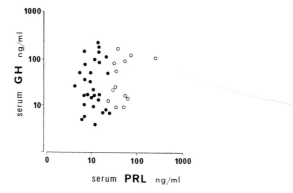

*Fig. 1.* Mean individual serum GH and PRL levels in basal conditions in 42 acromegalics. The open circles indicate PRL levels greater than normal values.

## TRH

TRH administration caused serum GH to rise in 17 cases (40%). GH-responders were 13 (45%) in the normoprolactinemic group (A) and 4 (31%) in the hyperprolactinemic group (B). GH-non responders were 16 (55%) and 9 (69%) in the two groups respectively.

*Responsiveness to TRH: PRL versus GH* (Table I). Serum PRL increased after TRH in the same proportion in GH-responders and non-responders of group A (46 and 44% respectively). In group B, all (100%) GH-responsive patients increased serum PRL, while only 11% of GH-non responders did.

## Bromocriptine

Bromocriptine administration lowered serum GH in 48% and serum PRL in 93% of patients. GH-responders were 14 (48%) in group A and 7 (54%) in group B; GH-non responders were 15 (52%) and 6 (46%) in the two groups.

*GH-responsiveness to bromocriptine versus TRH.* Among the GH-responders to bromocriptine, 76.5% were also GH-responders to TRH and vice versa; among the GH-non-responders to bromocriptine, 75% were GH-non-responders to TRH.

*PRL-responsiveness to TRH versus GH-suppressibility to bromocriptine.* (Table I). TRH increased serum PRL in 45% of GH-responders to bromocriptine and in 25% of GH-non-responders in group A. On the contrary, 80% of the hyperprolactinemic patients of group B whose GH was suppressed by bromocriptine had increased serum PRL after TRH, while no patient who was a GH-non-responder to bromocriptine did.

## Sulpiride (Table I).

Serum PRL increased in patients of group A, independently of their GH-responsiveness to TRH or bromocriptine. In group B, 25% of GH-responders to

Table I. Percentage of PRL responsiveness (PRL +) and unresponsiveness (PRL −) to TRH or sulpiride (SULP) in normoprolactinemic (A) and hyperprolactinemic (B) acromegalics, subdivided according to the GH-responsiveness to TRH or bromocriptine (brom.).

| | A | | B | | A | | B | |
| | resp. to TRH (n = 13)[a] | non-resp. to TRH (n = 16) | resp to TRH (n = 4) | non resp. to TRH (n = 9) | resp. to brom. (n = 14) | non-resp. to brom. (n = 15) | resp. to brom. (n = 7) | non-resp. to brom. (n = 6) |
|---|---|---|---|---|---|---|---|---|
| **TRH** | | | | | | | | |
| PRL (+) | 46 | 44 | 100 | 11 | 45 | 25 | 80 | 0 |
| PRL (−) | 54 | 56 | 0 | 89 | 55 | 75 | 20 | 100 |
| **SULP** | | | | | | | | |
| PRL (+) | 69 | 62 | 25 | 11 | | | | |
| PRL (−) | 31 | 38 | 75 | 89 | | | | |

[a] number of patients.

*Table II.* Effects of TRH, sulpiride (SULP), TRH injection during dopamine infusion (DA+TRH) and sulpiride injection during dopamine infusion (DA+SULP) on serum GH and PRL, expressed as percentage variations (Δ%) of basal values, in 6 normo- (A) and in 4 hyperprolactinemic (B) acromegalics.

| Patient No. | GH Basal ng/ml | GH TRH Δ% | GH SULP Δ% | GH DA+TRH Δ% | GH DA+SULP Δ% | PRL Basal ng/ml | PRL TRH Δ% | PRL SULP Δ% | PRL DA Δ% | PRL DA+TRH Δ% | PRL DA+SULP Δ% |
|---|---|---|---|---|---|---|---|---|---|---|---|
| **GH-responders to TRH:** | | | | | | | | | | | |
| 1 (A) | 13.3 | + 726 | −28 | −74 + 138 | −80 + 1500 | 16.5 | +700 | + 27 | −90 | +50 | −84 +666 |
| 2 (A) | 9.3 | +2087 | +20 | −29 +1750 | −20 + 393 | 22.5 | +460 | +212 | −68 | −62 | −56 + 33 |
| 3 (A) | 30.0 | + 169 | −11 | −82 − 46 | −76 + 61 | 15.6 | +500 | +232 | −72 | −26 | −81 +475 |
| 4 (A) | 10.1 | + 254 | 0 | −60 + 28 | −89 + 61 | 9.7 | +420 | + 66 | −77 | −77 | −80 +165 |
| 5 (B) | 51.7 | + 136 | −14 | −46 + 154 | −40 + 307 | 37.7 | +100 | + 54 | −50 | + 7 | −57 + 60 |
| **GH-non responders to TRH:** | | | | | | | | | | | |
| 6 (B) | 108.0 | + 11 | | −50 − 27 | −67 + 57 | 29.0 | + 40 | | −69 | −58 | −80 +310 |
| 7 (B) | 10.3 | + 5 | − 6 | −50 + 7 | −61 +108 | 28.3 | + 36 | + 64 | −75 | −50 | −80 +460 |
| 8 (B) | 104.2 | + 10 | | − 3 + 50 | −2 + 26 | 77.0 | + 12 | | −10 | −32 | − 0 + 13 |
| 9 (A) | 9.4 | + 14 | + 7 | −50 − 40 | −85 + 76 | 22.0 | + 41 | +318 | −83 | −65 | −81 +194 |
| 10 (A) | 29.5 | − 3 | −29 | − 6 − 8 | −14 + 8 | 6.4 | + 50 | − 7 | −68 | −46 | −50 0 |

TRH increased serum PRL after sulpiride, while no GH-non-responders showed any rise in serum PRL. Serum GH levels remained unchanged in most patients. However, a trend downwards was observed in 3 cases and slight rise in 1.

### Chlorpromazine

Chlorpromazine did not elicit any definite increment in serum PRL levels, except in 2 cases (1 normo- and 1 hyperprolactinemic).

### Dopamine

The infusion of dopamine lowered serum PRL in all patients tested except 2 (85%) and serum GH in 7 of 13 (54%).

*TRH administration during dopamine infusion* (Table II). No patient (irrespective of serum PRL responsiveness to TRH alone) showed any significant serum PRL increase after TRH injection during dopamine infusion, except for 1 (No. 1) whose PRL response was, however, actually reduced. On the contrary, 2 of 5 GH-responders to TRH continued to show a similar GH response to TRH

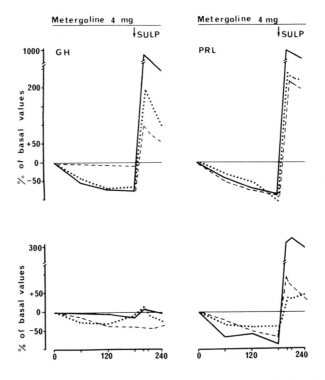

*Fig. 2.* Effect of acute metergoline administration (4 mg p.o.) followed by i.m. injection of sulpiride (100 mg) at 180 min on serum GH and PRL, in 3 GH-responding to TRH (upper part) and in 3 non-responding (lower part) acromegalics.

(Nos. 2, 5) and another 2 showed a blunted response (Nos. 1, 4), while in one case dopamine prevented any GH rise (No. 3). One GH-non-responder to TRH (No. 8) showed serum GH increase after TRH given during dopamine infusion.

### Sulpiride administration during dopamine infusion (Table II)

During dopamine infusion, sulpiride provoked a sustained serum PRL increase in 6 of 10 patients tested (Nos. 1, 3, 4, 6, 7, 9). However, 2 of them (Nos. 3, 9) had already shown serum PRL increases when sulpiride alone was injected. One patient (No. 2) had a blunted PRL response during dopamine infusion and another 3 (Nos. 5, 8, 10) did not show significant increases. Serum GH rose significantly in 8 patients (Nos. 1, 2, 3, 4, 5, 6, 7, 9) and remained unchanged in 2 (Nos. 8, 10). All the GH-responders to TRH and 3 non-responders had enhanced serum GH levels after sulpiride during dopamine infusion. No patient had been previously found GH-responsive to sulpiride alone.

### Metergoline (Fig. 2)

Metergoline administration lowered PRL levels in all patients but one and GH levels only in the GH-responders to TRH, except for one case. The subsequent administration of sulpiride was followed by an increase in serum PRL levels in all patients tested except in that patient whose PRL levels were not reduced by metergoline. Serum GH levels rose in all GH-responders to TRH, although one of them did not have lower serum GH after metergoline.

### DISCUSSION

The interrelationships between GH and PRL secretions in acromegaly have not been clarified as yet. In fact, in basal conditions, we did not find any overall correlation between GH and PRL levels in 42 patients with active acromegaly. This finding could result from the different secretory patterns of the two hormones, since PRL cells usually display a greater turnover and a smaller storage of the hormone than GH cells (Zimmermann *et al.*, 1974).

Moreover, the study of PRL and GH secretion in response to provocative and inhibitory stimuli suggests that some relationships do exist, at least in hyperprolactinemic acromegalics. In hyperprolactinemic patients, a strict correlation (100%) between GH and PRL responsiveness to TRH was found in GH-responders to TRH, while in GH-non-responders the percentage of PRL responsiveness to TRH was very low (11%).

Conversely, among normoprolactinemic patients, serum PRL increments after TRH were observed regardless of GH-responsiveness to TRH, in a percentage similar to that found in patients with "functionless" tumor (Faglia *et al.*, this volume). As also reported by Liuzzi *et al.* (1974), a good correlation was found between GH-responsiveness to TRH and to bromocriptine. In our series, TRH responsiveness and bromocriptine suppressibility were mutually correlated in about 75% of cases. However, dopaminergic drugs do not suppress GH and PRL secretions in the same proportions (48 and 93% respectively). When comparing the GH-suppressibility by bromocriptine and the PRL-responsiveness to TRH, a good correlation was observed: in fact, 80% of the hyperprolactinemic GH-responders to bromocriptine increased serum PRL after TRH, while none of the hyperprolactinemic GH-non-responders to bromocriptine did. These results are similar to those obtained correlating PRL- and GH-responsiveness to TRH. The ability to modify GH secretion after TRH, bromocriptine and dopamine, peculiar to some acromegalic patients, seems to be related to the presence of altered GH-secreting cells apparently reacting to the same stimuli as PRL-secreting cells. However, GH secretion in acromegaly is not unimodally influenced by antidopaminergic drugs such as chlorpromazine and sulpiride. As reported by Crosignani *et al.* (1977), sulpiride administration enables PRL to increase during dopamine infusion in hyperprolactinemic patients unresponsive to sulpiride. The same procedure influenced GH secretion too in 7 of 10 patients, particularly in all GH-responders to TRH. The administration of metergoline, a PRL-lowering agent, the effects of which on monoaminergic systems of hypothalamic-pituitary axis have not been fully clarified (Fuxe *et al.*, 1975; Sastry *et al.*, 1977; Chiodini *et al.*, 1976), was also effective in lowering GH levels. Furthermore, metergoline pretreatment not only failed to prevent the serum PRL increase after sulpiride, but also made it effective in stimulating GH release. Though this experiment points to a dopaminergic influence of metergoline, it is not clear whether metergoline acts directly on the pituitary, or whether it enhances the dopamine pool of the hypothalamic–pituitary system. On the other hand, its antiserotoninergic properties cannot be excluded, since serotonin stimulates GH secretion in normal subjects (Smythe and Lazarus, 1977). However, this procedure reveals a further PRL-like behaviour of GH secretion in some acromegalics. Based on these observations, GH secretion can be correlated to PRL secretion despite some dissociations. The previous findings of Guyda *et al.* (1973), Zimmermann *et al.* (1974) and Corenblum *et al.* (1976) of mixed tumors, in the postoperative morphological study of some acromegalics, strongly suggest that adenomatous GH cells which behave like PRL cells may derive from a single stem cell, able to differentiate into two cells (GH and PRL secreting), which share some common characteristics. However, Zimmermann *et al.* (1974) and Ishibashi and Yamaji (1975) reported that mixed tumors can also be found in normoprolactinemic acromegalics. Further investigations are needed to clarify the regulation of PRL secretion in acromegaly.

## REFERENCES

Camanni, F., Massara, F., Belforte, L., Rosatello, A. and Molinatti, G. M. (1977). *J. Clin. Endocr. Metab.* **44**, 465–473.

Chiodini, P. G., Liuzzi, A., Müller, E. E., Botalla, L., Cremascoli, G., Oppizzi, G., Verde, G. and Silvestrini, F. (1976). *J. Clin. Endocr. Metab.* **43**, 356–363.

Corenblum, B., Sirek, A. M. T., Horvath, E., Kovacs, K. and Ezrin, C. (1976). *J. Clin. Endocr. Metab.* **42**, 857–863.

Crosignani, P. G., Reschini, E., Peracchi, M., Lombroso, G. C., Mattei, A. and Caccamo, A. (1977). *J. Clin. Endocr. Metab.* **45**, 841–846.

Faglia, G., Paracchi, A., Beck-Peccoz, P. and Ferrari, C. (1975). *Acta Endocr. (Copenh.)* Suppl. **199**, 323.

Franks, S., Jacobs, H. S. and Nabarro, J. D. N. (1976). *Clin. Endocr.* **5**, 63–69.

Fuxe, K., Agnati, L. and Everitt, B. (1975). *Neurosci. Lett.* **1**, 283–290.

Guyda, H., Robert, F., Colle, E. and Hardy, J. (1973). *J. Clin. Endocr. Metab.* **36**, 531–547.

Ishibashi, M. and Yamaji, T. (1975). *Abstr. Am. Endocr. Soc.*, 57th Annual Meeting. New York June 18–20, 255.

Liuzzi, A., Chiodini, P. G., Botalla, L., Silvestrini, F. and Müller, E. E. (1974). *J. Clin. Endocr. Metab.* **39**, 871–876.

Liuzzi, A., Panerai, A. E., Chiodini, P. G., Secchi, C., Cocchi, D.; Botalla, L., Silvestrini, F. and Müller, E. E. (1975). *In* "Growth Hormone and Related Peptides" (A. Pecile and E. E. Müller, eds) pp. 236–251. Excerpta Med, Amsterdam.

Sastry, B. S. R. and Phillis, J. M. (1977). *Can. J. Physiol. Pharmac.* **55**, 130–133.

Schwinn, G., Dirks, H., McIntosh, C. and Köbberling, J. (1977). *Europ. J. Clin. Invest.* **7**, 101–107.

Smythe, G. A. and Lazarus, L. (1977). *Clin. Endocr.* **7**, 325–341.

Winkelmann, W., Fricke, U., Hadam, W., Heesen, D. and Mies, R. (1978). *In* "European Workshop on Treatment of Pituitary Adenomas" (R. Fahlbush and K. von Werder, eds) pp. 87–90. G. Thieme Verlag, Stuttgart.

Zimmermann, E. A., Defendini, R. and Frantz, A. G. (1974). *J. Clin. Endocr. Metab.* **38**, 577–585.

# SOMATOMEDIN LEVELS IN PATIENTS WITH PITUITARY MICROADENOMAS

E. M. Spencer, R. Mims and K. O. Uthne

*General Clinical Research Center, University of California,*
*San Francisco J4143, USA*

## INTRODUCTION

Somatomedin was discovered by Salmon and Daughaday (1957) and is the name for a group of polypeptide hormones of about 7500 daltons that are thought to be true mediators of the growth-promoting, but not all, actions of growth hormone (Rinderknecht and Humbel, 1978). Somatomedins (SM) have several characteristics in common: they are all growth hormone-dependent, in that growth hormone (GH) is the primary regulator of their plasma level. They are potent cell growth factors that directly stimulate the proliferation of a wide variety of cells in tissue culture in serum free-media. They possess insulin-like activity. They are produced in the liver and are uniquely transported in the plasma bound to a large carrier protein (Daughaday, 1971; Hall, 1972; Van Wyk *et al.*, 1973). SM can be measured by bioassay and recently in a few labs by radio-receptor and radioimmunoassays. Bioassays usually use the incorporation of labelled sulfate into cartilage, hence the older name for SM of "sulfation factor". In this paper we wish to report on plasma SM activity in patients with micro-adenomas associated with acromegaly and hyperprolactinemia.

Since in acromegaly SM may not be increased by traditional bioassays and since there is not a large body of experience with radioreceptor (Hall *et al.*, 1974; Megyesi *et al.*, 1975; D'Ercole *et al.*, 1977) and radioimmunoassays (Furlanetto *et al.*, 1977), we measured SM by all methods in a group of acromegalic patients before and after therapy. Our objectives in acromegaly were to:
(1) Use a radioreceptor assay to:
    (a) Establish whether the SM level was increased.

257

(b) Correlate SM and GH levels with each other and the activity of the disease.

(c) Present new data on the dynamics of the serum SM level in acromegaly and the potential use of SM levels diagnostically and to evaluate therapy.

(2) Use a radioimmunoassay and a new mitogenic bioassay for SM to evaluate these as alternate methods for measuring SM.

Although GH is the primary regulator of serum SM, prolactin has been shown to elevate depressed SM levels in GH-deficient animals (Bala *et al.*, 1976; Holder and Wallis, 1977) and to be a potent stimulus of SM generation in perfused livers (Francis and Hill, 1975). Therefore, we measured SM levels by radioreceptors and radioimmunoassays in male and female patients with prolactin secreting adenomas.

## METHODS

The human placental membrane radioreceptor assay for SM used followed the method of Hall *et al.* (1974). The radioligand used was SM-A (neutral SM). The assay is a measure of the total SM because all SM's cross react with the receptor. Specific binding averaged 23% and non-specific binding less than 2%. Interassay variability was 0.16 units/ml. Serum samples were obtained in the morning after an overnight fast unless otherwise noted. All values were compared to a standard pool of serum harvested from normal adults and arbitrarily assigned a value of 1.0 unit/ml.

The radioimmunoassay used an antibody developed against a basic SM (Reber and Liske, 1976) and subsequently determined to be the SM IGF-I (Rinderknecht and Humbel, 1978). IGF-I was iodinated by lactoperoxidase and purified on a CM-52 column. Assay conditions followed the nonequilibrium method of Furlanetto *et al.* (1977) with sample volumes of 200 $\mu l$ and a final antibody titer of 1:6000. Specific binding averaged 36%, and non-specific less than 1.5%. Because neutral SM (SM-A) cross-reacted in the radioimmunoassay, results were expressed relative to a pool of normal serum assigned a value of 1.0 unit per ml, analogous to the radioreceptor assay. In the radioimmunoassay 1 mg of IGF-I corresponded to 2500 units of this standard serum.

The mitogenic bioassay for SM used the stimulation of $GH_3$ cell growth by SM to measure SM (Hayashi and Sato, 1976). Serum (50 $\mu l$) was added in triplicate to 5 ml of Dulbecco's modified Eagle's medium supplemented with glucose to 4 g/1. Falcon 25 $cm^2$ flasks were seeded with $5 \times 10^5$ $GH_3$ cells and cultured at $37°C$ under a 5% $CO_2$ atmosphere for 5 days, then trypsinized and counted in a hemocytometer. Stimulation was expressed as per cent of cells observed with the test serum compared to a normal human standard serum made from a pool of 10 healthy adult sera. Maximal stimulation was observed with 12.5% horse plus 2.5% fetal calf sera and was 250 ± 13% (s.e.m.) compared to 1% normal human serum. The addition of exogenous SM at 5 and 0.5 units/ml to 1% normal serum significantly potentiated the mitogenic effect by 208 and 199%, respectively.

Patients were from the General Clinical Research Centers of the University of Southern California and the University of California San Francisco.

## RESULTS AND DISCUSSION

Figure 1 shows the results obtained with our radioreceptor assay. The mean ± s.e.m. SM was 1.06 ± 0.24 in normals, 0.35 ± 0.04 in GH-deficient children and 3.21 ± 0.4 units/ml in acromegalic patients. All 12 acromegalic patients had serum SM levels above the upper limit of normal. These results agree with those previously published by Hall *et al.* (1974) but differ from those of Megyesi *et al.* (1975) who found no increase in acromegaly. This discrepancy can probably be explained by the fact that the SM receptor assay cross reacts extensively with the other SM's and thus probably better measures the total SM level, while the liver receptor assay used by Megyesi is more specific and may "see" an SM that is less GH-dependent. Results similar to ours have been reported with a radioreceptor assay for SM-C (D'Ercole *et al.*, 1977).

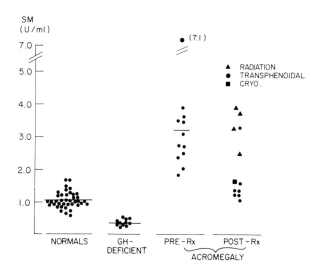

*Fig. 1.* Serum somatomedin levels measured by a human placental membrane radioreceptor assay in normal, growth hormone-deficient, and acromegalic subjects.

Since there were no data in the literature on SM levels measured by radio-receptor assay after therapy, we investigated this point. We found that after therapy for acromegaly, the serum SM fell to within the normal range in 7 patients (Fig. 1). However, the SM level in 5 patients 4 – 8 y post therapy and in one 6 months post therapy remained elevated, suggesting continuing activity of the disease. This was confirmed in one patient who subsequently had a trans-sphenoidal hypophsectomy. It is interesting that 4 of the 5 patients with continuing activity by the criterion of an increased serum SM had been treated by radiation. The significance of an increased SM serum level post therapy could be

that the conventional ways of assessing the completeness of therapy in acromegaly
are inadequate, and thus continuing activity might be the cause of the decreased
life expectancy of patients even after "successful" therapy. Consequently, we
believe that the SM level post therapy should be investigated in relation to the
adequacy of therapy and long term survival. SM lends itself to this kind of use
because of the lack of diurnal and day-to-day fluctuation of its serum level (data
not shown).

Oral glucose had no effect on SM levels in normal subjects and acromegalic
patients pre- and post-therapy (data not shown). The latter conclusion is in contrast to the report by Megyesi *et al.* (1975) that glucose increased the SM level.
This difference could also be due to different specificities of the respective assays.
We also found that L-DOPA had no effect on the SM level in normals and acromegaly (data not shown).

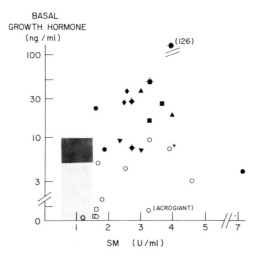

*Fig. 2.* Basal, fasting growth hormone levels plotted as a function of the serum SM level
determined in the same sample. Solid circles, acromegalic subjects prior to therapy. Open
circles, acromegalic subjects post therapy. The shaded areas represent the overlap of the two
ranges of normal. The darker area outlines the range that includes the upper limit of normal
for growth hormone.

Figure 2 shows the correlation between the basal, fasting serum GH and SM
levels measured in the same sample. Although the SM was always and the GH
generally increased in acromegaly, there was no correlation between the two
either before or after therapy. A similar result was obtained when mean GH
levels were correlated to SM levels (data not shown).

In our series there were three acromegalic patients with persistent basal GH
values in the 5 - 10 ng/ml range, levels usually accepted as within the normal
range. In an additional patient the GH level was below 5 ng/ml. All four patients
had active disease and elevated SM levels. The highest SM we have ever measured
was in the patient with the GH less than five. Had the SM level been considered on
this patient, therapy might not have been withheld for so long. These four
patients suggest that the serum SM may be of considerable diagnostic usefulness in

unusual cases of acromegaly with GH levels persistently in the upper range of normal. (They also serve to redefine the normal GH level.) However, the true incidence of these cases is not accurately reflected by this highly selected series.

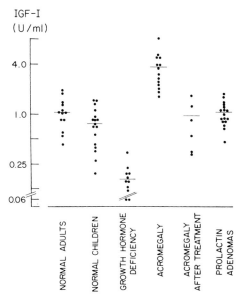

*Fig. 3.* Serum somatomedin levels measured by radioimmunoassay in several groups of patients. The antibody used in the assay was raised against the basic somatomedin IGF-I.

Although we have not studied this possibility, another use for the SM radioreceptor assay could be to screen subjects for an early diagnosis of acromegaly. Hopefully, this would improve the long term survival of acromegalic patients.

Preliminary observations have also been made on SM levels in acromegaly measured by radioimmunoassay (Fig. 3). Acromegalic patients had significantly elevated SM levels which fell to normal after therapy in those cases where the radioreceptor measurement also fell to the range of normal.

SM assays are not readily available to the average investigator. Radioreceptor- and radioimmunoassays are restricted to those laboratories that have highly pure SM and for the radioimmunoassay antibodies too. Cartilage bioassays are time consuming, difficult to perform and limited in the number of samples that can be processed. Therefore, a new bioassay was developed based on the mitogenic property of SM. This bioassay is simple and capable of handling large numbers of samples with ease. It uses $GH_3$ cells which are a line of SM-dependent rat pituitary tumor cells that can be cultured in a serum free medium if SM and 6 other factors are present. We found that in 1% serum the SM content was the limiting factor in the growth of these cells, which could therefore be used to bioassay serum for its SM content. Figure 4 shows that the stimulation index of acromegalic sera was significantly greater than in normals (176 ± 15% (s.e.m.) versus 96 ± 7%) and fell to normal after successful therapy as defined by a normal SM by radioreceptor assay (95 ± 8%). It appears that this bioassay may be very useful for laboratories where specific methodologies are lacking.

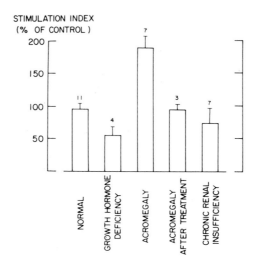

*Fig. 4.* Mitogenic bioassay for somatomedin using the growth stimulation of $GH_3$ cells as a measure of the serum SM.

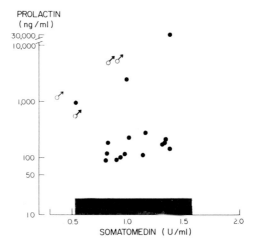

*Fig. 5.* Serum prolactin levels and serum somatomedin levels in patients with prolactin secreting adenomas. Prolactin was measured by radioimmunoassay and somatomedin by radioreceptor assay.

Figure 5 shows the relation of serum prolactin to SM in patients with prolactin secreting microadenomas. Although all the prolactin measurements were elevated (90 to 30 000 ng/ml) SM levels were normal (mean = 1.04 units/ml). Figure 3 also shows that SM measured by radioimmunoassay was also normal.

## REFERENCES

Bala, R. M., Bohner, H. G., Carter, J. N. and Friesen, H. G. (1976). *Clinical Res.* **24**, 655A.

Daughaday, W. H. (1971). *Adv. Intern. Med.* **17**, 237–263.

D'Ercole, A. M., Underwood, L. E. and Van Wyk, J. J. (1977). *J. Paediatric.* **90**, 375–381.

Francis, M. J. O. and Hill, D. J. (1975). *Nature* **255**, 167–168.

Furlanetto, R. W., Underwood, L. E., Van Wyk, J. J. and D'Ercole (1977). *J. Clin. Invest.* **60**, 648–657.

Hall, K. (1972). *Acta Endocrinol. (Copenh.)* Suppl. **163**, 1–62.

Hall, K., Takano, K. and Fryklund, L. (1974). *J. Clin. Endocrinol. Metab.* **39**, 973–976.

Hayashi, I. and Sato, G. H. (1976). *Nature* **259**, 132–134.

Holder, A. T. and Wallis, M. (1977). *J. Endocrinol* **74**, 223–229.

Megyesi, K., Kahn, C. R., Roth, J. and Gorden, P. (1975). *J. Clin. Endocrinol. Metab.* **41**, 475–485.

Reber, K. and Liske, R. (1976) *Hormone Res.* **7**, 201–213.

Rinderknecht, E. and Humbel, R. E. (1978). *J. Biol. Chem.* **253**, 2769–2776.

Salmon, W. D. and Daughaday, W. H. (1957). *J. Lab. Clin. Med.* **49**, 825–836.

Van Wyk, J. J., Underwood, L. W., Lister, R. C. and Marshall, R. N. (1973). *Am. J. Dis. Child.* **126**, 705–711.

# THE ENDOCRINOLOGY OF PROLACTIN-SECRETING MICROADENOMAS

J. Kellett and H. G. Friesen

*Department of Physiology, University of Manitoba, Winnipeg, Manitoba, Canada*

## INTRODUCTION

In reviewing the endocrinology of prolactin-secreting microadenomas we propose to discuss some of the clinical features of patients with hyperprolactinemia and to examine the pathogenesis of the symptoms and signs which these patients exhibit.

Tumours of less than 10 mm have been defined as "microadenomas" and can now be detected radiologically, using polycycloidal tomography. Although discussion initially will focus on endocrine changes in hyperprolactinemic females, distinctive clinical features observed in males with hyperprolactinemia will also be considered.

It is not yet clear whether prolactin exerts its primary effects at the hypothalamic or gonadal level. We have, therefore, reviewed the changes in gonadotropin secretion and ovarian function that occur in hyperprolactinemia in more detail.

## CLINICAL PRESENTATION OF HYPERPROLACTINEMIA

In the female, the three principal clinical features of hyperprolactinemia are galactorrhea, menstrual irregularities or a combination of these. It is now recognized that hyperprolactinemia causes a variety of menstrual disorders ranging from luteal insufficiency to anovulatory cycles, meno-metrorrhagia, oligomenorrhea and amenorrhea (Del Pozo *et al.*, 1977). Del Pozo showed that the higher the pro-

265

lactin levels, the more likely the occurrence of amenorrhea as a symptom. Serum prolactin levels over 60 ng/ml were almost invariably associated with amenorrhea, while other menstrual disorders were usually seen with lower prolactin levels. There are, of course, exceptions to this. Gomez et al. (1977) have reported patients with oligomenorrhea with levels higher than 60 ng/ml while patients with pituitary tumours treated with radiation often show a return of menses at a time when prolactin levels are still elevated. The reason for the imprecise correlation between prolactin levels and symptomatology is not clear. One explanation might be that all radioimmunoassayable forms of prolactin are not biologically active and patients with pituitary tumours that only secrete a "big" form of prolactin have been described (Guyda, 1975).

It should be stressed that galactorrhea is not a universal finding in hyperprolactinemia. In Jacobs' experience over 70% of patients with hyperprolactinemic amenorrhea do not have this symptom (Jacobs et al., 1976). Conversely, galactorrhea can be present without associated amenorrhea. In Kleinberg's series of 235 patients with galactorrhea, 32% of the women did not have amenorrhea (Kleinberg et al., 1977). Eighty-six per cent of these galactorrheic patients who did not have amenorrhea had normal prolactin levels.

Prolactinomas have been reported to cause delayed puberty (Koenig et al., 1977) and menarche (Ginsberg et al., 1977) when they arise prepubertally. Hyperprolactinemia has also been implicated in the pathogenesis of the premenstrual edema syndrome (Benedek-Jaszmann and Hearn-Sturtevant, 1976).

Hyperprolactinemic patients may have mild hirsutism, and a link with polycystic ovaries and hyperprolactinemia has been suggested. Adrenal cells possess prolactin receptors and some workers have shown an increased production of adrenal androgens in hyperprolactinemia (Carter et al., 1977; Vermeulen et al., 1977). Vermeulen and Ando (1978) have recently shown that ACTH increases dehydroepiandrosterone sulphate in patients with hyperprolactinemia but not in normals. When these patients were given cortisol, DHAS levels returned to normal despite a continued elevation of prolactin.

In 1954 Forbes observed that galactorrhea was associated with mild virilism and dysfunctional uterine bleeding. More recently Thorner et al. (1974) and Seppala and Hirvonen (1975) have noted that patients with hyperprolactinemia may present as the polycystic ovary syndrome. In Yen's experience, however, PRL levels are normal in this syndrome (Yen, 1978). Jaffe et al. (1978) have recently studied twelve patients with polycystic ovary syndrome, five of whom had abnormally high basal prolactin levels. It is tempting to attribute the development of polycystic ovaries to prolactin induced elevation of adrenal androgens. However, whether or not altered prolactin secretion is a primary or secondary defect in this syndrome remains to be determined.

The incidence of hyperprolactinemia in post-pill amenorrhea is not clear. In a study of 106 women with amenorrhea, Franks et al. (1975) found 16 cases that occurred after stopping the "pill". Only one of these women had elevated prolactin. Campenhout et al. (1977), however, discovered a high incidence of hyperprolactinemia and galactorrhea in women with post-pill amenorrhea (26 out of 82 patients). There was also a high incidence of pituitary tumour (10 out of 26 patients). It is well known that estrogen stimulates prolactin synthesis and release and Raymond and Lemarchand-Beraud (1976) have shown that sequential birth control pills significantly elevate prolactin. A number of investigators (Furth and Clifton, 1966; Gardner *et al.*, 1959; Jacobi *et al.*, 1975; Waelbroeck-Van Gaver and Potvliege, 1964) have shown that rodents invariably develop pituitary tumours when treated with estrogens over long periods of time. The possibility that birth control pills might stimulate the growth of prolactin secreting micro-adenoma must therefore be seriously considered.

In males with prolactin secreting pituitary tumours at the time of clinical pre-sentation, the tumours are much larger than those observed in females. Only a small proportion of these tumours could properly be classified as microadenomas, the majority presenting as macroadenomas, often with extrasellar extension of the tumour. Consequently, headaches and visual field impairment are prominent symptoms, while endocrine disturbances are often unrecognized. However, impo-tence is usually found when appropriate inquiry is made. Franks *et al.*, (1978) found that 16 of 20 men with hyperprolactinemia not only had an abnormal sella but also suprasellar extension. Prominent clinical findings in his patients were impotence, obesity, diminished facial and body hair, and small, soft testicles. We have recently studied 22 men with hyperprolactinemia, all of whom had pituitary tumours (Carter *et al.*, 1978). Twenty of these patients complained of decreased libido and potency. Visual impairment was present in nine patients, eight of whom had reduced visual fields and two of whom had diplopia. Only six com-plained of headaches and three had galactorrhea. The mean pretreatment serum prolactin level (3622 ng/ml) was higher than that usually found in women with prolactin-secreting adenomas. The administration of LHRH increased gonadotro-pin levels in all our patients, although basal LH levels were either normal or low, while basal FSH levels were low, normal or high. The increase in serum testoster-one levels after the administration of hCG was normal in all the patients we tested. The higher incidence of suprasellar extension, later age of diagnosis and higher prolactin levels than those in the women are probably due to the fact that the onset of impotence is more gradual than amenorrhea or goes unnoticed longer.

Gynecomastia is not a major feature and if present at all is only mild. Kleinberg *et al.* (1977) have described 13 men with galactorrhea, six of whom had pituitary tumours and markedly elevated serum prolactin levels. Of the seven men without tumours, most were probably drug induced and had normal prolactin levels. In our study of 22 men, all the patients treated with bromocryptine showed an improvement in potency (Carter *et al.*, 1978). Others have reported equally encouraging responses to drug therapy.

In those patients with hyperprolactinemia from whom semen specimens could be obtained the sperm count, motility and morphology were normal. The volume of the ejaculate, however, is reduced (Thorner, 1977). Elevated prolactin levels in oligospermic men have been reported (Segal *et al.*, 1976; Saidi *et al.*, 1977). Others, however, have reported that oligospermia is associated with low prolactin levels (Pierrepoint *et al.*, 1978). Goldhaber *et al.* (1977) have studied the prolac-tin response to TRH in men with azoospermia, Klinfelter's syndrome and Sertoli cell only syndrome. Although their basal PRL levels were normal, the increase in serum prolactin after TRH was somewhat reduced.

Clearly the role of PRL in the male has to be further investigated. The report by Besser and Thorner (1978) of five males with normal tomograms of the pituitary fossa suggests that microadenomas similar to those in women are almost certainly present in men. The earlier the diagnosis of prolactinoma is made the more favorable the outcome after transsphenoidal hypophysectomy. Therefore any male complaining of reduced libido or potency should have his prolactin level measured. This should allow the detection of tumours while still at the micro-adenoma stage.

Although the majority of patients with prolactinomas hypersecrete only pro-lactin, there are patients who have tumours composed of two cell types and indeed Tolis *et al.* (1978) have recently reported the coexistence of two pituitary tumours, each secreting excessive amounts of growth hormone and prolactin. The clinical features reflected the excessive secretion of these two hormones. In some series of patients with acromegaly from 30–50% of the patients exhibited hyper-prolactinemia (Tolis *et al.*, 1978). Similarly, in patients with Nelson's syndrome hyperprolactinemia is found occasionally.

## CONTROL OF PROLACTIN SECRETION

The secretion of prolactin is influenced by a great many hypothalamic factors, the dominant hypothalamic effect being an inhibitory one. Prolactin has been shown to inhibit its own secretion by a feedback effect on the hypothalamus which increases dopamine turnover (Meites *et al.*, 1972).

Recently prolactin receptors have been demonstrated in the choroid plexus and median eminence, but not in the hypothalamic ventro-medial nucleus (VMN) or dorsomedial nucleus (DMN) (Walsh *et al.*, 1978). This is a most unexpected finding, since the short-loop negative feedback effect of prolactin on its own secretion was thought to be due to neurons in the VMN or DMN.

Van Loon (1978) has shown that when bromocryptine is given to normal subjects their plasma dopamine, norepinephrine and epinephrine are reduced by more than 50%. In patients with hyperprolactinemia, however, there was no reduction of any of these catecholamines. He postulated that these patients had a widespread catecholamine defect which might cause uncontrolled prolactin release and stimulate the growth of adenomas.

## DIAGNOSIS OF PROLACTINOMAS

In view of the large number of drugs affecting prolactin secretion, either direc-tly or indirectly, it is hardly surprising that a normal serum prolactin value must be defined with considerable care. In a recent study we compared serum prolactin values in samples obtained from volunteers at a blood donor clinic, with values found in hospitalized patients (Fig. 1). It is immediately evident that the mean and range of serum prolactin in the hospital patient group differs considerably from that observed in a more "normal" group. Thus it is imperative that normal values should be carefully defined to establish the upper limit of normal. Since prolactin release is stimulated by estrogens, basal levels of prolactin are higher in females than in males, except prior to puberty and after the menopause. During the menstrual cycle, serum prolactin is higher in the luteal than in the pre-

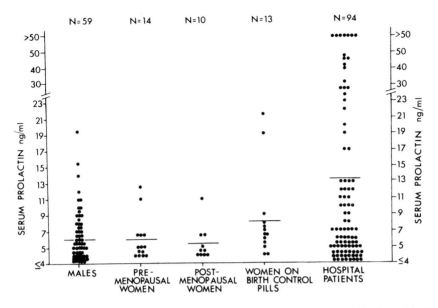

*Fig. 1.* Serum prolactin determinations in samples taken from normal individuals at a blood donor clinic compared with samples from hospitalized patients. It is apparent that the range of values in the latter group is much greater than in the "normal" group. Indeed, in seven patients values greater than 50 ng/ml were found.

ovulatory phase, and some investigators have shown a mid-cycle surge of prolactin coincident with FSH and LH peaks.

It should be emphasized, however, that these physiological variations are not major and seldom give rise to diagnostic confusion. Stress and minor discomforts, such as venepuncture, may cause a slight increase in prolactin levels. Pelvic examination can cause a substantial rise in serum prolactin levels (Koninckx, 1978), and this fact should be recognized because not infrequently blood samples are taken after the gynecologist has examined the patient.

Over the past few years a variety of dynamic tests have been described that attempt to distinguish between idiopathic hyperprolactinemia and hyperprolactinemia caused by tumour. In retrospect the reason why none of these tests work is because it was originally thought that dopamine and dopamine antagonists e.g. chlorpromazine, acted only at the hypothalamic level (Friesen *et al.*, 1972). Since both dopamine and dopamine antagonists are now known to act on both the hypothalamus and pituitary, it is unlikely that any test that works through dopamine will be helpful diagnostically.

It is now generally accepted that the two diagnostic tests which are the most informative in the differential diagnosis of hyperprolactinemia are a basal prolactin level and polycycloidal tomograms.

Basal prolactin values greater than 200 ng/ml make the diagnosis of a tumour more certain. Unfortunately, though, the majority of patients (both tumorous and non-tumorous) have values ranging between the upper limit of normal and 200

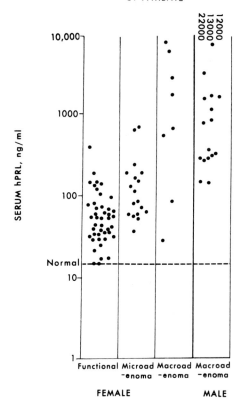

Fig. 2. Comparison of serum prolactin values of female and male patients with hyperprolactinemia. The prolactin values of female patients in the "functional" and microadenoma categories exhibit a great deal of overlap with the major difference being that fewer values in the microadenoma group cluster between 15 and 50 ng/ml. There are very few males who present with microadenomas and, as can be seen, the serum prolactin values are very comparable to those observed in females with macroadenomas. The dashed horizontal line indicates the upper limit of normal in our laboratory, which is equal to 15 ng/ml.

ng/ml (Friesen and Tolis, 1977). As can be seen in Fig. 2, men with prolactin secreting tumours have much higher mean prolactin levels than do women when first seen, which reflects the much larger tumours which are present.

## DIFFERENTIAL DIAGNOSIS

There are, of course, many causes of hyperprolactinemia, as outlined in Table I. In order to establish a diagnosis in an individual case, each of the entities listed should be excluded by appropriate means. However, the disorders listed in Table II constitute the most difficult clinical group. In actual practice, however, there

*Table 1.* Etiology of hyperprolactinemia.

1. Drugs
2. Hypothyroidism
3. Hypothalamic disorders leading to a decrease in PIF
   (a) Functional, e.g. Chiari-Frommel
   (b) Organic, e.g. tumour
4. Prolactin secreting pituitary tumours
   (a) with galactorrhea
   (b) without galactorrhea
5. Renal failure
6. Ectopic production by malignant tumours

*Table II.* Diagnostic difficulties in hyperprolactinemia.

1. Psychoneuroendocrine factors
2. Regulatory neurotransmitter disorders of the hypothalamus
3. Microadenomas
4. Empty sella syndrome

are only a few possibilities that have to be seriously considered. Drug induced hyperprolactinemia is probably the most common. Hypothyroidism is important to rule out, since even very mild reductions of thyroid function can elevate prolactin. Prolactin elevation can occur as a result of head injury and also is seen in empty sella syndrome. In the latter case the presence of an associated microadenoma has been described (Tolis, 1978). The possibility that "idiopathic" hyperprolactinemia may have a psychoneuroendocrine cause has been suggested by Tyson (1978).

## CHANGES IN GONADOTROPINS AND OVARIAN FUNCTION ASSOCIATED WITH HYPERPROLACTINEMIA

Prolactin could derange menstruation either by a direct effect on the ovary or by interfering with gonadotropin release. Several studies have now been published in which gonadotropin and estradiol levels have been examined in hyperprolactinemia (Franks *et al.*, 1977, 1975; Jacobs *et al.*, 1976; Gomez *et al.*, 1977; Kleinberg *et al.*, 1977).

### Response to LHRH

Boyar (1976) reported two cases in which both basal levels and 24 h production of FSH, LH and estradiol were normal. The responses of the gonadotropins to LHRH were also normal. Spark *et al.* (1976) studied 15 patients with galactorrhea. All the patients showed some response to LHRH and in eight of them this response was normal. In two of the patients who had tumours the response was blunted. Zarate *et al.* (1973) reported similar results. Wiebe *et al.* (1978)

described 11 patients, all with pituitary tumours and all but one had normal basal gonadotropin levels. Their responses to LHRH were also normal except for two patients who had "borderline low" results. Spark feels that a poor LHRH response is only seen in patients with tumours that have presumably destroyed the gonadotropin reserve.

On the other hand, Thorner et al. (1974) have found an exaggerated response to LHRH in hyperprolactinemia. They feel that this shows that there is an increased gonadotropin reserve and argue that this has come about because prolactin has impaired the responsiveness of the ovary to gonadotropin. Bergh et al. (1977) have also found an enhanced response to LHRH. However, they found that this only occurred in patients with an abnormal sella — those with "idiopathic" hyperprolactinemia and normal sellas had normal LHRH responses. The explanation for this may be related to the estrogen status of the patients.

### Estrogen levels

The levels of estradiol present in hyperprolactinemia vary from one report to another. Gomez et al. (1977) found levels comparable to those found in the early follicular range. Bohnet et al. (1976) also found low normal levels and most of their patients showed gestagen withdrawal bleeding. Most of Jacobs' patients, however, had low estradiol levels, in the post-menopausal range, and withdrawal bleeding only occurred in 2 of 21 patients (Jacobs, 1976). Davajan et al. (1978) have recently noted that the higher the prolactin the lower the estradiol level.

Corbey et al. (1977) have studied the responses of patients to LHRH and TRH and compared them to the responses of normal women on the third day of their cycle. They reasoned that this is a good time for comparison since after the third day of the cycle normal women are capable of the initiation of follicular growth and maturation. They showed that hyperprolactinemic patients could be divided into two groups — those that had an increased response to LHRH and those who had a reduced response. Those with an enhanced response tended to have high estradiol levels. The low estrogen poor LH responders tended to have higher prolactin levels, hyperprolactinemia of longer duration and were more likely to have tumours. These findings are consistent with Jacobs' view that the failure of basal gonadotropin levels to rise to post-menopausal levels when estradiol levels are low suggests an abnormality at the hypothalamic-pituitary level (Jacobs, 1976).

It is clear from these reports that the LHRH response and estrogen status in hyperprolactinemia are interdependent. It would also seem that these determinations are of limited diagnostic or therapeutic value, but they may be helpful in identifying those patients in whom a large tumour has destroyed all gonadotropin function.

## RESPONSE TO CLOMIPHENE AND LOSS OF
## POSITIVE FEEDBACK OF ESTROGENS

Aono et al. (1976) and Glass et al. (1975) have demonstrated that hyperprolactinemia impairs the positive feedback effect of estrogens on LH release. It has been recognized for some time that it is very difficult to induce menses in patients with galactorrhea by using clomiphene. Jacobs (1976) was unable to induce ovulation with clomiphene in 19 out of 20 hyperprolactinemic patients and others have had similar experience. It would seem that this derangement of gonadotropin regulation is the most consistent finding in hyperprolactinemia and many feel that it primarily is this abnormality that results in prolactin-induced amenorrhea. Hyperprolactinemia also appears to have an inhibitory effect on ovarian function.

## EXPERIMENTAL HYPERPROLACTINEMIA

In order to investigate the mechanisms by which hyperprolactinemia affects ovarian function, elevations of prolactin levels have been induced experimentally.

Sulpiride is a dopamine blocking drug that has been shown to release prolactin from the lactotroph *in vitro* and *in vivo*. It does not appear to have any direct effect on circulating LH, FSH and TSH (Robyn *et al.*, 1977). Hyperprolactinemia induced by the drug led to amenorrhea. If the drug was not given until mid-cycle, ovulation still occurred in some cases; however, the luteal phase was considerably shortened and the LH, FSH and progesterone levels during the luteal phase were reduced. Although LH levels were low they were often in the normal range. The most marked effect noted was on the LH surges, which were considerably reduced. It could be postulated that the inadequate LH surges do not stimulate the granulosa cells adequately, resulting in luteal insufficiency. However, severe luteal insufficiency was still observed even after an LH surge of normal amplitude which occurred several days after the interruption of the sulpiride induced hyperprolactinemia. This suggests that the granulosa cell's capacity to produce an adequate corpus luteum is interfered with by prolactin very early on in the follicular phase. In those patients in whom sulpiride induced amenorrhea, the endocrine changes immediately after the last period were of interest. In some the FSH and estradiol levels were greater than in the control cycles and normal LH surges were seen. Presumably, however, the granulosa cells were unable to respond, resulting in lack of ovulation and amenorrhea. Subsequently the LH surges disappeared and the positive feedback of estradiol on LH was lost. From this it would appear that the first abnormality in hyperprolactinemia is at the granulosa cell level, resulting in luteal insufficiency and then unresponsiveness to LH surges. This would be in keeping with the *in vitro* work of McNatty and Sawers (1975), who showed that excess PRL inhibits the production of progesterone by granulosa cells.

## CONCLUSION

In summary, therefore, it would appear that hyperprolactinemia in the female is associated with a variable response to LHRH, which is to some extent a reflection of the estrogen status of the patient and the size of the tumour, but may also be an effect of prolactin *per se*. The loss of positive feedback to estrogens and clomiphene appears to be a fairly consistent finding. Studies on drug induced hyperprolactinemia suggest that granulosa cell insensitivity to gonadotropins occurs early during the development of hyperprolactinemia, but impaired release of LH surges also occurs. Whether the impaired gonadotropin release is due to reduced production of ovarian steroids or to a prolactin induced hypothalamic derangement, or both, is not clear.

In the male, since both the testes and pituitary respond appropriately to stimulating agents, we favour the view that diminished LHRH secretion is responsible for both the gonadotropin and testosterone deficiency. The effects of prolactin in the male, however, may not be exactly analogous to those in the female. Rubin *et al.* (1978) have demonstrated a small but significant rise of testosterone levels following haloperidol-induced elevation of prolactin concentration and Ambrosi *et al.* (1976) have reported higher testosterone responses to human chorionic gonadotropin in volunteers with sulpiride-induced hyperprolactinemia.

Impotence is not solely related to diminished testosterone production, since impotence persisted in two of our patients despite adequate testosterone replacement, and subsequently improved when prolactin levels were lowered with bromocryptine. Moreover, impotence was present in patients with circulating testosterone values that in our experience are not usually associated with this symptom in normoprolactinemic men (Carter *et al.*, 1978). In guinea pigs (Mawhinney *et al.*, 1975) prolactin has been demonstrated to inhibit $5\alpha$-reductase activity, the enzyme converting testosterone to the metabolically more active dihydrotestosterone. There is some recent indirect evidence to suggest a similar response in man (Magrini *et al.*, 1976). Thus, a defect in conversion of testosterone to dihydrotestosterone in hyperprolactinemic states may serve to explain the diminished libido and impotence. Admittedly, this concept is highly speculative, especially since data from animals suggest that dihydrotestosterone is considerably less effective in influencing sexual behaviour than is testosterone (Clemens, 1974). An alternative explanation is that impotence may result from a direct effect of prolactin on the central nervous system.

## REFERENCES

Ambrosi, B. *et al.* (1976). *J. Clin. Endocr. Metab.* **43**, 700–703.
Aono, T. *et al.* (1976). *J. Clin. Endocr. Metab.* **42**, 696–702.
Benedek-Jaszmann, L. J. and Hearn-Sturtevant, M. D. (1976). *Lancet* 1095–1098.
Bergh, T. *et al.* (1977). *Acta Endocrinologica* **86**, 683–694.
Bohnet, H. *et al.* (1976). *J. Clin. Endocr. Metab.* **42**, 132–143.
Boyar, R. M. (1976) *New Eng. J. Med.* **294**, 263–265.
Campenhout, J. V. *et al.* (1977). *Fertl. Steril.* **28**, 728
Carter, J. N. *et al.* (1977). *J. Clin. Endocr. Metab.* **45**, 973–980.
Carter, J. N. *et al.* (in press). *New Eng. J. Med.*
Clemens, L. G. (1974). *In* "Reproductive Behaviour" (W. Montagna and W. A. Sadler, eds) pp. 29–30., Plenum Press, New York and London.
Corbey, R. S. *et al.* (1977). *In* "Prolactin and Human Reproduction" (P. G. Crosignani and C. Robyn, eds) pp. 203–316. Academic Press, London and New York.
Davajan, V. *et al.* (1978). *Am. J. Obst. Gynecol.* **130**, 894–904.
Del Pozo, E. *et al.* (in press). Proceedings of the Prolactin Symposium, Nice.
Forbes, A. *et al.* (1954). *J. Clin. Endocr. Metab.* **14**, 265–271.
Franks, S. *et al.* (1975). *Clin. Endocrinol.* **4**, 597–607.
Franks, S. *et al.* (1977). *Br. J. Obstet, Gynec.* **84**, 241.

Franks, S. *et al.* (1978). *Clin. Endocrinol.* **8**, 277–287.
Friesen, H. G. and Tolis, G. (1977). *Clin. Endocrinol. Suppl.* **6**, 91s–99s.
Friesen, H. G. *et al.* (1972). *J. Clin. Invest.* **51**, 706–709.
Furth, J. and Clifton, K. (1966). *In* "The Pituitary Gland" (G. W. Harris and B. T. Donovan, eds) pp. 460–497. Butterworth, London.
Gardner, W. *et al.* (1959). *In* "The Physiology of Cancer" (Homburger, ed) pp. 152–237. Harper (Hoeber), New York.
Ginsberg, J. *et al.* (1977). *Br. Med. J.* **2**, 32–35.
Glass, M. R. *et al.* (1975). *Br. Med. J.* **3**, 274–275.
Goldhaber, G. *et al.* (1977). *J. Reprod. Fert.* **49**, 135–137.
Gomez, F. *et al.* (1977). *Amer. J. Med.* **62**, 648–660.
Guyda, H. (1975). *J. Clin. Endocr. Metab.* **41**, 953.
Jacobi, J. *et al.* (1975). *Horm. Metab. Res.* **7**, 228.
Jacobs, H. S. *et al.* (1976). *Clin. Endocrinol.* **5**, 439–454.
Jaffee, W. *et al.* (1978). Abst. No. 71, Endocrine Society Annual Meeting, Miami, 1978.
Kleinberg, D. *et al.* (1977). *New Eng. J. Med.* **296**, 589–600.
Koenig, M. P. *et al.* (1977). *J. Clin. Endocrin. Metab.* **45**, 825–828.
Koninckx, P. (1978). *Lancet* **I**, 273.
Magrini, G. *et al.* (1976). *J. Clin. Endocr. Metab.* **43**, 944–947.
Mawhinney, M. G. *et al.* (1975). *J. Pharmacol. Exp. Ther.* **192**, 242–249.
McNatty, K. P. and Sawers, R. S. (1975). *J. Endocrinol.* **66**, 391.
Meites, J. *et al.* (1972). *Rec. Prog. Horm. Res.* **28**, 471.
Pierrepoint, C. G. *et al.* (1978). *J. Endocrinol.* **76**, 171–172.
Reymond, M. and Lemarchand-Beraud, T. H. (1976). *Clin. Endocrinol.* **5**, 429–437.
Robyn, C. *et al.* (1977). *In* "Prolactin and Human Reproduction" (P. C. Crosignani and C. Robyn, eds) pp. 71–96. Academic Press, London and New York.
Rubin, R. T. *et al.* (1978). *J. Clin. Endocr. Metab.* **47**, 447–452.
Saidi, K. *et al.* (1977). *Lancet* **I**, 250–251.
Segal, S. *et al.* (1976). *Fertil. Steril.* **26**, 1425–1427.
Seppala, M. and Hirvonen, E. (1975). *Br. Med. J.* **4**, 144–145.
Spark, R. F. *et al.* (1976). *Ann. Intern. Med.* **84**, 532–537.
Thorner, M. O. (1977). *In* "Clinical Neuroendocrinology" (L. Martini and G. M. Besser, eds) pp. 320–363., Academic Press, New York and London.
Thorner, M. O. (1978). *Acta Endocrinologica Suppl. 216*, **88**, 131–146.
Thorner, M. O. *et al.* (1974). *Br. Med. J.* **2**, 419–422.
Tolis, G. (1978). Abst. No. 95, Royal College of Physicians and Surgeons of Canada, Annual Meeting, Vancouver, 1978.
Tolis, G. *et al.* (1978). *Ann. Intern. Med.* **89**, 345–348.
Tyson, J. *et al.* (1978). *In* "Human Fertility Control" (J. J. Sciarra and G. I. Zatuchni, eds). Harper and Row, New York.
Van Loon, C. R. (1978). Abst. No. 190, Endocrine Society Annual Meeting, Miami, 1978.
Vermeulen, A. *et al.* (1977). *J. Clin. Endocr. Metab.* **44**, 1222–1225.
Vermeulen, A. and Ando, S. (1978). *Clin. Endocrinol.* **8**, 295–303.
Waelbroeck-Van Gaver, C. and Potvliege, P. (1969). *Europ. J. Cancer* **5**, 99.
Walsh, R. J. *et al.* (1978). *Science* **201**, 1041–1042.
Wiebe, R. H. *et al.* (1978). *Fertil. Steril.* **29**, 282–286.
Yen, S. C. (1978). *In* "Reproductive Endocrinology" (S. C. Yen and R. B. Jaffee, eds) pp. 297–323. W. B. Saunders, Philadelphia.
Zarate, A. *et al.* (1973). *J. Clin. Endocr. Metab.* **37**, 855–859.

# ANTERIOR PITUITARY HORMONES,
# OTHER THAN THOSE HYPERSECRETED, IN PATIENTS
# WITH FUNCTIONING MICROADENOMAS

G. Faglia, P. Travaglini, P. Beck-Peccoz, B. Ambrosi,
P. Moriondo, R. Elli and M. Rondena

*Second Medical Clinic, Endocrine Unit, University of Milan, Italy*

## INTRODUCTION

Anterior pituitary function so far has been extensively investigated only in patients with both secreting and non-secreting macroadenomas (Nieman *et al.*, 1967; Nelson *et al.*, 1974; Snyder *et al.*, 1974; Joplin *et al.*, 1975; Weisberg *et al.*, 1976). Only a little information is presently available about patients with pituitary microadenomas (Jaquet *et al.*, 1978).

In macroadenomas, the impairment of pituitary hormone secretion is generally believed to be secondary to compression of the normal pituitary tissue or to alterations in microcirculation caused by the expanding tumour mass or to hypothalamic involvement due to the suprasellar extension of the tumour. These mechanisms are of little or no importance in pituitary microadenomas. In this case, the alterations in pituitary hormone secretion might be regarded as a consequence of an effect of the hypersecreted hormones on the regulatory processes for other anterior pituitary hormones or, alternatively, as a consequence of a hypothalamic disorder causing changes in trophin secretion.

Furthermore, since the major goal of pituitary surgery is to remove the tumour without affecting pituitary function, the study of the modifications in pituitary function is of particular importance (Cross *et al.*, 1972; Giovanelli *et al* , 1976; Guitelman *et al.*, 1977; Jaquet *et al.*, 1978).

The present paper will consider the incidence of anterior pituitary hormone impairment in functioning microadenomas as compared with functioning and non-functioning macroadenomas, before and after transsphenoidal microsurgery, and the possible effects of hypersecreted hormones on the regulation of secretion of other pituitary trophic hormones.

## MATERIALS AND METHODS

### Patients

The incidence of altered secretion of the anterior pituitary hormones, other than those hypersecreted was investigated in 63 untreated patients with functioning pituitary microadenomas. Thirty-eight were women with microprolactinoma (serum PRL 47 - 487 ng/ml); 18 (5 men and 13 women) were acromegalics (serum GH 13.5 - 82 ng/ml); 7 (1 man and 6 women) had Cushing's disease (plasma ACTH 60 - 260 pg/ml).

Data obtained in 98 patients with pituitary macroadenomas, matched for age and sex with patients with microadenomas, were used for comparison. Fourteen patients were women with PRL-secreting tumours (serum PRL 46 - 800 ng/ml), 53 (20 men and 33 women) were acromegalics (serum GH 13 - 420 ng/ml), and 31 were women with non-secreting pituitary tumours. The endocrine function after transsphenoidal pituitary surgery was re-evaluated in 38 patients with microadenomas (26 PRL-secreting, 9 GH-secreting and 3 ACTH-secreting) and in 65 subjects with pituitary macroadenomas (13 PRL-secreting, 32 GH-secreting and 20 non-secreting). Patients with functioning pituitary tumours were subdivided according to whether or not the surgical treatment was successful in reducing the hypersecreted hormone to within the normal range.

The existence of a microadenoma was assumed when fine alterations were seen by pituitary fossa tomography [the sellar volume, calculated by the method of Busch (1951) and Tori (1953), not exceeding 1500 mm$^3$] and was documented in all patients who underwent surgery.

### Functional studies

*Gonadotrophic function*

Gonadotrophic function was studied by determining serum LH and FSH in basal conditions and after the following tests:
(i)   i.v. injection of 25 μg of LRH (Relisorm L$^®$ − Serono, Rome, Italy), blood being drawn at − 20, 0, 20, 30, 60, 90 and 120 min. The results were compared with those obtained in 10 normally menstruating women in the early follicular phase and in 12 normal males;
(ii)   i.m. injection of 1 mg oestradiol benzoate, blood being taken at 0, 24, 48, 72 and 96 h. This test was carried out on 11 patients with microprolactinoma and was repeated in 6 after normalization of serum PRL levels obtained by surgical treatment;
(iii)   i.m. injection of 1 mg oestradiol benzoate followed, 36 h later, by 25 mg progesterone i.m. This test was carried out in 4 patients with microprolactinoma, blood being taken at 0, 24, 48, 72 and 96 h;

(iv)   oral administration of clomiphene citrate (100 mg/day for 5 consecutive days). This test was carried out in 6 patients with microprolactinoma. LH, FSH, PRL, 17-$\beta$ oestradiol, and progesterone were determined every other day over a 20 day period.

In addition, a time study was made of LH and FSH secretory patterns in 8 patients with microprolactinoma. Blood was withdrawn every 20 min from 08.00 to 12.00 h.

## Thyrotrophic function

Thyrotrophin secretion was evaluated by measuring basal and TRH-stimulated (200 $\mu$g i.v., Biodata-Serono, Rome, Italy) plasma TSH (blood being drawn at $-20, 0, 20, 30, 60, 90$ and 120 min) and by determining serum $T_3$ increases over basal values 120–180 min after TRH injection. The criteria for interpretation of the TRH test were those previously described (Faglia *et al.*, 1973b; Faglia *et al.*, 1975). Thyroid function was assessed by measuring serum $T_3$ and $T_4$ and the per cent $T_3$ uptake on a resin column.

## Corticotrophic function

Corticotrophic function was evaluated indirectly by measuring plasma cortisol concentrations in basal conditions and after insulin induced hypoglycaemia (ITT) (blood glucose less than 40 mg/dl) and by determining the increase in urinary 17-OHCS after oral administration of metyrapone (4.5 g over 24 h, divided in 6 doses). The criteria of interpretation were previously published elsewhere (Faglia *et al.*, 1973a).

## Growth hormone

Growth hormone secretion was investigated by evaluating the serum GH levels in the basal state and after ITT. An increase of serum GH concentration over the basal value of at least 10 ng/ml was defined as normal.

## Prolactin

Serum PRL was determined in basal conditions and after TRH stimulation. An increase of 100% over basal values of at least 25 ng/ml was defined as normal. In order to study PRL secretion in acromegaly, the serum PRL response to sulpiride (100 mg i.m.) to chlorpromazine (0.7 mg/kg b.w.), and the serum PRL and GH responses to TRH were evaluated in 42 acromegalics. PRL responses to these stimuli were compared with those obtained in 38 patients with microprolactinoma and in 20 cases of non-secreting pituitary tumours.

## Methods

Serum LH and FSH concentrations were determined by radioimmunoassay (RIA) by the methods of Midgley (1966, 1967), using as reference standard the second International Reference Preparation for human menopausal gonadotrophin (2nd IRP-HMG). In our assay system, 1 mIU of the 2nd IRP-HMG was equivalent to 4.0 ng of LH and 25.0 ng of FSH of the human pituitary gonadotrophin reference preparation LER 907. Plasma 17$\beta$-oestradiol and serum progesterone were determined by the methods of Hotchkiss *et al.* (1971) and Abraham *et al.* (1972), respectively, using specific reagents supplied by Dow-Lepetit Ltd. (Milan, Italy) and

Biodata-Serono (Rome, Italy). Serum TSH was estimated as described by Odell *et al.* (1967), using as standard the reference preparation 68/38 (NIMR, Mill Hill, London, GB) and specific antisera and hTSH for labelling supplied by NIH (Bethesda, USA) and Dow-Lepetit Ltd (Milan, Italy). Serum $T_4$, $T_3$ and the resin per cent $T_3$ uptake were determined with commercial kits (RIA-$T_4$ and RIA-$T_3$, Dow-Lepetit Ltd. Milan, Italy, Trilute®, Ames Co. Yssum, Jerusalem, Israel). Plasma cortisol was determined by RIA (RIA-Cortk, Sorin, Saluggia, Italy) urinary 17-OHCS were measured by the method of Silber and Porter (1954). Serum growth hormone was determined by hGH Kit (Dow-Lepetit Ltd, Milan, Italy) and serum prolactin by the method of Sinha *et al.* (1973), using reference standard hPRL VLS 1 and labelled HPRL and antiserum supplied by Biodata-Serono (Rome, Italy).

## RESULTS

*Gonadotrophins*

In microadenomas, the basal serum LH concentration appeared to be more often affected (35% of the patients) than that of FSH (3%), the most frequent impairment being observed in patients with Cushing's disease (LH, 57%, FSH, 28%). Low basal LH concentrations were found in 28% of microprolactinomas and in 17% of GH-secreting microadenomas. In macroadenomas, low LH values were seen in 36% and low FSH values in 24% of PRL-secreting and low values for both in 42% of non-secreting tumours. In acromegalic patients, LH was low in 32% of cases and FSH in only 9% (Table I).

All the patients with pituitary microadenomas increased serum gonadotrophins after LRH except 5 women with microprolactinoma who had impaired LH responses. Exaggerated FSH elevations after LRH were seen in 24% of patients with PRL-secreting microadenoma and in about 10% of acromegalics; excessive increases in serum LH in 16 and 5%, respectively. The incidence of reduced or absent LH and FSH responses to LRH was much higher in macroadenomas (56 and 36% respectively), particularly in patients with non-secreting pituitary tumours (71 and 61% respectively).

Pituitary LH reserve was reduced after surgery in a relatively high proportion of patients with microadenoma (Table II), although it improved in two cases. However, in three patients with impaired LH response to LRH after operation, a progressive improvement in the LH reserve was demonstrated by later endocrine evaluation (Fig. 1).

In 11 patients with microprolactinoma, oestradiol benzoate administration (Fig. 2) caused a significant fall in serum FSH and LH within 24 h, but failed to induce any increase in serum gonadotrophins except in one patient. However, a definite increase in serum LH concentration was obtained in six cases retested after serum PRL normalization. No significant modification in serum PRL occurred throughout the test. Progesterone administration 36 h after oestradiol benzoate injection induced a definite LH peak in 4 patients with PRL-secreting microadenoma who previously did not respond to oestradiol benzoate alone (Fig. 2). All patients but one treated with clomiphene showed normal rises in LH, FSH and

Table I. Per cent of impaired secretion of pituitary trophic hormones, other than those hypersecreted, in patients with pituitary microadenomas as compared to patients with macroadenomas.

| Cases (n) | HPG[a] | | | | HPT | | | | HPA | | | | GH | PRL | |
| | LH | | FSH | | T$_4$ | T$_3$ | | TSH | Cortisol | | 17-OHCS | | | | |
| | Bas. % | after LRH % | Bas. % | after LRH % | Bas. % | Bas. % | after TRH % | after TRH % | Bas. % | after ITT % | Bas. % | after Metyr. % | after ITT % | Bas. % | after TRH % |
|---|---|---|---|---|---|---|---|---|---|---|---|---|---|---|---|
| *Microadenomas* (63) | 35 | 8 | 3 | 0 | 10 | 12 | 36 | 36 | 5 | 32 | 13 | 7 | 40 | 32[b] | 28 |
| PRL-secreting (38) | 28 | 13 | 0 | 0 | 3 | 3 | 34 | 24 | 0 | 32 | 10 | 3 | 29 | – | – |
| GH-secreting (18) | 17 | 0 | 0 | 0 | 17 | 17 | 33 | 39 | 17 | 33 | 17 | 17 | – | 28[b] | 33 |
| ACTH-secreting (7) | 57 | 0 | 28 | 0 | 28 | 42 | 57 | 100 | – | – | – | – | 100 | 43[b] | 14 |
| *Macroadenomas* (98) | 36 | 56 | 24 | 36 | 36 | 14 | 36 | 36 | 12 | 35 | 23 | 28 | 89 | 23[b] | 46 |
| PRL-secreting (14) | 36 | 57 | 36 | 36 | 43 | 14 | 36 | 43 | 14 | 36 | 14 | 28 | 85 | – | – |
| GH-secreting (53) | 32 | 45 | 9 | 21 | 29 | 12 | 34 | 26 | 15 | 34 | 23 | 23 | – | 32[b] | 55 |
| Non-secreting (31) | 42 | 71 | 42 | 61 | 45 | 19 | 39 | 48 | 7 | 35 | 29 | 35 | 90 | 10 | 32 |

[a] HPG: Hypothalamic-pituitary-gonadotropic function; HPT: hypothalamic-pituitary-thyroid function; HPA: hypothalamic-pituitary-adrenal; GH: growth hormone secretion; PRL: prolactin secretion.

[b] Elevated basal serum PRL values.

Table II. Impaired trophic hormone secretion before and after transsphenoidal surgery in patients with pituitary microadenomas as compared to patients with macroadenomas.

| Cases (n) | HPG LH after LRH | | HPT Basal T$_4$, T$_3$ | | HPT TSH after TRH | | HPA Cortisol after ITT | | GH GH after ITT | | PRL Basal | | PRL after TRH | |
|---|---|---|---|---|---|---|---|---|---|---|---|---|---|---|
| | Before | After | Before | After | Before | After | Before | After | Before | After | Before | After | Before | After |
| *Microadenomas* (38) | 1 | 14 | 2 | 4 | 9 | 7 | 7 | 5 | 11 | 12 | 1[a] | 0 | 2 | 4 |
| PRL-secreting (26) | 1 | 8 | 1 | 2 | 4 | 3 | 6 | 3 | 8 | 10 | – | – | – | – |
| successful (19) | 1 | 4 | 0 | 1 | 2 | 2 | 5 | 2 | 5 | 7 | – | – | – | – |
| unsuccessful ( 7) | 0 | 4 | 1 | 1 | 1 | 1 | 1 | 1 | 3 | 3 | – | – | – | – |
| GH-secreting ( 9) | 0 | 4 | 1 | 2 | 2 | 2 | 1 | 2 | – | – | 1[b] | 0 | 2 | 4 |
| successful ( 7) | 0 | 4 | 1 | 2 | 1 | 2 | 0 | 1 | – | – | 1[b] | 0 | 2 | 4 |
| unsuccessful ( 2) | 0 | 0 | 0 | 0 | 1 | 0 | 1 | 1 | – | – | 0 | 0 | 0 | 0 |
| ACTH-secreting ( 3) | 0 | 2 | 0 | 0 | 3 | 2 | – | – | 3 | 2 | 1[b] | 0 | 0 | 0 |
| successful ( 1) | 0 | 0 | 0 | 0 | 1 | 0 | – | – | 1 | 0 | 1[b] | 0 | 0 | 0 |
| unsuccessful ( 2) | 0 | 2 | 0 | 0 | 2 | 2 | – | – | 2 | 2 | 0 | 0 | 0 | 0 |
| *Macroadenomas* (65) | 37 | 43 | 23 | 19 | 22 | 28 | 20 | 17 | 28 | 28 | 13 | 5[b] | 21 | 21 |
| PRL-secreting (65) | 8 | 13 | 5 | 5 | 6 | 9 | 3 | 4 | 11 | 11 | – | – | 21 | 21 |
| successful ( 1) | 1 | 1 | 0 | 0 | 1 | 1 | 1 | 0 | 1 | 1 | – | – | – | – |
| unsuccessful (12) | 7 | 12 | 5 | 5 | 5 | 8 | 2 | 4 | 10 | 10 | – | – | – | – |
| GH-secreting (32) | 11 | 12 | 9 | 5 | 7 | 10 | 12 | 7 | – | – | 13 | 2[b] | 12 | 12 |
| successful (13) | 5 | 3 | 2 | 0 | 3 | 4 | 4 | 2 | – | – | 4[b] | 2[b] | 6 | 6 |
| unsuccessful (19) | 6 | 9 | 7 | 5 | 4 | 6 | 8 | 5 | – | – | 6[b] | 0 | 6 | 6 |
| Non-secreting (20) | 18 | 18 | 9 | 9 | 9 | 9 | 5 | 6 | 17 | 17 | 3 | 3 | 9 | 9 |

[a] Elevated basal serum PRL values.

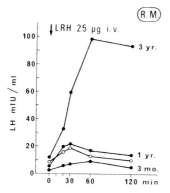

*Fig. 1.* Progressive recovery of LH responsiveness to LRH after operation, in one patient with microprolactinoma.

    ○ : before operation,  ● : after operation.

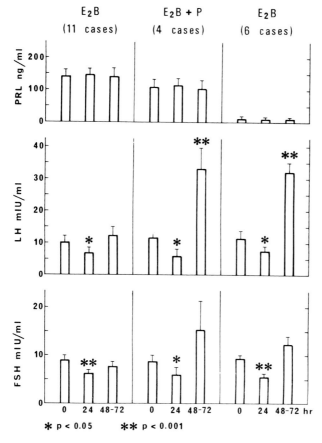

*Fig. 2.* Oestradiol benzoate ($E_2B$) administration (1 mg i.m.) in 11 patients with prolactinoma caused inhibition of serum gonadotrophins not followed by LH increase. In four cases oestradiol benzoate followed by 25 mg progesterone ($E_2B + P$) caused LH to rise. In six patients, retested after PRL normalization, $E_2B$ alone provoked serum LH increase.

**EFFECT OF CLOMIPHÉNE (100 mg p.o. × 5 days)**

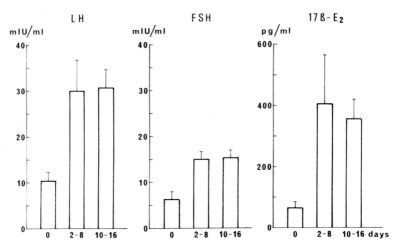

*Fig. 3.* Effect of clomiphene administration on serum LH, FSH and 17β-oestradiol in six patients with microprolactinoma.

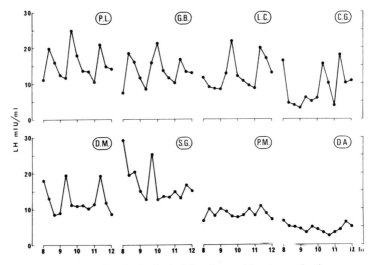

*Fig. 4.* Pulsatile serum LH episodes in 6 of 8 patients with microprolactinoma.

17 β-oestradiol on days 2–8, followed by a second LH peak on days 10–16 (Fig. 3). None of these was responsive to oestradiol benzoate.

Normal pulsatile serum LH, according to the criteria reported by Yen *et al.* (1972), was observed in 6 of 8 patients with microprolactinoma (Fig. 4).

### Thyrotrophin

Thyroid function, as indicated by basal serum $T_4$ and $T_3$ levels, appeared to be altered in only a minority of patients with microadenomas if we exclude a patient suffering from primary thyroid failure and the patients with Cushing's disease in whom thyroid hormone concentration was influenced by hypercorticism and was not accompanied by any alteration of the free thyroid hormone indices (Table I).

In patients with macroadenomas, thyroid failure was present in 36% of cases, and the incidence was particularly elevated in non-secreting (43%) and PRL-secreting (45%) tumours.

Impaired or absent TRH-stimulated TSH secretion was detected with the same incidence (36% of cases) in micro- and macroadenomas, with no clear relationship to the basal thyroid status. A number of alterations in the pattern of TSH response to TRH were observed in both micro- and macroadenomas, normal and regular responses being seen in only about half the cases (Table III). The incidence of various patterns of response was about the same in micro- and macroadenomas except for some exaggerated responses which were recorded only in patients with macroadenomas.

*Table III.*   Patterns of serum TSH response to TRH (classified according to Faglia *et al.*, 1973b), in patients with pituitary micro- and macroadenomas.

| Pattern of TSH response to TRH | Microadenomas % | Macroadenomas % |
|---|---|---|
| Normal and regular | 55.0 | 51.8 |
| Absent | 8.5 | 8.6 |
| Impaired | 27.5 | 27.5 |
| Delayed | 4.0 | 5.2 |
| Prolonged | 4.0 | 1.7 |
| Exaggerated | 0.0 | 5.2 |

After operation, two patients with microprolactinoma and one with acromegaly manifested transient hypothyroidism; the plasma TSH response to TRH was normalized in three cases and became impaired in one (Table II).

### Corticotrophin

Hypothalamic-pituitary adrenal function was found to be impaired in a minority of patients with microadenomas (excluding the ACTH-secreting) in basal conditions and after the metyrapone test, as compared with patients with macroadenomas, where the incidence of negative metyrapone tests reached 28%. However, alterations in the plasma cortisol response to hypoglycaemia had the same incidence in micro- and macroadenomas (Table I). After operation, the cortisol response to ITT normalized in three patients with microprolactinoma and disappeared in one acromegalic. Normalization of this test was also observed in five acromegalic patients with macroadenoma, while one patient with PRL-secreting macroadenoma and one with non-secreting pituitary tumour became unresponsive to insulin (Table II).

### Growth hormone

Growth hormone secretion in response to hypoglycaemia was impaired or absent in 40% of patients with microadenomas (excluding acromegalics); among these were all the patients with Cushing's disease and 29% of the cases with micro-

*Table IV.* Serum PRL responsiveness to TRH, sulpiride and chlorpromazine in 42 acromegalic patients classified according to their basal serum PRL levels and GH-responsiveness to TRH.

| Cases (n) | TRH | | Sulpiride | | Chlorpromazine | |
|---|---|---|---|---|---|---|
| | Respond. | Non-resp. | Respond. | Non-resp. | Respond. | Non-resp. |
| Acromegaly (42) | 18 (43%) | 24 (57%) | 21 (50%) | 21 (50%) | 0 (0%) | 42 (100%) |
| *Normo-PRL* (29) | 13 (45%) | 16 (55%) | 19 (66%) | 10 (34%) | | |
| GH-resp. (13) | 6 (46%) | 7 (54%) | 9 (69%) | 4 (31%) | | |
| GH-non-resp. (16) | 7 (44%) | 9 (56%) | 10 (62%) | 6 (38%) | | |
| *Hyper-PRL* (13) | 5 (38%) | 8 (62%) | 2 (15%) | 11 (85%) | | |
| GH-resp. (4) | 4(100%) | 0 ( 0%) | 1 (25%) | 3 (75%) | | |
| GH-non-resp. (9) | 1 (11%) | 8 (89%) | 1 (11%) | 8 (89%) | | |
| Microprolactinoma (38) | 4 (11%) | 34 (89%) | 3 ( 8%) | 35 (92%) | 0 (0%) | 38 (100%) |
| Non-secreting ad. (20) | 9 (45%) | 11 (55%) | 2 (10%) | 18 (90%) | 1 (5%) | 19 ( 95%) |

For comparison serum PRL responsiveness to the same stimuli in patients with microprolactinomas and non-secreting pituitary adenomas are also reported.

prolactinoma. This figure is much smaller than that observed in patients with macroadenomas (89%) (Table I). After operation, two patients with microprolactinoma become unresponsive, while in the successfully operated patient with Cushing's disease a normal responsiveness was restored (Table II).

*Prolactin*

Alterations in PRL secretion observed in patients with prolactinoma are not reported here. No patient with microadenoma had low serum PRL levels, while serum PRL concentrations below the sensitivity of our method (0.5 ng/ml) were observed in about 10% of patients with non-secreting pituitary macroadenomas. Elevated basal serum PRL levels were seen in 28% of patients with GH- and in 43% of patients with ACTH-secreting microadenomas, and in 32% of GH-secreting macroadenomas. Absent or impaired responses to TRH were more frequently observed in macro- than in microadenomas.

After operation two acromegalic patients with microadenoma became unresponsive to TRH. In 42 acromegalic patients with either micro- or macroadenomas, PRL secretion was more extensively investigated and the results compared with those obtained in microprolactinomas and in non-secreting pituitary tumours (Table IV). Basal serum PRL levels were normal in 29 cases and slightly elevated in 13 (PRL 38 – 68 ng/ml). A normal PRL response to TRH was observed in 18 (43%) normoprolactinaemic patients and was unrelated to the responsiveness of serum GH to TRH. The incidence of impaired PRL responses to TRH in this subgroup of acromegalics was similar to that found in those with non-secreting pituitary tumours. Five of 13 hyperprolactinaemic acromegalics increased serum PRL normally after TRH; four of them were also GH- responsive to TRH. All GH-responsive hyperprolactinaemic acromegalics had increased serum PRL after TRH, while only one GH-unresponsive did. The incidence of impaired PRL responses to TRH in GH-unresponsive hyperprolactinaemic acromegalics was similar to that found in patients with microprolactinomas. Sulpiride administration caused serum PRL to rise in only a minority of hyperprolactinaemic acromegalics as well as in microprolactinomas and in non-secreting pituitary tumours, while it evoked a normal response in 66% of normoprolactinaemic patients. Chlorpromazine failed to induce any serum PRL increase in any of the acromegalics, in microprolactinomas and in all but one patient with non-secreting pituitary tumours.

## DISCUSSION

In microadenomas, the incidence of endocrine abnormalities as revealed by multiple pituitary function tests appears to be much greater than suspected on clinical grounds and on the basis of previous reports (Jaquet *et al.*, 1978). In macroadenomas, the incidence we found of impaired endocrine function tests is in general agreement with that of other series (Nieman *et al.*, 1967; Snyder *et al.* 1974; Joplin *et al.*, 1975; Weisberg *et al.*, 1976).

The relative frequencies with which the various pituitary hormone secretions appeared to be affected after provocative tests were, in descending order, growth hormone, gonadotrophins, thyrotrophin and corticotrophin in macroadenomas, while in microadenomas gonadotrophin secretion was the least impaired. However this sequential order might be more apparent than real, depending on the different modalities and degrees of precision of the procedures used for assessing the secretion of each hormone. Pituitary gonadotrophin reserve investigated by a single LRH administration seems not to be significantly affected in either microprolactinomas or GH-secreting microadenomas, in contrast with the high incidence of impairment recorded in macroadenomas. Thus it appears that gonadotrophin reserve is not influenced by high serum PRL or GH levels. In fact, the gonadotrophic reserve was found to be enhanced in some cases, and independent of the levels of serum PRL or GH. Exaggerated FSH or LH responses to LRH in hyperprolactinaemic women had been previously reported by Thorner *et al.* (1974), Glass *et al.* (1975a), Archer *et al.* (1976), Aono *et al.* (1976), Asfour *et al.* (1977) and Kletzky *et al.* (1977), but not satisfactorily explained as yet, though probably mediated by altered ovarian steroid levels. However, Lachelin *et al.* (1977) and Kletzky *et al.* (1977) recently reported a diminished pituitary LH reserve, using repeated LRH stimulation, in patients with amenorrhoea-galactorrhoea and pituitary tumours. In acromegalic patients exaggerated FSH responses were also observed. This confirms the previous reports by Lindholm *et al.* (1976) and by Charro *et al.* (1973), who described high FSH/LH ratios and a greater increase in serum FSH than in LH after clomiphene administration to acromegalics.

In patients with Cushing's syndrome there was a high incidence of low basal gonadotrophin levels, the pituitary gonadotrophin reserve being always normal. Very little is known of the hypothalamic control of gonadotrophin secretion in Cushing's disease and conflicting results have been reported (Franchimont *et al.*, 1971; Demura *et al.*, 1972; Codaccioni *et al.*, 1973; Boccuzzi *et al.*, 1975). It appears unlikely that the reduction in serum gonadotrophin levels is caused by ACTH hypersecretion, since FSH and LH are not low in Addison's disease (Franchimont *et al.*, 1971) or in patients given ACTH (Beitins *et al.*, 1973). Possible interference of adrenal androgen and glucocorticoid excesses with gonadotrophin secretion has been considered, but at the present time no definite evidence has been obtained in man.

In recent years a number of alterations of hypothalamic-pituitary-ovarian function have been described in hyperprolactinaemic patients. A failure to respond to oestrogen-induced positive feedback has been previously demonstrated (Shaw *et al.*, 1975; Glass *et al.*, 1975a; Aono *et al.*, 1976; Travaglini *et al.*, 1978) and confirmed by the data presented here, which also show that the normalization of serum PRL levels restores normal response to oestrogenic positive feedback (Fig. 2). However, an LH surge was seen in microprolactinomas when progesterone was administered 36 h after oestradiol benzoate injection. This might be due to a triggering action of progesterone (Glass *et al.*, 1975b) on oestrogen-induced positive feedback. Since McNatty *et al.* (1977) demonstrated that high prolactin concentrations inhibit progesterone production by human granulosa cells in culture, our data suggest that the failure to respond to oestrogen-induced positive feedback in hyperprolactinaemic patients might be due to low progesterone secretion and that elevated serum prolactin has no direct effect on this hypothalamic regulatory mechanism.

Thorner *et al.* (1974) and Bohnet *et al.* (1976) described a high incidence of impaired clomiphene tests in hyperprolactinaemic patients, suggesting an alteration in the negative feedback mechanism: on the contrary, Mortimer *et al.* (1973) observed an increase in serum gonadotrophins after clomiphene administration to six cases. In our series of microprolactinomas the persistence of normal sensitivity to the oestrogenic negative feedback mechanism in spite of elevated serum PRL levels is documented by the rise in serum gonadotrophins after clomiphene in 5 of 6 patients tested and receives further support from the finding of a significant reduction in serum gonadotrophins 24 h after oestradiol benzoate administration (Fig. 2). Boyar *et al.* (1976) and Bohnet *et al.* (1976) observed absent or dampened serum LH pulsatility in patients with amenorrhoea-galactorrhoea syndrome. In our patients with PRL-secreting microadenomas, normal LH pulsatility was seen in 6 out of 8 cases.

Taken together, the data from our laboratory suggest that hyperprolactinaemia does not have a direct effect on the gonadotrophs and that PRL-induced alterations in gonadotrophin secretion are exerted at the hypothalamic level and are, at least in part, mediated by a peripheral effect of prolactin on ovarian steroidogenesis.

Reduced thyroid function was observed in a minority of patients with pituitary microadenomas and except in one woman with microprolactinoma, primary thyroid failure was excluded. The finding of undetectable basal plasma TSH levels is of no value in assessing deficient TSH secretion. However, undetectable plasma TSH levels were found in 25 and 26% of patients with micro- and macroadenomas, respectively, while in a normal population the incidence of undetectable values was 7.4%. The frequency of impaired or absent TSH responses to TRH was, however, greater than we expected in patients with microadenomas and in several cases was not accompanied by thyroid failure. It is likely that the small amount of TSH secreted is sufficient to ensure normal thyroid function. The incidence of absent or impaired TSH responses to TRH has been reported to be higher in acromegaly than in other pituitary tumours (Hall *et al.*, 1972; Schalch *et al.*, 1972; Samaan *et al.*, 1974; Lamberg *et al.*, 1976). This was also found in our acromegalic patients with microadenoma but not in those with macroadenoma. On the other hand, Snyder *et al.* (1974) and McLaren *et al.* (1974) did not find any significant difference in TSH responsiveness to TRH between acromegalics and patients with other pituitary tumours. Plasma TSH responses to TRH appeared to be always impaired in patients with ACTH-secreting microadenomas. These data are in agreement with those previously reported by Otsuki *et al.* (1973) and Lamberts *et al.* (1977) for patients with Cushing's syndrome, and by ourselves (Faglia *et al.*, 1973c) for normal subjects given dexamethasone. This TSH hyporesponsiveness to TRH is probably due to a glucocorticoid effect directly exerted on the pituitary. Low serum $T_4$ (2 cases) and $T_3$ (3 cases) concentrations are probably due to the effect of glucocorticoids on thyroid synthesis and peripheral metabolism of thyroid hormones (De Groot and Hoye, 1976), the free thyroid hormones indices being within the normal range in all cases. After our prior observations (Faglia *et al.*, 1971, 1973b), several reports (Pickardt *et al.*, 1972; Schalch *et al.*, 1972; Patel and Burger 1973; McLaren *et al.*, 1974) described abnormal patterns of TSH response to TRH in patients with hypothalamic-pituitary disorders, including pituitary tumours. Those alterations, consisting of delayed, prolonged and exaggerated increases in plasma TSH after TRH administration, have been described in detail elsewhere (Faglia *et al.*, 1973b), and have been generally considered to be due to the time required to restore TSH synthesis and secretion by thyro-trophs which had lacked adequate TRH stimulation for long time (delayed res-ponses) or to hypothalamic involvement caused by suprasellar extension of the tumour. However, as shown in Table III, the incidence of abnormal patterns of response to TRH is not significantly different in micro- and macroadenomas except for exaggerated responses that were observed only in macroadenomas. These data suggest that the exaggerated responses might be considered to be the consequence of the pressure on the stalk or hypothalamus from suprasellar exten-sion of huge pituitary tumours, whereas delayed and prolonged responses would be indicative of some functional impairment of TRH secretion. The finding of slightly elevated basal plasma TSH in patients with secondary hypothyroidism, normally or supranormally TSH-responsive to TRH but with inadequate increases in serum $T_3$, has been interpreted as indicative of reduced biological activity of the secreted TSH (Faglia *et al.*, 1975; Hall *et al.*, 1975). This was not observed in any patient with microadenomas, but was seen in four macroadenomas.

Previous studies showed a variable incidence of impaired ACTH secretion in pituitary tumours: Niemann *et al.* (1967) reported impaired secretion in 88% of cases, Jenkins and Else (1968) in 54%, Snyder *et al.* (1974) in 37%. On the con-trary, Jaquet *et al.* (1978) did not find any impairment in ACTH secretion in 18 intrasellar adenomas and 15 pituitary tumours with supra-sellar extension. In the present series, none of the patients with microprolactinoma and only two cases of GH-secreting microadenomas had low basal plasma cortisol, and 4 and 3 patients, respectively, had low urinary 17-OHCS. Insulin-induced hypoglycaemia caused insufficient plasma cortisol increases in about 30% of microadenomas while only a minority of patients showed impaired urinary 17-OHCS increases after metyrapone. Thus urinary 17-OHCS measurement seems to better reflect adrenocortical insufficiency in basal conditions, while plasma cortisol after ITT appears to be more sensitive in detecting fine abnormalities of corticotrophin secretion than are the 17-OHCS after metyrapone. Impaired plasma cortisol responses after ITT occurred with almost the same incidence in microadenomas and in macroadenomas, while the metyrapone test was more frequently impaired in macroadenomas. As in the present study, a lower incidence (12%) of impaired ACTH secretion, as judged by the metyrapone test, in patients with intrasellar pituitary tumours versus patients with supra-sellar extension of the adenoma (53%) was previously described (Faglia *et al.*, 1973a), while the incidence of impaired plasma cortisol responses was nearly the same in the two groups. This confirms that ITT is a more sensitive test for disclosing alterations in the regu-lation of ACTH secretion and that these alterations are not dependent on the size of the tumour.

Impaired or absent serum GH responses to ITT were found in 29% of patients with microprolactinoma and in all the cases of Cushing's disease. Jaquet *et al.* (1978), however, did not find any impairment of growth hormone secretion in 18 PRL-secreting microadenomas investigated by ITT and sleep studies. Reduced or absent GH responses to ITT have been previously reported by James *et al.* (1968) in patients with Cushing's syndrome of different etiology. Those alterations are probably due to cortisol rather than to ACTH excess. In fact, corticotrophin has been proved to have a stimulatory effect on GH secretion (Zahnd *et al.*, 1969). Furthermore, altered GH-responses to ITT have been observed in normal subjects after glucorticoid treatment (Frantz and Rabkin, 1964) and in patients with ACTH-independent Cushing's syndrome the serum GH response to ITT reverted to normal after cure of the hypercorticism (Krieger and Glick, 1972). In one patient of the present series, serum GH responsiveness to ITT normalized after successful microadenomectomy. GH secretion was impaired in a very high percentage of macroadenomas, as previously demonstrated by Nieman *et al.* (1967), Nelson *et al.* (1974), and many other investigators, and appears to be the anterior pituitary hormone secretion which is most frequently altered in pituitary tumours.

Reduced serum PRL levels were seen only in a minority of cases of non-secreting macroadenomas. The elevated basal serum PRL levels observed in patients with ACTH-secreting microadenomas were associated in only one patient with impaired response to TRH. The existence of alterations in PRL secretion in Cushing's disease have been described by Krieger *et al.* (1978), who observed an absence of the nocturnal PRL rise. On the contrary, Lamberts *et al.* (1977) described normal basal and TRH-stimulated PRL levels in three cases in whom, however, ITT did not induce an adequate PRL rise. This was also confirmed in 2 of 3 cases of ours. However, it is questionable whether high basal PRL values and impaired PRL responses to TRH in Cushing's disease can be attributed to hypercorticism: in fact, Copinschi *et al.* (1975) found blunted serum PRL responses to TRH in normal subjects given 4 mg dexamethasone daily for two days, while Re *et al.* (1976) did not observe any variation in PRL responsiveness to TRH after administration of 16 mg of dexamethasone for two days.

The question of whether in hyperprolactinaemic acromegalics the serum PRL excess is due to the presence of mixed adenoma or is the consequence of hypothalamic imbalance has not been fully clarified as yet. Guyda *et al.* (1973) and Corenblum *et al.* (1976) described the presence of two distinct cytotypes with different immunoreactivity in some GH- and PRL-secreting adenomas. However, Furth and Clifton (1966) and Tashjian *et al.* (1970) induced in rats pituitary adenomas consisting of only one cytotype that secretes two or more pituitary hormones.

Undoubtedly there are some differences in PRL secretion, in prolactinomas and in acromegaly. The present studies have demonstrated that the incidence of impaired responses to TRH in hyperprolactinaemic acromegalics whose GH is unresponsive to TRH is similar to that found in microprolactinoma patients while all GH-responsive patients normally increased serum PRL. Possible explanations are that in GH-non-responders two distinct types of adenomatous cells secrete GH and PRL, while in GH-responders hyperprolactinaemia may by due to "functional" disconnection of normal lactotrophs from hypothalamic control, or alternatively that GH and PRL are secreted by cells arising from a common progenitor.

In conclusion, the impairment of anterior pituitary hormones other than those hypersecreted appears to be due to pituitary damage in only a minority of patients with functioning microadenomas, whereas in most cases it appears to be secondary to alterations of hypothalamic regulation or to peripheral and/or central effects of the hypersecreted hormones.

The modifications seen in microadenoma patients in pituitary hormone secretion after surgery are of minor importance except for the gonadotrophins, for which the reserve was sometimes lowered after surgery. This is of importance to women with microprolactinomas who wish to become pregnant and one must consider carefully for these patients whether to recommend pharmacological or surgical treatment.

## REFERENCES

Abraham, G. E., Swerdloff, R., Tulchinsky, D. and Odell, W. D. (1972). *J. Clin. Endocr. Metab.* **35**, 458.

Aono, T., Myake, A., Shioji, T., Kinugasa, T., Onishi, T. and Kurachi, K. (1976). *J. Clin. Endocr. Metab.* **42**, 696.

Archer, D. F., Sprong, J. W., Nankin, H. R. and Josimovich, J. B. (1976). *Fertil. Steril.* **27**, 1158.

Asfour, M., L'Hermite, M., Hedouin-Quincampoix, M. and Fossati, P. (1977). *Acta endocr. (Copenh.)* **84**, 738.

Beitins, I. B., Bayard, F., Kowarski, A. and Migeon, C. J. (1973). *Steroids* **21**, 553.

Boccuzzi, G., Angeli, A., Bisbocci, D., Fonzo, D., Gaidano, G. P. and Ceresa, F. (1975). *J. Clin. Endocr. Metab.* **40**, 892.

Bohnet, M. G., Dahlen, H. G., Wuthke, W. and Schneider, M. P. G. (1976). *J. Clin. Endocr. Metab.* **42**, 132.

Boyar, R. M., Kapen, S., Weitzman, E. D. and Hellman, L. (1976). *New Engl. J. Med.* **294**, 263.

Busch, W. (1951). *Virshows Arch. Path. Anat.* **320**, 437.

Charro, A. L., Levin, S. R., Becker, N., Hofeldt, F. D., Friedman, S. and Forsham, P. H. (1973). *J. Clin. Endocr. Metab.* **36**, 502.

Codaccioni, J. L., Mattei, A., Djian, R. and Ruf, N. (1973). *In* "Syndromes polyendocriniens et Relations Interglandulaires" (M. J. Decourt and M. Gilbert-Dreyfus, eds) p. 267. L'Expansion Scientifique Française, Paris.

Copinschi, G., L'Hermite, M., Leclerq, R., Goldstein, J., Vanhaelst, L., Virasoro, E. and Robyn, C. (1975). *J. Clin. Endocr. Metab.* **40**, 442.

Corenblum, B., Sirek, A. M. T., Horvath, E., Kovacs, K. and Ezrin, C. (1976). *J. Clin. Endocr. Metab.* **42**, 857.

Cross, J. N., Glinne, A., Grossart, K. W. M., Jennet, W. B., Kellet, R. J., Lazarus, J. H., Thomson, J. A. and Webster, M. H. C. (1972). *Lancet* i, 215.

De Groot, L. J. and Hoye, K. (1976). *J. Clin. Endocr. Metab.* **42**, 978.

Demura, R., Demura, H., Nunokawa, T., Baba, H. and Miura, K. (1972). *J. Clin. Endocr. Metab.* **34**, 852.

Faglia, G., Beck-Peccoz, P., Ambrosi, B., Ferrari, C. and Neri, V. (1971). *J. Clin. Endocr. Metab.* **33**, 999.

Faglia, G., Ambrosi, B., Beck-Peccoz, P. and Travaglini, P. (1973a). *Acta endocr. (Copenh.)* **73**, 223.

Faglia, G., Beck-Peccoz, P., Ferrari, C., Ambrosi, B., Spada, A., Travaglini, P. and Paracchi, S. (1973b). *J. Clin. Endocr. Metab.* **37**, 595.

Faglia, G., Ferrari, C., Beck-Peccoz, P., Spada, A., Travaglini, P. and Ambrosi, B. (1973c). *Horm. Metab. Res.* **5**, 289.

Faglia, G., Beck-Peccoz, P., Ferrari, C., Spada, A. and Paracchi, A. (1975). *Clin. Endocr.* **4**, 585.

Franchimont, P. (1971). "Secretion normal et pathologique de la Somatotrophine et des Gonadotrophines humaines" p. 202. Masson et Cie. Paris.

Frantz, A. G. and Rabkin, M. T. (1964). *N. Engl. J. Med.* **271**, 1375.

Furth, J. and Clifton, K. H. (1966). *In* "The Pituitary Gland" (G. W. Harris and B. T. Donovan, eds) Vol. 2. 460–497. Butterworth and Co., London.

Giovanelli, M. A., Motti, E. D. F., Paracchi, A., Beck-Peccoz, P., Ambrosi, B. and Faglia, G. (1976). *J. Neurosurg.* **44**, 677.

Glass, M. R., Shaw, R. W., Butt, W. R., Edwards, R. L. and London, D. R. (1975a). *Brit. Med. J.* **2**, 274.

Glass, M. R., Shaw, R. W., Williams, J. W., Butt, W. R., Logan-Edwards, R. and London, D. R. (1975b). *Clin. Endocr.* **5**, 521.

Guitelman, A., Aparicio, N. J., Mancini, A., Encinas, M. T., Levalle, O. and Schally, A. V. (1977). *J. Clin. Endocr. Metab.* **45**, 810.

Guyda, H., Robert, F., Coll, E. and Hardy, J. (1973). *J. Clin. Endocr. Metab.* **36**, 531.

Hall, R., Ormston, B. J., Besser, G. M., Cryer, R. J. and McKendrick, M. (1972). *Lancet*, i, 759.

Hall, R., Smith, B. R. and Mukhtar, E. D. (1975). *Clin. Endocr.* **4**, 213.

Hotchkiss, J., Atkinson, L. E. and Knobil, E. (1971). *Endocrinology* **89**, 177.

James, V. H. T., Landon, J., Wynn, V. and Greenwood, F. C. (1968). *J. Endocrinol.* **34**, 192.

Jaquet, P., Grisoli, F., Guibout, M., Lissitzky, J. C. and Carayon, P. (1978). *J. Clin. Endocr. Metab.* **46**, 459.

Jenkins, J. S. and Else, W. (1968). *Lancet* ii, 940.

Joplin, G. F., Jackson, R. A., Arnot, R. N., Burke, C. V., Doyle, F. H., Harsoulis, P., Lewis, P. D., MacErlean, D. P., Marshall, J. C., Van Noorden, S. and Russel Fraser, T. (1975). *Clin. Endocr.* **4**, 139.

Kletzky, O. A., Davajan, V., Mishell, D. R., Nicoloff, J. T., Mims, R., March, C. M. and Nakamura, R. M. (1977). *J. Clin. Endocr. Metab.* **45**, 631.

Krieger, D. T. (1978). *Med. Clin. N. Amer.* **62**, 261.

Krieger, D. T. and Glick, S. M. (1972). *Amer. J. Med.* **52**, 25.

Lachelin, G. C. L., Abu-Fadil, S. and Yen, S. S. C. (1977). *J. Clin. Endocr. Metab.* **44**, 1163.

Lamberg, B.-A., Pelkonen, R., Aro, A. and Grahne, B. (1976). *Acta endocr.' (Copenh.)* **82**, 254.

Lamberts, S. W. J., Timmermans, H. A. T., De Jong, F. M. and Birkenhager, J. C. (1977). *Clin. Endocr.* **7**, 185.

Lindholm, J., Rasmussen, P. and Korsgaard, O. (1976). *Europ. J. Clin. Invest.* **7**, 141.

McLaren, E. H., Hendriks, S. and Pimstone, B. L. (1974). *Clin. Endocr.* **3**, 113.

McNatty, K. P., McNeilly, A. S. and Sawers, R. S. (1977). *In* "Prolactin and Human Reproduction" (P. G. Crosignani and C. Robyn, eds) pp. 109–117. Serono Symposia Vol. 11. Academic Press, London and New York.

Midgley, A. R. Jr. (1966). *Endocrinology* **79**, 10.

Midgley, A. R. Jr. (1967). *J. Clin. Endocr. Metab.* **27**, 295.

Mortimer, C. H., Besser, G. M., McNeilly, A. S., Marshall, J. C., Harsoulis, P., Turnbridge, W. M. G., Gomez-Pan, A. and Hall, R. (1973). *Brit. Med. J.* **4**, 73.

Nelson, J. C., Kollar, D. J. and Lewis, J. E. (1974). *Arch. Intern. Med.* **133**, 459.

Nieman, E. A., Landon, J. and Wynn, V. (1967). *Quart, J. Med.* **36**, 357.

Odell, W. D., Rayford, P. L. and Ross, G. T. (1967). *J. Lab. Clin. Med.* **70**, 973.

Otsuki, M., Dakoda, M. and Baba, S. (1973). *J. Clin. Endocr. Metab.* **36**, 95.

Patel, Y. C. and Burger, H. G. (1973). *J. Clin. Endocr. Metab.* **37**, 190.

Pickardt, C. R., Geiger, W., Fahlbusch, R. and Scriba, P. S. (1972). *Klin. Wochenschr.* **50**, 42.

Re, R. H., Kourides, I. A., Ridgway, E. C., Weintraube, B. D. and Maloof, F. (1976). *J. Clin. Endocr. Metab.* **43**, 338.

Samaan, N. A., Leavens, M. E. and Jesse, R. H. (1974). *J. Clin. Endocr. Metab.* **38**, 957.

Schalch, D. S., Gonzales-Barcena, D., Kastin, A. J., Schally, A. V. and Lee, L. A. (1972). *J. Clin. Endocr. Metab.* **35**, 609.

Shaw, R. W., Butt, W. R., London, D. R. and Marshall, J. C. (1975). *Clin. Endocr.* **4**, 267.

Silber, R. H. and Porter, C. C. (1954). *J. biol. Chem.* **210**, 923.

Sinha, Y. N., Selby, F. W., Lewis, V. F. and Vanderlaan, W. P. (1973). *J. Clin. Endocr. Metab.* **36**, 509.

Snyder, P. J., Jacobs, C. S., Rabello, M. M., Sterling, F. H., Shore, R. N., Utiger, R. D. and Daughaday, W. H. (1974). *Ann. Int. Med.* **81**, 751.

Tashjian, A. H. Jr., Bancroft, F. C. and Levine, L. (1970). *Cell. Biol.* **47**, 61.

Tori, G. (1953). *Boll. Sci. Med.* **125**, 251.

Thorner, M. O., McNeilly, A. S., Hagen, G. and Besser, G. M. (1974). *Brit. Med. J.* **2**, 419.

Travaglini, P., Ambrosi, B., Beck-Peccoz, P., Elli, R., Rondena, M., Bara, R. and Weber, G. (1978). *J. endocrinol. Invest.* **1**, 39.

Weisberg, L. A., Zimmermann, E. A. and Frantz, A. G. (1976). *Am. J. Med.* **61**, 560.

Yen, S. S. C., Tsai, C. C., Naftolin, F., Vandenberg, G. and Ajabor, L. (1972). *J. Clin. Endocr. Metab.* **34**, 671.

Zahnd, G. R., Nadeau, A. and Von Mühlendahl, K. E. (1969). *Lancet* ii, 1278.

# THE LH MICROADENOMA HYPOTHESIS.
## POST CLIMACTERIC FORMS?

S. Geller[1] and R. Scholler[2]

[1] Laboratoire d'Hormonologie C.E.F.E.R., 21, rue Ed. Rostand
F 13006, Marseille, France
[2] Fondation de Recherche en Hormonologie, 67, Bd. Pasteur,
F 94260, Fresnes, France

In previous work, we have reported sella turcica micro-enlargements associated with pituitary LH hyperactivity for which the hypothesis of pituitary LH microadenoma has been forwarded (Geller et al., 1976).

The patho-physiology of this disease suggested a LH inappropriate secretion stemming from a supposedly partial rupture of the estrogen/LH physiologic feedback and resulting in hypothalamic LH-RH, secondarily pituitary LH, and ovarian estrogen hyperactivity (Geller and Scholler, 1977).

These microenlargements, hypothetically labelled pituitary LH microadenomas had been indeed reported in premenopausal patients, notably with polycystic ovaries, and in premenopausal patients, where this combined estrogen + LH hyperproduction, so-called hyperovarism, can be encountered (Geller et al., 1979).

However, similar sella turcica microenlargements have also been encountered in postmenopausal patients, notably those with a past history of hyperovarism. These radiological aspects were apparently associated with a special pattern of response to the LH-RH test in postmenopausal patients, characterized by a preferential LH release (Geller and Scholler, 1979). So a statistical study was undertaken in postmenopausal patients to check whether these sella turcica microenlargements could be considered to be the post climacteric form of the so-called "LH microadenomas" previously reported in premenopausal patients.

## MATERIAL AND METHODS

All the patients included in this study have been investigated by the classical LH-RH test. LH-RH 100 $\mu$g is given intravenously as a bolus injection at $t = 0$; FSH and LH, assayed by R.I.A. (Roger et al., 1975) are estimated on plasma samples taken at regular intervals. FSH and LH total cumulative responses (T.C.R.), as estimated from the area encompassed by FSH (S1) and LH (S2) tracings, have been calculated by planimetry.

Sella turcica hypocycloidal tomographs have been carried out according to a technique adapted from Velina (Kandelman et al., 1976).

Appropriate investigations, notably prolactin estimations prior to and following TRH administration, have also been carried out in each patient, in order to rule out a possible micro-enlargement of other origin, notably prolactin or TSH adenoma.

## RESULTS

Eighty-nine postmenopausal patients without special gynaecological past history (called normal postmenopausal patients), 31 patients castrated for fibroids, 24 patients castrated for other gynaecological conditions, chiefly of infectious origin, 49 postmenopausal patients with breast cancer, and 26 patients castrated for breast cancer have been studied (Tables I – III and Fig. 1).

(1)   In *normal postmenopausal patients,* high S2/S1 values are statistically prevalent in the 1st age group, characterized by still appreciable estradiol levels (Fig. 1, Table I, line 1). The responses to the LH-RH test have been arbitrarily ranged into 3 types according to the value of the S2/S1 ratio:
type I : S2/S1 $< 0.8$; type II : $0.8 \leqslant$ S2/S1 $< 1$; type III : S2/S1 $\geqslant 1$.

In these normal postmenopausal patients the incidence of type III responses to LH-RH (i.e. "LH preferential release" pattern) is also maximal in the first age group and reduces thereafter with increasing menopausal age (and lowered estradiol levels), and type I responses then become prevalent (Table II, line 1).

In these same normal menopausal patients, type III responses to LH-RH, i.e. LH preferential release pattern, are generally associated with indisputable or at least suspected sella turcica microenlargements (Table III, bottom line) and conversely type I responses are generally associated with radiological by normal sella turcica (Table III, top line).

(2)   *Patients castrated for fibroids* also display higher values of S2/S1 ratio in the first age group, although estradiol levels are significantly lower in these patients than in the postmenopausal patients of the same age group (Fig. 1, Table I, line 2).

(3)   *Patients castrated for other gynaecological conditions,* in contrast, do not display such high values of S2/S1 ratio, even in the first age group (Fig. 1, Table I, line 3).

(4)   *In patients with breast cancer* high S2/S1 values are maintained beyond the first age group, notably in castrated patients, where highest values of this ratio are reached in the third age group (Fig. 1, Table I, line 4 and 5). Moreover, postmeno-

*Table I.* S2/S1 ratio and plasma estradiol (E2 pg/ml) in postmenopausal and castrated patients.

| Patient group | | < 2 years | | | 2 – 5 years | | | 5 – 10 years | | | ≥ 10 years | | |
|---|---|---|---|---|---|---|---|---|---|---|---|---|---|
| | | $n$ | $\bar{x}$ | Sm | $n$ | $\bar{x}$ | Sm | $n$ | $\bar{x}$ | Sm | $n$ | $\bar{x}$ | Sm |
| Normal postmenopausal | S2/S1 | 39 | 1.29 | 0.11 | 29 | 0.92 | 0.05 | 13 | 0.87 | 0.05 | 8 | 0.85 | 0.12 |
| | E2 | 31 | 72.7 | 14.7 | 25 | 20.8 | 7.1 | 12 | 18.2 | 4.2 | 5 | 25.2 | 9.5 |
| Castrated for fibroids | S2/S1 | 9 | 1.36[a] | 0.05 | 7 | 0.99 | 0.10 | 8 | 1.13[a] | 0.13 | 7 | 0.65 | 0.06 |
| | E2 | 7 | 10.1 | 0.4 | 5 | 9.3 | 0.7 | 6 | 11.2 | 0.6 | 5 | 8.5 | 0.7 |
| Castrated for other gynaecological conditions | S2/S1 | 6 | 0.74[c] | 0.10 | 7 | 0.80 | 0.07 | 6 | 0.77[a] | 0.10 | 5 | 0.65 | 0.08 |
| | E2 | 5 | 9.3 | 0.6 | 5 | 8.7 | 0.8 | 4 | 11.5 | 0.9 | 4 | 10.2 | 1.9 |
| Postmenopausal + breast cancer | S2/S1 | 8 | 1.23[a] | 0.18 | 13 | 1.16 | 0.17 | 8 | 1.17[a] | 0.18 | 20 | 1.10 | 0.12 |
| | E2 | 7 | 63.8 | 17.9 | 10 | 18.3 | 9.4 | 9 | 21.5 | 6.8 | 16 | 15.3 | 5.3 |
| Castrated for breast cancer | S2/S1 | 6 | 1.04[a] | 0.07 | 8 | 1.15 | 0.20 | 8 | 1.43[b] | 0.23 | 4 | 0.77 | 0.10 |
| | E2 | 5 | 9.2 | 0.5 | 6 | 8.7 | 0.6 | 5 | 10.4 | 0.7 | 4 | 7.6 | 0.9 |

[a]Non significant; [b]$P \leqslant 0.05$ (borderline significance); [c]$P < 0.01$ (highly significant), as compared to the corresponding normal postmenopausal subgroup.

Statistical calculations have been made using Sukhatme's test (Morice, E. and Chartier, F., Methode Statistique II, pp. 204–238), Cochran's test (Cochran, W. G., (1964). Approximate significance levels of the Behrens–Fisher test (*Biometrics* **20**, 191–195), Welch and Aspin's test (Bennet, C. A. and Franklin, N. L. (1954) "Statistical Analysis in Chemistry and the Chemical Industry" p. 177. John Wiley, New-York.)

*Table II.* Distribution of responses to **LH-RH** test in 89 normal postmenopausal patients and in 49 postmenopausal patients with breast cancer.

| Patients group | < 2 years | | | | | | 2 – 5 years | | | | | | 5 – 10 years | | | | | | ≥ 10 years | | | | | |
|---|---|---|---|---|---|---|---|---|---|---|---|---|---|---|---|---|---|---|---|---|---|---|---|---|
| | Type I | | Type II | | Type III | | Type I | | Type II | | Type III | | Type I | | Type II | | Type III | | Type I | | Type II | | Type III | |
| | n | % | n | % | n | % | n | % | n | % | n | % | n | % | n | % | n | % | n | % | n | % | n | % |
| Normal post-menopausal patients | 7 | 17.9 | 17 | 43.6 | 15 | 38.5 | 9 | 31 | 15 | 51.7 | 5 | 17.2 | 4 | 30.7 | 8 | 61.5 | 1 | 7.8 | 5 | 62.5 | 2 | 25 | 1 | 12.5 |
| Post-menopau-sal patients with breast cancer | 1 | 12.5 | | | 6 | 75 | 6 | 46.2 | 1 | 7.6 | 6 | 46.2 | 3 | 37.5 | 1 | 12.5 | 4 | 50 | 7 | 35 | 6 | 30 | 7 | 35 |

Type I : S2/S1 < 0.8; Type II : 0.8 ≤ S2/S1 < 1; Type III : ≥ S2/S1 ≥ 1.

*Table III.* Relation between response to LH-RH test and radiological findings in 62 patients.

|  |  | Radiological findings | | | |
|---|---|---|---|---|---|
|  |  | A | B | C | |
| Responses to LH-RH Test | Type I (S2/S1 < 0.8) | 10 | 3 | 3 | 16 |
|  | Type II (0.8 ≤ S2/S1 < 1) | 3 | 9 | 14 | 26 |
|  | Type III (S2/S1 ≥ 1) | 3 | 6 | 11 | 20 |
|  |  |  |  |  | 62 |

A : normal radiological aspect
B : doubtful microenlargement
C : undisputable microenlargement.

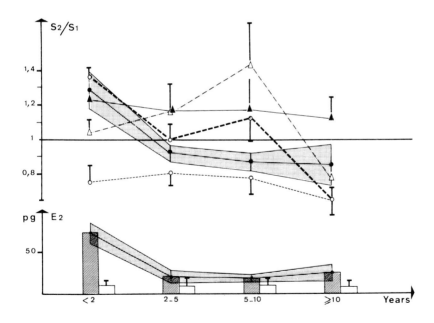

*Fig. 1.* Top panel: S2/S1 ratio in 89 postmenopausal patients (●—●), 31 patients castrated for fibroids (○--○), 24 patients castrated for other gynaecologic conditions (○.--.○), 49 postmenopausal patients with breast cancer (▲—▲) and 26 patients castrated for breast cancer (△.--.△).

Bottom panel : estradiol levels (E2) in 89 normal postmenopausal patients (hatched bars) and 31 patients castrated for fibroids (open bars).

pausal patients with breast cancer display a higher incidence of type III responses to LH-RH (LH preferential release) than the corresponding normal postmenopausal patients of the same age group (Table II, line 2).


## DISCUSSION

It may be deduced from these findings that sella turcica microenlargements found in postmenopausal patients are indeed associated with postmenopausal LH preferential release and higher estradiol levels, such as are normally found in early menopause. Still appreciable E2 levels associated with high LH responses to LH-RH, that is to say, all the conditions required for the development of the so-called LH microadenoma, are thus found in these patients. These postmenopausal sella turcica microenlargements may then be logically considered indeed as the postclimacteric form of the so-called LH microadenomas previously reported in premenopausal patients.

One may speculate that estrogens would favour LH-RH receptors in the pituitary gonadotroph cell, which would explain why they enhance the pituitary response to LH-RH (Arimura and Schally, 1971; Eshkol et al., 1975; Labrie et al., 1977a) and might also account for the well known LH-RH self-priming effect (Vasquez and McCann, 1976; Wang et al., 1976). It is true that such an effect of the estrogens upon the pituitary LH-RH receptors does not appear to have been reported thus far, at least to our knowledge. However, estrogen-induced enhancement of TSH response to TRH, which is comparable, mutatis mutandis, to estrogen induced enhancement of LH response to LH-RH, appears to be mediated through such an effect upon TRH pituitary receptors (Labrie et al., 1977b). At any rate, the statistical prevalence of "preferential LH release" (and associated sella turcica microenlargements) in the first postmenopausal age group, associated with still appreciable estrogen levels and its disappearance thereafter along with the lowering of estrogen levels, would be in agreement with this hypothesis.

This peculiar outcome with increasing menopausal age and estrogen fate suggests that these sella turcica microenlargements are probably not true adenomas but rather, presumably, "functional hyperplasia", with possible radiologic expression, which, in normal patients, would fade away with the disappearance of the pathophysiologic link, namely the estrogens.

High S2/S1 values in patients castrated for fibroids, in spite of very low estradiol levels seem apparently to be at variance with this patho-physiological scheme. However, as is well known, fibroids and related lesions, such as polycystic ovaries, endometrial hyperplasia and endometriosis, are admittedly associated with a rich estrogen "milieu". So, the efficient factor might be, not so much the present estrogen status, but the previous long-standing estrogen over-saturation extended over years and years. That would account at any rate for the persistence of relatively high S2/S1 values in these patients even beyond the first age group, and for the final dropping off of this ratio in the older age group.

The persistence of high S2/S1 values in postmenopausal patients with breast cancer and the prevalence of LH preferential release in these patients as compared to normal postmenopausal patients suggests that such a mechanism would also be at play in these patients. A statistical study of estrogen receptors is presently in progress in these patients. The first available results seem to indicate that there would indeed be a relation between LH preferential release (and associated sella turcica microenlargements) and high estrogen receptor levels, which would be in agreement with this hypothesis. Should these results be confirmed, postmenopausal LH preferential release and sella turcica associated microenlargements could then be considered as the witness of previous long-standing estrogen over-saturation, with all the prognostic and therapeutic implications involved by this statement.

At this time, the above findings in postmenopausal and castrated patients, taken as a whole, seem to provide an additional support to the LH microadenoma hypothesis previously put forward for premenopausal patients.

However, it must be stressed that, though the trend of the means is indeed suggestive, the differences in S2/S1 ratio, notably in the third age group are at the limit of statistical significance. Firm conclusions can be drawn only when larger populations have been studied.

## REFERENCES

Arimura, A. and Schally, A. V. (1971). *Proc. Soc. exp. Biol. Med.* **136**, 290–293.

Eshkol, A., Lunenfeld, B. and Insler, V. (1975). *J. Steroid Biochem.* **6**, 1061–1066.

Geller, S. and Scholler, R. (1977). *VIth International Seminar on reproductive physiology and sexual endocrinology*, Brussels May 1976, *Prog. Reprod. Biol.* **2**, 176–179.

Geller, S. and Scholler, R. (1979). *2nd International Congress on the Menopause*, Jerusalem, June 4–9, 1978.

Geller, S., Ayme, Y., Lemasson, C., Kandelman, M., Grisoli, F. and Scholler, R. (1976). *Annales Endocr. (Paris)* **37**, 281–282.

Geller, S., Ayme, Y., Kandelman, M., Grisoli, F., Lemasson, C. and Scholler, R. (1979). *International Symposium on Ovarian function*, Paris-Fresnes Oct. 1976.

Kandelman, M., Grisoli, F. and Jaquet, P. (1976). *C. R. du Congrès International de Tomographie*, Gênes 9 Sept. 1976 in *Excerpta Medica* 1978.

Labrie, F., Drouin, J., Lagace, L. and Ferland, L. (1977a). *VIth International Seminar on Reproductive Physiology and Sexual Endocrinology*, Brussels, May 1976, *Prog. Reprod. Biol.* **2**, 96–104.

Labrie, F., Lagace, L., Drouin, J., Delean, A., Kelly, A. P., Ferland, L., Beaulieu, M., Raymond, V., Dupont, A. and Cusan, L. (1977b). "Les Oestrogènes", pp. 3–23. Masson, Paris.

Roger, M., Veinante, A., Soldat, M. C., Tardy, J., Tribondeau, S. and Scholler, R. (1975). *Nouv. Presse Med.* **4**, 2173–2178.

Vasquez, C. A. and McCann, S. M. (1975). *Endocrinology* **97**, 13–19.

Wang, C. F., Lasley, B. F., Lein, A. and Yen, S. S. C. (1976). *J. Clin. Endocr. Metab.* **42**, 718–726.

# RELATIONSHIP BETWEEN PITUITARY TUMOR SIZE, HORMONAL PARAMETERS AND EXTRASELLAR EXTENSION IN PATIENTS WITH PROLACTINOMAS

J. G. M. Klijn[1], S. W. J. Lamberts[1], F. H. de Jong[1], R. Docter[1],
K. J. van Dongen[2] and J. C. Birkenhäger[1]

[1]*Department of Internal Medicine (III) and of Clinical Endocrinology,
University Hospital "Dijkzigt", Erasmus University, Rotterdam,
The Netherlands*
[2]*Department of Neuroradiology, University Hospital "Dijkzigt",
The Netherlands*

## INTRODUCTION

Generally pituitary tumors are divided into microadenomas with asymmetrical or localized alterations of the sella turcica and macroadenomas with an enlarged sella; extrasellar extension can occur in supra-, infra- and/or parasellar directions (Vezina, 1978; Hardy *et al.*, 1978; Chang *et al.*, 1977; Wilson and Dempsey, 1978; Jaquet *et al.*, 1978). Impaired endocrine functions can also exist in the presence of pituitary adenomas (Zarate *et al.*, 1973; Faglia *et al.*, 1973; Snyder *et al.*, 1974; Franchimont *et al.*, 1975). It is not known, however, whether there is a critical tumor size at which these problems are going to occur. We studied the significance of tumor size in 62 patients with prolactin-secreting tumors in relation to extrasellar extension, prolactin level and hormonal insufficiency.

## MATERIAL AND METHODS

### Patients

Sixty-two patients were selected on the basis of elevated basal prolactin levels and evidence of a pituitary (micro) adenoma. In 58 patients the sella turcica was enlarged or asymmetrical on plain radiography and/or tomography. Four female patients with galactorrhea and secondary amenorrhea had a normal sella without radiologically detectable abnormalities. Primary hypothyroidism and use of medication were excluded. This group of 62 patients consists of 38 females (61%) and 24 males (39%). The mean age of the female patients was 32 years and of the male patients 35 years. We found a fairly even distribution of the male patients with regard to age in contrast to a frequency peak in the female patients between 25 and 35 years.

### Radiological and ophthalmological examination

All patients were investigated by lateral radiography, sellar polytomography and complete ophthalmological evaluation. Further radiological examinations consisted of pneumoencephalography (with or without cisternography) and in most cases angiography of the carotid artery.

The largest lateral area of the sella turcica or, in the case of extrasellar extension, of the pituitary tumor was measured with a planimeter. In patients without suprasellar extension of the tumor the upper limit of sellar content was taken as a straight line between the tuberculum sellae and the tip of the dorsum sellae. The measurement of sellar or tumor size was carried out in all patients at least six times and the average standard deviation of this investigation was 3.4%. With this method we obtained a normal range of 0.7 - 1.4 cm$^2$ in 20 patients without pituitary pathology.

### Endocrine investigations

The dynamics of the secretion of LH, FSH, TSH and ACTH were investigated only in untreated patients ($n = 40$, $n = 39$, $n = 41$ and $n = 46$, respectively) by the LHRH-test (100 $\mu$g i.v.), the TRH-test (400 $\mu$g i.v.) and the metyrapone-test (6 × 750 mg orally).

### Assays

Prolactin, LH, FSH and TSH were measured using previously described radioimmunoassay techniques (Kwa *et al.*, 1973; Lamberts *et al.*, 1978; Odell *et al.*, 1965). Materials for determination of gonadotrophins and TSH were supplied by KABI AB (Stockholm) and Calbiochem AG (Lucerne). The preparations 69/104 and 68/38 (MRC, Mill Hill) were used as a standard for human LH, FSH and TSH. Plasma 11-desoxycortisol (S) was measured by the method of Meikle *et al.* (1969).

### Normal values

Normal basal plasma PRL levels are up to 12 ng/ml in men and up to 15 ng/ml in women. Normal basal LH levels are between 0.6 - 2.8 U/l and basal FSH levels are between 1.2 - 4.2 U/l in the early to mid-proliferative phase of the menstrual cycle while $\Delta$ LH varied between 3 and 12 U/l and $\Delta$ FSH between 2 and 8 U/l. In 9 normal males basal levels of LH and FSH varied from 0.6 to 2.5 U/l and from 0.7 to 3.3 U/l resp, while LH varied between 3.7 and 8.8 U/l and $\Delta$ FSH between

1.3 and 5.5 U/l. Normal basal values of TSH are lower than 4.9 mU/l (95% range of 71 controls). The maximal increment of TSH after TRH in 16 control females (aged 28-60 years) varied between 7.1 and 38.7 mU/l (Smeulers *et al.*, 1977), while in 8 normal men the variation in maximal increment was between 6.1 and 13.1 mU/l. Our normal values for S after metyrapone exceed 15 μg/dl, while the range of 10 to 15 μg/dl may be regarded as borderline.

## RESULTS

### Radiological findings

There was a normal sella in 6%, an asymmetrical sella in 19%, and enlarged sella without extrasellar extension in 31% and extrasellar extension as determined by radiological and perimetrical examination in 43% of the 62 patients. Tumor size varied between 1 and 25 cm$^2$. In our male patients the average tumor size was considerably larger than in the female patients (6.08 ± 5.15cm$^2$ *vs* 2.88 ± 2.74 cm$^2$; mean ± S.D.; $P < 0.01$). No correlation was found between age and tumor size.

In the group of 36 patients with pituitary adenoma sizes of 3 cm$^2$ or less, only a 14 year old boy with a chromophobe adenoma that was located mainly above the sellar diaphragm showed radiological evidence of suprasellar extension of the tumor (Fig. 1). Three other patients had slight visual field defects without radiologically evident suprasellar extension. One of these three patients had a partially empty sella, which probably caused tension of the optic nerves.

In the group of 26 patients with a (para) sagittal planimetric surface of the pituitary tumor greater than 3 cm$^2$, 21 patients showed radiologically suprasellar extension (8 with infrasellar extension too). One patient showed only infrasellar extension and 2 patients (tumor size 4.9 and 10.1 cm$^2$) only impairment of the visual fields without radiologically detectable extrasellar extension of the tumor.

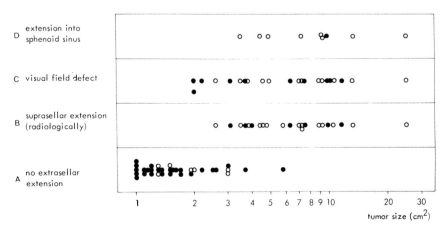

*Fig. 1.* Tumor size in relation to the presence of extrasellar extension by radiological or perimetrical criteria (*n* = 62). It may be pointed out that there is some overlap of the groups of patients represented in the upper three panels (B, C, D) whereas all patients represented in the lowest panel (A) are separate. Solid dots represent female patients.

### Hormonal studies

*Prolactin levels* in the whole group of 62 patients basal PRL levels varied
between 17–27 000 ng/ml. The range in 47 as-yet-untreated patients was 17–5000
ng/ml. A positive correlation existed between log tumor size and log basal PRL in
these patients (Fig. 2, $P < 0.0005$).

*Pituitary–thyroidal axis (TRH-test)*

In 41 untreated patients log basal TSH and log $\Delta$TSH showed a negative correlation with log tumor size (Fig. 3; $P < 0.025$ and $P < 0.01$, resp.). Above a tumor

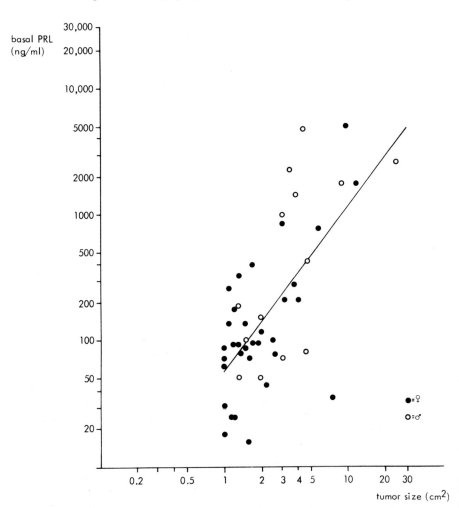

*Fig. 2.* Correlation between log tumor size and log basal prolactin levels in 47 untreated
patients ($r = 0.68$; $P < 0.0005$). Solid dots represent female patients.

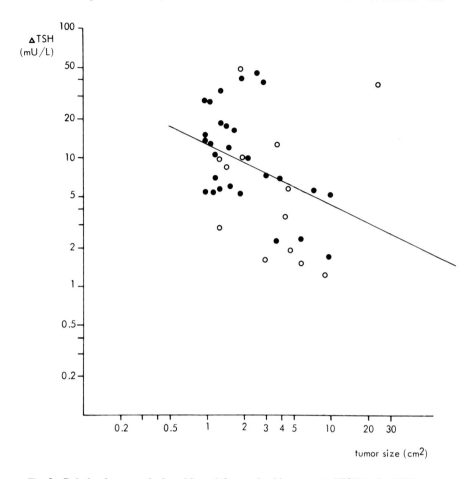

*Fig. 3.* Relation between the logarithm of the maximal increment of TSH in the TRH-test ($\Delta$TSH) and log tumor size in 41 untreated patients with prolactinoma ($r = 0.36$; $P < 0.01$). Solid dots represent female patients.

size of 3 cm², 11 of the 14 patients (79%) had a disturbed response of TSH, while only 7 of the 27 patients (26%) with a tumor size of or less than 3 cm² showed a diminished TSH reserve.

*Pituitary–gonadal axis (LHRH-test)*

Log basal plasma LH and FSH levels showed a negative correlation with log tumor size (both $P < 0.005$). A similar negative correlation existed also for the maximal increment in LH and FSH (Fig. 4a, b; $P < 0.0005$ and $P < 0.005$, resp.). In the presence of a pituitary tumor with a size greater than 3 cm² a disturbed FSH response was found in all 6 women and in 4 of 6 men (83% of 12 patients), and a disturbed LH response in 7 of all 13 patients (54%).

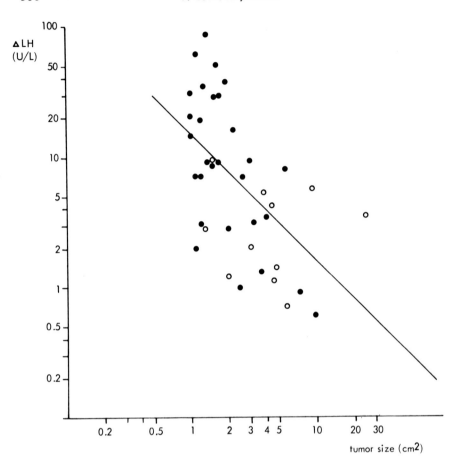

**Fig. 4a.** Relationship between the logarithm of the maximal increment of LH in the LHRH-test (ΔLH) and the log tumor size in untreated patients with prolactinoma. Solid dots represent female patients.

$$n = 40; r = 0.56; P < 0.0005.$$

*Pituitary–adrenal axis (metyrapone-test)*

A negative correlation was also observed between pituitary tumor size and plasma desoxycortisol level 4 h after the last dose of 6 × 750 mg metyrapone in 36 patients ($P < 0.025$). Of the 46 untreated patients in whom the integrity of the pituitary–adrenal axis was judged either by the plasma desoxycortisol level or the increase of urinary 17-OHCS excretion after metyrapone, 16 patients had tumor or sellar size of 3 cm² or larger. Seven of these 16 patients (44%) had an impaired reactivity in contrast to only one patient with a disturbed metyrapone-test in the 30 patients with a tumor size of less than 3 cm².

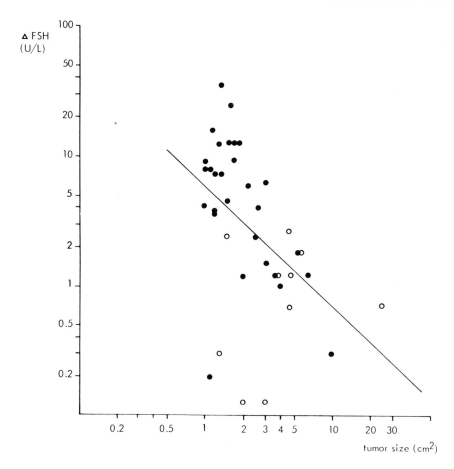

*Fig. 4b.* Relationship between the logarithm of the maximal increment of FSH in the LHRH test (ΔFSH) and the log tumor size in untreated patients with prolactinoma. Solid dots represent female patients.

$$n = 39; r = 0.47; P < 0.005.$$

## DISCUSSION

Vezina (1978) has never found suprasellar expansions in patients with "grade 1" microadenomas. Chang (1977) reported suprasellar expansions in patients with microadenomas ( ≤ 1 cm in diameter). Studying the incidence of extrasellar extension in relation to the size of prolactin secreting adenomas we found that an area of 3 cm$^2$ is rather critical. Below this value extrasellar extension of the tumor occurs very seldomly. When tumor size exceeded 3 cm$^2$, however, extrasellar extension (by radiological and perimetrical examination) occurred in 92% of the patients.

As to the relationship between the size of prolactinomas and the secretory activity, Child *et al.* (1975) described a positive correlation between log tumor size (range 0.5 - 3.0 cm$^2$) and log basal prolactin level. Our data confirmed this for a larger group of untreated patients with a wider variation in tumor size (1-25 cm$^2$) and basal prolactin levels (17-5000 ng/ml).

More important is the relationship between tumor size and the occurrence of endocrine deficiencies. Hormonal deficiencies are reported frequently in patients with clear evidence of a pituitary tumor. We know of no previous data, however, on the relationship of tumor size to the incidence of endocrine deficiencies. In this study we found that a tumor size of 3 cm$^2$ is not only important with regard to the incidence of extrasellar extension of the tumor but also with regard to the incidence of loss of pituitary functional reserve. We demonstrated that above a tumor size of 3 cm$^2$ the incidence of a disturbed response to TRH, LHRH and metyrapone is greatly increased.

When we compared the results of the TRH test with those of a control group, a disturbed response of TSH to TRH was observed in 11 of 14 patients (79%) with a tumor size above 3 cm$^2$ as opposed to an incidence of 7 in 27 patients (26%) with a tumor size below 3 cm$^2$. Some authors reported a normal value of TSH of (less than) 5mU/l (Faglia *et al.*, 1973; McLaren *et al.*, 1974; Snyder *et al.*, 1974; Sowers *et al.*, 1976; Krassas *et al.*, 1977). Taking a value of TSH of 5 mU/ml as the normal lower limit, subnormal values occurred in 7 of 14 patients (50%) with a tumor size above 3 cm$^2$. This was only found in 1 of 26 patients with a tumor size of 3 cm$^2$.

A very high degree of correlation was noted between $\Delta$ LH and $\Delta$ FSH ($P <$ 0.0005). We observed hyperresponses of FSH and LH in women with a tumor size below 2.5cm$^2$ only.

The pronounced increased incidence of supra- or extrasellar extension of the tumor and of secondary endocrine deficiencies at prolactinoma sizes greater than 3 cm$^2$ is probably of great importance in the management of these patients. We showed before that an impaired response of LH and FSH to LHRH in patients with prolactinomas greatly diminished the possibility of obtaining ovulatory cycles after normalization of circulating PRL levels during bromocriptine therapy (Lamberts *et al.*, 1978). On the basis of the data presented here it appears to be desirable to perform a transsphenoidal hypophysectomy or preferably an adenomectomy before the size of the adenoma has exceeded 3 cm$^2$.

We thank H. G. Kwa for the determination of the prolactin levels; Dr. W. van Rijn from Hoechst, Amsterdam, the Netherlands, for generous supply of TRH and LHRH; Miss A. de Graaff for expert administrative help.

## REFERENCES

Chang, R. J., Keye, W. R., Young, J. R., Wilson, G. B. and Jaffe, R. B. (1977). *Am. J. Obstet. Gynec.* **128**, 356–363.

Child, D. F., Nader, S., Mashiter, K., Kjeld, M., Banks, L. and Russell Fraser, T. (1975). *Br. Med. J.* **1**, 604–606.

Faglia, G., Beck-Peccoz, P. Ferrari, C., Ambrosi, B., Spada, A., Travaglini, P. and Paracchi, S. (1973). *J. Clin, Endocrinol. Metab.* **37**, 595–601.

Franchimont, P., Demoulin, A. and Bourguignon, J. P. (1975). *Hormone Res.* **6**, 177–191.

Hardy, J., Beauregard, H. and Robert, F. (1978). *In* "Progress in Prolactin Physiology and Pathology" (C. Robijn and M. Harter, eds) pp. 361–370. Elsevier/North-Holland Biomedical Press, Amsterdam and New York.

Jaquet, P., Grisoli, F., Guibout, M., Lissitzky, J. and Carayou, P. (1978). *J. Clin. Endocrinol. Metab.* **46**, 459–466.

Krassas, G., McHardy-Young, S., Ramsay, I. and Florin-Christensen, A. (1977). *Clin. Endocrinol.* **6**, 145–151.

Kwa, H. G., Engelsman, E. and van der Gugten, A. A. (1973). *In* "Human Prolactin" (J. L. Pasteels and C. Robyn, eds) pp. 102–106.

Lamberts, S. W. J., Docter, R., de Jong, F. H., Birkenhäger, J. C. and Kwa, H. G. (1978). *Fert. Steril.* **29**, 287–290.

McLaren, E. H., Hendricks, S. and Pimstone, B. L. (1974). *Clin. Endocrinol.* **3**, 113–122.

Meikle, A. W., Jubiz, W., Hutchings, M. P., West, C. D. and Tyler, F. H. (1969). *J. Clin. Endocrinol. Metab.* **29**, 985–987.

Odell, W. D., Wilber, J. F. and Paul, W. E. (1965). *J. Clin. Endocrinol.* **25**, 1179–1183.

Smeulers, J., Docter, R., Visser, T. J. and Hennemann, G. (1977). *Clin. Endocrinol.* **7**, 389–397.

Snyder, P. J., Jacobs, L. S., Rabello, M. M., Sterling, F. H., Shore, R. N., Utiger, R. D. and Daughaday, W. H. (1974). *Ann. Int. Med.* **81**, 751–757.

Sowers, J. R., Hershman, J. M. and Pekary, J. M. (1976). *J. Clin. Endocrinol. Metab.* **43**, 741–748.

Vezina, J. L. (1978). *In* "Progress in Prolactin Physiology and Pathology" (C. Robyn and M. Harter, eds) pp. 351–360. Elsevier/North-Holland, Biomedical Press, Amsterdam and New York.

Wilson, C. B. and Dempsey, L. C. (1978). *J. Neurosurg.* **48**, 13–22.

Zarate, A., Jacobs, L. S., Canales, E. S., Schally, A. V., de la Cruz, A., Soria, J. and Daughaday, W. H. (1973). *J. Clin. Endocrinol. Metab.* **37**, 855–859.

# RADIOLOGIC EVALUATION OF PITUITARY
# MICROADENOMAS*

T. H. Newton and I. Richmond

*Department of Radiology, University of California,
School of Medicine, San Francisco, California 94143, USA*

Pituitary microadenomas (tumors less than 10 mm in diameter) present an increasingly important diagnostic problem to the endocrinologist, gynecologist, neurosurgeon and neuroradiologist. In most cases early recognition of the tumor is possible because of the presence of endocrine abnormalities such as galactorrhea and amenorrhea. The clinical diagnosis of a secreting pituitary adenoma is ordinarily confirmed by hormonal assays and radiographic findings.

This investigation is divided into two parts: (1) a radiologic assessment of sellar changes in pituitary microadenomas and (2) a correlation of the radiographic with the surgical findings in prolactin-secreting pituitary adenomas.

## RADIOLOGIC ASSESSMENT OF SELLAR CHANGES
## IN PITUITARY MICROADENOMAS

In an attempt to evaluate the role of sellar changes in the diagnosis of pituitary microadenomas, we reviewed skull radiographs and thin section tomograms of 146 consecutive patients who had had pituitary adenomas removed via the transsphenoidal approach (Robertson and Newton, 1979). The adenomas were classified as secreting or non-secreting on the basis of clinical presentation, laboratory analysis and light and electron microscopy. Secreting adenomas were subdivided

---

*Addendum-portions of this manuscript were previously published *in* Robertson, W. D. and Newton, T. H. Radiologic assessment of pituitary microadenomas, *Am. J. Roentgenol.* to be published.

into those that secreted adrenocorticotrophic hormone (ACTH), those secreting
growth hormone (GH), and those secreting prolactin. Non-secreting adenomas
were frequently associated with pituitary hypofunction but were also often
asymptomatic and were then noted as an incidental finding in skull radiographs.

The area and volume of the sella were determined in each instance from plain
frontal and lateral radiographs of the skull and from anteroposterior (AP) and
lateral tomograms of the sella obtained at 2 mm intervals, using the hypocycloidal
motion of the Polytome (Di Chiro, 1960; Di Chiro and Nelson, 1962). The upper
limits for normal length and height of the sella were considered to be 16 mm and
13 mm respectively and the upper limit of normal area was considered to be
208 mm$^2$ (Vezina and Sutton, 1974). The upper limit of normal volume of the
sella was considered to be 1500 mm$^3$ (Busch, 1951; Tori, 1953). In those patients
in whom the sella was normal in area and volume, the tomograms of the sella were
further analyzed for localized expansion or abnormal configuration.

Table I.  Classification of 146 microadenomas.

|  |  | No. (%) |
|---|---|---|
| Secreting |  | 110 (75) |
| ACTH | 21 (14) |  |
| prolactin | 31 (21) |  |
| GH | 58 (40) |  |
| Nonsecreting |  | 36 (25) |

Table II.  Sellar area measured in 146 patients with pituitary microadenomas.

|  | Patients | Normal area < 208 mm$^2$ | Abnormal area > 208 mm$^2$ |
|---|---|---|---|
| Secreting adenomas |  |  |  |
| ACTH | 21 | 20 (95%) | 1 ( 5%) |
| prolactin | 31 | 23 (74%) | 8 (26%) |
| GH | 58 | 16 (28%) | 42 (72%) |
| Nonsecreting adenomas | 36 | 10 (28%) | 26 (72%) |

*Table III.* Sellar volume in 146 patients with pituitary microadenomas.

| | Patients | Di Chiro's[a] Normal $< 1100$ mm$^3$ | Tori-Busch[b] Normal $< 1500$ mm$^3$ | Abnormal $> 1500$ mm$^3$ |
|---|---|---|---|---|
| Secreting adenomas | | | | |
| ACTH | 21 | 18 (86%) | 20 (95%) | 1 ( 5%) |
| prolactin | 31 | 18 (58%) | 24 (77%) | 7 (23%) |
| GH | 58 | 13 (22%) | 16 (28%) | 42 (72%) |
| Nonsecreting adenomas | 36 | 9 (25%) | 13 (36%) | 23 (64%) |

[a]From Di Chiro and Nelson (1962).
[b]From Tori (1953) and Busch (1951).

*Table IV.* Location of changes in sellar configuration seen on lateral tomograms of 73 patients with normal sellar area and volume.

| Microadenoma | Sellar location Anterior | Posterior | General | Normal configuration |
|---|---|---|---|---|
| Secreting | | | | |
| ACTH | 11 | 1 | 5 | 3 |
| prolactin | 10 | 2 | 12 | |
| GH | 11 | 1 | 4 | |
| Nonsecreting | 4 | 2 | 7 | |

Seventy-five per cent of the 146 pituitary adenomas studied were secreting while 25% were non-secreting (Table I). The non-secreting adenomas tended to be larger at the time of diagnosis. Seventy-two per cent of the non-secreting adenomas had a greater than normal sellar area and 64% had an abnormally large sellar volume (greater than 1500 mm$^3$)(Tables II and III). Of the secreting adenomas, patients with acromegaly tended to have the largest sellar size. Seventy-two per cent of these patients had an abnormal sellar area and an abnormal sellar volume. Patients with Cushing's disease and patients with prolactin-secreting adenomas tended to have small sellas at the time of diagnosis. Among the patients with prolactin-secreting tumors, 26% had an abnormal sellar area and only 23% had an abnormal sellar volume. Of the patients with Cushing's disease, an abnormal sellar area and volume were noted in only 5%.

Of the 146 patients with pituitary adenomas, 73 (50%) had sellas of normal area and volume. Thin section tomograms of the sella, however, demonstrated abnormal configurations in all but three. Changes in the configuration of the sella were most commonly noted in lateral tomograms (Table IV). Bulging or localized expansion of the sella was usually present along the anterior or anteroinferior margins of the sella (Figs 1–4). These changes in configuration were usually seen in two adjacent tomographic sections (i.e. separated by 2 mm). The configuration

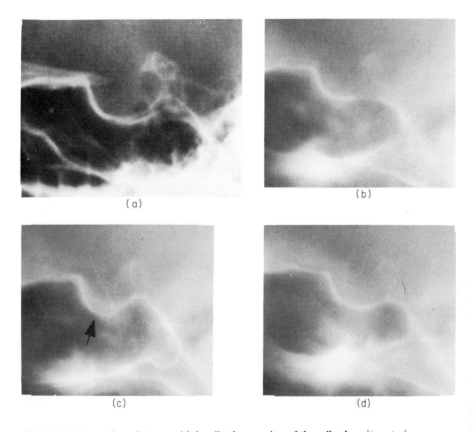

(a)

(b)

(c)

(d)

*Fig. 1.* Pituitary microadenoma with localized expansion of the sella along its anterior–inferior margin. (a) Lateral film of the sella shows no abnormality. (b–d) Lateral tomographic sections of the sella separated by 4-mm intervals. Localized bulging (arrow) of the sella floor is visible.

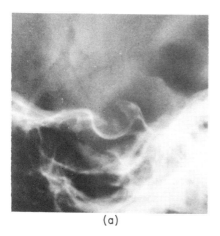
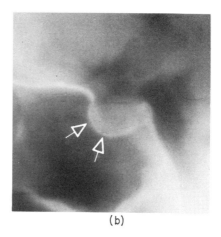

(a)                                    (b)

*Fig. 2.* Pituitary microadenoma with minimal expansion of the anterior–inferior wall of the sella. (a) Lateral film of the sella shows no abnormality. (b) Lateral tomographic section shows slight expansion (arrows) of the anterior–inferior wall of the sella.

of the anterior wall or floor of the sella may sometimes be changed by septae in the sphenoid sinus. These changes should not be confused with those caused by pituitary adenoma. Frontal tomograms of the sella often showed no abnormality even when lateral tomograms were abnormal (Table V). The sellar floor as seen on frontal projections is normally straight or slightly convex inferiorly. The lateral corners of the floor are normally rounded and smooth. Microadenomas may depress the floor on one side and cause the lateral corners to change to a more acute angle. Thirty-three of the 73 patients with normal sellar area and volume had normal configuration of the sella as noted on frontal tomograms. Of these 33 patients, 30 showed expansion along the anterior or anteroinferior portions of the sella in lateral tomograms. Frontal tomograms, therefore, were noted to be less sensitive in demonstrating changes in these locations.

The study indicated that measurements of the sellar area and volume are insensitive indicators of the presence of a pituitary microadenoma. Ninety-five per cent of the ACTH-secreting adenomas and approximately 75% of the prolactin-secreting adenomas in our series would not have been detected if measurements of the sellar area and volume were used. However, 72% of the acromegalic patients and about 70% of the non-secreting adenomas would have been diagnosed simply by an analysis of sellar area and volume.

The most sensitive radiologic means of detecting pituitary microadenomas was thin-section (hypocycloidal) tomography performed at 2 mm intervals. Of the 73 patients considered to have a normal sellar area and volume, all except three ACTH-secreting adenomas showed an abnormal sellar configuration on the tomograms. Tomography is therefore indicated in all instances of clinically suspected pituitary adenoma in which the sella appears normal in routine frontal and lateral radiographs of the skull.

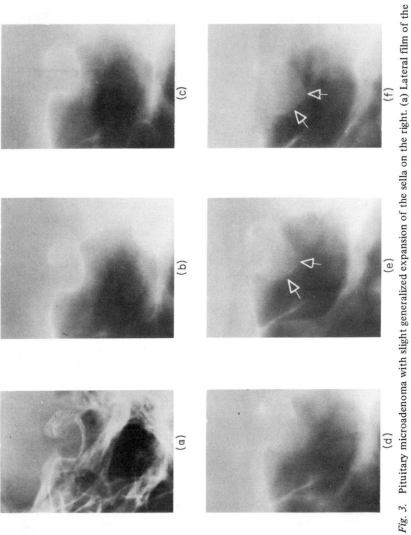

*Fig. 3.* Pituitary microadenoma with slight generalized expansion of the sella on the right. (a) Lateral film of the sella shows no abnormality. (b–f) Lateral tomographic sections of the sella at 2-mm intervals. Slight generalized expansion of the sella and demineralization of the floor are noted in *e* and *f*.

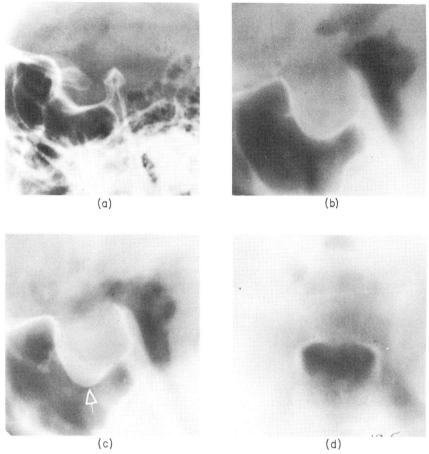

*Fig. 4.* Pituitary microadenoma with localized expansion of the anterior–inferior wall. (a) Lateral film of the sella shows no abnormality. (b) Hypocycloidal tomographic section through the midportion of the sella, at the time of pneumoencephalography. The anterior–inferior portion of the sella appears slightly expanded. (c) Hypocycloidal section obtained 3-mm lateral to *b*. A localized expansion of the sellar floor is now evident (arrow). No suprasellar mass is noted. (d) Frontal tomographic section of the sellar floor shows no abnormality.

*Table V.* Location of changes in sellar configuration seen in anteroposterior tomograms of 73 patients with normal sellar area and volume.

| Microadenoma | Sellar location | | | Normal configuration |
| --- | --- | --- | --- | --- |
| | Lateral | Central | General | |
| Secreting | | | | |
| ACTH | 3 | 2 | 2 | 13 |
| prolactin | 3 | 9 | 3 | 9 |
| GH | 2 | 5 | 5 | 4 |
| Nonsecreting | 2 | 2 | 2 | 7 |

## CORRELATION BETWEEN RADIOGRAPHIC
## AND SURGICAL FINDINGS IN
## PROLACTIN SECRETING ADENOMAS

The second part of the study reviewed the radiologic findings in 100 patients with suspected prolactin-secreting pituitary adenomas who underwent transsphenoidal resection (Richmond *et al.*, to be published). Of these, 96 proved to have adenomas while four were found to have pituitary hyperplasia on pathologic examination. The radiologic studies included frontal and lateral hypocycloidal tomograms of the sella, pneumoencephalograms with polytomography of the sellar region and bilateral internal carotid arteriograms. The arteriograms, usually performed using 2:1 magnification and subtraction techniques, included frontal, lateral and basal projections.

*Table VI.*   Prolactin secreting adenomas staging (after Guiot) 100 cases.

| | | |
|---|---|---|
| H. | Hyperplasia | 4 |
| *Enclosed adenomas:* | | |
| I. | < 10 mm Intracapsular<br>sellar volume normal | 53 |
| II. | > 10 mm Intracapsular<br>sellar volume increased | 15 |
| *Extracapsular adenomas:* | | |
| III. | Extension inferiorly or laterally | 23 |
| IV. | Diffusely invasive (more than one direction<br>of dural penetration) | 5 |

The adenomas were found to be totally intracapsular in 68 out of the 96 patients (Table VI). Fifty-three of the 68 patients had normal sellar volume and tumors less than 10 mm in diameter. In all 15 patients with intracapsular adenomas in whom the sellar volume was increased, the tumor measured more than 10 mm in diameter. In 28 patients, the tumor had broken through the capsule.

Although the sellar volume was normal in 72 patients, the sellar shape as judged by hypocycloidal tomography showed abnormalities in all but four patients. The most frequent abnormality noted was an anteroinferior bulge in the outline of the sella as shown in lateral tomograms (Table VII). Although the cortical margin was often thin, it usually remained intact. The location of the lesion within the sella was exactly predicted by means of tomography alone in 88% of the patients. In no instance, however, was there complete disagreement between the radiologic prediction of tumor location and the surgical findings.

*Table VII.*   Prolactin secreting adenomas.

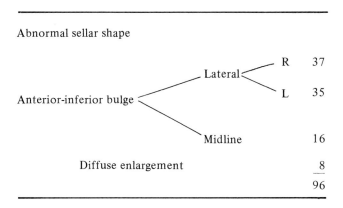

Abnormal sellar shape

Anterior-inferior bulge — Lateral — R   37
                                    L   35
                        — Midline      16

Diffuse enlargement                     8
                                       96

*Table VIII.*   Pneumoencephalographic findings: prolactin secreting adenomas

| | |
|---|---|
| Suprasellar extension | 19 |
| encroachment of suprasellar cisterns only | 10 |
| deformity of third ventricle | 9 |
| Partially empty sella | 24 |

Pneumoencephalographic examination disclosed suprasellar extension in 19 of the 100 patients (Table VIII). Extension of the tumor into the suprasellar compartment was noted in five of the 53 Stage I patients with normal sellar volumes, and intracapsular tumors less than 10 mm in diameter (Hardy, 1973). Suprasellar extension was noted in 11 of the 15 Stage II patients with intracapsular tumors larger than 10 mm and increased sellar volume. There was excellent correlation between the radiographic and the surgical staging of the tumor. All 19 of the patients found by pneumoencephalography to have suprasellar extension had this finding confirmed at operation.

Partially empty sellas, ranging from 10 to 80% of sellar volume, were demonstrated in 24 patients. Such an extension of the suprasellar cistern into the sella was noted in all four patients in whom only pituitary hyperplasia was found pathologically. It was noted in 11 of the 53 patients with Stage I tumors but in only one of the 15 patients with Stage II tumors. Partially empty sellas were noted in eight of the 28 patients with extracapsular adenomas.

Bilateral carotid arteriography proved to be of little diagnostic help in the evaluation of prolactin secreting pituitary adenomas (Table IX). Arteriography was performed primarily to evaluate lateral extension of the tumor and to rule out

*Table IX.* Prolactin-secreting pituitary adenomas.

| Angiographic findings | |
|---|---|
| Normal angiograms | 72 |
| Lateral displacement IC | 21 |
| Anterior cerebral elevation | 1 |
| Tumor blush | 7 |
| Siphon irregularity | 1 |
| Siphon encasement | 1 |
| Medial bowing | 1 |
| Open siphon | 3 |
| Posterior extension | 1 |

vascular anomalies. Evaluation of lateral extension by basal internal carotid views proved to be unreliable. Of the 21 patients showing lateral displacement of the internal carotid artery, 13 had no lateral extensions at surgery. Moreover, an additional 12 patients with normal arteriograms were found at exploration to have lateral extension. Only seven studies showed tumor blush in magnification subtracting views; all of these were in patients harboring large lesions. No aneurysms were encountered. Large dural venous sinuses significantly compromised operative exposure in three patients. Such venous anomalies were not demonstrated even with bilateral carotid angiograms including basal views and subtractions.

## REFERENCES

Busch, W. (1951). *Virchows Arch. Path. Anat.* **320**, 437–458.
Di Chiro, G. (1960). *Am. J. Roentgenol.* **84**, 26–37.
Di Chiro, G. and Nelson, K. B. (1962). *Am. J. Roentgenol.* **87**, 989–1008.
Hardy, J. (1973). *Excerpta Medica.* International Congress Series No. **303**, 179–198.
Richmond, I., Newton, T. H. and Wilson, C. B. "Correlation Between Radiographic and Surgical Findings in Prolactin Secreting Pituitary Adenomas". *To be published.*
Robertson, W. D. and Newton, T. H. (1979). *Am. J. Roentgenol., to be published.*
Tori, G. (1953). *Bull Sci. Med. (Bologna)* **125**, 251–269.
Vezina, J. L. and Sutton, T. J. (1974) *Am. J. Roentgenol.* **120**, 46–54.

# PROLACTIN-SECRETING PITUITARY
## MICROADENOMAS: TOMOGRAPHIC ASSESSMENT
## OF NORMAL SELLA IN PLAIN SKULL FILMS

V. Bernasconi, A. Bettinelli and U. Vaccari

*Department of Radiology, Chair of Neuroradiology,
University of Milan, Italy*

It is well-known that it is possible to find a normal sella turcica in patients with pituitary adenoma. The sella turcica can be considered to be normal in plain skull films when it has the following characteristics:
(1)  round, oval or flat shape,
(2)  maximum size of 16 mm in the sagittal diameter, 13 mm in the vertical and 10-15 mm in the transverse diameter; surface of no more than 208 mm$^2$ (Vezina and Maltais, 1973) and volume of no more than 1092 mm$^3$ (Di Chiro and Nelson, 1962),
(3)  thickness and density of the lamina dura,
(4)  lack of double floor contour.
As far as the last characteristic is concerned, it should be noted that sometimes a non-pathological double floor contour may be encountered.

According to Taveras and Wood (1976), a non-pathological double floor contour can be due to:
(1)  a central concave depression of the floor not exceeding 2 mm (seen in frontal view),
(2)  a slightly tilted floor, with a gradient not exceeding 1 mm (seen in frontal view) and integrity of the lamina dura,
(3)  asymmetrical development of the sphenoid sinus,
(4)  prominent carotid grooves.
Tomography is necessary in most cases in order to document these anatomical conditions.

Our study concerns a group of prolactin-secreting pituitary microadenomas with normal sella in plain skull films. We did not consider the ACTH-secreting microadenomas because they were limited in number, nor the GH-secreting ones because they constantly showed pathological sellar shapes in plain skull films.

## MATERIALS AND METHODS

Two hundred and fifty patients with hyperprolactinemia and amenorrhea, with or without galactorrhea, were studied in the Neuroradiological Department of the University of Milan between 1976 and 1977. All patients had plain skull films with straight postero–anterior view, lateral view, antero–posterior half-axial view, axial view and tomography of the sella in the frontal and lateral projections. For tomographic investigation we use an unidirectional linear movement tomographic equipment with limiting conus 4 cm across, 50° pendular angle and sections at 2 mm intervals. We tried to overcome the limits of linear tomography by moving the patient's head (for the lateral tomograms) in order to have the pendular plane of the X-ray tube perpendicular to the portion of the floor concerned in the expansive process.

Of the 250 patients examined, 65 showed sellar changes in plain skull films that suggested the presence of microadenoma (pathological double floor contour, localized bulging with thinning of the lamina dura). Tomography confirmed the changes and localized them in the frontal plane. Among these patients, 40 underwent surgical treatment while 25 had medical treatment.

The plain skull films of the remaining 185 patients showed normal sellas according to the criteria mentioned before. In 14 of these patients, the tomograms showed changes related to a microadenoma which was then surgically confirmed. Preoperatively, tomopneumoencephalography was also carried out, but it never showed suprasellar expansion of the adenoma.

The ages of the patients varied from 17 to 44 years, with an average of 22 years. The serum prolactin levels varied from 59 to 500 ng/ml. Tomographic examination of the sella turcica of these 14 patients showed three types of changes. The first type (six cases) consists of a slight ballooning of one side of the sella with thinning of the lamina dura, while the other side is oval-shaped and has a well preserved lamina dura. This change is mainly seen in lateral tomograms. It does not appear in plain skull films as a double floor contour because of the smallness of the morphological change (Fig. 1 a, b, c).

The second type (six cases) is characterized by a localized erosion of the floor, more frequently in its lateral and antero–inferior portion. This change fails to appear in plain skull films because of the superimposition of the contiguous normal portions (Fig. 2 a, b, c).

The third type of tomographic change (two cases) consists of a gross inferior bulging of the floor, a well-known change that generally can already be found in plain films. In these two cases, the change failed to appear because it was hidden by the bony septa of the sphenoidal sinus (Fig. 3 a, b, c).

At surgery, a close relation between the location of the adenoma and the tomographic change was found.

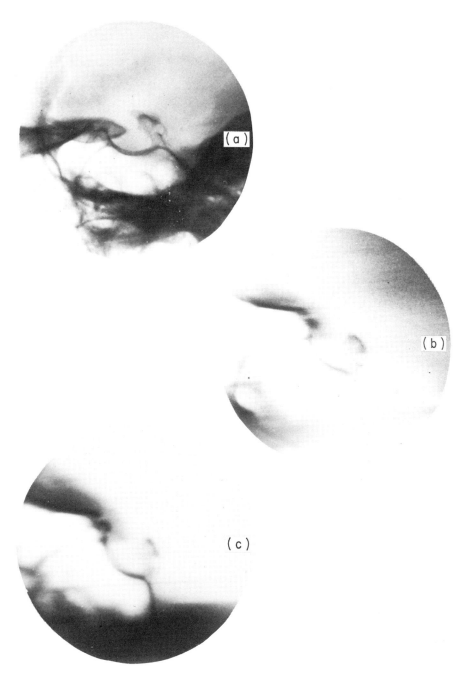

*Fig. 1.* S. T. 28 years old. Amenorrhea, galactorrhea. Serum prolactin level: 110 ng/ml.
(a) Lateral projection: sella with normal shape, width, contour thickness.
(b) Lateral tomogram of left hemisella: normal outline.
(c) Lateral tomogram of right hemisella: ballooning of the antero–inferior contour with thinning of the cortex.

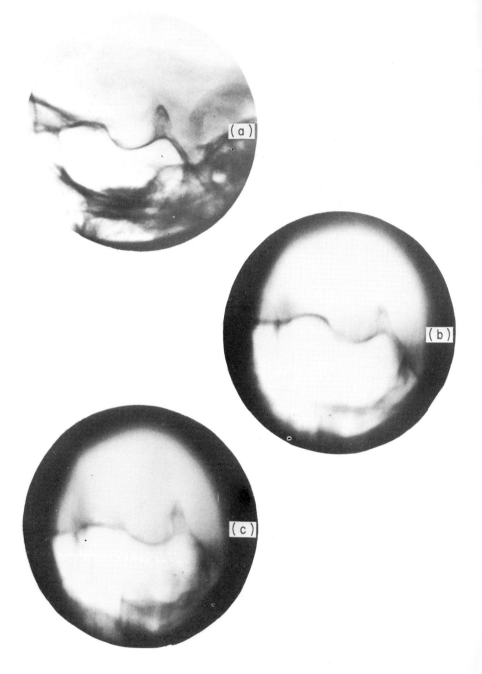

*Fig. 2.* M.A. 26 years old. Amenorrhea, obesity. Serum prolactin level: 55 ng/ml.
(a) Lateral projection: sella with normal shape, width, contour thickness.
(b) Lateral tomogram of left hemisella: localized erosion of the antero–inferior portions of the left side floor.
(c) Lateral tomogram of right hemisella: normal outline.

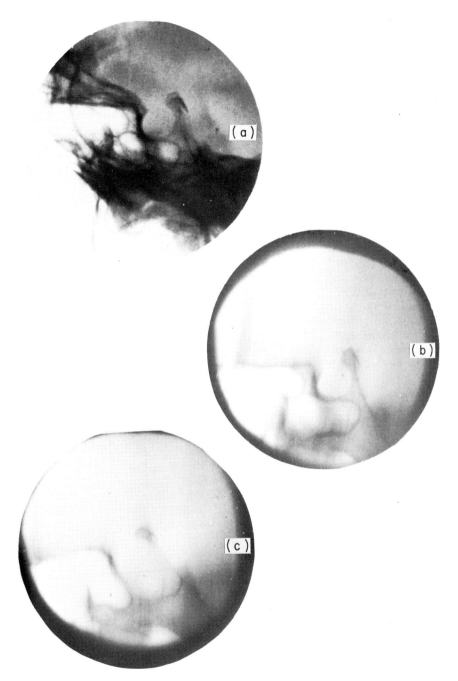

*Fig. 3.* B.A. 31 years old. Amenorrhea, galactorrhea. Serum prolactin level: 440 ng/ml.
(a) Lateral projection: sella with normal shape, width, contour thickness.
(b) Lateral tomogram of left hemisella: normal outline.
(c) Lateral tomogram of right hemisella: postero–inferior bulging masked in plain skull film by the septa of the sphenoidal sinus.

While the changes of the third type do not present diagnostic problems, the tomographic changes of types 1 and 2 must be discussed.

Swanson and Du Boulay (1975) examined the tomopneumoencephalographic studies (linear tomography) of 85 subjects without clinical evidence of pituitary lesion and found sellar changes similar to those seen in our first and second types (thinning or erosion of the lamina dura, slight ballooning of a sellar side) in 31.7% of the cases. They were not sure whether these signs should be considered as indicative of clinically silent microadenomas. However, in 1976 Besser remarked that such subjects, examined only from a clinical point of view, could not be considered free from pituitary lesions, since endocrinological essays were not carried out. The same author noticed that in an important anatomopathological study Costello (1936) had found clinically silent microadenomas in 22.5% of the cases and this percentage rose to 31.5% when subjects from 20 to 70 years were considered, as in the Swanson and Du Boulay study. Therefore, Besser refuses to accept the conclusions of those authors who do not admit to so high a percentage of unrecognized pituitary tumors.

In conclusion, we think that the tomographic changes seen in patients with a normal sella in plain skull films are certainly due to microadenomas when they are associated with clinical and endocrinological signs of hyperprolactinemia. According to our experience, the cases presented in previous studies (McLachlan et al., 1970; Vezina and Maltais, 1973; Vezina and Sutton, 1974) which stressed the importance of the tomographic technique for the diagnosis of microadenomas, had normal-sized sellae in plain skull films but showed changes in shape (double floor contour, lateralized bulging), or in structure (thinning or erosion of the lamina dura), that already led to suspicion of the presence of microadenoma. In these cases tomography confirmed the lesion and localized it exactly.

On the other hand, in the fourteen cases we just presented, tomography was of fundamental importance for the diagnosis of microadenomas, since the sella was completely normal in plain skull films.

Our results, which were surgically confirmed, stress the effectiveness of linear tomography for the diagnosis of pituitary microadenomas, even though it has some limits as compared with hypocycloidal tomography.

The size of the surgically removed microadenomas varied from 5 to 10 mm diameter. There was no relation between the tomographic changes, the volume of the adenoma and the serum prolactin level.

## REFERENCES

Besser, G. M. (1976). Brit. J. Radiol. 49, 652–653.
Costello, R. T. (1936). Am. J. Path. 12, 205–215.
Di Chiro, G. and Nelson, K. B. (1962). Am. J. Roentg. 87, 989–1008.
McLachlan, M. S., Wright, A. D. and Doyle, F. H. (1970). Brit. J. Radiol. 43, 360–369.
Swanson, H. A. and Du Boulay, G. (1975). Brit. J. Radiol. 48, 366–369.
Taveras, M. Y. and Wood, E. H. (1976). "Diagnostic Neuroradiology". Williams and Wilkins, Baltimore.
Vezina, J. L. and Maltais, R. (1973). Neurochirurgie Suppl. 2, 33–56.
Vezina, J. L. and Sutton, T. J. (1974). Am. J. Roentg. 120, 46–54.

# CT EVIDENCE OF FUNCTIONING
# MICROADENOMAS OF THE PITUITARY

M. Leonardi[1] , F. Bertolissi[2] , T. Penco[1] , G. Fabris[1] and F. De Nardi[3]

[1] *Sezione di Neuroradiologia, I Istituto di Radiodiagnostica,*
*Ospedale Generale Regionale di Udine, Italia*
[2] *Sezione di Endocrinologia, III Divisione di Medicina Generale*
*Ospedale Generale Regionale di Udine, Italia*
[3] *Divisione di Neurochirurgia, Ospedale Generale Regionale di Udine, Italia*

A number of endocrine disorders are associated with an adenoma of the pituitary that can not be visualized with standard X-ray techniques including tomography, angiography and pneumoencephalography.

Endocrine diseases due to functioning microadenomas of the anterior hypophyseal lobe without any appreciable sellar change include cases of Cushing's disease (Bigos *et al.*, 1977; Ganguly *et al.*, Tyrrel *et al.*, 1978) acromegaly and, more frequently, hyperprolactinemia with or without nonpuerperal galactorrhea-amenorrhea syndrome or anovulatory cycles (Metzger *et al.*, 1976).

The possibility of a selective resection of pituitary microadenomas by transsphenoidal microsurgery (Bigos *et al.*, 1977; Tyrrell *et al.*, 1978) makes the identification of such intrasellar growth of the utmost importance in the course of endocrine evaluation of patients with disorders of the pituitary function. Furthermore, some of the above-mentioned endocrinopathies can be associated with an empty sella or, possibly, with a non-adenomatous hyperplasia or over-activity of the hormone-producing pituicytes, making a differential diagnosis extremely difficult on the basis of clinical and laboratory findings.

Microadenomas of the pituitary have been previously identified by a few investigators by employing newer CT systems (Belloni *et al.*, 1978; Gyldensted and Karle, 1977; Leonardi *et al.*, 1978; Vignaud, 1978).

Since computerized tomography (CT) became available to us, we have been able to identify an abnormal intrasellar image suggestive of a microadenoma of the anterior pituitary in 7 of 17 patients with nonpuerperal amenorrhea–galactorrhea syndrome, in one with Cushing's disease and in one with inactive acromegaly.

CT images consistent with an empty sella have been found in two patients with untreated, longstanding primary hypothyroidism, in one with Cushing's disease and one with amenorrhea-galactorrhea and hyperprolactinemia. All but two had perfectly normal sellas by standard X-ray techniques.

## METHODS AND CASE REPORTS

CT examinations have been carried out with an Artronix Neurological CAT system with fan beam, 128 cell Xeron multidetector, 256 × 256 matrix, 1 × 1 × 3 mm pixel with 3 mm slice thickness. The standard examination of the sella was accomplished with 15–20 contiguous cuts parallel to the Frankfurt horizontal plane.

The different computer presentation of the image pixels allows sagittal and coronal reconstruction. A scan was performed after an i.v. infusion of 100–150 ml of aqueous solution of $N$-methylglucosamine iodamine salt (Uromiro® 300, Bracco) in 10 min following a preliminary examination without contrast medium injection.

The ages of patients with nonpuerperal amenorrhea–galactorrhea syndrome and evidence of a pituitary microadenoma ranged between 19 and 39 years. None of them had received previous medication that could be responsible for the hyperprolactinemia. The symptoms were restricted to amenorrhea, galactorrhea and infertility of 1–12 years duration. The physical examination was negative; the endocrine evaluation did not show an impairment of the pituitary function, except an excessive prolactin (PRL) secretion. Basal blood levels of PRL ranged between 50 and 300 ng/ml with a mean of 126 ng/ml (normal values: < 25 ng/ml). After i.v. injection of TRH (200 μg) blood PRL levels did not change in 5 patients and showed a significant but percentage-wise subnormal rise in 3. Serum LH and FSH levels were normal and showed a normal rise after Gn-RH stimulation.

The patients with Cushing's disease were aged 27, 48 and 47, and showed the classical features of acquired bilateral adrenal hyperplasia.

The patient with inactive acromegaly was a 40-year-old man with somatic changes typical of the disease. At the time of this study blood GH levels were normal with a blunted response to arginine, insulin and bromocriptine stimulation.

The patients with untreated primary hypothyroidism were a 38-year-old male, hypothyroid from childhood, with a hypoplastic lingual thyroid and a female of 29 with an acquired idiopathic myxedema. Basal TSH values were > 80 and > 100 μU/ml (normal values: < 5 μU/ml) and PRL values were 24 and 22 ng/ml, with an exaggerated rise after TRH stimulation.

## RESULTS AND CONCLUSION

An intrasellar area of augmented density suggestive of a microadenoma of the pituitary has been observed in 9 patients with evidence of pituitary dysfunction. Following the injection of the contrast medium, in 7 cases we noted an intrasellar

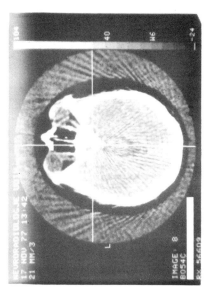

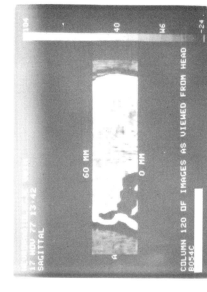

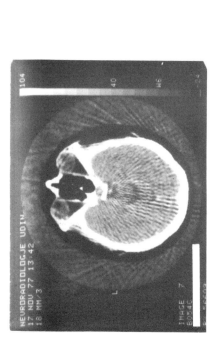

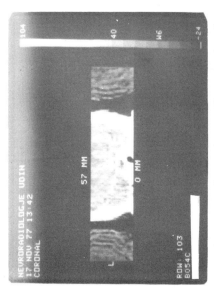

*Fig. 1.* Amenorrhea–galactorrhea syndrome. CT examination after contrast enhancement. A hyperdense nodule is evident in the superior portion of the pituitary: (a) axial view, (b) selection of sagittal and coronal planes of reconstruction, (c) sagittal and (d) coronal view.

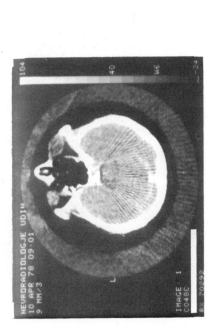

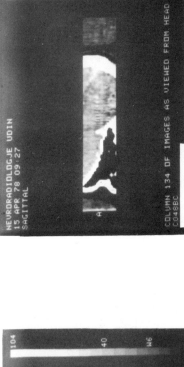

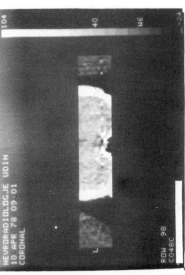

*Fig. 2.* Amenorrhea–galactorrhea syndrome. (A) CT standard examination: no intrasellar abnormalities. After contrast enhancement an intrasellar hyperdense area is evident close to a lowering of the sellar floor: (B) axial view, (C) coronal and (D) sagittal

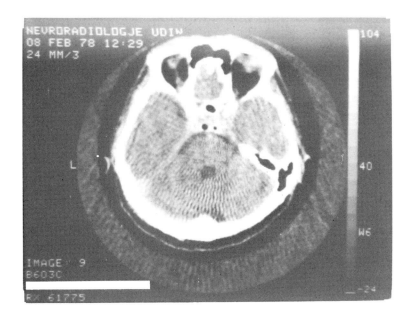

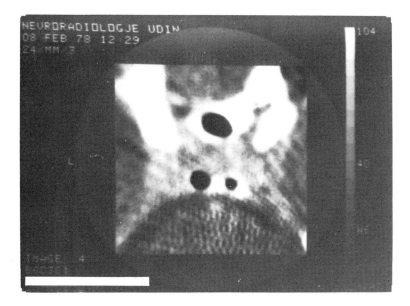

*Fig. 3.* Inactive acromegaly. (A) CT examination after contrast enhancement, (B) magnification of × 3. An irregularly spotted intrasellar area is suggestive of micronodules.

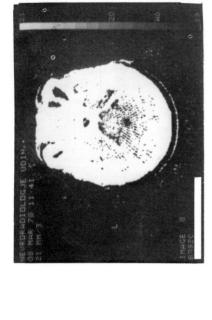

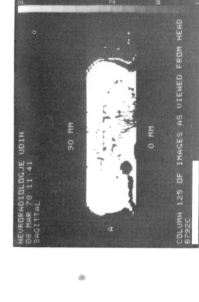

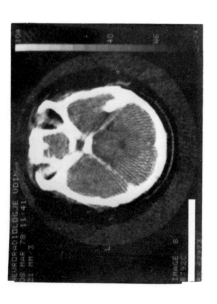

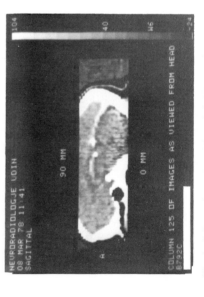

*Fig. 4.* Primary hypothyroidism. (A) CT examination after contrast enhancement, axial view, (B) densitometry, (C) sagittal view, on the midline, (D) densitometry. The sella turcica is occupied by a CSF pocket: empty sella.

micronodule of marked and uniform opacity; in 2 the increased density appeared as an irregularly spotted area. In 3 patients findings consistent with an empty sella were present. In 8 patients with CT evidence for microadenoma the sella was of normal appearance by standard computed tomography before the injection of the contrast medium. Only one patient (with amenorrhea-galactorrhea syndrome) showed a slightly lowered floor on the right side.

In conclusion, the intrasellar densitometry by CT following the i.v. injection of a suitable contrast medium appears to make possible the detection of abnormalities not detectable with conventional diagnostic tools; it makes CT the method of choice for direct or indirect visualization of the pituitary gland in clinical endocrinology.

The identification of a small intrasellar adenoma can modify the therapeutic approach to several endocrine disorders, as far as small tumors can be removed successfully by selective transsphenoidal microsurgery and an empty sella image does not encourage a surgical approach. Furthermore, repeated CT examinations allow a follow-up of suspected or proven intrasellar adenomas before the onset of signs and symptoms of compression of the contiguous intracranial structures, such as a visual field defect.

## REFERENCES

Belloni, G., Baciocco, A., Borelli, P., Sangui, G., Di Rocco, C. and Maira, G. (1978. *Neuroradiology* **15**, 179.
Bigos, S. T., Robert, F., Peletier, G. and Hardy, J. (1977). *J. Clin. Endocr. Metab.* **45**, 1251.
Ganguly, A., Stanchfield, J. B., Roberts, T. S., West, C. D. and Tyler, F. H. (1976). *Am. J. Med.* **60**, 306.
Gyldensted, C. and Karle, A. (1977). *Neuroradiology* **14**, 5.
Leonardi, M., Fabris, G. and Penco, T. (1978). Studio tridimensionale della sella — Tomodensitometria endosellare. 2° Convegno di Tomografia Computerizzata, Firenze, maggio.
Metzger, J., Bugault, R. and Bonneville, J. P. (1976). "Traitè de Radiodiagnostic", Vol. 14, 278. Massons, Paris.
Tyrrell, J. B., Brooks, R. M., Fitzgerald, P. A., Cofoid, P. B., Forsham, P. H. and Wilson, C. B. (1978) *N. Eng. J. Med.* **298**, 753.
Vignaud, J. (1978). La 3me dimension in tomodensitometrie. Atti 2° Convegno di Tomografia Computerizzata, Firenze, maggio.

# MINOR STRUCTURAL CHANGES IN INTRASELLAR PATHOLOGY: A RADIOLOGICAL DIAGNOSTIC PROBLEM

G. Belloni[1] and G. Maira[2]

[1] Istituto di Radiologia, Università Cattolica, Roma, Italia
[2] Istituto di Neurochirurgia, Università Cattolica, Roma, Italia

A detailed radiological analysis of the sella turcica may lead to a very early diagnosis of endosellar expansive lesions, as has been pointed out by several authors in recent years (Vezina and Maltais, 1973; Vezina and Sutton, 1974; MacErlean and Doyle, 1976). In order to quantify bony changes and to define exact diagnostic criteria, different radiological signs have been established. Nevertheless, many doubts still remain when minor radiological changes occur. In this circumstance, some authors, including Swanson and Du Boulay (1975), tend to consider these minimal alterations to be normal variants.

The aim of this work is first to verify in our own material the real diagnostic value of the minor changes in patients presenting clinical and endocrinological signs of hypophyseal dysfunction; second, to present and discuss the limitations of current radiological investigations.

## MATERIAL AND METHODS

The data we intend to present have been obtained in 19 surgically verified patients. The main clinical and endocrinological signs are reported in Table I.

These patients belong to a group of 54 patients with pituitary dysfunction due to endosellar expansive pathology—which were successfully treated in the last two years in the Neurosurgical Institute of the Catholic University of Rome. A transsphenoidal approach was used in all the cases (Hardy, 1971).

*Table I.* Minor sellar changes (19 surgically verified cases): clinical and hormonal data.

| Cases | Age sex | Clinical syndrome | Main hormonal data | | Histology |
|---|---|---|---|---|---|
| 1 M.G. | 32 ♀ | amenorrhea galactorrhea | PRL | 50 ng/ml | eosinophilic adenoma |
| 2 P.C. | 32 ♀ | amenorrhea galactorrhea | PRL | 70 ng/ml | eosinophilic adenoma |
| 3 M.M. | 26 ♀ | amenorrhea galactorrhea | PRL | 80 ng/ml | eosinophilic adenoma |
| 4 D.A. | 28 ♀ | amenorrhea galactorrhea | PRL | 100 ng/ml | eosinophilic adenoma |
| 5 D.M.F. | 30 ♀ | amenorrhea galactorrhea | PRL | 195 ng/ml | eosinophilic adenoma |
| 6 O.E. | 35 ♀ | amenorrhea galactorrhea | PRL | 200 ng/ml | eosinophilic adenoma |
| 7 G.M.R. | 32 ♀ | amenorrhea galactorrhea | PRL | 200 ng/ml | eosinophilic adenoma |
| 8 M.M. | 27 ♀ | amenorrhea galactorrhea | PRL | 660 ng/ml | eosinophilic adenoma |
| 9 V.G. | 25 ♀ | amenorrhea galactorrhea | PRL | 50 ng/ml | Rathke's pouch cyst |
| 10 F.R. | 37 ♀ | amenorrhea galactorrhea | PRL | 75 ng/ml | arachnoidal diverticulum |
| 11 G.N. | 12 ♂ | growth failure | GH | 0.4 ng/ml | cromophobe adenoma |
| 12 S.S. | 10 ♂ | growth failure | GH | 0.5 ng/ml | cromophobe adenoma |
| 13 S.G. | 7 ♂ | growth failure | GH | 1.2 ng/ml | cromophobe adenoma |
| 14 A.A. | 7 ♀ | growth failure | GH | 2.2 ng/ml | cromophobe adenoma |
| 15 V.G. | 15 ♂ | failure of sexual maturation | FSH LH | 0.7 m UI/ml 0.7 m UI/ml | cromophobe adenoma |
| 16 B.M.L. | 19 ♀ | failure of sexual maturation | FSH LH | 1.2 m UI/ml 0.8 m UI/ml | cromophobe adenoma |
| 17 C.C. | 23 ♀ | failure of sexual maturation | FSH LH | 2.5 m UI/ml 5 m UI/ml | cromophobe adenoma |
| 18 J.A. | 35 ♀ | hyperthyroid-ism | TSH | 40 $\mu$ UI/ml | trabecular adenoma |
| 19 M.R. | 42 ♀ | Cushing's disease | ACTH | 250 pg/ml | trabecular adenoma |

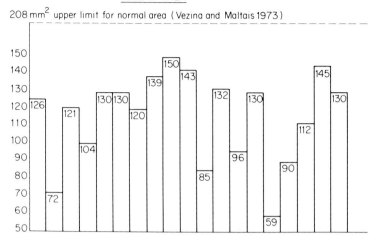

SELLAR AREA

208 mm² upper limit for normal area (Vezina and Maltais 1973)

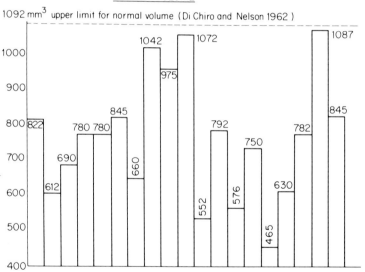

SELLAR VOLUME

1092 mm³ upper limit for normal volume (Di Chiro and Nelson 1962)

*Fig. 1.* Sellar area and volume in 19 cases of pituitary microadenoma.

Among these, 35 patients had obviously pathologic sella: in 15 the sella was increased in size, in 20 clear structural and morphological changes were present in spite of normal size.

The remaining 19 patients were selected for discussion because of the paucity of the abnormalities found by radiological examination. In particular, in all of these the surface and volume were within normal limits, according to the most

*Table II.* Radiological findings.

| Cases | Sellar surface mm² | Sellar volume mm³ | Floor asymmetry (lateral proj.) | Floor asymmetry (A.P. proj.) | Structural changes | CT Scan |
|---|---|---|---|---|---|---|
| 1 | 126 | 822 | antero-basal double contour <2 mm | obtuse angle 137° | thinning left side of floor and dorsum | |
| 2 | 72 | 612 | antero-basal double contour <2 mm | obtuse angle 155° | thinning left side of dorsum | |
| 3 | 121 | 690 | antero-basal double contour <2 mm | localized depression | thinning left side of floor and dorsum | |
| 4 | 104 | 780 | anterior double contour <2 mm | normal | thinning right side of dorsum and anterior wall | |
| 5 | 130 | 780 | antero-basal double contour 1 mm | smooth central depression | thinning left side of dorsum | |
| 6 | 130 | 845 | basal double contour <2 mm | left tilting 10° | thinning left side of dorsum and floor | pathologic |
| 7 | 120 | 660 | antero-basal double contour <2 mm | obtuse angle 154° | thinning left side of dorsum | |
| 8 | 139 | 1042 | antero-basal double contour <2 mm | left tilting 10° | thinning left side of dorsum | |

| | | | | | | |
|---|---|---|---|---|---|---|
| 9 | 150 | 975 | antero-basal double contour 1 mm | right tilting 1° | thinning right side of dorsum | |
| 10 | 143 | 1072 | normal | left tilting 5° | thinning left side of dorsum | |
| 11 | 85 | 552 | normal | normal | normal | pathologic |
| 12 | 132 | 792 | anterior double contour 2 mm | smooth central depression | pointed posterior clinoids | pathologic |
| 13 | 96 | 576 | basal double contour 1 mm | localized central depression | antero basal increased density (sinus "congha" type) | pathologic |
| 14 | 130 | 750 | normal | normal | pointed posterior clinoids | pathologic |
| 15 | 59 | 465 | normal | normal | thinning right side of dorsum | pathologic |
| 16 | 90 | 630 | posterior double contour 1 mm | left side localized depression | thinning left side of dorsum | |
| 17 | 112 | 782 | basal double contour 1 mm | localized central depression | thinning of dorsum | pathologic |
| 18 | 145 | 1087 | anterior double contour 2 mm | mild left side depression | porous dorsum | |
| 19 | 130 | 845 | antero-basal double contour 1 mm | localized central depression | diffuse osteoporosis | pathologic |

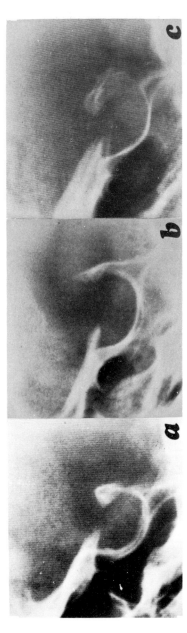

*Fig. 2.* Plain lateral films of sella turcica. a (Case n.5), antero-based double contour < 2 mm. b (Case n.17), localized double contour < 2 mm. c (Case n.10), normal sellar morphology; thinning of dorsum.

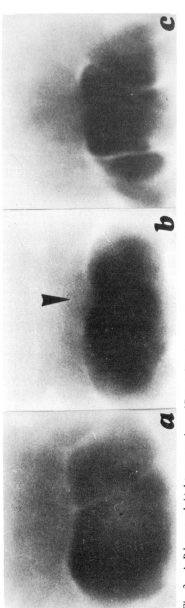

*Fig. 3.* A–P hypocycloical tomography. a (Case n.2), obtuse angle open upwards. b (Case n.3), localized depression. c (Case n.9), regular inclination of the floor towards right.

reliable criteria reported in the literature (Vezina and Maltais, 1973; Di Chiro and Nelson, 1962) (Fig. 1). Morphological and structural changes were minimal or even absent.

In 8 of these cases a CT scan study was performed (Belloni *et al.*, 1978).

## RESULTS OF THE RADIOLOGICAL STUDY OF
## THE SELLA TURCICA (TABLE II)

### Morphological alterations

These mainly consisted of a slight asymmetry of the sellar profile which in no case was greater than 2 mm on the plain film (Table III). In 8 cases the so-called double contour affected both floor and anterior wall (Fig. 2a). In 7 cases it was localized (Fig. 2b). In 4 cases no asymmetries could be seen in the lateral films (Fig. 2c).

In the A.P. view (Table III) the asymmetry can be seen as a regular inclination towards one side (tilted floor) (Fig. 3c), a localized depression (Fig. 3b) or as an obtuse angle open upwards (Fig. 3a).

Minor deformities of this type were detected in 15 patients. In the remaining 4, the sellar floor was normal.

*Table III.* Sellar morphology and structure in 19 cases of pituitary microadenomas.

|  | No. of cases |
|---|---|
| *Sellar morphology* (lateral view) | |
| Antero-basal double contour $<$ 2 mm | 8 |
| Localized double contour $<$ 2 mm | 7 |
| Normal | 4 |
| *Sellar morphology* (A.P. view) | |
| Floor tilted $<$ 10° | 4 |
| Obtuse angle $\geqslant$ 137° | 3 |
| Localized depression | 8 |
| Normal | 4 |
| *Sellar structure* | |
| Thickening of floor | 1 |
| Thinning of dorsum and floor | 5 |
| Thinning of dorsum | 12 |
| Normal | 1 |

### Structural abnormalities (Table III)

Hypocycloidal tomography enabled us to detect even minor structural changes with no doubts. Demineralization and thinning of the dorsum, are in our view, the most valuable signs of endosellar expansive pathology in the great majority of

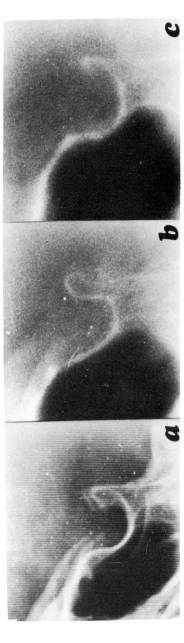

*Fig. 4.* (Case n.15). a, Pain lateral film of sella turcica. b, Left hypocycloidal tomography. c, Right hypocycloidal tomography.

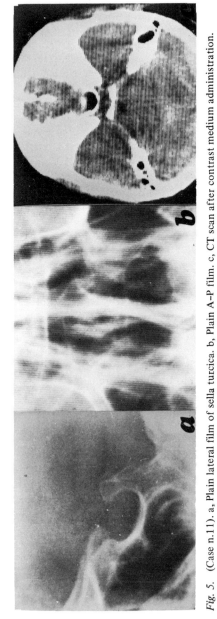

*Fig. 5.* (Case n.11). a, Plain lateral film of sella turcica. b, Plain A–P film. c, CT scan after contrast medium administration.

the cases. We have found these changes in 17 of our patients and in every case they mostly affected the side of the sella where the lesion was discovered afterwards (Fig. 4a, b, c). An associated and localized thinning of the floor was found in five patients. On the contrary, a thickened floor was present in a little girl of seven years with a congha type sphenoid. This aspect, which is probably due to the presence of the adenoma above, has already been described in the literature.

In one case (n. 11) the sellar structure was completely normal (Fig. 5a, b).

## CT SCAN

The examination was performed on eight patients. In all these cases it was possible to recognize a localized nodular area of increased density within the sella turcica after administration of the contrast medium; it corresponded in location and volume to the adenoma found at surgery.

In one case (n.11) it was the only positive examination result (Fig. 4c).

## DISCUSSION

Sellar surface and volume certainly are very variable aspects of sellar morphology; all the patients with intrasellar pathology considered by us had a sellar surface and volume contained within the so-called normal limits.

In the patients considered here the diagnostic meaningfulness of the sellar asymmetries was independent of their entity (as expressed in millimeters or degrees); therefore, even quite slight asymmetries can be of diagnostic importance. However, in three of our cases (11, 14, 15) there were none.

The structural changes observed, mainly the thinning of the dorsum sellae, seem to be the most reliable minor sellar changes in intrasellar pathology. Our findings suggest that they are the consequence of an "endosellar hypertension", as indicated by the immediate eruption of the pituitary adenomatous tissue when the sella turcica is opened. The structural changes were present in 18 of our 19 patients.

No relation was found between the nature of the endosellar space-occupying pathology (pituitary adenomas, arachnoidal diverticulum, Rathke pouch cyst) and the type and entity of sellar deformity.

The utilization of the CT scan for the diagnosis of pituitary microadenoma has permitted us to make evident the endosellar pathology in all the eight cases in which it was performed. Actually, it was this examination which enabled us to reach a correct diagnosis in our radiologically negative case 11. Furthermore, the CT scan can discriminate among endosellar space-occupying pathologies of different natures, such as pituitary adenoma and arachnoidal diverticulum, which can produce similar radiological deformities of the sella turcica.

## CONCLUSIONS

(1)  The radiological finding of even minor deformities of the sella in subjects showing clinical and endocrinological signs of hypophyseal dysfunction are highly indicative of intrasellar pathology.

(2) The association of radiological and endocrinological abnormalities does not necessarily indicate a pituitary adenoma. In fact, other pathologic processes can show similar clinical and radiological pictures.

(3) The absence of detectable structural changes of the sella in radiological examination in subjects showing clinical and endocrinological signs of hypophyseal dysfunction does not rule out intrasellar pathology.

(4) The C.T. seems to permit an early and unequivocal diagnosis of minor intrasellar pathology.

## REFERENCES

Belloni, G., Baciocco, A., Borrelli, P., Sagui, G., Di Rocco, C. and Maira, G. (1978). *Neuroradiology* **15**, 179–181.

Di Chiro, G. and Nelson, K. B. (1962). *Roentgenol.* **87**, 989–1008.

Hardy, J. (1971). *J. Neurosurg.* **34**, 581–594.

MacErlean, D. P. and Doyle, F. H. (1976). *Br. J. Radiol.* **49**, 820–826.

Swanson, H. A. and Du Boulay, G. (1975). *Br. J. Radiol.* **48**, 366–369.

Vezina, J. and Maltais, R. (1973). *Neurochirurgie supp.* **2**, 33–56.

Vezina, J. L. and Sutton, T. J. (1974). *Am. J. Roentgenol.* **1**, 46–54.

# NEUROPHARMACOLOGIC APPROACH TO THE DIAGNOSIS AND TREATMENT OF SECRETING PITUITARY ADENOMAS*

E. E. Müller[1], A. R. Genazzani[2], F. Camanni[3], D. Cocchi[4], F. Massara[3], E. Picciolini[2], V. Locatelli[4] and G. M. Molinatti[3]

[1] *Institute of Pharmacology and Pharmacognosy, University of Cagliari, Italy,*
[2] *Chair of Obstetric Pathology, University of Siena, Italy*
[3] *Chair of Endocrinology, University of Turin and* [4] *Department of Pharmacology, University of Milan, Italy*

## INTRODUCTION

The introduction of a more sophisticated technology for the assessment of even minor radiologic alterations of the pituitary fossa, e.g. hypocycloidal polytomography and computerized cranial tomography (CCT) (Fineberg *et al.,* 1977) has provided in recent years an important screening test for the diagnosis of pituitary tumors. However, proof has also been presented for the existence of small prolactin (PRL)-secreting adenomas in patients who have the clinical manifestations of the disease but radiologically normal pituitary fossae (Jacobs and Franks, 1975) and, conversely of minor radiologic "abnormalities" in up to 30% of apparently normal subjects (Swanson and De Boulay, 1975). Extrapolation of data showing the existence of a positive correlation between the area of the fossa (as judged from lateral tomographic projections) and the logarithm of the PRL concentration (Child *et al.,* 1975) showed that a serum PRL level of 50 ng/ml or lower is compatible with a small pituitary tumor which may cause no radiologic expansion of the fossa (Jacobs and Franks, 1975). In addition, the CCT approach, due to the high technology and cost involved, cannot be considered a routine test to use in patients suspected of bearing pituitary microadenomas.

*This work was supported in part by Progetto Finalizzato "Biologia della Riproduzione," C.N.R. Rome, Italy.

The first part of this paper will consider how the acquired knowledge about the neurotransmitter control of anterior pituitary (AP) hormones, coupled with the development of drugs capable of altering selective aspects of neurotransmitter function (Müller *et al.*, 1978a), can be properly exploited for the diagnosis of PRL-secreting pituitary tumors. The second part is devoted to considering the rationale for a therapeutic approach with direct dopamine (DA) agonist drugs in the treatment of patients with GH-secreting adenomas.

## PROLACTIN-SECRETING PITUITARY ADENOMAS

In the last few years, studies of the mechanisms involved in the neuroendocrine regulation of PRL secretion have led to the introduction of several functional tests into clinical practice. These tests have been used mainly with the aim of differentiating between hyperprolactinemia due to pituitary tumors and so-called "functional" hyperprolactinemia (Crosignani and Robyn, 1977).

These tests are mainly based on the use of (1) central nervous system (CNS)–acting compounds capable of affecting neurotransmitter function and/or metabolism and hence of altering the secretion of AP hormones, and (2) hypothalamic neurohormones which exert their effects directly at the AP level. On purely theoretical grounds, combined application of neuroactive drugs and hypothalamic hormones should be able to distinguish the CNS from the pituitary origin of the endocrine disorder. This is not always the case, either because of the ability of the CNS-active compounds used to act also at the level of AP receptor sites or because the hyperplastic or tumoral pituitary unmasks neurotransmitter receptors normally inactive in the physiologic states. Finally, the altered AP tissue may respond normally to hypophysiotropic stimuli. Therefore, either the diagnosis of the site and type of alteration, of great importance for the prognosis and therapy of the disease, is not made properly or by the time it is made, the alteration has already progressed considerably.

As the matter stands, it is obvious that it would be useful to have neuroactive drugs capable of influencing the central monoaminergic neurotransmission but unable to act directly on monoamine receptors present on normal or pathologic pituitary cells. Such drugs should be (1) capable of modifying the altered secretory pattern in case of the presence of a "functional" alteration in neurotrans-

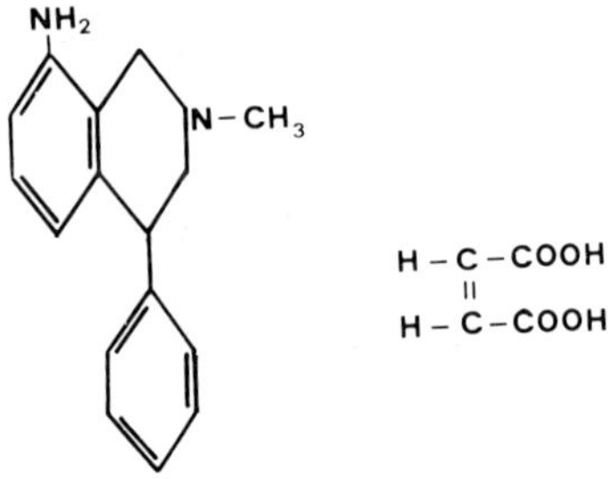

*Fig. 1.* Nomifensive, 8-amino-2-methyl-4-phenyl-1, 2, 3, 4-tetrahydroisoquinoline hydrogenmaleate.

mission or of prompting a normal secretory response when there is a sluggish reactivity of the monoaminergic systems, and (2) unable to modify an altered secretory pattern resulting from primary pituitary hypo- or hyperfunction.

Nomifensine, Psicronizer® Hoechst S.p.A., Italy, (Fig. 1), is an antidepressant drug which activates DA neurotransmission mainly by inhibiting DA re-uptake (Hunt *et al.*, 1974) but has no ability to directly affect DA receptors (Gerhards *et al.*, 1974). We propose here that this drug may be a useful neuropharmacological tool for discriminating "functional" from tumorous hyperprolactinemia.

## DIAGNOSTIC USE OF NOMIFENSINE IN HYPERPROLACTINEMIC STATES

### Animal studies

Before assessment of nomifensine (Nom) as a research tool for studies in the human, the PRL-lowering effect of the drug was tested in the rat in conditions of either basal or stimulated PRL secretion. These studies, which are beyond the scope of this presentation, will be published elsewhere (Cocchi *et al.*, in preparation). Here they are only summarized, to offer an idea of the mechanism of the PRL-inhibiting properties of the drug. Nom (5 and 10 mg/kg, i.p.) reduced baseline plasma PRL levels in untreated male and in ovariectomized-estrogen-primed female rats; Nom altered neither plasma PRL levels in reserpinized male rats and in hypophysectomized female rats bearing AP transplants under the kidney capsule nor PRL release from pituitaries incubated *in vitro*. In all, these data indicate that the drug does not act directly at the level of pituitary dopaminergic receptors but requires the presence of an intragranular pool of DA available for release (see also below). Supporting this view are behavioral studies showing that Nom-induced (Braestrup and Scheel-Krüger, 1976) but not amphetamine-induced (Braestrup, 1977) stereotyped behaviour is blocked by reserpine.

### Human studies

This PRL-lowering effect of Nom manifested in conditions of either basal or stimulated PRL secretion of the rat fostered studies aimed at ascertaining the drug effect in normal and hyperprolactinemic subjects.

Although no general agreement exists on this topic, the main causes for the presence of hyperprolactinemia in the human are those listed below.

## HYPERPROLACTINEMIC STATES

(1) Alterations of the hypothalamo-pituitary system:
    (a) hypothalamic lesions (traumatic, inflammatory and neoplastic hypothalamic disorders),
    (b) stalk section,
    (c) PRL-secreting tumors (prolactinoma, acromegaly, mixed forms),
    (d) iatrogenic,

(e) primary hypothyroidism,
(f) hyper-hypo-cortisolism,
(g) functional? (idiopathic, post-partum, post-pill etc.).
(2) PRL-secreting extrapituitary tumors.
(3) Chronic infiltrative processes of the mammary gland and the chest.
(4) Chronic renal failure, liver cirrhosis.

Several tests have been proposed for discriminating between hyperprolactinemia due to pituitary tumor and so-called "functional" hyperprolactinemia.
So far the most frequently used "stimulation" tests include administration of
hypothalamic hormones, e.g. TRH, or CNS-active drugs, e.g. DA-receptor
blockers such as chlorpromazine or sulpiride. The "inhibition" tests consist in
the administration of DA precursor or agonist drugs, e.g. L-DOPA or bromocriptine (Faglia *et al.*, 1977; Kleinberg *et al.*, 1977). None of these tests discriminates
accurately between tumorous and functional hyperprolactinemia (Frantz, 1978),
though negative responses are more frequently observed in patients with PRL-
secreting tumors. Also, concomitant evaluation of the other pituitary trophic
hormone secretions (e.g. gonadotropins) in the resting state or following administration of LRH has been discouraging with regard to this differentiation (L'Hermite
*et al.*, 1977). The differential diagnosis is further compounded by the fact that many
cases originally classified as functional because of the finding of a radiologically
normal pituitary fossa may be due to pituitary microadenoma (Jacobs and Franks,
1975).

We report here data on the PRL-lowering effect of Nom in normal and hyperprolactinemic human subjects.

## MATERIALS AND METHODS

### Subjects

On the basis of clinical, radiologic and biochemical data the 79 subjects who
were investigated were divided into four major groups.

*Group A—control subjects*
This group consisted of 23 normal female volunteers, ranging in age from 18 to
32 years. On the basis of baseline PRL levels equal to or lower than 12 ng/ml or
between 13 and 20 ng/ml, Group A subjects were subdivided into Groups $A_1$ and
$A_2$, respectively.

*Group B—puerperal subjects*
This group consisted of 11 volunteers, ranging in age from 20 to 33 years,
with physiologic puerperal hyperprolactinemia (post-partum day 2).

*Group C—pathological hyperprolactinemia*
*With proven pituitary tumors* ($C_1$). This group consisted of 19 patients with
pituitary PRL-secreting tumors. In these patients, the diagnosis of pituitary tumor
was made at surgery by the selective removal through transsphenoidal microsurgical exploration of the sella and histological examination of an adenoma.

*With suspected pituitary tumors* ($C_2$). This group was composed of 18 subjects in whom, on the basis of alterations of the sella of varying degrees and/or basal PRL levels > 100 ng/ml, the presence of a PRL-secreting adenoma was suggested.

*With no evidence of pituitary tumor* ($C_3$). This group was composed of 10 patients with a normal sella turcica and plasma PRL levels which on several occasions were found to be moderately elevated (range 22-75 ng/ml; mean ± s.e.m. 31 ± 4.9 ng/ml).

Irrespective of the underlying pathological process, all Group C patients had different types of menstrual disorders (amenorrhea, oligomenorrhea or polymenorrhea), which were very often associated with galactorrhea.

None of the subjects received medication during the studies. In the menstruating subjects, neuropharmacological testing was performed in the early follicular phase.

Standard X-ray and tomographic studies of the sella turcica (in 24 cases with the use of hypocycloidal movement) were obtained for all 47 subjects of Group C.

### Neuropharmacological testing

All tests were performed in the morning after an overnight fast. Blood samples were collected via an indwelling needle, inserted into an antecubital vein at least 30 min before drug administration and kept patent by the slow infusion of saline. Starting at 08.30-09.00, subjects received Nom (200 mg) orally, in a single administration. Group C patients (31 subjects) also underwent on separate days acute testing with bromocriptine (CB 154, Sandoz, 2.5 mg, p.o.) on a different day. Seven puerperal women and 7 $C_3$ patients were also given a placebo to evaluate spontaneous fluctuations in plasma PRL. After two baseline blood samples were taken (−30 and 0 min), further blood samples were obtained at 30-60 min intervals for 5 hours.

The criterion adopted to define "responsiveness" to Nom in pathological hyperprolactinemia was that basal PRL levels be suppressed more than 30% in at least 3 consecutive samples collected within the 120-240 min post-treatment interval. This criterion was based on results gathered in puerperal hyperprolactinemia where the minimum plasma PRL fell after the drug had this magnitude and timing.

Because of the large variations in initial basal PRL levels, plasma PRL for each subject was expressed as a percentage of the initial value (mean of −30 and 0 min). Data were analyzed using unpaired or paired *t*-tests.

## RESULTS AND DISCUSSION

### Normal and puerperal subjects

In all Group A subjects, acute administration of Nom induced a significant decrease in basal PRL levels (Biodata, Milan, Italy) (Genazzani *et al.,* 1977). Evaluation of the fall in plasma PRL in each sub-group shows that this was more marked (about 50% at 210 min) and prompt (30 min) in Group $A_2$ than in

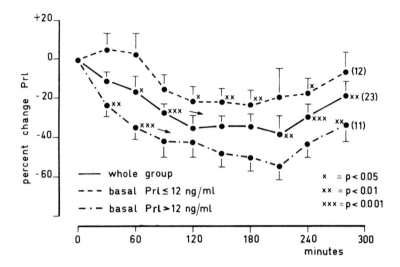

*Fig. 2.* Plasma PRL levels in normal women given nomifensine (200 mg, p.o.). Number of subjects is in parentheses. On the ordinate, values are expressed as per cent change from baseline (−30 and 0 min) ± s.e.m. The patterns of the PRL-lowering by Nom in all 23 subjects are indicated, as well as those occurring in subjects with PRL levels lower or higher than 12 ng/ml. Symbols denote significant differences *vs* baseline levels. Arrow denotes the degree of significance as indicated by the last symbol. The same description applies to Figs 3, 4, 7, 8.

Group $A_1$ subjects (about 20% at 120–240 min) (Fig. 2). In all Group A subjects, there was a direct correlation between basal PRL levels and the maximal percent fall after Nom ($r = 0.522; P < 0.02$).

In group B subjects, administration of 200 mg Nom, p.o., was also followed by a clear-cut lowering from basal PRL levels, which started at 30 min (20% inhibition) and reached nadir values at 150–180 min (about 60% inhibition). No significant changes from basal PRL were induced by administration of placebo to 7 puerperal subjects (Fig. 3).

### Pathological hyperprolactinemia

#### With proven or suspected PRL-secreting tumor ($C_1$ and $C_2$)

In none of the 19 patients in whom the existence of a PRL-secreting tumor was established at surgery, and in 17 of 18 subjects with a diagnosis of suspected PRL tumor, did Nom alter plasma PRL levels (Fig. 4). In contrast, bromocryptine resulted in a striking fall in plasma PRL levels in these subjects (not shown).

#### Without evidence of PRL secreting tumor ($C_3$)

In the 10 patients with no evidence of PRL-secreting tumor, administration of Nom was followed by a prompt and clear-cut reduction in plasma PRL levels

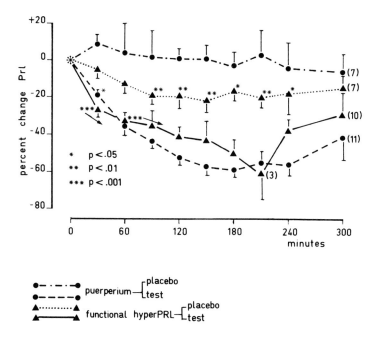

*Fig. 3.* Plasma PRL levels in puerperal subjects or in hyperprolactinemic subjects with no evidence of PRL-secreting tumor (functional) given nomifensine (200 mg, p.o.). Also shown are the patterns of plasma PRL in 7 puerperal subjects and in 7 "functional" hyperprolactinemic subjects given placebo.

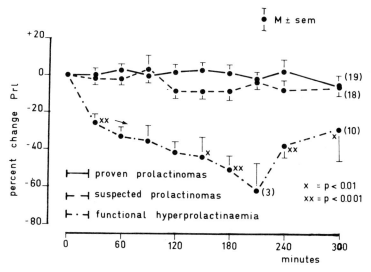

*Fig. 4.* Plasma PRL levels in subjects with proven or suspected PRL-secreting tumors given nomifensine (200 mg, p.o.). For comparison, the pattern of the PRL-lowering effect of Nom in "functional" hyperprolactinemia is also shown.

(about 50% at 180 min) (Figs 3 and 4), similar to that observed in post-partum women (Fig. 3). In 7 of the same subjects, administration of placebo was also followed by a significant decrease in basal PRL (about 20% inhibition from 90 to 240 min), which was, however, significantly less than that induced by Nom ($P < 0.01$ at all time intervals) (Fig. 3).

No untoward side effects were noticed in any subject after drug administration.

Nomifensine was effective in lowering plasma PRL levels in normal subjects, in subjects with the functional hyperprolactinemia of the puerperium and in those with non-puerperal hyperprolactinemia without evidence of PRL-secreting tumor.

In normal subjects, the effect was directly related to the resting PRL levels because the more marked and prompt falls in plasma PRL after the drug occurred in those individuals with higher basal PRL. Since nomifensine facilitates dopaminergic neurotransmission at post-synaptic sites (Hunt *et al.*, 1974), the greater susceptibility of subjects with higher basal PRL may indicate the existence of a greater post-synaptic dopaminergic sensitivity, resulting from diminished pre-synaptic function (Gianutsos *et al.*, 1974).

Nomifensine also had a marked inhibitory effect on plasma PRL in subjects with the functional hyperprolactinemia of the puerperium, a fact which, like the pattern in normal subjects with "high" basal PRL, would indicate that in puerperium, even though the CNS dopaminergic tone is probably diminished (Ben-Jonathan *et al.*, 1978) because of the damping effect of high estrogen levels (Euvrard *et al.*, 1978), DA neurotransmission is nevertheless preserved. Interestingly enough, nomifensine also elicited marked PRL-lowering effects in estrogen-primed rats (see page 349), an animal model in which hyperprolactinemia apparently results from the same events as those occurring in puerperium.

In contrast to what it does in normal and puerperal women and in hyperprolactinemic subjects without evidence of PRL-secreting tumor, and in agreement with earlier data in a small population of tumorous subjects (Müller *et al.*, 1978b), nomifensine did not alter plasma PRL in 19 subjects with proven pituitary adenomas and in 17 of 18 subjects in whom the presence of a pituitary adenoma was suggested (Group $C_2$). The ineffectiveness of the drug was related neither to the magnitude of the basal PRL levels, which ranged between 28.0 and 800 ng/ml, nor to an insufficient drug dose, considering both the sensitivity of DA receptor sites located in the tumorous gland (Mashiter *et al.*, 1977) and the finding that in 2 subjects even a dose of 300 mg p.o., was completely ineffective to lower plasma PRL (data not shown). On the other hand, in the tumorous subjects, bromocriptine, which directly activates pituitary DA receptors (MacLeod and Lehmeyer, 1974) induced a striking suppression of plasma PRL titers.

Thus it seems likely that rather than being related to one of the reasons cited above, non-supressibility of plasma PRL by nomifensine in patients with PRL-secreting adenomas may result both from the ability of the drug to affect CNS-DA receptors exclusively and the existence of a central defect in catecholaminergic neurotransmission (Fig. 5). Supporting this view are recent reports in the literature (Van Loon, 1978; Fine and Frohman, 1978).

In sum, it would appear that nomifensine may be a simple, safe, inexpensive and rapid test for discriminating between individuals with and without pituitary adenoma. Its use might be particularly useful for the early detection of pituitary tumors when basal PRL levels are still moderately elevated and there are not even

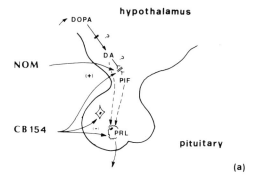

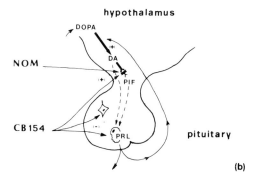

*Fig. 5.* Hypothetical scheme to explain the absence of a suppressive effect of Nom in patients with PRL-secreting tumors. In the upper part (a) is depicted the possibility that in patients with pituitary tumor there is a primary impairment in the central dopaminergic control either because DOPA cannot be converted to DA and/ or because of alteration of DA receptors located on the PIF neuron (//). In the lower part (b), it is proposed that hypersecretion of PRL by the tumorous pituitary via a short-loop feedback to the CNS alters secondarily the central dopaminergic control, most likely by increasing DA turnover, with ensuing desensitization of DA receptors (//). Given the main mechanism of action of Nom, i.e. blockade of DA reuptake, its inability to activate DA neurotransmission in both (a) and (b) is evident. In contrast, bromocriptine is able to inhibit PRL secretion in both (a) and (b) via direct stimulation of DA receptors located on the tumorous gland. DA, Dopaminergic neurons; PIF, prolactin-inhibiting factor neuron; PRL, tumorous PRL-secreting cell; (+) refers to activation of DA neurotransmission by Nom or bromocriptine or by the positive feedback effect of PRL; (−) refers to the inhibitory effect of bromocriptine on PRL secretion on both nontumorous and tumorous tissue (a) (b).

minor alterations of the sella turcica (Jacobs and Franks, 1975). In this vein the findings obtained in one subject of this study are highly promising. At a first examination, performed a few years after the beginning of polymenorrhea, she had a negative nomifensine test, in the presence of a sella turcica within normal limits and PRL values slightly exceeding 40 ng/ml. One year later, when the sella had developed a double profile and PRL values had risen to over 100 ng/ml, the diagnostic value of nomifensine testing was confirmed at surgery.

### DA-receptor blockers in hyperprolactinemic states

In the preceding section, mention was made of the inability of anti-dopaminergic drugs to distinguish between tumoral and functional hyperprolactinemia. In the study of Faglia *et al.* (1977), intramuscular injection of 100 mg of sulpiride did not cause an increase in serum PRL greater than 75% over basal values in 12 patients with PRL-secreting tumors, elicited a positive response in only 2 "functional" cases out of 5, and in one acromegalic out of 5. Chlorpromazine (0.75 mg/kg) was ineffective in increasing serum PRL in patients with PRL-secreting tumors and elicited positive responses in only 2 of 8 "functional" cases and in 1 of 4 acromegalics. Although other interpretations can be offered, these drugs lack discriminating ability probably because they demand integrity of both the CNS and the pituitary for their PRL-releasing effect. The availability of DA-receptor blockers which do not cross the blood brain barrier (BBB), and therefore exert their action only on "peripheral" DA receptors, should provide a neuropharmacological means capable of better differentiating between organic and "functional" cases of enhanced PRL secretion.

We report data on the PRL-releasing effect of a recently developed anti-dopaminergic compound which does not readily cross the BBB, i.e. domperidone. Both the results of some animal experiments and of preliminary observations made in hyperprolactinemic states of the human are given.

### Effect of domperidone on plasma prolactin in animals and man

Domperidone (Janssen Pharmaceutica, Beerse, Belgium) (Fig. 6) is a specific, powerful, fast-acting and safe anti-dopaminergic receptor blocker, which due to its poor penetrability through the BBB (see below) is virtually devoid of central sedative or autonomic effects at dose levels below 10 mg/kg b. wt, independent of

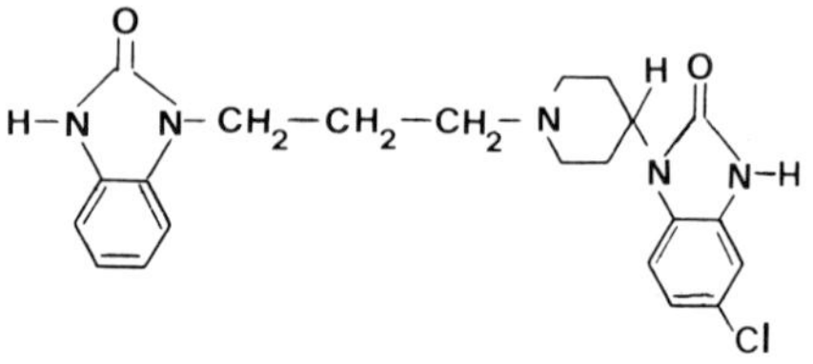

*Fig. 6.* Domperidone (5-chloro-1 1-/3-1, 5-dihydro-2-oxo-2H-benzimidazol-1) propyl-4-piperidinyl 1, 3-dihydro-2H-benzimidazol-2-one.

the route of administration. Its potent anti-emetic effect in dogs contrasts with its very weak antagonism of apomorphine-induced stereotypy in rats, an action which involves CNS dopamine receptors. Domperidone (Dom) possesses a relatively high affinity for DA-receptors when tested by the $[^3H]$-haloperidol binding assay *in vitro,* but binding experiments suggest that *in vivo* it cannot reach striatal DA receptors. Similarly, domperidone at very high doses *in vivo* does not notably change the homovanillic acid (HVA) content of rat and rabbit brains, an index of DA turnover, whereas haloperidol and metoclopramide induce striking increases (Martres *et al.,* 1978).

All these findings support the view that Dom does not readily cross the BBB; in connection with our problem it should be able to affect DA receptors located in

*Table I.*    Effect of domperidone (Dom) and haloperidol (Hal) on $[^3H]$-spiroperidol binding in rat striatal and pituitary tissue.[a]

| | Striatum | | Pituitary | |
|---|---|---|---|---|
| Drug | Dom | Hal | Dom | Hal |
| None | 100 ± 6 | 100 ± 6 | 100 ± 7 | 100 ± 7 |
| $5 \times 10^{-9}$ | – | – | 76 ± 3 | – |
| $1 \times 10^{-8}$ | 66 ± 5[b] | 69 ± 6 | 68 ± 6 | – |
| $5 \times 10^{-8}$ | 37 ± 3 | 40 ± 5 | 41 ± 5 | 48 ± 4 |
| $1 \times 10^{-7}$ | 24 ± 4 | 28 ± 3 | 27 ± 5 | 38 ± 6 |
| $5 \times 10^{-7}$ | 17 ± 7 | 13 ± 6 | 16 ± 4 | – |

[a] From Gil-Ad *et al.,* unpublished results.

[b] Values represent % ± s.e. of binding values determined in the absence of any drug.

*Table II.*    Effect of different doses of domperidone on plasma prolactin levels in the male rat: comparison with haloperidol [a]

| Treatment | Plasma PRL (ng/ml) | | |
|---|---|---|---|
| | $t = 30$ min | $t = 60$ min | $t = 120$ min |
| Diluent | 23.3 ± 4.2[b] | 19.5 ± 6.3 | 22.4 ± 7.9 |
| Domperidone 0.01 mg/kg s.c. | 24.2 ± 5.5 | 43.8 ± 9.3[c] | 21.5 ± 6.5 |
| Domperidone 0.05 mg/kg s.c. | 43.7 ± 7.8[d] | 55.6 ± 7.2[f] | 34.6 ± 2.8 |
| Domperidone 0.1 mg/kg s.c. | 78.2 ± 7.6[f] | 65.4 ± 6.2[f] | 53.7 ± 5.8[f] |
| Haloperidol 0.1 mg/kg s.c. | 50.0 ± 5.0[e] | 43.1 ± 7.7[f] | 30.2 ± 5.5 |
| Haloperidol 0.5 mg/kg s.c. | 62.2 ± 9.4[f] | 49.9 ± 7.7[f] | 37.5 ± 5.8[d] |
| Haloperidol 1.0 mg/kg s.c. | 102.8 ± 9.9[f] | 74.3 ± 3.2[f] | 60.0 ± 6.1[f] |

[a] From Gil-Ad *et al.,* unpublished results.
[b] Each point represents the mean ± s.e.m. of 6 determinations. Blood samples were obtained from unanesthetized rats by puncture of the orbital vein.
[c] $P \leqslant 0.01$ *vs* diluent.
[d] $P \leqslant 0.02$ *vs* diluent.
[e] $P \leqslant 0.005$ *vs* diluent.
[f] $P \leqslant 0.001$ *vs* diluent.

areas of the CNS outside the BBB, i.e. the pituitary and the median eminence (ME). Table I shows that *in vitro* Dom was at least as effective as Hal in displacing [$^3$H]-spiroperidol from DA-binding sites in the rat AP and striatum. In the pituitary, Dom ($5 \times 10^{-8}$ M) induced a displacement of 59% *vs* a 51% displacement induced by Hal. Table II shows that s.c. administration of Dom induced a rise in plasma PRL which was visible at a dose of 10 μg/kg. Comparison with Hal showed that Dom was 5 times as potent as Hal as a PRL releaser (Dom $ED_{250} = 0.084$ mg/kg; Hal $ED_{250} = 0.42$ mg/kg). Both apomorphine (5 mg/kg s.c.) and CB 154 (5 mg/kg, s.c.), given 15 min after administration of Dom (0.1 mg/kg s.c.), were capable of counteracting the PRL-releasing effect of the latter, thus showing that Dom was releasing PRL through blockage of DA-receptors (not shown).

The observed efficacy of Dom as a PRL-releasing agent coupled with the inability of the compound to influence DA-receptor sites located in the CNS and, eventually, playing a role in the control of PRL secretion, led to its use in human hyperprolactinemia.

Domperidone (4 mg i.v.) administered to 5 normoprolactinemic subjects elicited a 10–15 fold rise from baseline PRL 15–30 min later (not shown). Dom, administered at the same dose to 7 puerperal women (post-partum day 2) elicited peak PRL rises ranging from 50 to 300% of baseline in 5 of these subjects, whereas in 2 subjects it induced only an inconsistent rise in plasma PRL. In contrast with this pattern, in none of 6 subjects with biochemical and/or radiologic evidence of pituitary tumor was Dom capable of eliciting further rises over baseline PRL (Fig. 7).

These studies are only preliminary and no definitive conclusions can be drawn at present, so that their extension to a larger population of subjects is warranted.

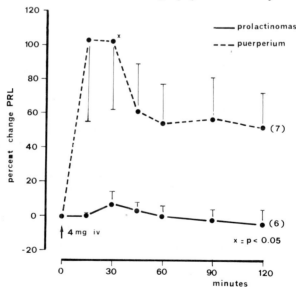

*Fig. 7.* PRL-releasing effect of domperidone in puerperal women and in hyperprolactinemic subjects with evidence of PRL-secreting tumors.

However, from the overall findings, it would appear that PRL responsiveness to the drug was present in both normoprolactinemic and puerperal subjects. In view of the ability of the compound to act mainly at the level of pituitary DA receptors, its use may be foreseen for the assessment of the pituitary PRL reserve.

Domperidone proved to be ineffective in individuals bearing prolactinomas, a fact that is difficult to understand should this prove to be the situation in a larger group of subjects. The possibility that tumorous patients did not respond to the drug since they were already secreting PRL maximally is not tenable: no PRL rise was present in three subjects with basal PRL levels as low as 35–56 ng/ml and, conversely, a rise in plasma PRL was induced in most of the puerperal women despite the presence of higher or equally elevated baseline PRL levels.

Antagonists of DA receptors such as Dom act by depressing a receptor which is modulated by dopamine. Thus an inherent dopaminergic tone at the receptor level is needed for their action to occur. In view of the postulated and indirectly proved defect in central dopaminergic neurotransmission in tumorous subjects (see above), it may be hypothesized that unresponsiveness to Dom in patients with a PRL-secreting tumor reflects the lack of a sufficient modulation of the tumorous lactotrophs by DA transported via the portal blood. Interestingly, in hyperoprolactinemic subjects unresponsive to sulpiride, infusion of DA was effective in restoring an evident response to the drug (Crosignani *et al.*, 1977). In keeping with this view is also the finding that sulpiride, which *per se* does not affect DA-sensitive adenylate cyclase of tumorous lactotrops, is able to counteract the inhibition of the cyclase induced by DA (De Camilli *et al.*, this Volume).

## DIRECT DA AGONIST DRUGS: RATIONALE TO THEIR USE IN ACROMEGALY

Even though the physiopathology of acromegaly is still incompletely understood, irrefutable evidence has been produced that in this disease dopaminergic compounds, in contrast to the stimulatory effect they exert in normal subjects (Müller *et al.*, 1977), induce a consistent suppression of the elevated hGH levels. It was first observed in 1972 that acute administration of L-DOPA markedly lowered hGH levels in plasma of some acromegalics (Liuzzi *et al.*, 1972), a finding which has been subsequently extended to include other DA-stimulant drugs, i.e. apomorphine (Chiodini *et al.*, 1974), bromocriptine (Liuzzi *et al.*, 1974a; Camanni *et al.*, 1975a), piribedil (Camanni *et al.*, 1975b), lisuride (Liuzzi *et al.*, 1978) and lergotrile (Thorner *et al.*, 1978). Of the compounds tested so far, acute administration of bromocriptine (2.5 mg po) appears to cause the more striking and long-lasting decreases in about 60% of the patients, so that chronic administration of this compound has been proposed as a new valid and safe pharmacological approach to the treatment of acromegaly when other means have been tried and have failed (Sachdev *et al.*, 1975; Liuzzi *et al.*, 1976; Belforte *et al.*, 1977). In this context, promising results have also been obtained with short-term treatment with lisuride, although more side effects appear to be characteristic of its action than with bromocriptine (Liuzzi *et al.*, 1978), and with lergotrile (Kleinberg *et al.*, 1978).

The possible site(s) of action of dopaminergic compounds, e.g. the pituitary or suprapituitary locations of the receptor sites invoived, has been widely discussed (Müller *et al.*, 1977; Camanni *et al.*, 1977). It is generally accepted that dopaminergic compounds affect the GH control at loci within the CNS (Müller *et al.*, 1977) and a function imbalance between excitatory (GRF) and inhibitory (GIF) inputs which regulate pituitary GH release has been invoked as a possible cause of the paradoxical fall observed in some patients (Liuzzi *et al.*, 1976). However, the evidence so far presented makes a direct action of these compounds on DA receptors located on somatotrophs more likely the pituitary as site of action is favored by (1) the almost complete dissociation observed in the same patient between the GH response elicited by ergot drugs, i.e. bromocriptine, and the responses evoked by CNS-acting stimuli, such as insulin hypoglycemia, arginine infusion, etc. (Liuzzi *et al.*, 1974b); (2) the observation that DA, which does not cross the BBB (Broadwell and Brightman, 1976) and does not stimulate GH secretion in normal subjects, lowers GH levels when infused into "responsive" acromegalics (Verde *et al.*, 1976; Camanni *et al.*, 1977); (3) the findings that bromocriptine inhibits GH release from human pituitary tumor in culture (Mashiter *et al.*, 1977) and that $\alpha$ and $\beta$ adrenergic blockers, for which no evidence has been obtained indicating a pituitary site of action (Müller *et al.*, 1978a), failed to modify in acromegalics the qualitatively abnormal suppression by L-DOPA of GH secretion (Cryer and Daughaday, 1977); (4) the fact that the competence of a given dopaminergic compound to suppress the release of GH from the tumorous or hyperplastic pituitary appears to be related to its ability to stimulate DA receptors directly. Indirect DA-agonist drugs, e.g. amphetamine, amantadine and nomifensine, whose actions rely on presynaptically released DA, while active in releasing GH in the normal subjects are ineffective in lowering GH levels in acromegaly (Müller *et al.*, 1977) (Table III).

*Table III.* Dopaminergic stimulation and GH levels in acromegaly.

| Drug | Mechanism of action[a] | Effect on GH release | Authors |
|---|---|---|---|
| DA | Direct receptor stimulant | ↓ | Verde *et al.*, 1976 |
| Apomorphine | Direct receptor stimulant | ↓ | Chiodini *et al.*, 1974 |
| C B 154 | Direct receptor stimulant[b] | ↓ | Liuzzi *et al.*, 1974 |
| Piribedil | Direct receptor stimulant | ↓ | Camanni *et al.*, 1975 |
| Lisuride | Direct receptor stimulant | ↓ | Liuzzi *et al.*, 1978 |
| Lergotrile | Direct receptor stimulant | ↓ | Thorner *et al.*, 1978 |
| L-DOPA | Conversion to DA by L-AAAD[c] | ↓ | Chiodini *et al.*, 1974 |
| Amantadine | Inhibition of DA reuptake | → | Camanni *et al.*, 1975 |
| D-145 | Release of DA stores | → | Camanni *et al.*, 1975 |
| Amphetamine | Release of DA stores | → | Müller *et al.*, 1977 |
| Nomifensine | Inhibition of DA reuptake | → | Scanlon *et al.*, 1977 |

[a]Refers to main action.
[b]Possible presynaptic mechanism.
[c]L-Amino acid aromatic decarboxylase.
→ Means no effect.
↓ Means inhibition.

The ability of L-DOPA to inhibit GH secretion in responder acromegalics also appears to be due to peripheral conversion of this precursor to DA and not to activation of central DA neurotransmission, as discussed below.

Five women and three men with clinically active acromegaly underwent acute L-DOPA testing before and after pretreatment with carbidopa, a drug which inhibits the peripheral conversion of L-DOPA to DA (Porter, 1971). Treatment with carbidopa (100 mg orally, 3 times daily for 3 days) neither significantly modified baseline DA levels nor induced significant changes in baseline GH (and PRL) titers. Infusion with L-DOPA induced a striking rise in plasma DA levels, which was maximum at 30 min; this was paralleled by a clearcut but short-lived reduction in GH levels (Fig. 8, upper panel). Following L-DOPA, there was also a marked and long-lasting suppression of plasma PRL (Fig. 8, lower panel). A different pattern was present when the test was repeated after carbidopa administration. In this instance the rise in plasma DA levels induced by the DA precursor was strikingly less and there was no significant decrease in GH and PRL from the baseline levels (Fig. 8).

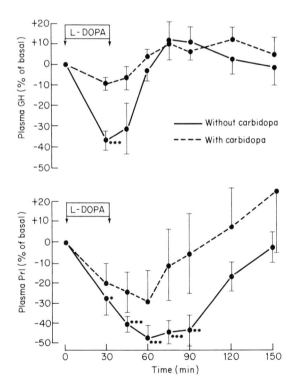

*Fig. 8.* GH (upper part) and PRL (lower part) suppressive effects of L-DOPA (1.25 mg/kg bw, in 30 min) in 6 acromegalic subjects before and after treatment with carbidopa (100 mg, p.o. 3 times daily for 3 days) (Reproduced with permission from Camanni *et al.*, 1978).

In all, these data do indicate that in acromegaly the inhibitory effect of L–DOPA on GH (and PRL) secretion depends upon its decarboxylation to DA at a site or sites outside of the BBB, i.e. the pituitary and/or the ME. Were DA receptor sites in the CNS, above the ME, involved in the inhibitory effect of L-DOPA on GH and PRL secretion, exacerbation of L-DOPA's suppressive effects would have occurred. It is known in fact that after peripheral dopa-decarboxylase inhibition, L-DOPA loading results in a greatly enhanced activation of DA neurotransmission (Bartholini and Platscher, 1968). In contrast to the above findings, there are few acromegalics in whom L-DOPA elicits significant increases in hGH levels (Camanni et al., 1975b). Since this response is the one that also occurs in normal subjects, persistence of a CNS-dependent control of GH secretion has been postulated for these cases (Camanni et al., 1975b).

The precise reason why responder acromegalics develop or unmask "receptors" sensitive to dopaminergic stimulation on the hyperplastic or tumorous somato-trophs is still unknown. The view that this may be due to interruption of the functional links between the CNS and the pituitary, although supported by the similar responsiveness to TRH of both responder acromegalics (Irie and Tsushima, 1972) and animal models of CNS-AP disconnection (Udeschini et al., 1976; Gil-Ad et al., 1976), is not consistent with the ineffectiveness of dopaminergic compounds to lower GH secretion in vivo from pituitaries devoid of CNS influence (Liuzzi et al., 1976; Müller and Locatelli, unpublished results). Also, in pathologic conditions in the human, such as liver cirrhosis, in which TRH elicits a GH rise (Panerai et al., 1977), infusion of DA is unable to affect baseline GH levels or to blunt the TRH-induced GH rise (Müller, Locatelli, Salerno, unpublished results), events which instead occur in acromegaly (Camanni et al., 1977). Thus, it would appear that the "anomalous" GH response to dopaminergic stimulation does not merely reflect the existence of a "denervation" supersensitivity to DA, such as the one described for lactotrophs devoid of CNS influences (Cheung and Weiner, 1976), since the amine is apparently inactive on "intact" somatotrophs. However, it has been reported recently that both DA and apomorphine inhibited GH release from normal pituitary tissues obtained from a patient undergoing hypophysectomy for a breast tumor or from normal fetuses (Goodyer et al., 1978). To elucidate these aspects more studies are needed.

## CONCLUSIONS

New knowledge about neurotransmitter control of anterior pituitary hormones permits fruitful exploitation of drugs capable of altering selected aspects of neuro-transmitter function for the diagnosis and treatment of neuroendocrine disorders.

Application of nomifensine, an indirect DA agonist drug which activates DA neurotransmission in the CNS but has no ability to affect the pituitary DA receptor sites directly, proved capable of discriminating between individuals with and without pituitary adenomas. The use of nomifensine provides a new, safe, inexpensive, valuable adjunct to the more traditional diagnostic armanentarium for hyperprolactinemia. Preliminary results with domperidone, a DA receptor blocker, whose action preferentially involves DA receptor sites located on struct-ures outside the blood brain barrier, showed the drug to be capable of enhancing plasma PRL levels in normal or puerperal subjects but unable to rise the elevated baseline PRL levels of subjects with PRL-secreting adenomas further. Direct DA agonist drugs, by acting on dopaminergic "receptors" located on pituitary somatorophs, offer the rationale for a medical approach to the cure of acromegaly.

## ACKNOWLEDGMENTS

We gratefully acknowledge Drs Laura Belforte and Clara Frigerio for participation in these studies; Miss Rosaria Scirea for preparation of the manuscript; Dr M. Sesso, Hoechst Italia SPA, and Dr De Martin, Janssen Farmaceutici S. P. A., Italia for supplying nomifensine and domperidone, respectively; Dr Piero Angeletti Merck Sharp and Dhome (Italia) and Dr Paolo Priore, Hoffman La Roche (Italia) for the generous supply of carbidopa and Larodopa, respectively.

## REFERENCES

Bartholini, G. and Platscher, A. (1968). *J. Pharmacol. exp. Ther.* **161**, 14.

Belforte, C., Camanni, F., Chiodini, P. G., Liuzzi, A., Massara, F., Molinatti, G. M., Müller, E. E. and Silvestrini, F. (1977). *Acta Endocrinol.* **85**, 235.

Ben-Jonathan, N., Neill, M. A., Arbogast, L. A., Peters, L. L. and Hoefer, M. T. (1978). *60th Ann. Meet. Endocr. Soc., Miami, Fla. Abs.* **238**.

Braestrup, C. (1977). *J. Pharm. Pharmacol.* **29**, 463.

Braestrup, C. and Scheel-Krüger, J. (1976). *Europ. J. Pharmacol.* **38**, 305.

Broadwell, R. D. and Brightman, M. W. (1976). *J. Comp. Neurol.* **166**, 257.

Camanni, F., Massara, F., Belforte, L. and Molinatti, G. M. (1975a). *J. Clin. Endocr. Metab.* **40**, 363.

Camanni, F., Massara, F., Fassio, V., Molinatti, G. M. and Müller, E. E. (1975b). *Neuroendocrinology* **19**, 227.

Camanni, F., Massara, F., Belforte, L., Rosatello, A. and Molinatti, G. M. (1977). *J. Clin. Endocr. Metab.* **44**, 465.

Camanni, F., Picotti, G. B., Massara, F., Molinatti, G. M., Mantegazza, P. and Müller, E. E. (1978). *J. Clin. Endocr. Metab.* **47**, 647.

Cheung, C. Y. and Weiner, R. I. (1976). *Endocrinology* **99**, 914.

Child, D. F., Gordon, H., Mashiter, K. and Joplin, G. F. (1975). *Brit. Med. J.* **4**, 87.

Chiodini, P. G., Liuzzi, A., Botalla, L., Cremascoli, G., and Silvestrini, F. (1974). *J. Clin. Endocr. Metab.* **38**, 200.

Crosignani, P. G. and Robyn, C. (eds) (1977). "Prolactin and Human Reproduction". Academic Press, New York.

Crosignani, P. G., Reschini, E., Peracchi, M., Lombroso, G. C., Mattei, A. and Caccamo, A. (1977). *J. Clin. Endocr. Metab.* **43**, 841.

Cryer, P. E. and Daughaday, W. H. (1977). *J. Clin. Endocr. Metab.* **44**, 977.

De Camilli, P., Spada, A., Beck-Peccoz, P., Moriondo, P., Giovanelli, M. and Faglia, G. (1980). This Volume.

Euvrard, C., Boissier, J. R., Labrie, F. and Raynaud, J.-P. (1978). *7th Int. Congr. Pharmacol. Paris. Abs.* 1133.

Faglia, G., Beck-Peccoz, P., Travaglini, P., Ambrosi, B., Rondena, M., Paracchi, A., Spada, A., Weber, G., Bara, R. and Rouzin, A. (1977). *In* "Prolactin and Human Reproduction" (P. G. Crosignani and C. Robyn, eds) pp. 225-238. Academic Press, New York and London.

Fine, S. A. and Frohman, A. (1978). *J. Clin. Invest.* **61**, 973.

Fineberg, H. V., Bauman, R. and Sosman, P. (1977). *J. Am. Med. Ass.* **238**, 224.

Frantz, A. G. (1978). *N. Engl. J. Med.* **298**, 201.

Genazzani, A. R., Magrini, G., Facchinetti, P., Romagnino, S., Pintor, C., Felber, G. P. and Fioretti, P. (1977). *In* "Androgens and Antiandrogens" (L. Martini and M. Motta, eds) pp. 247-261. Raven Press, New York.

Gehards, H. G., Carenzi, A. and Costa, E. (1974). *Naunyn Schmiedebergs Arch. Pharmacol.* **284**, 49.

Gianutsos, G., Drawbaugh, R. B., Hynes, M. D. and Lal, H. (1974). *Life Sci.* **14**, 887.

Gil-Ad, I., Cocchi, D., Panerai, A. E., Locatelli, V., Mantegazza, P. and Müller, E. E. (1976). *Neuroendocrinology* **21**, 336.

Goodyer, C. G., Marcovitz, S., Guyda, H., Giroud, C. J. P., Hardy, J., Gardiner, R. J. and Martin, J. B. (1978). *Ann. Meet. Endocr. Soc. Miami, Fla, Abs.* **143**.

Hunt, P., Kannengiesser, M. -H. and Raynaud, J. -P. (1974). *J. Pharm. Pharmacol.* **26**, 370.

Irie, M. and Tsushima, T. J. (1972). *J. Clin. Endocr. Metab.* **35**, 97.

Jacobs, H. S. and Franks, S. (1975). *Brit. Med. J.* **2**, 141.

Kleinberg, D. L., Noel, G. L. and Frantz, A. (1977). *New Engl. J. Med.* **296**, 589.

Kleinberg, D. L., Schaaf, M. and Frantz, A. G. (1978). *Fed. Proc.* **37**, 2198.

L'Hermite, M., Caufriez, A. and Robyn, C. (1977). *In* "Prolactin and Human Reproduction" (P. G. Crosignani and C. Robyn, eds) pp. 179-202. Academic Press, New York and London.

Liuzzi, A., Chiodini, P. G., Botalla, L., Cremascoli, G. and Silvestrini, F. (1972). *J. Clin. Endocr. Metab.* **35**, 941.

Liuzzi, A., Chiodini, P. G., Botalla, L., Cremascoli, G. Müller, E. E. and Silvestrini, F. (1974a). *J. Clin. Endocr. Metab.* **38**, 910.

Liuzzi, A., Chiodini, P. G., Botalla, L., Silvestrini, F. and Müller, E. E. (1974b). *J. Clin. Endocr. Metab.* **39**, 871.

Liuzzi, A., Panerai, A. E., Chiodini, P. G., Secchi, C., Cocchi, D., Botalla, L., Silvestrini, F. and Müller, E. E. (1976). *In* "Growth Hormone and Related Peptides" (A. Pecile and E. E. Müller, eds) pp. 236-251. Excerpta Medica Found., Amsterdam.

Liuzzi, A., Chiodini, P. G., Opizzi, G., Botalla, L., Verde, G., De Stefano, L., Colussi, G., Gräf, K. J. and Horowski, R. (1978). *J. Clin. Endocr. Metab.* **47**, 196.

MacLeod, R. M. and Lehmeyer, J. E. (1974). *Endocrinology* **94**, 1077.

Martres, M. P., Baudry, M. and Schwarz, J. C. (1978). Abstract Book, Symposium on "Receptors of Dopamine Antagonists: New Biochemical approaches" Janssen Pharmaceutica, Beerse, Belgium, p. 51.

Mashiter, K., Adams, E., Beard, M. and Holley, A. (1977). *Lancet* **2**, 197.

Müller, E. E., Liuzzi, A., Cocchi, D., Panerai, A. E., Opizzi, G., Locatelli, V., Silvestrini, F., Mantegazza, P. and Chiodini, P. G. (1977). *In* "Advances in Biochemical Psychopharmacology" (E. Costa and G. L. Gessa, eds) Vol. 16, pp. 127-138. Raven Press, New York.

Müller, E. E., Nisticò, G. and Scapagnini, U. (1978a). "Neurotransmitters and Anterior Pituitary Function." Academic Press, New York and London.

Müller, E. E., Genazzani, A. R. and Murru, S. (1978b). *J. Clin. Endocr. Metab.* **47**, 1352.

Panerai, A. E., Salerno, F., Manneschi, M., Cocchi, D. and Müller, E. E. (1977). *J. Clin. Endocr. Metab.* **45**, 134.

Porter, C. C. (1971). *Fed. Proc.* **30**, 871.

Sachdev, Y., Turnbridge, W. M. G., Weightman, D. R., Gomez-Pan, A., Duns, A. and Hall, R. (1975). *Lancet* **2**, 1164.

Scanlon, M. F., Gomez-Pan, A., Mora, B., Cook, D. B., Deward, J. H., Hildyard, A., Weightman, D. R., Evered, D. C. and Hall, R. (1977). *Brit. J. Clin. Pharmacol.* **4**, 191.

Swanson, H. A. and Du Boulay, G. (1975). *Brit. J. Radiology.* **48**, 366.

Thorner, M. O., Ryan, S. M., Wass, J. A. H., Jones, A., Bouloux, P., Williams, S. and Besser, G. M. (1978). *J. Clin. Endocr. Metab.* **47**, 372.

Udeschini, G., Cocchi, D., Panerai, A. E., Gil-Ad, I., Rossi, G. L., Chiodini, P. G., Liuzzi, A. and Müller, E. E. (1976). *Endocrinology.* **98**, 807.

Van Loon, G. R. (1978). *60th Ann. Meet. Endocr. Soc. Miami, Fla, Abs.* 190.

Verde, G., Oppizzi, G., Colussi, G., Cremascoli, G., Botalla, L., Müller, E. E., Silvestrini, F., Chiodini, P. G. and Liuzzi, A. (1976). *Clin. Endocr.* **5**, 419.

# EFFECTS OF NEUROACTIVE DRUGS ON GROWTH HORMONE AND PROLACTIN SECRETION IN ACROMEGALY

A. Liuzzi, P. G. Chiodini, F. Silvestrini, R. Cozzi, G. Oppizzi, L. Botalla and
G. Verde

*Center of Endocrinology-Ente Ospedaliero di Niguarda, Milano, Italy*

The pioneer studies of Cryer and Daughaday (1969) and of Lawrence and Kirsteins (1970) showed that the secretion of growth hormone (GH) in acromegaly can be modified by drugs acting at the central nervous system (CNS) level. Since then the effects of neuroactive drugs on GH, and later on prolactin (PRL) secretion, in this disease have been widely investigated. This paper will summarize the present knowledge about this problem, with more extensive consideration of some topics at present under investigation by our group. The effects of drugs affecting neurotransmitters and of neurohormones on GH and PRL secretion in acromegaly will be considered first. On the basis of these data will be discussed some pathophysiological implications and examined the new approaches to the medical treatment of acromegaly which derive from these studies.

## EFFECTS OF DRUGS ACTING ON NEUROTRANSMITTERS

As in the normal subject, the secretion of GH and PRL in acromegalics is under the influence of brain neurotransmitters. Peculiarities exist, however, which distinguish the neural control of the two hormones in acromegalics from that in normal subjects. In addition to the classical neurotransmitters (i.e. monoamines) evidence is emerging that many other substances can behave as neurotransmitters in regulating the secretion of GH and PRL. Their roles however are still unclear in the normal subject, and in acromegaly, data on the effect of these substances (e.g. GABA, histamine, substance P) are still lacking. For these reasons we will limit our exposition to the studies on drugs affecting monoamine activity.

367

## Dopamine

Since the first demonstration of a paradoxical inhibitory effect of L-dopa on GH secretion in some acromegalic patients (Liuzzi *et al.*, 1972), evidence has been accumulated that drugs capable of stimulating the dopaminergic system can reduce GH levels in a substantial portion of acromegalics. Indeed, drugs with indisputable dopaminergic activity, such as apomorphine (Anden *et al.*, 1967), bromocriptine (Corrodi *et al.*, 1973) and lisuride (Horowski and Wachtel, 1976). have been shown by us (Chiodini *et al.*, 1974a; Liuzzi *et al.*, 1974a) to be effective in reducing GH levels in those acromegalic patients thus defined as responders. These patients are characterized by the suppressibility of their GH levels when tested with any of the previously mentioned dopamine agonists. On the contrary, there are patients defined as nonresponders, who do not reduce their GH levels when given either L-dopa, apomorphine, bromocriptine or lisuride. The distinction between responders and nonresponders is not a clear-cut one. Indeed, it has been made on the basis of an arbitrary parameter (i.e. reduction in GH levels of at least 50% of the basal value) after acute administration of a dopamine agonist. In acromegalic patients there is a great variability, ranging from maximal suppression (100%) of GH levels to no reduction at all. The distinction between responders and nonresponders does not apply to PRL release, the suppressibility of this hormone being the same in responder and nonresponder patients. Since L-dopa, apomorphine, bromocriptine, and lisuride can stimulate dopaminergic receptors both at the CNS and at the pituitary level, their use does not give information as to the site of the GH-lowering effect of the dopaminergic stimulation in acromegaly. For this reason, we have performed studies with dopamine agonists with different sites of action. Drugs capable of releasing dopamine at the CNS level, such as amphetamine (Glowinski and Axelrod, 1966) or pemoline (Everett, 1975), do not reduce GH levels in responder acromegalics.

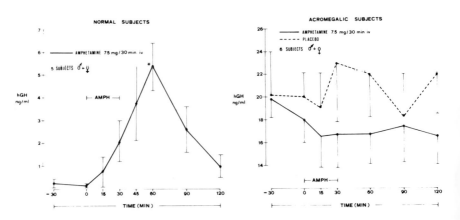

*Fig. 1.*   Plasma GH levels during amphetamine (AMPH) infusion into six acromegalic patients.

Similar results have been obtained with nomifensine, an inhibitor of dopamine reuptake (Hunt *et al.*, 1974). In addition, nomifensine does not potentiate the inhibitory effect of L-dopa on GH release. Thus, neuropharmacological manipulations expected to increase dopaminergic activity at the CNS level are ineffective both in reducing GH levels and in potentiating the GH-lowering effect of a dopamine precursor. On the contrary, the infusion of dopamine, a drug which, unlike L-dopa, does not readily cross the blood brain barrier (BBB) and is ineffective in increasing GH levels in normal subjects, is a very powerful inhibitor of GH release in acromegalic patients (Verde *et al.*, 1976). Since the median eminence is also considered to lie outside the BBB, an effect of dopamine at the level of the median eminence cannot be ruled out by this experiment. However, the lack of dopaminergic receptors at this level (Brown *et al.*, 1976) indicates the pituitary to be the site of the GH-lowering effect of dopamine. By analogy, it would be possible to conclude that apomorphine, bromocriptine and lisuride also exert their GH-lowering effects by acting on the pituitary. This view is supported by *in vitro* observations (Mashiter *et al.*, 1977) and by the finding that the selective removal of a GH-secreting adenoma not only abolishes the inhibitory effect of L-dopa on GH secretion but leads to the appearance of a GH-releasing effect of the drug, like that in the normal subject (Hoyte and Martin, 1975). This latter result, indicating the persistence of a stimulatory dopaminergic control at the hypothalamic level, is in agreement with the conclusion that may be drawn after comparing the effects of bromocriptine and of dopamine on GH release in a group of 50 acromegalic patients. Although the inhibitory effect of the two drugs was highly correlated in the whole group of patients

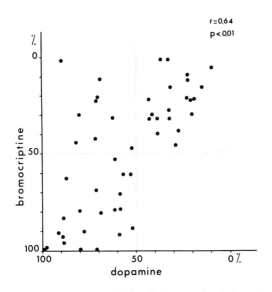

*Fig. 2.* Correlation between bromocriptine (2.5 mg p.o.) and dopamine (0.5 mg/min i.v.) induced GH inhibition (% of basal levels) in 50 acromegalic patients.

($r = 0.64, P < 0.01$), in 9 patients there was a clear-cut GH lowering effect (i.e. reduction of GH levels of more than 50% of the basal value) of dopamine but not of bromocriptine. Since the doses of the two drugs were chosen to give the maximal inhibitory effect, this discordance suggests differences in the mechanisms of the two drugs, possibly attributable to their capability of acting at the CNS level or not. We hypothesize that in acromegaly bromocriptine and other drugs which cross the BBB act at both the hypothalamic level to stimulate and at the pituitary level to inhibit GH release. Thus the inhibitory effect on the pituitary would be counteracted by the stimulatory effect on the hypothalamus. The level of plasma GH recorded after drug administration would be the resultant of these two opposite effects. In the case of dopamine, the stimulatory effect would be lacking, thus allowing the unopposed inhibitory effect on the pituitary to take place. That dopaminergic drugs such as bromocriptine can also affect GH release in acromegaly through a CNS site of action is supported by the data of Chihara *et al.* (1977) which show that the sleep-related GH increase, lacking in acromegalics, is restored by the drug.

Since dopaminergic drugs inhibit GH release in acromegaly, an opposite effect by antidopaminergic drugs would be expected. Pretreatment with pimozide was able in our studies to counteract the GH-lowering effects of L-dopa, bromocriptine (Chiodini *et al.*,1974b) and lisuride (Liuzzi *et al.*, 1978). Similarly, pretreatment with pimozide (Müller *et al.*, 1977) sulpiride or haloperidol (our unpublished observations) lessened the inhibitory effect of dopamine on GH release. However a few studies have envisaged the possibility of a more complex situation. Schaison *et al.*, (1974) reported on some acromegalic patients whose GH levels fell during chronic treatment with sulpiride. These data were confirmed in acute

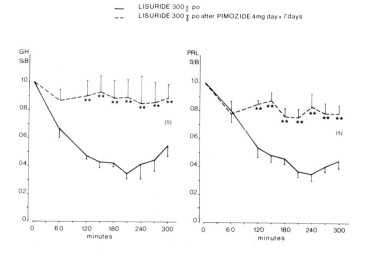

*Fig. 3.*    Effect of lisuride administration on plasma GH and PRL levels before and after treatment with pimozide. Values are expressed as ratio of suppressed (S) to baseline (B) levels ± s.e.m. Asterisks indicate significant ($P < 0.01$) differences.

experiments by Schwinn *et al*. (1977) showing that pimozide reduced GH levels in a few patients, both responders and nonresponder. Moreover, Paracchi *et al*. (1977) demonstrated that the acute administration of sulpiride lowered GH levels in 5 responders of the 13 patients tested. These unexpected results prompted us to investigate the problem. The administration of pimozide did not change basal GH levels during either acute or chronic administration to either responder or nonresponder patients, whereas it was able to increase GH levels which were lowered by chronic treatment with bromocriptine. In none of 33 patients tested did the acute administration of sulpiride (100 mg i.m.) lower GH levels. On the contrary, in three of these patients, clear-cut and repeatable increases in GH levels were observed. In these three patients, the sulpiride-induced GH release was unchanged when the stimulus was carried out during an infusion of somatostatin (0.33 $\mu$g/min) or of dopamine (0.5 mg/min). Since *in vitro* studies (MacLeod and Robyn, 1977) have shown that sulpiride does not release PRL unless dopamine is added to the incubation medium, we have given 18 patients unresponsive to sulpiride the same dose of the drug 30 min after beginning an infusion of dopamine. In accordance with the experimental data, GH levels were now significantly increased ($P < 0.01$) not only versus the preinjection but also versus the basal levels. The meaning of these experiments is not easy to explain. On the basis of the data of MacLeod and Robyn (1977), we might speculate that dopamine is lacking in the nonresponders to sulpiride. However, since PRL levels increase after sulpiride in these patients, this hypothesis is not fully satisfactory. Whatever the pathophysiological interpretation of these results may be, our studies do not confirm that antidopaminergic drugs can inhibit GH release in acromegaly but rather indicate that they can increase GH levels provided that the experimental conditions are adequate.

### Serotonin

The effect of the serotoninergic system on GH release is still questionable even in the normal subject (Müller *et al*., 1974; Smythe *et al*., 1975), possibly owing to the lack of specificity of the drugs commonly used to affect the serotoninergic system. Most of the present evidence, however, (see for review Smythe, 1977), favors the view that serotonin stimulates the release of GH in the normal subject. In acromegaly, the data are still scanty. The infusion of tryptophan seems at present to be the most specific tool for increasing the activity of the serotoninergic system. This drug, unlike 5OH-tryptophan, is taken up and converted into serotonin only by the serotoninergic neurons (Green and Grahame-Smith, 1976). In our experience tryptophan did not change GH levels when infused at the dose of 10-20 g in 30 min into acromegalic patients (Oppizzi *et al*., 1976). Our results do not necessarily imply difference in reactivity to tryptophan in normal subjects and acromegalic patients, since in some studies (Müller *et al*., 1974; Woolf and Lee, 1977) the administration of tryptophan to normal individuals failed to increase GH levels. The use of drugs with antiserotoninergic activity has given contradictory results in acromegalic patients, as in normal subjects. Acute or chronic administration of cyproheptadine leaves the levels of GH unaffected (Winkelman *et al*., 1975; Chiodini *et al*., 1976). On the contrary, methysergide

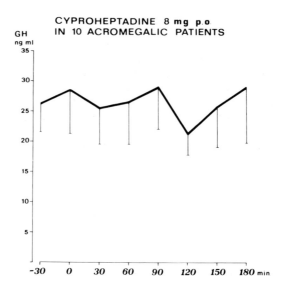

*Fig. 4.*　　Failure of administration of cyproheptadine to affect GH levels in acromegalic patients.

and metergoline have been reported to be effective in reducing GH levels in acromegalics (Feldman *et al.*, 1976; Delitala *et al.*, 1976; Oppizzi *et al.*, 1977) leading to the suggestion that serotonin can play an inhibitory role against GH secretion in acromegaly. In our opinion, the GH-lowering effects of either drug can be better explained on the basis of a dopaminergic mechanism. We have shown (Chiodini *et al.*, 1976; Oppizzi *et al.*, 1977) that these two ergot derivatives reduce PRL levels in all patients tested but lower GH levels only in those patients in whom the secretion of the hormone is also reduced by a drug with indisputable dopaminergic activity such as bromocriptine. Moreover the GH and PRL lowering effects of both drugs are inhibited by pretreatment with antidopaminergic drugs. In the case of methysergide, *in vitro* studies (MacLeod, 1977) support the view that the drug possesses a dopaminergic activity. It has been proposed by Smythe *et al.* (1975) that the GH lowering effect of dopamine agonists is brought about by their interaction with the serotoninergic receptors. According to this hypothesis, dopamine agonists would displace serotonin from its receptors and, being less active in stimulating them, would reduce the stimulatory effect of serotonin on GH release thus leading to lower GH levels. Our data showing that the inhibitory effect of bromocriptine is unaffected by cyproheptadine (Oppizzi *et al.*, 1976) indicate that such an interaction is not required to explain the GH lowering effect of the dopamine agonists.

### Noradrenaline

In normal subjects the administration of phentolamine, an alpha-adrenergic blocking drug, reduces the GH responsiveness to several provocative stimuli; on the contrary the administration of propranolol, a beta-adrenergic blocking agent, potentiates it (see Martin, 1976 for review). Cryer and Daughaday (1974) demonstrated that in acromegaly the infusion of high doses of phentolamine can reduce GH levels in some acromegalics and that this effect can be antagonized by insoproterenol. Accordingly, in 5 of 15 patients tested with 90 mg of phentolamine infused over 180 min we have noticed appreciable falls in GH levels, whereas PRL release was unaffected in all patients. It is worth noting that although some experimental data indicate an alpha-adrenergic blocking activity of bromocriptine (Gibson and Samini, 1978), we have not found a strict correlation between the GH lowering effects of the two drugs, since phentolamine can reduce GH levels in patients not responsive to bromocriptine and vice versa thus suggesting differences

| CB 154 + PHENTOLAMINE + decrease of GH >50% | | |
| CASES | CB154 | PHENTOLAMINE |
|---|---|---|
| 2 | + | + |
| 8 | − | − |
| 3 | + | − |
| 2 | − | + |

*Fig. 5.* Comparison between the GH-lowering activity of bromocriptine (2.5 mg, p.o.) and of phentolamine (90 mg/180 min, i.v.) in 15 acromegalic patients.

in their GH lowering mechanism. Similar conclusions were reached by Cryer and Daughaday (1977). It has been hypothesized (Cryer and Daughaday, 1974) that the blockade of alpha-adrenoreceptors can inhibit GH release through a hypothalamic mechanism (i.e. reduction of GRF tone). This view is supported by our data showing that noradrenaline, which like dopamine does not readily cross the blood brain barrier, did not change GH levels even in patients responsive to phentolamine. According to this hypothesis, GH suppressibility by phentolamine would identify those acromegalics in whom the hypersecretion of GH is due to an excess of hypothalamic GRF.

## EFFECTS OF NEUROHORMONES

### Somatostatin

The infusion of somatostatin is able to reduce GH levels in most patients with acromegaly when given at doses varying between 250 and 500 µg (Chiodini *et al.*, 1975). The degree of GH suppressibility is highly variable in different patients, however. Indeed, the same dose of the neurohormone can either completely suppress or only slightly reduce GH levels. Thus in the case of somatostatin a distinction between responder and nonresponder patients would also be possible. This finding would suggest variable impairments in the sensitivity of GH-secreting cells rather than a deficiency of somatostatin at the hypothalamic level. The fact that both somatostatin and dopamine inhibit GH release, at the pituitary level with variable effectiveness, prompted us to a comparative study between the effects of the two drugs with maximal inhibitory activity on GH release. In the 33 patients studied, the effects of the two drugs were significantly correlated ($r = 0.48$;

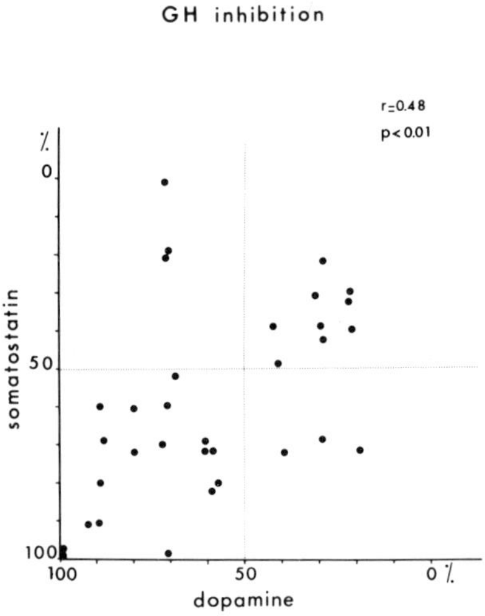

*Fig. 6.* Correlation between dopamine (0.5 mg/min) and somatostatin (0.33 μg/min) induced GH inhibition (% of basal level) in 33 acromegalic patients.

$P < 0.01$). In particular, in 17 patients both drugs caused a GH inhibition greater than 50% and in 4 of them a complete suppression of GH. In 10 patients neither drug achieved a reduction in GH levels of at least 50% below basal levels. In three patients dopamine, but not somatostatin, reduced GH levels and in another three cases opposite behavior was observed. Since some patients exhibit a complete suppression of their GH levels by both dopamine and somatostatin, we can suggest that a single GH-secreting cell can sense both somatostatin and dopamine. Admittedly, this could be due either to the presence of different receptors on the same cell or to a single receptor activated by both dopamine and somatostatin. The observation that in some patients GH levels are suppressed by dopamine but not by somatostatin and vice versa favors the conclusion that on a single GH-secreting cell separate receptors for dopamine and somatostatin exist. This view is supported by the data showing that pretreatment with sulpiride counteracts the inhibitory effect on GH release of dopamine but not that of somatostatin in patients who respond equally to both drugs.

## MRIP–I

On the basis of experimental studies suggesting a dopamine-like effect of MRIP-I, Faglia *et al.* (1976) tested the acute administration of this drug in acromegalic patients and showed that this peptide was able to reduce GH levels. Since PRL values were not lowered by the drug, the authors excluded dopaminergic activity of MRIP–I and speculated that a mechanism involving the pineal hormone melatonin might be implicated, since MRIP–I is accumulated in the pineal. We cannot confirm these data since in our tests infusion of MRIP–I was not able to appreciably change GH levels in a group of six acromegalics.

## TRH

An anomalous GH-releasing effect of TRH is present in about 50% of acromegalic patients (Saito *et al.*, 1971; Irie and Tsuchima, 1972; Schalch *et al.*, 1972; Faglia *et al.*, 1973; Liuzzi *et al.*, 1974 b). The lack of responsiveness to TRH in nonresponder patients does not seem to be related to the dose of TRH, since doses of 400 $\mu$g of TRH are as ineffective as 200 $\mu$g. The possibility has been advanced that this effect of TRH is due to the presence on the tumoral cells of nonspecific receptors which can be activated by releasing factors other than GRF (Faglia *et al.*, 1973; von Werder *et al.*, 1976). This hypothesis has been challenged by studies showing that in other pathological conditions, i.e. anorexia nervosa and depression (Maeda *et al.*, 1975, 1976), primary hypothyroidism (Hamada *et al.*, 1976), renal failure (Gonzalez-Barcena *et al.*, 1973) and hepatic cirrhosis (Panerai *et al.*, 1977a), a GH-releasing effect of TRH occurs which often disappears with the recovery from the disease. Experimental studies have shown that the GH-releasing activity of TRH present in the intact rat (Chihara *et al.*, 1976) is magnified when the pituitary is disconnected from the hypothalamus either by lesions

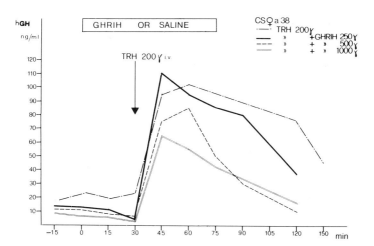

*Fig. 7.* Failure of different doses of somatostatin (GHRIH) to suppress the TRH-induced GH release in one acromegalic patient.

placed in the median eminence (Chihara *et al.*, 1976) or by transplanting the pituitary under the renal capsule (Udeschini *et al.*, 1976). Panerai *et al.* (1977 b) hypothesized that the GH responsiveness to TRH appears when the pituitary is released from inhibitory influences coming from the hypothalamus. Since a magnification of the GH-releasing effect of TRH could be obtained in intact rats treated with an antisomatostatin antiserum, these authors identify the hypothalmic inhibitory influences with somatostatin. This interesting hypothesis is not supported in the case of acromegaly by the experiments showing that in most of the patients tested, somatostatin was ineffective in suppressing the stimulatory effect of TRH on GH release even when infused in the very high and unphysiological doses of 1000 μg. The possibility that the GH-releasing effect of TRH may appear in acromegaly as a consequence of a derangement of brain catecholamines, as has been postulated for other pathological conditions (Collu *et al.*, 1977), prompted us to study whether drugs with either antidopaminergic or antiserotoninergic activity can affect the TRH-induced GH release. In our experiments, treatment with pimozide (4 mg/day for 7 days) or cyproheptadine (16 mg/day for 7 days) neither changed the stimulatory effect of TRH on GH release in responder patients nor led to the appearance of a GH reactivity to TRH in either non-responder patients or in normal subjects. It has also been investigated whether hormonal factors can affect the TRH-induced GH release in acromegaly. The administration of triiodothyronine has been reported either not to affect (Faglia *et al.*, 1973) or to reduce (Pawlikowski and Owcrarczyk, 1977) this effect. Similarly, the administration of glucocorticoids was able to reduce the TRH-induced GH release in the study of Tolis *et al.* (1975) but not in ours. The reported similarity between the stimulatory effects of TRH and the bromocriptine induced inhibition of GH release present in most acromegalic patients (Liuzzi *et al.*, 1974b) led to the observation that in responder patients the secretion of GH exhibits a PRL-like behavior (Liuzzi *et al.*, 1975). To point out other similarities in the regulation of GH and PRL secretion in these patients, the interaction between the effects of dopamine agonists and TRH on GH and PRL release has been investigated: the injection of TRH into responsive patients chronically treated with dopaminergic drugs such as L-dopa, bromocriptine or lisuride was followed by suppression of PRL release, whereas the release of GH was not significantly reduced. When TRH was injected during a dopamine infusion a significant reduction of both hormones was observed. However, some patients exhibited the same GH reactivity as under basal conditions. Thus, it appears that the regulation of GH and PRL in the responder patients is not superimposable.

## LHRH

LHRH is also able to release GH in some acromegalic patients (Rubin *et al.*, 1973; Faglia *et al.*, 1973 b). There is no homogeneity of the GH responses to TRH or LHRH (Faglia *et al.*, 1973) and, like that of TRH, the LHRH-induced GH release is not inhibited by somatostatin (Cantalamessa *et al.*, 1976).

### alpha–MSH

Since it has been shown that alpha–MSH can release GH in normal subjects by a pituitary mechanism of action (Zahnd and Versey, 1977), we have studied whether this effect is also present in acromegalic patients. The acute administration of 1 mg of alpha–MSH, i.v., failed to change GH levels in any of the patients tested.

## PATHOPHYSIOLOGICAL IMPLICATIONS

The absence of the sleep-related GH increase (Chihara *et al.*, 1977) and the paradoxical response to glucose load (Beck *et al.*, 1966) indicate the presence of a hypothalamic derangement in the control of GH secretion in acromegaly. An excess of GRF (Cryer and Daughaday, 1969) or, later on, a deficiency of somatostatin have been hypothesized (Besser *et al.*, 1974). The latter possibility was supported by showing that somatostatin could inhibit the paradoxical response to glucose load (Besser *et al.*, 1974). Adjunct support for this view derived from the study of Patel *et al.* (1977) showing the presence of normal levels of somatostatin in the cerebro-spinal fluids of acromegalics in spite of the presence of elevated plasma GH concentrations. The finding of the variable degree of responsiveness to somatostatin, the paradoxical inhibitory effect of dopamine agonists and the GH-releasing effect of unspecific neurohormones (i.e. TRH and LHRH) clearly indicate the existence of a pituitary derangement. The similarity in the responsiveness to TRH and dopaminergic drugs, which suggests a PRL-like behavior of GH in about 50% of the acromegalic patients, led us to speculate (Chiodini *et al.*, 1975; Liuzzi *et al.*, 1975) on existence in these patients of a mammosomatotropic cell, i.e. a cell able to synthesize both GH and PRL and to respond to stimuli specific for either GH or PRL. This hypothesis is supported by some histological data (Guyda *et al.*, 1973) and by the finding of significantly higher PRL levels in responder patients than in non-responders (Chiodini *et al.*, 1975). However there is a difference in reactivity to neuroactive drugs (e.g. somatostatin or alpha-adrenergic blocking agents) between GH and PRL in the responder patients, so that at present we feel that in some acromegalic patients a tumoral GH-secreting cell with the receptor properties of the PRL-secreting cell is present. Hypothalamic and pituitary alterations of GH control in acromegaly might not be separate phenomena: it is possible that abnormalities of the hypothalamic control of GH secretion might induce alterations of the functional properties of the somatotropes; alternatively, the presence of tumoral cells in the pituitary might induce some derangement in the hypothalamic mechanisms which govern the secretion of the hormone.

## THERAPEUTIC IMPLICATIONS

The demonstration of Chiodini *et al.* (1974b) that chronic bromochriptine administration results in a stable reduction of GH levels in acromegaly provided the first effective means for the medical treatment of this disease. At present the effectiveness of this drug in the medical treatment of acromegaly is supported by

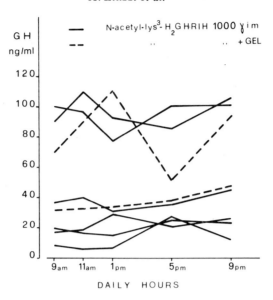

*Fig. 8.*    Effect of a somatostatin analog on plasma GH levels in eight acromegalic patients. In two patients the drug was administered in gelatine (GEL).

a great number of studies even though disagreements still exist about the percentage of the patients who benefit from the treatment and the doses to be employed. Besides bromocriptine, other drugs have been used to obtain a stable reduction of GH levels in acromegaly. Our attempts to prolong the very short-lived action of somatostatin to make this powerful inhibitor of GH-release suitable for therapeutic use have been so far unsuccessful. Indeed, somatostatin administered either with zinc-protamine, with gelatine, or in the form of a modified molecule, or as nasal drops never displayed an appreciable or prolonged GH-lowering effect. Drugs interfering with the serotoninergic system have also been used. Cyproheptadine has been completely ineffective in reducing GH levels during prolonged administration (Feldman *et al.*, 1976; Chiodini *et al.*, 1976). Both methysergide (Feldman *et al.*, 1976) and methergoline (our unpublished observations) have reduced GH levels when chronically administered to some patients. We have previously discussed the reasons why, in our opinion, the GH-lowering effects of these two ergot derivatives are mediated through a dopaminergic effect. Neuropharmacological studies have demonstrated that another semisynthetic ergot derivative, lisuride hydrogen maleate, is a powerful dopamine agonist which possesses some peculiarities in its mechanism of action in comparison with bromocriptine. In particular, it has been shown (Horowski and Wachtel, 1976) that unlike bromocriptine, the dopaminergic activity of lisuride is still present in rats depleted of catecholamines. In acute experiments we have shown (Liuzzi *et al.*, 1978) that this drug is as effective as bromocriptine in reducing GH levels in acromegalic patients. The chronic administration of lisuride to 18 acromegalics also resulted in a GH-lowering effect like that of bromocriptine. The drug was effective in daily doses as low as 600 $\mu$g, which in some patients kept GH levels markedly lower than pretreatment values. In patients with very high GH values, doses of 2 mg/day had to be administered to obtain the maximal GH inhibitory effect. As in the case of bromocriptine the responsiveness to an acute test performed with a dose of 300–400 $\mu$g is, in our experience, predictive of the effectiveness of the treatment. In non-responders to the acute test, even the administration of 2 mg/day of lisuride failed to reduce GH levels. The clinical advantages, the metabolic effects and the side effects of lisuride are the same as those of bromocriptine.

Although the effectiveness of long-lasting dopamine agonists in lowering GH levels during treatments prolonged up to three years (Silvestrini *et al.*, 1978) is well-established, it should be stressed that in many patients GH levels are not normalized or lowered at all by these drugs. For these reasons, the problem of the medical treatment of acromegaly is not yet solved and we feel that the study of other neurotransmitters involved in the regulation of GH secretion will give rise to more satisfactory results.

## REFERENCES

Anden, N. E., Rubensson, E., Fuxe, K. and Hokfelt, T. (1967). *J. Pharm. Pharmac* **19**, 627–629.

Beck, P., Parker, M. L. and Daughaday, W. H. (1966). *J. Clin. Endocr. Metab.* **26**, 463–469.

Besser, G. M., Mortimer, C. H., McNeilly, A. S., Thorner, M. O., Batistoni, G. A., Bloom, S. R., Kastrup, K. W., Hanssen, K. F., Hall, R., Coy, D. H., Kastin, A. J. and Schally, A. V. (1974). *Br. Med. J.* **4**, 622–627.

Brown, G. M., Seeman, P. and Lee, T. (1976). **99**, 1407–1410.

Cantalamessa, L., Reschini, E., Catania, A. and Giustina, G. (1976). *Acta Endocrinol.* **83**, 673–683.

Chihara, K., Kato, Y., Ohgo, S., Iwosaki, Y., Abe, H., Maeda, K. and Imura, H. (1976). *Endocrinology* **98**, 1047–1053.

Chihara, K., Kato, Y., Abe, H., Furomoto, M., Maeda, K. and Imura, H. (1977). *J. Clin. Endocr. Metab.* **44**, 78–84.

Chiodini, P. G., Liuzzi, A., Botalla, L., Cremascoli, G. and Silvestrini, F. (1974a). *J. Clin. Endocr. Metab.* **38**, 200–206.

Chiodini, P. G., Liuzzi, A., Cremascoli, G., Botalla, L., Silvestrini, F. and Muller, E. E. (1974b). *56th Meet. Endocr. Soc. Abst.* 206.

Chiodini, P. G., Liuzzi, A., Müller, E. E., Botalla, L., Oppizzi, G. and Cremascoli, G. (1975). *In* "Atti del Secondo Convegno sui Metodi Radioimmunilogici in Endocrinologia", pp. 71–82, Serono Symposia, Milan.

Chiodini, P. G., Liuzzi, A., Müller, E. E., Botalla, L., Cremascoli, G., Oppizzi, G., Verde, G. and Silvestrini, F. (1976). *J. Clin. Endrocr. Metab.* **45**, 356–363.

Collu, R., Leboeuf, G., Letarte, J. and Ducharme, J., R. (1977). *J. Clin. Endocr. Metab.* **44**, 743–747.

Corrodi, H., Fuxe, K., Hokfelt, T., Lidbrink, P. and Ungerstedt, U. (1973). *J. Pharm. Pharmac.* **25**, 409–412.

Cryer, P. E. and Daughaday, W. H. (1969). *J. Clin. Endocr. Metab.* **29**, 386–393.

Cryer, P. E. and Daughaday, W. H. (1974). *J. Clin. Endocr. Metab.* **39**, 658–663.

Cryer, P. E. and Daughaday, W. H. (1977). *J. Clin. Endocr. Metab.* **44**, 977–999.

Delitala, G., Masala, A., Alagna, S., Devilla, L. and Lotti, G. (1976). *J. Clin. Endocr. Metab.* **42**, 1382–1385.

Everett, G. M. (1975). *Pharmacologist* **17**, 227–232.

Faglia, G., Beck-Peccoz, P., Ferrari, C., Travaglini, P., Ambrosi, B. and Spada, A. (1973a). *J. Clin. Endocr. Metab.* **36**, 1259-1262.

Faglia, G., Beck-Peccoz, P., Travaglini, P., Paracchi, A., Spada, A. and Lewin, A. (1973b). *J. Clin. Endocr. Metab.* **37**, 338-340.

Faglia, G., Paracchi, A., Ferrari, C., Beck-Peccoz, P., Ambrosi, P., Travaglini, P., Spada, A. and Oliver, C. (1976). *J. Clin. Endocr. Metab.* **42**, 991-994.

Feldman, J. M., Plonk, J. W. and Bivens, C. H. (1976). *Clin. Endocrinol.* **5**, 71-78.

Gibson, A. and Samini, M. (1978). *J. Pharm. Pharmac.* **30**, 314-19.

Glowinski, J. and Axelrod, J. (1966). *Pharmacol. Rev.* **18**, 775-782.

Gonzalez-Barcena, D., Kastin, A. J., Schalch, D. S., Torres-Zamora, M., Perez-Paten, E., Kato, A. and Schally, A. V. (1973). *J. Clin. Endocr. Metab.* **36**, 117-120.

Green, A. R. and Grahame-Smith, D. G. (1976). *Nature* **260**, 487-491.

Guyda, H., Robert, F., Colle, E. and Hardy, J. (1973). *J. Clin. Endocr. Metab.* **36**, 531-547.

Hamada, N., Uoi, K., Nishizawa, Y., Okamoto, T., Hasegawa, K., Morri, H. and Wada, M. (1976). *Endocrinol. Jpn.* **23**, 5-10.

Horowski, R. and Wachtel, H. (1976). *Eur. Pharmacol.* **33**, 373-360.

Hoyte, K. M. and Martin, J. B. (1975). *J. Clin. Endocr. Metab.* **41**. 656-659.

Hunt, P., Kannengiesser, M. K. and Raynaud, J. P. (1974). *J. Pharm. Pharmac.* **26**, 371-377.

Irie, M. and Tsushima, T. (1972). *J. Clin. Endocr. Metab.* **30**, 646-652.

Lawrence, A. M. and Kirsteins, L. (1970). *J. Clin. Endocr. Metab.* **30**, 646-652.

Liuzzi, A., Chiodini, P. G., Botalla, L., Cremascoli, G. and Silvestrini, F. (1972). *J. Clin. Endocr. Metab.* **35**, 941-943.

Liuzzi, A., Chiodini, P. G., Botalla, L., Cremascoli, G., Müller, E. E. and Silvestrini, F. (1974a). *J. Clin. Endocr. Metab.* **38**, 910-912.

Liuzzi, A., Chiodini, P. G., Botalla, L., Silvestrini, F. and Müller, E. E. (1974b). *J. Clin. Endocr. Metab.* **39**, 871-876.

Liuzzi, A., Panerai, A. E., Chiodini, P. G., Secchi, C., Cocchi, D., Botalla, L., Silvestrini, F. and Müller, E. E. (1975). *In* "Growth Hormone and Related Peptides" (E. Pecile and E. E. Müller, eds) pp. 236-251. Excerpta Medica, Amsterdam.

Liuzzi, A., Chiodini, P. G., Oppizzi, G., Botalla, L., Verde, G., De Stefano, L., Colussi, G., Graf, K. J. and Horowski, R. (1978). *J. Clin. Endocr. Metab.* **46**, 196-205.

MacLeod, R. M. (1977). *Progr. Reprod. Biol.* **2**, 54-68

MacLeod, R. M. and Robyn, C. (1977). *J. Endocrinol.* **72**, 273-278.

Maeda, K., Kato, Y., Ohgo, S., Chihara, K., Yoshimoto, Y., Yamaguchi, N., Kuromaru, S. and Imura, H. (1975). *J. Clin. Endocr. Metab.* **40**, 501-505.

Maeda, K., Kato, Y., Yamaguchi, N., Chihara, K., Ohgo, S., Awasaki, Y., Yoshimoto, Y., Moridera, K., Kuromaru, S. and Imura, H. (1976). *Acta Endocrinol.* **81**, 1-8.

Martin, J. B. (1976). *In* "Frontiers in Neuroendocrinology" (L. Martini and W. F. Ganong, eds) pp. 129-168. Raven Press, New York.

Mashiter, K., Adams, E., Beard, M. and Holley, A. (1977). *Lancet.* **2**, 197.

Müller, E. E., Brambilla, F., Cavagnini, F., Peracchi, M. and Panerai, A. (1974). *J. Clin. Endocr. Metab.* **39**, 1-5.

Müller, E. E., Liuzzi, A., Cocchi, D., Panerai, A. E., Oppizzi, G., Locatelli, V., Mantegazza, P., Silvestrini, F. and Chiodini, P. G. (1977). *In* "Nonstriatal Dopaminergic Neurons" (E. Costa and G. L. Gessa, eds) pp. 127-138. Raven Press, New York.

Oppizzi, G., Cremascoli, G., De Stefano, L., Colussi, G., Verde, G., Liuzzi, A., Chiodini, P. G. and Botalla, L. (1976). 16th Congr. Soc. It. Endocr., *Abst.* **31**.

Oppizzi, G., Verde, G., De Stefano, L., Cozzi, R., Botalla, L., Liuzzi, A. and Chiodini, P. G. (1977). *Clin. Endocrinol.* **7**, 267–272.

Panerai, A. E., Salerno, F., Manneschi, M., Cocchi, D. and Müller, E. E. (1977a). *J. Clin. Endocr. Metab.* **45**, 134–140.

Panerai, A. E., Giannattasio, G., Zanini, A., Meldolesi, I., Rossi, G. L. and Müller, E. E. (1977b). *59th Meet. Endocr. Soc. Abst.* **144**.

Paracchi, A., Ferrari, C. and Faglia, G. (1977). *11th Acta Endocrinologica Congr., Lausanne, Abst.* **274**.

Patel, Y. C., Krishna, R. and Reichlin, S. (1977). *N. Engl. J. Med.* **296**, 529–533.

Pawlikoski, M. and Owcrarczyk, I. (1977). *Endokrinol. Pol.* **6**, 497–501.

Rubin, A. L., Levin, S. R., Bernstein, R. I., Tyrrell, J. B., Noacco, C. and Forsham, P. H. (1973). *J. Clin. Endocr. Metab.* **37**, 160–162.

Saito, S., Abe, K., Yoshida, H., Kaneko, T., Nakamura, E., Shimuzu, N. and Yanaihara, N. (1971). *Endocrinol. Jpn.* **17**, 101–108.

Schaison, G., Croisier, J. C., Nathan, C. and Dreyfus G. (1974). *Annls. Endocr.* **35**, 103–110.

Schalch, D. S., Gonzalez-Barcena, D., Kastin, A. J., Schally, A. V. and Lee, L. A. (1972). *J. Clin. Endocr. Metab.* **35**, 609–615.

Schwinn, G., McIntosh, C., Blossey, C. and Kobberling, I. (1977). *Acta Endocrinol. Suppl.* **208**, Abst. 26.

Silvestrini, F., Liuzzi, A. and Chiodini, P. G. (1978). *Pharmacology*, Suppl. 1, 78–87.

Smythe, G. A. (1977). *Clin. Endocrinol.* **7**, 325–341.

Smythe, G. A., Compton, P. J. and Lazarus, L. (1975). *In* "Growth Hormone and Related Peptides" (E. Pecile and E. E. Muller, eds) pp. 222–235. Excerpta Medica, Amsterdam.

Tolis, G., Kovacs, L., Friesen, H. and Martin, J. B. (1975). *Acta Endocrinol.* **78**, 251–257.

Udeschini, G., Cocchi, D., Panerai, A. E., Gil-Ad, I., Rossi, G., Chiodini, P. G., Liuzzi, A. and Müller, E. E. (1976). *Endocrinology* **98**, 807–814.

Verde, G., Oppizzi, G., Colussi, G., Cremascoli, G., Botalla, L., Müller, E. E., Silvestrini, F., Chiodini, P. G. and Liuzzi, A. (1976). *Clin. Endocrinol.* **5**, 419–423.

von Werder, K., Fahlbusch, R., Gay, R., Pickhardt, C. R. and Schultz, B. (1976). *Klin. Wochenschr.* **54**, 335–8.

Winkelmann, W., Schorn, H., Hadam, W. R., Heesen, D. and Mies, R. (1975). *Int. Symp. on Growth Hormone and Related Peptides, Milan, Abst.* **99**.

Woolf, P. D. and Lee, L. (1977). *J. Clin. Endocr. Metab.* **45**, 123–133.

Zahnd, G. R. and Vecsey, A. (1977). *11th Acta Endocrinologica Congr., Lausanne, Abst.* **144**.

# MEDICAL THERAPY OF HYPERPROLACTINEMIA AND CUSHING'S DISEASE ASSOCIATED WITH PITUITARY ADENOMAS

K. von Werder, C. Brendel, T. Eversmann, R. Fahlbusch, O. A. Müller
and H. K. Rjosk

*Medizinische Klinik Innenstadt, Neurochirurgische Klinik Grosshadern,
I. Frauenklinik, University of Munich, Munich, FRG*

Patients with pituitary adenomas have to be treated for either an expanding lesion in the sella turcica which leads to visual problems and pituitary insufficiency or for pituitary hormone excess. In recent years, there are apparently more endocrinologically active than inactive pituitary adenomas (Franks *et al.*, 1977; Frantz and Kleinberg, 1978). Among the hormone-secreting pituitary adenomas, the prolactinoma is the most common, followed by growth hormone (GH) and ACTH producing adenomas (Frantz and Kleinberg, 1978).

There is little doubt about the mode of treatment of large pituitary adenomas, leading to marked changes of the osseous structure of the sella turcica and suprasellar extension. The treatment must be directed toward diminishing adenoma mass, which can best be achieved by surgical procedures (Guiot, 1978). When the pituitary adenoma is small, i.e. has a diameter of less than 10 mm, there is no immediate need for diminishing adenoma mass by surgical procedures. The main therapeutic aim is directed toward abolishing the hormone excess caused by a hypersecreting microadenoma. Thus attention has been focused on possible medical treatment of pituitary hormone excess. There are several reasons why pharmacotherapy may be particularly indicated for the treatment of pituitary hormone hypersecretion:

(1) Drug therapy can selectively inhibit pituitary hormone hypersecretion without influencing residual anterior pituitary function, which cannot always be preserved in surgical and radiotherapeutical procedures.

(2) Ideal drug therapy leads to suppression of excess hormone secretion *and* should have an antiproliferative effect on adenoma growth ("medical adenomectomy").

(3) Residual hormone excess after pituitary surgery and radiotherapy for an expanding adenoma can be normalized by post-operative drug therapy.

(4) Since the pituitary hormone excess might be only a secondary consequence of a primary hypothalamic lesion, only total hypophysectomy could lead to abolition of the hormone excess. In these cases pharmacological manipulation of hypothalamic function would be the therapy of choice.

Because medical therapy of pituitary hormone excess is so valuable, many agents have been investigated for the treatment of hyperprolactinemia, acromegaly and Cushing's disease. Our increasing knowledge about neuroendocrine regulation of anterior pituitary function has stimulated this field to a great extent. Particularly in patients with hyperprolactinemia, medical therapy has become a real alternative to invasive procedures (Bergh *et al.*, 1978; del Pozo *et al.*, 1972; Mornex *et al.*, 1978; von Werder *et al.*, 1978a). In contrast to the accepted medical therapy of hyperprolactinemia, drug therapy of Cushing's disease is still controversial (Orth, 1978). Medical therapy of acromegaly will be discussed elsewhere (Liuzzi and Chiodini, 1979).

## TREATMENT OF PATIENTS WITH HYPERPROLACTINEMIA

Since the radioimmunoassay for human prolactin has become available, more and more patients with hyperprolactinemia have been discovered. Particularly in females, hyperprolactinemia with or without enlargement of the sella turcica has been frequently shown to be the cause of galactorrhea, amenorrhea or anovulatory menstrual cycles (Gomez *et al.*, 1977; Kleinberg *et al.*, 1977; Rjosk *et al.*, 1976). But also in the male, where galactorrhea is usually absent, it has been shown that many pituitary tumors formerly thought to be hormonally inactive were in fact producing prolactin (Franks *et al.*, 1977; von Werder *et al.*, 1978a,b).

It is well known that PRL secretion is under chronic inhibitory control by the hypothalamus. It has been shown that dopamine inhibits prolactin secretion, whereas dopaminergic receptor blockers lead to an increase in serum prolactin levels. Thus, phenothiazine and metoclopramide stimulate prolactin secretion, whereas L-dopa, a dopamine precursor, inhibits prolactin secretion (Frantz, 1978). The inhibitory effect of L-dopa on prolactin secretion has also been demonstrated for hyperprolactinemic patients with pituitary adenomas (Frantz and Kleinberg, 1978). The disadvantage of the short biological half-life of L-dopa has been overcome by the longer-acting dopamine agonists bromocriptine (del Pozo *et al.*, 1972) and lisuride (Liuzzi *et al.*, 1978). In particular bromocriptine has been shown to be capable of normalizing hyperprolactinemia and restoring gonadal function (Rjosk *et al.*, 1976; von Werder *et al.*, 1978a). It has thus become an established primary therapy in hyperprolactinemic patients without evidence of pituitary enlargement, whereas its primary use in pituitary tumor patients is still controversial (Thorner, 1977).

In the last five years we have been following more than 300 patients with hyperprolactinemia in our endocrine clinic. The patients were referred to us because of amenorrhea and galactorrhea, because of clinical evidence for pituitary insufficiency, or because of visual field problems. All patients with evidence of pituitary enlargement were admitted to the hospital before initiation of surgical or medical therapy in order to perform the endocrine evaluation. The patients with enlargement of the sella turcica were subdivided into those with minute changes of the sella turcica, suggestive of a microadenoma, and those with large pituitary tumors, sometimes breaking into the sphenoid sinus and extending into the supra-sellar space.

Serum prolactin was measured by radioimmunoassay using VLS-hPRL (NIH, Bethesda, Md.) or hPRL from KABI, Stockholm, for labeling. As standard we used pooled pregnancy serum, which was calibrated with the MRC-Research-Standard A-71/222 (Cotes, 1973). 20 $\mu$U of the MRC-standard A-71/222 are equivalent to 1 ng VLS-hPRL from the NIH. As hPRL-antibody we used a rabbit antiserum raised against the "little" fragment of serum hPRL as described previously (von Werder *et al.*, 1978b).

The endocrine evaluation consisted of TRH-LHRH-stimulation tests and insulin-induced hypoglycemia, as described previously (von Werder *et al.*, 1978a). All patients had lateral skull X-rays as well as sellar tomography. Most of the patients with an enlarged sella turcica had computer-tomography (CT) of the skull. In all patients with an enlargement of the sella turcica visual fields were examined.

## RESULTS AND DISCUSSION

Prolactin levels in 133 hyperprolactinemic female patients without any radiological evidence for a pituitary adenoma ranged from 560 to 3000 $\mu$U/ml. Since other causes of hyperprolactinemia, such as hypothyroidism and therapy with PRL-secretion-stimulating agents had been excluded, it is most likely that the elevation of PRL in these patients is due to a microadenoma which has not led to changes in the osseous structure and is therefore not detectable by our present methods. This is also suggested by the rather uniform response of PRL secretion to stimulation and suppression in all patients with hyperprolactinemia, those with a normal and those with an enlarged sella turcica (Frantz and Kleinberg, 1978; Tolis, 1977).

In 68 female patients with hyperprolactinemia who had minute changes of the sella turcica, such as a double floor demonstrated by tomography, suggestive of a microadenoma, prolactin levels ranged from 690 to 9800 $\mu$U/ml (Fig. 1).

In 57 female patients with large adenomas, the PRL levels were sometimes extremely elevated, ranging from 2000 to 150 000 $\mu$U/ml, demonstrating the reported correlation between tumor size and PRL level (Fahlbusch *et al.*, 1978). In contrast to the females, we observed only four males with moderate hypogonadism who had elevated PRL levels associated with a completely normal sella turcica, though we measured PRL regularly in all patients from a psychiatric impotence clinic as well as from an andrological infertility clinic for one year, in addition to our own hypogonadal patients. We observed only two other male patients with evidence of a microadenoma and mild hyperprolactinemia (Fig. 1) and clinical symptoms of hypogonadism. In contrast to the rarity of hyperpro-

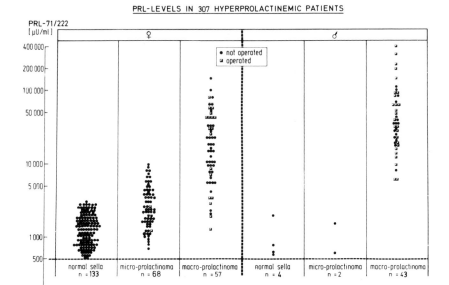

*Fig. 1.* PRL levels in 307 hyperprolactinemic patients with hypogonadism, with or without radiological evidence of enlargement of the sella turcica. The mean ages of all groups were not significantly different.

lactinemia in males associated with only minor or no changes in the osseous structure of the sella turcica, 43 male patients with large pituitary adenomas had extremely elevated PRL levels. Although 26 of these patients were investigated only postoperatively, the PRL levels were still above 5000 $\mu$U/ml, ranging up to 400 000 $\mu$U/ml in one patient after several transfrontal and transsphenoidal operations. These findings demonstrate that the pituitary macroprolactinoma, the most frequent endocrine active pituitary adenoma (Frantz and Kleinberg, 1978), is almost evenly distributed among the sexes. This is in obvious contrast to the microprolactinoma, which seems to occur almost exclusively in females. It suggests that microprolactinomas may not be regarded generally to be precursors of the macroprolactinomas, particularly since the mean age of the two groups was not significantly different. Micro- and macroprolactinoma may be different entities, one of which occurs in female and males alike, the other being a female disease for the development of which circulating estrogens may be essential (Peillon *et al.*, 1970).

The general therapeutic approach has been outlined before (von Werder *et al.*, 1978a). All patients with pituitary macroadenomas and those patients with microadenomas who had PRL levels above 5000 $\mu$U/ml were operated on. The therapeutic results have been reported by Fahlbusch *et al.* (1979). Patients without any abnormality of the sella turcica, as well as those with microadenomas and PRL levels below 5000 $\mu$U/ml and no evidence of altered pituitary function, were treated with bromocriptine only. Bromocriptine was also started in those patients whose postoperative PRL levels remained elevated, i.e. all patients with macroprolactinomas. When postoperative PRL levels were above 20 000 $\mu$U/ml or there was evi-

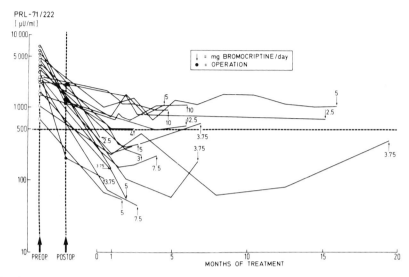

*Fig. 2.* Effect of bromocriptine on PRL levels in 19 female patients with microprolactinomas. The patients who showed no normalization after bromocriptine therapy still had regular menses. The upper limit of normal is 500 μU/ml.

dence of enhanced proliferation of the resected adenoma on histological examination, radiotherapy with 5000 rad followed the operative procedure (von Werder *et al.*, 1978c).

Figure 2 shows the response to bromocriptine therapy in 19 females with microadenomas and hyperprolactinemia, with and without prior operation. The few patients who did not normalize their PRL secretions had normal menstrual cycles, which we have sometimes also observed in untreated patients with mild hyperprolactinemia. Since basal body temperatures were not always obtained and progesterone measurements were not performed, we cannot be sure that these patients had normal ovulations.

In 16 hyperprolactinemic patients with no radiological evidence of a microadenoma and in 6 patients with radiological changes suggesting a microadenoma, pregnancies after bromocriptine therapy occurred without prior operation (Rjosk *et al.*, 1979). In an additional 6 patients with postoperatively persisting hyperprolactinemia, uneventful pregnancies were observed after bromocriptine therapy (Rjosk *et al.*, 1979).

In female patients with macroprolactinomas postoperatively persisiting hyperprolactinemia could be normalized if the postoperative PRL level was below 12 000 μU/ml (Fig. 3). Higher PRL levels were only normalized when additional radiotherapy or very large bromocriptine dosages, up to 60 mg per day, were employed (Fig. 3). In 23 male patients, bromocriptine therapy led to normalization of postoperatively elevated PRL levels, except in seven. The latter patients all had PRL levels above 50 000 μU/ml and some of them received bromocriptine in only moderate dosages (Fig. 4). Though PRL levels did not normalize in these patients, all experienced improvement of such symptoms as loss of sexual potency and libido when under bromocriptine treatment.

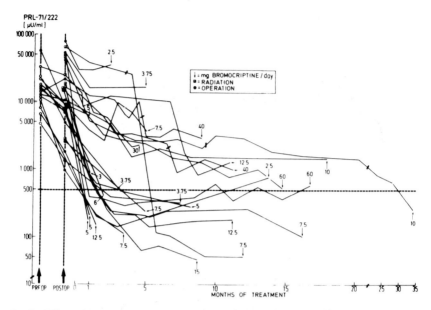

*Fig. 3.* Effect of bromocriptine on PRL levels in 27 female patients with macroprolactinomas. PRL levels under 12 000 μU/ml could be normalized by bromocriptine alone. Most patients with PRL levels above 20 000 μU/ml received postoperative radiotherapy.

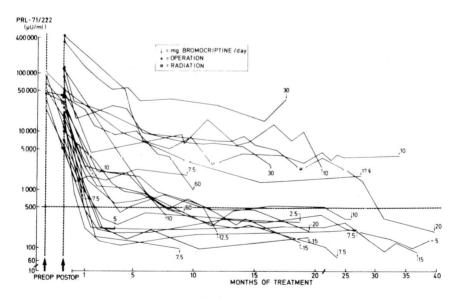

*Fig. 4.* Effect of bromocriptine on PRL levels in 23 male patients with macroprolactinomas. In contrast to female patients, PRL levels above 20 000 μU/ml could be normalized by bromocriptine therapy. This may be explained by the lower circulating estrogens in males.

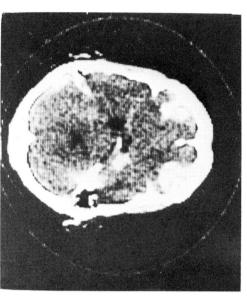

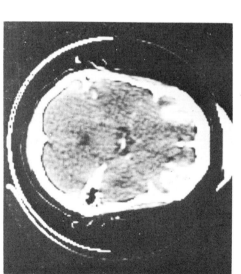

*Fig. 5.* Effect of long term bromocriptine therapy on a macroprolactinoma with parasellar extension in a male patient (M.H., 37 yr). Whereas the computer-tomography with contrast enhancement shows a right parasellar adenoma (left side) before therapy, the computer-tomography after one year of bromocriptine therapy (7.5 mg/day) shows no evidence of a pituitary adenoma extending into the parasellar area. The PRL level decreased at the same time from 13 082 μU/ml to 71 μU/ml.

We and others (Friesen and Tolis, 1977) have had the impression that bromocriptine might stop adenoma growth or even lead to actual shrinking of the adenoma. This was based mainly on clinical data, such as improvement of visual fields under bromocriptine and the long term follow-up of patients with invasively growing adenomas, who had been operated on several times, and subsequently had been considered inoperable, and who had improved clinically with bromocriptine alone (von Werder *et al.*, 1978a). An antiproliferative effect of bromocriptine has been demonstrated *in vitro* (Lloyd *et al.*, 1975). Recently, diminution of the adenoma mass extending into the sphenoid sinus has been reported in one patient under bromocriptine therapy, documented by X-ray (Sobrinho *et al.*, 1978). We have observed one patient who had a recurrent macroprolactinoma extending into the parasellar area, documented by computerized tomography (Fig. 5). Since he refused a second operation, he was treated with bromocriptine, which led to a fall in his PRL levels from 13 000 to 71 µU/ml. In computerized tomography after one year of treatment, we could no longer detect supra- or parasellar adenoma tissue (Fig. 5). These findings indicate that bromocriptine has an effect not only on PRL secretion but on the adenoma itself.

We have withdrawn bromocriptine for at least one month after long-term therapy in 9 male and 6 female patients with macroprolactinomas (Fig. 6). PRL levels were measured several times before initiation of therapy and just before therapy was reinstated. The PRL levels after bromocriptine withdrawal were

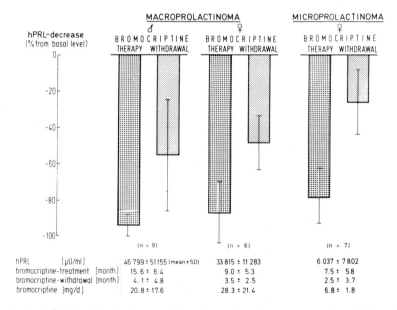

Fig. 6. Prolactin levels during bromocriptine therapy and after bromocriptine withdrawal in 9 male and 6 female patients with macroprolactinomas and 7 females with microprolactinomas. The decrease of prolactin levels during and after withdrawal of bromocriptine therapy is shown as per cent of the basal level before start of therapy. Despite the fact that bromocriptine had been withdrawn for at least one month, PRL levels were significantly lower in all groups compared to pretreatment level.

found to be significantly lower than pretreatment levels (Fig. 6). This effect was less pronounced in 7 females with microprolactinomas, who showed less permanent suppression after bromocriptine withdrawal. Since PRL levels correlate well with adenoma size (Fahlbusch *et al.*, 1978) and since it is not likely that the inhibitory effect on PRL secretion of bromocriptine is still present after one month, one is inclinded to attribute this phenomenon to the bromocriptine-induced diminution of adenoma tissue. Thus, the results of neurosurgical interventions are also determined by the postoperative PRL levels, which are comparable to the PRL levels after bromocriptine withdrawal. The differences between micro- and macroprolactinoma may be due to the different biology of these tumors, which is already apparent clinically.

## MEDICAL TREATMENT OF CUSHING'S DISEASE

According to Orth and Liddle (1971) more than 50% of all patients with Cushing's syndrome have a pituitary ACTH excess, and of these 15% have an enlarged sella turcica at the onset of the disease. In one quarter of all patients, Cushing's syndrome is due to an autonomous adrenal tumor and 16% have a non-pituitary tumor capable of secreting excessive amounts of ACTH ("ectopic ACTH syndrome"). There is no dispute about the operative treatment of benign adrenocortical tumors, leading to the complete disappearance of the disease (Orth and Liddle 1971). In case of adrenocortical cancers, which cannot be completely removed, additional medical therapy with adrenocorticolytic drugs such as ortho, para, dichlorodiphenyldichloroethane (o, p'DDD) or amino-glutethimide (Smilo *et al.*, 1967) may have a beneficial but only palliative effect on the symptoms caused by the steroid excess. The same is true for the treatment of ectopic ACTH syndrome, in which the primary ACTH-producing tumor often cannot be removed. Thus, only bilateral adrenalectomy or adrenocorticolytic therapy can correct the severe mineralocorticoid syndrome generally observed in these patients. In contrast to the above-mentioned cause of Cushing's syndrome, there is considerable divergence of opinion about the treatment of bilateral adrenal hyperplasia due to pituitary ACTH excess (Feldman, 1975). Most of the controversy about the therapy of Cushing's disease is based on the fact that we still do not know the etiology of this disease. Some investigators favor the idea that the primary lesion is a hypothalamic one leading to deranged control of pituitary ACTH secretion (Feldman, 1975; Krieger *et al.*, 1975; Krieger and Luria, 1976; Lamberts *et al.*, 1977), whereas others have evidence that the primary defect is an autonomous corticotrophic pituitary adenoma (Müller *et al.*, 1976; Tyrrell *et al.*, 1978). From the data that have been accumulated recently, particularly those concerning the response to medical (Krieger *et al.*, 1975) and operative therapy (Müller *et al.*, 1978a; Schnall *et al.*, 1978; Tyrrell *et al.*, 1978) it may be concluded that there are two different causes of Cushing's disease, one of hypothalamic origin and the other caused by an autonomous pituitary adenoma. Bilateral adrenalectomy, which until recently has been an established form of therapy in patients with a normal sella turcica, only abolishes excess steroidogenesis without correction of the basic defect of this disease. Thus, in 10–15% of patients with Cushing's disease treated in this fashion, an ACTH-producing pituitary adenoma can be encountered

Table I.  Drug therapy of pituitary dependent Cushing's syndrome.

| Drug | Site of action | Therapeutic result | Investigator |
|------|----------------|--------------------|--------------|
| Cyproheptadine | CNS | beneficial effect in Cushing's syndrome and Nelson's syndrome | Krieger et al. (1975 and 1976) |
| L-dopa | CNS | no effect | Krieger (1973) |
| Reserpine | CNS | partly beneficial effect combined with radiotherapy | Miura et al. (1975) |
| Bromocriptine | CNS | beneficial effect | Lamberts et al. (1977) |
| Somatostatin | pituitary | in acute experiments only lowering of ACTH | Tyrrell et al. (1975) |
| Bromocriptine and metyrapone | CNS and adrenal | beneficial effect | Besser et al. (1976) |
| Metyrapone | adrenal | beneficial effect | Jeffcoate et al. (1977) |
| Aminoglutethimide | adrenal | beneficial effect | Smilo et al. (1967) |
| Aminoglutethimide and metyrapone | adrenal | partly beneficial effect | Child et al. (1976) |
| o, p'-DDD | adrenal | beneficial effect in selected cases | Orth et al. (1971) |

(Moore et al., 1976). The same is true for adrenocorticolytic therapy (Table I), which may be indicated in some patients with severe symptoms of hypercortisolism in order to prepare the patient for final treatment (Child et al., 1976; Smilo et al., 1967).

Some authors favor treatment with o, p'-DDD or metyrapone (Jeffcoate et al., 1977) as permanent therapy. Since both drugs are not available for regular distribution in Germany, we have never been tempted to treat patients with Cushing's disease with these agents continuously. Considering the side effects which are encountered with these agents (Orth, 1978), and the fact that adrenocorticolytic therapy is not directed against the basic defect of Cushing's disease, we fail to see the advantages of this kind of therapy. The theoretical arguments against solely adrenocorticolytic therapy in pituitary ACTH-dependent bilateral adrenal hyperplasia have been pointed out recently in an editorial by Orth (1978).

In contrast to adrenocorticolytic therapy, pharmacological modulation of pituitary ACTH secretion seems to be of great importance, particularly if there is evidence of hypothalamic derangement as a cause of this disease. Unfortunately, the latter is difficult to prove without measurement of CRF, whose structure has not yet been elucidated. Though Krieger et al. (1975) have seen remission of Cushing's disease after cyprohcptadine treatment in three cases with pituitary ACTH excess, documented by quantitative normalization of cortisol secretion without restoration of regular diurnal variation, this experience has not been shared by other investigators (von Petrykowski *et al.*, 1977). The reason for treating patients with this primarily antiserotoninergic drug is the evidence that serotonin plays an important role in the regulation of ACTH secretion (Plonk and Feldman, 1976). Thus, Krieger and Luria (1976) also demonstrate that some patients with Nelson's syndrome show a fall in ACTH levels after cyproheptadine treatment. We also have observed a fall in ACTH in a patient with Nelson's syndrome to 50% of the pretreatment level after cyproheptadine, but the drug had to be withdrawn because of excessive weight gain in this patient, who already had severe osteoporosis.

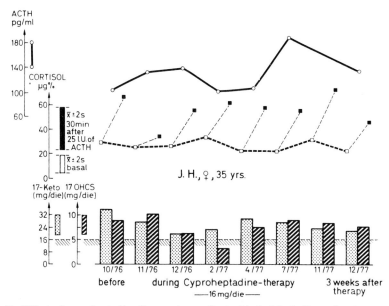

Fig. 7. Effect of cyproheptadine therapy in a patient with Cushing's disease in whom no microadenoma was found during transsphenoidal exploration of the sella turcia. No effect on ACTH and cortisol or on the excretion of steroid metabolites could be detected.

One patient with Cushing's disease, in whom no microadenoma could be found during exploration of the sella turcica, was also treated with cyproheptadine (Fig. 7) without any effect on ACTH levels, cortisol levels before and after exogenous ACTH, urinary 17-ketosteroids, or 17-OHCS. Another attempt to normalize increased ACTH secretion by administration of dopaminergic agents has been made. Though Krieger (1973) could not demonstrate any effect of L-dopa in Cushing's disease, surprisingly, Lamberts *et al.* (1977) induced normalization of cortisol secretion by administration of the dopamine agonist bromocriptine, in two of four patients, though the longest treatment period was only four months. Besser *et al.* (1976) have also reported a beneficial effect of bromocriptine in combination with metyrapone in patients with Cushing's disease. Our own experience again is limited. First we must say that in agreement with everybody else we have never seen inhibition of normal adrenal function in patients treated with bromocriptine, up to 60 mg per day, for other causes. One patient with bilateral adrenalectomy for Cushing's disease and elevated ACTH levels has been treated with 7.5 mg bromocriptine per day for more than a year for severe normoprolactinemic mastopathy, without any significant decrease in basal ACTH levels. In contrast to this finding, we have seen a significant fall of elevated ACTH levels in one patient who, after bilateral adrenalectomy in 1969 for Cushing's disease and pituitary operation for acromegaly shortly after the adrenalectomy still had several years

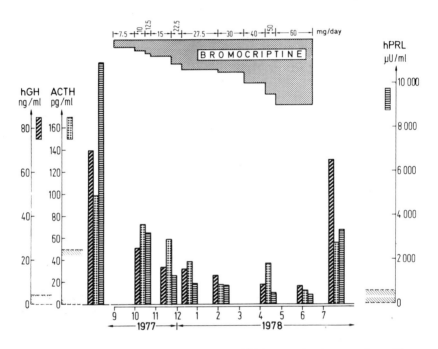

*Fig. 8.* Effect of bromocriptine on hGH, ACTH and hPRL secretion in one patient with a pituitary triple-hormone-excess. This patient had been treated by bilateral adrenalectomy for Cushing's disease and by transfrontal pituitary surgery for acromegaly 9 years ago. He now has recurrence of acromegaly and hyperprolactinemia whereas his ACTH levels are only slightly elevated. Bromocriptine leads to a suppression of all three hormones, which rise to pretreatment level after bromocriptine withdrawal, with the exception of prolactin, which again remains significantly lower compared to the pretreatment level.

later ACTH-, GH- and PRL-hypersecretion (Fig. 8). This patient has also responded acutely to somatostatin (Müller *et al.*, 1978b) with a fall of ACTH levels, as described by Tyrrell *et al.* (1975). The reason for long-term bromocriptine therapy in this patient is the recurrence of acromegaly and hyperprolactinemia.

## CONCLUSION

From our experience in the treatment of hyperprolactinemic patients with and without pituitary adenomas we can draw the following conclusions:

(1) Hyperprolactinemia associated with pituitary adenomas can be treated surgically, medically and with radiotherapy.

(2) The primary therapy in all patients with macroprolactinomas should be surgical.

(3) In females with macroprolactinomas or microprolactinomas with prolactin levels above 5000 $\mu$U/ml who want to become pregnant, a gentle neurosurgical procedure should induce nomalization or lowering of prolactin secretion without disturbing the gonadotropic function, so that postoperative treatment with bromocriptine therapy can lead to normal ovulatory cycles.

(4) In patients with microadenomas and prolactin levels below 5000 $\mu$U/ml, bromocriptine alone is indicated. If pregnancy occurs, these patients have to be monitored appropriately.

(5) There is good evidence that bromocriptine exerts an anti-proliferative effect on pituitary tumor growth, particularly in the larger adenomas. Bromocriptine should therefore be given not only to ameliorate the symptoms caused by hyperprolactinemia but also in order to prevent pituitary adenoma recurrence, if prolactin levels remain elevated after operation or rise again.

(6) It seems that postoperative radiotherapy and bromocriptine are equally effective. Whether they should be combined or one can replace the other form of therapy is still an open question.

Reviewing the present state of medical therapy of pituitary ACTH-dependent Cushing's disease and the tremendous advances in pituitary microsurgery (Müller *et al.*, 1978a; Tyrrell *et al.*, 1978) we feel that it is justified to subject to a transsphenoidal exploration every patient with this rather rare disease, even when there is a normal sella turcica. As has been shown in most instances, a microadenoma will be found and can be removed, thus curing the disease (Tyrrell *et al.*, 1978). These excellent operative results should not prevent us from looking for effective medical therapy, which may be particualrly indicated for the hypothalamus-induced ACTH hypersecretion, if we find methods to demonstrate that there is indeed such a disease.

So far, suffice it to say that medical therapy for pituitary ACTH-dependent Cushing's disease is still at an experimental stage.

## REFERENCES

Bergh, T., Nillins, S. J. and Wide, L. (1978). *Br. Med. J.* **1**, 875–880.
Besser, G. M., Jeffcoate, W. J. and Tomlin, S. (1976). *Vth Int. Congr. of Endocrinol., Hamburg. Abstr.* **494**, p. 202.
Child, D. F., Burke, C. W., Burley, D. M., Rees, L. H. and Fraser, T. R. (1976). *Acta Endocrinol.* **82**, 330–341.
Cotes, P. M. (1973). *In* "Human Prolactin" (P. G. Crosignani and C. Robyn, eds) pp. 97–101. Amsterdam, Excerpta Medica.

Fahlbusch, R., Rjosk, H. K. and von Werder, K. (1978). *In* "Treatment of Pituitary Adenomas" (R. Fahlbusch and K. von Werder, eds) pp. 225–237. Georg Thieme Publishers, Stuttgart.

Fahlbusch, R., Giovanelli, M., Crosignani, P. G., Faglia, G., Rjosk, H. K. and von Werder, K. (1980). This volume.

Feldman, J. M. (1975). *New Engl. J. Med.* 293, 930–931.

Franks, S., Nabarro, J. D. N. and Jacobs, H. S. (1977). *Lancet* I, 778–780.

Frantz, A. G. (1978). *New Engl. J. Med.* 298, 201–203.

Frantz, A. G. and Kleinberg, D. L. (1978). *Fed. Proc.* 37, 2192–2196.

Friesen, H. G. and Tolis, G. (1977). *Clin. Endocr.* 6, Suppl., 91–99.

Gomez, F., Reyes, F. I. and Faiman, C. (1977). *Am. J. Med.* 62, 648–660.

Guiot, G. (1978). *In* "Treatment of Pituitary Adenomas" (R. Fahlbusch, and K. von Werder, eds) pp. 202–213. Georg Thieme Publishers, Stuttgart.

Jeffcoate, W. J., Rees, L. H., Tomlin, S., Jones, A. E., Edwards, C. R. W. and Besser, G. M. (1977). *Br. Med. J.* 2, 215–217.

Kleinberg, D. L., Noel, G. L. and Frantz, A. G. (1977). *New Engl. J. Med.* 296, 589–600.

Krieger, D. T. (1973). *J. Clin. Endocrinol.* 36, 277–284.

Krieger, D. T., Amorosa, L. and Linick, F. (1975). *New Engl. J. Med.* 293, 893–896.

Krieger, D. T. and Luria, M. (1976). *J. Clin. Endocrinol.* 43, 1179–1182.

Lamberts, S. W. J., Timmermans, H. A. T., de Jong, F. H. and Birkenhäger, J. C. (1977). *Clin. Endocrinol.* 7, 185–193.

Liuzzi, A. and Chiodini, P. G. (1980). This volume.

Liuzzi, A., Chiodini, P. G., Oppizzi, G., Botalla, L., Verde, G., di Stefano, C., Colussi, G., Gräf, K. J. and Horowski, R. (1978). *J. Clin. Endocrinol.* 46, 196–202.

Lloyd, H. M., Meares, J. D. and Jacobi, J. (1975). *Nature* 225, 497–498.

Miura, H., Aida, M., Mihara, A., Kato, K., Ojima, M., Demura, R., Demura, H. and Okuyama, M. (1975). *J. Clin. Endocrinol.* 41, 511–526.

Moore, T. J., Dluhy, R. G., Williams, G. H. and Cain, J. P. (1976). *Ann. Int. Med.* 85, 731–734.

Mornex, R., Orgiazzi, J., Hugues, B., Gagnaire, J. C. and Claustrat, B. (1978). *J. Clin. Endocrinol.* 47, 290–295.

Müller, O. A. Marguth, F. and Scriba, P. C. (1976). *Vth Int. Congr. of Endocrinol., Hamburg. Abstr.* 491, p. 201.

Müller, O. A., Baur, X., Fahlbusch, R., Madler, M., Marguth, F., Uhlig, C. and Scriba, P. C. (1978a). *In* "Treatment of Pituitary Adenomas" (R. Fahlbusch and K. von Werder, eds) pp. 343–351. Georg Thieme Publishers, Stuttgart.

Müller, O. A., Fink, R., von Werder, K. and Scriba, P. C. (1978b). *Acta Endocrinol. (Kbh.)* 87 Suppl. 215, 4–5.

Orth, D. N. (1978). *Ann. Int. Med.* 89, 128–130.

Orth, D. N. and Liddle, G. W. (1971). *New Engl. J. Med.* 285, 243–247.

Peillon, F., Vila-Porcile, E., Olivier, L. and Radacot, J. (1970). *Ann. Endocrinol. (Paris)* 31, 259–270.

von Petrykowski, W., Brämswig, J., Girard, J., Beck, U. and Marquetand, D. (1977). *Acta Endocrinol. (Kbh)* Suppl. 208, 83–84.

Plonk, J. and Feldman, J. M. (1976). *J. Clin. Endocrinol.* 42, 291–295.

del Pozo, E., Brun del Re, R., Varga, L. and Friesen, H. (1972). *J. Clin. Endocrinol.* 35, 768–771.

Rjosk, H. K., von Werder, K. and Fahlbusch, R. (1976). *Geburtshilfe und Frauenheilkunde* 36, 575–587.

Rjosk, H. K., Fahlbusch, R., Huber, H. and von Werder, K. (1980). This volume.
Schnall, A. M., Brodkey, J. S., Kaufman, B. and Pearson, O. H. (1978). *J. Clin. Endocrinol.* **47**, 410–417.
Smilo, R. P., Earll, J. M. and Forsham, P. H. (1967). *Metabolism* **16**, 374–377.
Sobrinho, L. G., Nunes, M. C. P., Santos, M. A. and Mauricio, J. C. (1978). *Lancet* **II**, 257–258.
Thorner, M. O. (1977). *In* "Clinical Neuroendocrinology" (L. Martini and G. M. Besser, eds) pp. 319–361. Academic Press, New York and London.
Tolis, G. (1977). *Clin. Endocrinol. (Oxf.)* **6**, 81–89.
Tyrrell, J. B., Lorenzi, M., Gerich, J. E. and Forsham, P. H. (1975). *J. Clin. Endocrinol.* **40**, 1125–1127.
Tyrrell, J. B., Brooks, R. M., Fitzgerald, P. A., Coffoid, P. B., Forsham, P. H. and Wilson, C. B. (1978). *New Engl. J. Med.* **298**, 753–758.
von Werder, K., Fahlbusch, R., Landgraf, R., Pickardt, C. R., Rjosk, H. K. and Scriba, P. C. (1978a). *J. Endocrinol. Invest.* **1**, 47–58.
von Werder, K., Felixberger, F., Gottsmann, M., Kerner, W. and Glöckner, B. (1978b). *In* "Radioimmunoassay and Related Procedures in Medicine", pp. 43–57. Int. Atomic Energy Agency, Vienna.
von Werder, K., Gottsmann, J., Brendel, C., Landgraf, R., von Lieven, H., Rjosk, H. K. and Fahlbusch, R. (1978c). *Acta Endocr. (Kbh.), Suppl.* **215**, 1.

# INHIBITION OF PROLACTIN SECRETION BY ACUTE AND CHRONIC METERGOLINE TREATMENT IN HYPER-PROLACTINEMIC PATIENTS WITH PITUITARY MICROADENOMAS OR OTHER DISORDERS*

C. Ferrari[1], P. Travaglini[2], A. Mattei[3], R. Caldara[1], P. Moriondo[2], M. Romussi[1], and P. G. Crosignani[3]

[1] 2nd Department of Medicine, Fatebenefratelli Hospital, University of Milan, Milan, Italy [2] 2nd Medical Clinic, Endocrine Unit, University of Milan, Milan, Italy [3] Section of Endocrinology, Department of Obstetrics and Gynecology, University of Milan, Milan, Italy

## INTRODUCTION

Metergoline, an ergoline derivative with potent peripheral (Beretta *et al.*, 1965) and central (Fuxe *et al.*, 1975; Sastry and Phillis, 1977; Enjalbert *et al.*, 1978) antiserotoninergic properties, has been shown to inhibit prolactin (PRL) release during acute or short-term administration in normal subjects (Ferrari *et al.*, 1976, 1978), in puerperal women (Crosignani *et al.*, 1978), in acromegalics (Chiodini *et al.*, 1976), and in several hyperprolactinemic patients (Ferrari *et al.*, 1979a). Preliminary studies demonstrated that this drug may lower serum PRL concentration and/or restore ovarian function during chronic treatment in some subjects with hyperprolactinemic amenorrhea (Crosignani *et al.*, 1977a, b; Ferrari *et al.*, 1979b). The present study was designed to evaluate the effects of acute and chronic metergoline administration on serum PRL levels and on gonadal function in a large number of hyperprolactinemic patients with pituitary microadenomas or other disorders.

*We thank Farmitalia S.p.A., Milan, for the generous supply of metergoline (Liserdol). This study was partially supported by CNR, Special Program Biology of Reproduction.

## MATERIALS AND METHODS

Sixty-one hyperprolactinemic patients (56 females aged 18–41 and 5 males aged 18–44 years) were studied. Nine subjects (6 females and 3 males) were considered to have pituitary macroadenomas on the basis of enlarged sella turcica found by standard radiologic techniques and of pneumoencephalographic findings; this diagnosis was surgically confirmed in the 6 patients who were subsequently operated on. In 28 women, pituitary microadenomas were diagnosed by finding localized blister deformities and undermineralization of the sella in tomography, in the presence of normal standard X-ray studies (Hardy, 1973). The diagnosis was then confirmed at surgery in the 10 operated patients. No abnormalities were found in sellar tomographs of the remaining 24 subjects.

The PRL-lowering effect of acute metergoline administration (4 mg by mouth) was evaluated after an overnight fast in 36 patients (16 with pituitary microadenomas, 7 with macroadenomas, and 13 with normal sellar tomography) by determining the serum PRL levels in two basal samples taken at 30 min intervals

*Table I.* Effect of metergoline (MCE) treatment on serum PRL concentrations and ovarian function in 20 women with hyperprolactinemic secondary amenorrhea and pituitary microadenoma (patients No. 1 to 16) or macroadenoma (patients 17–20). The diagnosis was confirmed by surgery in patients 1–7 and 17–20.

| Case No. | Age | MCE treatment mg/day | Time (month) | Serum PRL ng/ml Before treatment | During treatment[a] | Clinical outcome |
|---|---|---|---|---|---|---|
| 1 | 31 | 12 | 6 | 155 | 59 | ovulatory menses[b] |
| 2 | 31 | 12 | 4 | 160 | 80 | no bleeding |
| 3 | 22 | 12 | 2 | 250 | 184 | no bleeding |
| 4 | 37 | 12 | 2 | 185 | 120 | one bleeding |
| 5 | 24 | 12 | 1 | 260 | 126 | no bleeding |
| 6 | 34 | 12 | 3 | 70 | 5 | one bleeding |
| 7 | 24 | 12 | 2 | 135 | 99 | no bleeding |
| 8 | 38 | 8–12 | 8 | 44 | 30 | ovulatory menses[b] |
| 9 | 29 | 12 | 4 | 101 | 19 | ovulatory menses[b] |
| 10 | 35 | 12 | 4 | 60 | 9 | pregnancy[c] |
| 11 | 30 | 12 | 2 | 96 | 10 | pregnancy |
| 12 | 26 | 12 | 3 | 84 | 10 | ovulatory menses[b] |
| 13 | 32 | 12 | 2 | 212 | 58 | no bleeding |
| 14 | 32 | 12 | 4 | 85 | 13 | ovulatory menses[b] |
| 15 | 34 | 12 | 3 | 150 | 32 | ovulatory menses[b] |
| 16 | 37 | 6–12 | 3 | 104 | 20 | ovulatory menses[b] |
| 17 | 35 | 12 | 2 | 116 | 20 | no bleeding |
| 18 | 21 | 12 | 3 | 45 | 2 | no bleeding |
| 19 | 41 | 8 | 3 | 1000 | 355 | no bleeding |
| 20 | 29 | 12 | 2 | 200 | 141 | no bleeding |

[a]Mean of at least 2 morning samples taken during the last month of treatment.
[b]As judged by serum progesterone levels above 3 ng/ml in the presumed luteal phase.
[c]A normal baby was delivered at term.

*Table II.* Effects of metergoline (MCE) treatment on serum PRL concentrations and ovarian function in 16 hyperprolactinemic women with normal sellar tomography.

| Case No. | Age | Clinical diagnosis | MCE treatment | | Serum PRL ng/ml | | Clinical outcome |
|---|---|---|---|---|---|---|---|
| | | | mg/day | Time (month) | Before treatment | During treatment[a] | |
| 1 | 19 | Primary amenorrhea | 8–12 | 21 | 95 | 12 | menarche after 15 months[b] |
| 2 | 33 | Secondary amenorrhea | 8 | 1 | 39 | 19 | no bleeding |
| 3 | 30 | Secondary amenorrhea | 12 | 3 | 80 | 4 | ovulatory menses[c] |
| 4 | 33 | Secondary amenorrhea | 8 | 2 | 183 | 50 | pregnancy[d] |
| 5 | 18 | Secondary amenorrhea | 12 | 3 | 32 | 4 | ovulatory menses[c] |
| 6 | 30 | Secondary amenorrhea | 12 | 3 | 112 | 53 | no bleeding |
| 7 | 31 | Secondary amenorrhea | 12 | 5 | 120 | 20 | two bleedings |
| 8 | 40 | Secondary amenorrhea | 12 | 3 | 90 | 36 | ovulatory menses[c] |
| 9 | 26 | Secondary amenorrhea | 12 | 4 | 200 | 20 | pregnancy[d] |
| 10 | 27 | Secondary amenorrhea | 12 | 2 | 50 | 10 | pregnancy[d] |
| 11 | 34 | Secondary amenorrhea | 12 | 2 | 54 | 48 | ovulatory menses[c] |
| 12 | 29 | Secondary amenorrhea | 12 | 3 | 60 | 19 | no bleeding |
| 13 | 19 | Anov. oligomenorrhea | 12 | 3 | 38 | 8 | ovulatory menses[c] |
| 14 | 39 | Anov. polymenorrhea | 6–12 | 5 | 56 | 15 | ovulatory menses[c] |
| 15 | 24 | Isolated galactorrhea | 8–12 | 2 | 39 | 13 | reduced galactorrhea |
| 16 | 27 | Isolated galactorrhea | 8–12 | 1 | 38 | 19 | reduced galactorrhea |

[a] Mean of at least 2 morning samples taken during the last month of treatment.
[b] Five other bleedings occurred during the 6 following months.
[c] As judged by serum progesterone levels above 3 ng/ml in the presumed luteal phase.
[d] A normal baby was delivered at term.

and 120, 180 and 240 min after drug ingestion. The same procedure had also been performed in 34 healthy subjects (Ferrari *et al.*, 1978) who served as controls. On separate days, the same 36 hyperprolactinemic patients were given bromocriptine, 2.5 mg by mouth, and serum PRL was measured at the same time intervals.

The effect of chronic metergoline treatment (6-12 mg/day in 3 divided doses for 1-21 months) on serum PRL concentrations and on ovarian function was investigated in 36 hyperprolactinemic women with secondary or primary amenorrhea, anovulation and/or galactorrhea. Sixteen of them had pituitary microadenomas, 4 had macroadenomas, and 16 had normal sellar tomography. The relevant clinical data are reported in Tables I and II. Serum PRL was determined in all patients in at least two morning samples before starting therapy and during the last month of treatment. Serum progesterone was measured in the presumed luteal phase whenever possible, and ovulation was presumed to have occurred when progesterone levels above 3 ng/ml were obtained (Israel *et al.*, 1972).

Serum PRL was evaluated by radioimmunoassay according to Sinha *et al.* (1973), using the reagents supplied by Biodata-Serono (Rome). In our laboratory the normal range is 2-15 ng/ml for males and 4-20 ng/ml for females. Serum progesterone was measured by the radioimmunoassay method of Hotchkiss *et al.* (1971).

The statistical analysis was performed by the two-tailed Student's $t$ test, for paired or unpaired data as appropriate.

## RESULTS

Acute metergoline administration was followed by highly significant decreases in mean serum PRL levels in all 3 groups of hyperprolactinemic patients as well as in normal subjects (Fig. 1). However, serum PRL was suppressed to below 50% of the basal level in only 25 of 36 patients (10 of 16 with pituitary microadenomas, 5 of 7 with macroadenomas, and 10 of 13 with normal sellas). After acute bromocriptine administration, serum PRL was decreased to below 50% of the basal level in 28 of the 36 patients (12 of 16 with microadenomas, 4 of 7 with macroadenomas, and 12 of 13 with normal sellas) (Fig. 2). Although there was no significant difference between the mean PRL-lowering effects of the two drugs in any group considered, the PRL-suppressive responses to metergoline and bromocriptine were dissociated in 7 patients, 2 of them being inhibited only by metergoline (1 with micro- and 1 with macroadenoma) and 5 by bromocriptine (3 with microadenomas and 2 with normal sellas). Chronic metergoline treatment (Tables I and II) was associated with a reduction of serum PRL concentration to below 50% of the basal level in 30 of 36 patients (12 of 16 with microadenomas, 3 of 4 with macroadenomas, and 15 of 16 with normal sellas), and with actual normalization (< 20 ng/ml) in 21 cases (7 with microadenomas, 2 with macroadenomas, and 12 with normal sellas). Of 29 patients with secondary amenorrhea who were treated for at least two months, pregnancy occurred in 5, presumptive evidence of ovulation was obtained in 11, and menses were restored in 3 others. Resumption of menstruation or pregnancy were observed after 1 to 4 months of

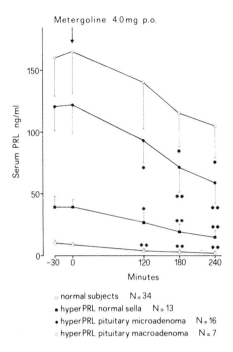

Metergoline 4.0 mg p.o.

□ normal subjects    N = 34
■ hyper PRL normal sella    N = 13
● hyper PRL pituitary microadenoma    N = 16
○ hyper PRL pituitary macroadenoma    N = 7

*Fig. 1.* Effect of acute metergoline administration on serum PRL concentrations in normal subjects and in hyperprolactinemic patients. Results are means ± s.e.m. Asterisks indicate significant differences from basal values (one asterisk, $P < 0.01$; two asterisks, $P < 0.001$).

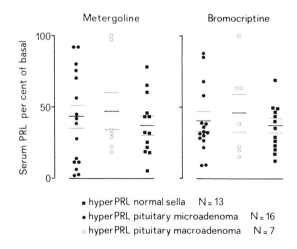

■ hyper PRL normal sella    N = 13
● hyper PRL pituitary microadenoma    N = 16
○ hyper PRL pituitary macroadenoma    N = 7

*Fig. 2.* Effect of acute metergoline (4 mg, p.o.) or bromocriptine (2.5 mg, p.o.) administration on serum PRL levels in individual hyperprolactinemic patients. Each point represents the nadir level in per cent of basal value. Mean and s.e.m. values are also indicated.

treatment. Two other patients suffering from anovulation had ovulatory menses during treatment. Galactorrhea was markedly reduced in 18 of 30 cases, and disappeared in 8. Menarche was induced after 15 months of treatment in a 19-year-old girl with hyperprolactinemic primary amenorrhea, and 5 other bleedings occurred in the 6 following months.

No consistent side effects were noticed by any patient. Hematologic values and blood chemistries including liver and kidney function tests were normal throughout the treatment period in all cases.

## DISCUSSION

The present study confirms in a larger series of patients our previous finding that metergoline acutely inhibits PRL release in hyperprolactinemic subjects in a manner similar to that of the dopamine agonist, bromocriptine (Ferrari *et al.*, 1979a). Although failure of PRL suppression by metergoline appears to be somewhat more frequent in patients with pituitary adenomas than in those with normal sellar tomography, the present findings indicate that metergoline administration has no greater value for differentiating tumoral and nontumoral hyperprolactinemia than other PRL inhibition tests, such as L-dopa (Kleinberg *et al.*, 1977), bromocriptine (Gomez *et al.*, 1977; Faglia *et al.*, 1977), and dopamine infusion (Reschini *et al.*, in preparation).

It was previously reported in preliminary or single case studies that chronic metergoline treatment may be of value in some patients with hyperprolactinemic secondary amenorrhea. Of 9 treated subjects, serum PRL was consistently reduced in 3, of whom one had resumption of menses and one became pregnant; menstruation and possibly ovulation also occurred in 2 other patients, in spite of only slight lowering of serum PRL (Crosignani *et al.*, 1977a, b; Ferrari *et al.*, 1979b). The present investigation demonstrates in a large number of hyperprolactinemic women that metergoline is an effective and safe PRL-lowering drug, both in patients with pituitary adenomas and in those with apparently normal sella, and that ovulation and menses can be restored in the majority of subjects without large pituitary tumors. As a matter of fact, there were only 2 treatment failures among 13 patients with hyperprolactinemic anovulation and normal sellar tomography, and 4 among 15 patients with pituitary microadenoma, while none of the 4 subjects with macroadenoma had resumption of menses with metergoline. These last patients had severely impaired gonadotropin secretion. The present data suggest that metergoline treatment is nearly as effective as bromocriptine (Crosignani *et al.*, 1977a; Thorner and Besser, 1977; Franks *et al.*, 1977; Kleinberg *et al.*, 1977) in the management of hyperprolactinemic states. Although restoration of ovarian function by metergoline is probably dependent on suppression of the elevated PRL levels, a direct stimulation of gonadotropin release might also be operating in some cases in whom PRL suppression was either minimal or undetectable in morning samples taken at various intervals during treatment (see Table I, Case No. 8; Table II, Case No. 11). Such an action of the drug could be explained on the basis of reports suggesting that serotonin is inhibitory to gonadotropin release, both in animals (Arendash and Gallo, 1978) and in man (Feldman *et al.*, 1974).

Based on the neuropharmacological profile of metergoline and on evidence implicating serotonin in the stimulation of PRL release in animals (see Lawson and Gala, 1978, for review) and in man, the PRL-lowering action of the drug has been attributed to its antiserotoninergic properties (Ferrari *et al.*, 1976, 1978, 1979a). Stimulation of dopamine receptors might also explain the PRL-suppressive effect of metergoline, as suggested by Chiodini *et al.* (1976) on the basis of studies performed in acromegalic patients. However, several arguments speak against this hypothesis. Metergoline blocks postsynaptic dopamine receptors in the rat brain (Enjalbert *et al.*, 1978). It does not inhibit PRL release by the rat pituitary *in vitro* (Cocchi *et al.*, 1979), an action which is a prerequisite for dopamine agonists (MacLeod and Lehmeyer, 1974). Its PRL-lowering effect is unaffected by blockade of dopamine receptors with pimozide in normal humans (Ferrari *et al.*, 1978), and it is frequently dissociated from that of bromocriptine in hyperprolactinemic patients, as shown by the present study. The drug does not stimulate GH release (Pontiroli *et al.*, 1975), nor does it reduce serum LH levels (Ferrari, unpublished data) and the TSH response to TRH (Ferrari *et al.*, 1976), all known properties of dopamine agonists (Müller *et al.*, 1977; Lachelin *et al.*, 1977; Spaulding *et al.*, 1972). Although this evidence indicates that metergoline does not possess dopaminergic properties *per se*, the possibility cannot be excluded that the drug might indirectly stimulate dopamine receptors, either via hypothetical metabolite(s) synthesized following *in vivo* administration, or as a result of blockade of serotoninergic neurotransmission (Caligaris and Taleisnik, 1974). These hypothetical actions of the drug could perhaps mediate some effects exerted by metergoline in pathological conditions associated with supersensitivity of pituitary dopamine receptors, such as acromegaly (Müller *et al.*, 1977) and hypothalamic diseases (Cheung and Weiner, 1978).

## REFERENCES

Arendash, G. W. and Gallo, R. V. (1978). *Endocrinology* **102**, 1199–1206.
Beretta, C., Ferrini, R. and Glasser, A. H. (1965). *Nature* **207**, 421–422.
Caligaris, L. and Taleisnik, S. (1974). *J. Endocr.* **62**, 25–33.
Cheung, C. Y. and Weiner, R. I. (1978). *Endocrinology* **102**, 1614–1620.
Chiodini, P. G., Liuzzi, A., Müller, E. E., Botalla, L., Cremascoli, G., Oppizzi, G., Verde, G. and Silvestrini, F. (1976). *J. Clin. Endocr. Metab.* **43**, 356–363.
Cocchi, D., Locatelli, V., Carminati, R. and Müller, E. E. (1979). *Life Sci.* (in press).
Crosignani, P. G., Peracchi, M., D'Alberton, A., Lombroso, G. C., Torjsi, L., Cammareri, G., Caccamo, A., Attanasio, A. and Reschini, E. (1977a). *In* "Prolactin and Human Reproduction" (P. G. Crosignani and C. Robyn, eds) pp. 273–283. Academic Press, New York and London.
Crosignani, P. G., Reschini, E., Peracchi, M., D'Alberton, A. and Lombroso, G. C. (1977b). *Br. J. Obstet. Gynaec.* **84**, 386–388.
Crosignani, P. G., Lombroso, G. C., Caccamo, A., Reschini, E. and Peracchi, M. (1978). *Obstet. Gynec.* **51**, 113–115.
Enjalbert, A., Hamon, M., Bourgoin, S. and Bockaert, J. (1978). *Mol. Pharmac.* **14**, 11–23.
Faglia, G., Beck-Peccoz, P., Travaglini, P., Ambrosi, B., Rondena, M., Paracchi, A., Spada, A., Weber, G., Bara, R. and Bouzin, A. (1977). *In* "Prolactin and

Human Reproduction" (P. G. Crosignani and C. Robyn, eds) pp. 225–238. Academic Press, New York and London.

Feldman, J. M., Plonk, J. W. and Bivens, C. E. (1974). *Am. J. Med. Sci.* **268**, 215–226.

Ferrari, C., Paracchi, A., Rondena, M., Beck-Peccoz, P. and Faglia, G. (1976). *Clin. Endocr.* **5**, 575–578.

Ferrari, C., Caldara, R., Romussi, M., Rampini, P., Telloli, P., Zaatar, S. and Curtarelli, G. (1978). *Neuroendocrinology* **25**, 319–328.

Ferrari, C., Caldara, R., Rampini, P., Telloli, P., Romussi, M., Bertazzoni, A., Polloni, G., Mattei, A. and Crosignani, P. G. (1979a). *Metabolism* (in press).

Ferrari, C., Caldara, R., Telloli, P., Rampini, P. and Bertazzoni, A. (1979b). *Fertil. Steril.* (in press).

Franks, S., Jacobs, H. S., Hull, M. G. R., Steele, S. J. and Nabarro, J. D. N. (1977). *Br. J. Obstet. Gynaec.* **84**, 241–253.

Fuxe, K., Agnati, L. and Everitt, B. (1975). *Neurosci. Lett.* **1**, 283–290.

Gomez, F., Reyes, F. I. and Faiman, C. (1977). *Am. J. Med.* **62**, 648–660.

Hardy, J. (1973). *In* "Diagnosis and Treatment of Pituitary Tumors" (P. O. Kohler and G. T. Ross, eds) pp. 179–194. Excerpta Medica, Amsterdam.

Hotchkiss, J., Atkinson, L. E. and Knobil, E. (1971). *Endocrinology* **89**, 177–184.

Israel, R., Mishell, D. R., Stone, S. C., Thorneycroft, I. H. and Moyer, D. L. (1972). *Am. J. Obstet. Gynec.* **112**, 1043–1046.

Kleinberg, D. L., Noel, G. L. and Frantz, A. G. (1977). *New Engl. J. Med.* **296**, 589–600.

Lachelin, G. C. L., Leblanc, H. and Yen, S. S. C. (1977). *J. clin. Endocr. Metab.* **44**, 728–732.

Lawson, D. M. and Gala, R. R. (1978). *Endocrinology* **102**, 973–981.

MacLeod, R. M. and Lehmeyer, J. E. (1974). *Endocrinology* **94**, 1077–1085.

Müller, E. E., Liuzzi, A., Cocchi, D., Panerai, A. E., Oppizzi, G., Locatelli, V., Mantegazza, P., Silvestrini, F. and Chiodini, P. G. (1977). *In* "Advances in Biochemical Psychopharmacology" (E. Costa and G. L. Gessa, eds) Vol. 16, 127–138. Raven Press, New York.

Pontiroli, A. E., Cavagnini, F., Peracchi, M., Bulgheroni, P., Panerai, A. E. and Pinto, M. (1975). *Horm. metab. Res.* **7**, 95–96.

Sastry, B. S. R. and Phillis, J. W. (1977). *Can. J. Physiol. Pharmac.* **55**, 130–133.

Sinha, A. N., Selby, F. W., Lewis, U. J. and Vanderlaan, W. G. (1973). *J. clin. Endocr. Metab.* **36**, 509–516.

Spaulding, S. W., Burrow, G. N., Donabedian, R. and Van Woert, M. (1972). *J. clin. Endocr. Metab.* **35**, 182–185.

Thorner, M. O. and Besser, G. M. (1977). *In* "Prolactin and Human Reproduction" (P. G. Crosignani and C. Robyn, eds) pp. 285–301. Academic Press, New York and London.

# BROMOCRIPTINE-INDUCED REGRESSION OF A PROLACTIN-SECRETING PITUITARY TUMOUR

S. J. Nillius, T. Bergh, P. O. Lundberg, J. Stahle and L. Wide

*Departments of Obstetrics and Gynaecology, Neurology, Otorhinolaryngology and Clinical Chemistry, University Hospital, Uppsala, Sweden*

Dopamine agonists, like the ergot alkaloid derivative bromocriptine, can effectively suppress prolactin hypersecretion in patients with prolactin-secreting pituitary adenomas. These drugs may also affect the growth of such tumours. In experimental animals, ergot alkaloids can inhibit growth and even cause regression of hormone-producing pituitary tumours (Quadri *et al.*, 1972; MacLeod and Lehmeyer, 1973). Bromocriptine has been shown to reduce mitotic activity and inhibit oestrogen-induced proliferation of the pituitary prolactin cells in rats (Lloyd *et al.*, 1975). Several reports on improvement of visual field abnormalities during bromocriptine treatment of patients with prolactin-secreting pituitary adenomas have appeared (Corenblum *et al.*, 1975; Friesen and Tolis, 1977; Bergh *et al.*, 1978a; Besser, 1978; Vaidya *et al.*, 1978), suggesting that bromocriptine may have an anti-tumour effect.

We have recently reported possible bromocriptine-induced tumour regression in a woman with clear clinical, endocrinological and radiological evidence of a prolactin-secreting pituitary adenoma (Nillius *et al.*, 1978). The history of this patient is reviewed below.

## CASE REPORT

The patient was 31 years old and had had 12 years of amenorrhoea-galactorrhoea when bromocriptine treatment was instituted in 1975. Menarche had occurred at age 14, followed by irregular menstrual periods. Amenorrhoea developed at age 19 in connection with a change in residence and working conditions.

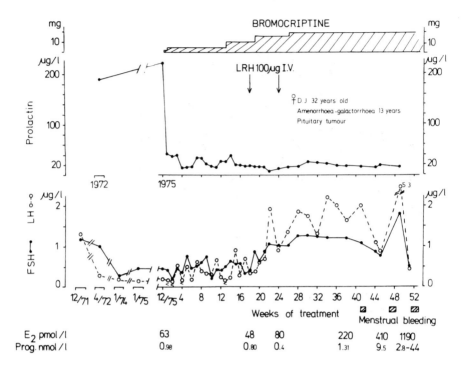

*Fig. 1.* Basal levels of prolactin, FSH and LH before and during the first year of bromocriptine therapy. From Bergh *et al.* (1977). Reproduced with permission of the publisher of *Acta Endocrinologica*.

In an investigation of the amenorrhoea three years later (1966), X-ray of the sella turcica was judged to be normal. The patient received two treatment courses with combined oral contraceptives (2–6 months). She did not return for follow-up.

Five years later, she replied to a postal questionnaire on the epidemiology of amenorrhoea and was offered a clinical examination. She was then found to have galactorrhoea. She had normal thyroid and adrenal function, normal basal serum concentrations of follicle-stimulating hormone (FSH) and luteinizing hormone (LH) but low endogenous oestrogen production. She had no desire for pregnancy and did not receive any treatment until hyperprolactinaemia was diagnosed four years later. The basal gonadotrophin concentrations gradually decreased during this four-year-period (Fig. 1).

X-ray of the sella turcica in 1971 showed a marked asymmetric enlargement of the pituitary fossa (Fig. 2). The visual fields were normal. Re-examination of the sellar X-ray from 1966 revealed that there was a small asymmetry already at that time. The asymmetry was more pronounced on the new X-ray and the sellar volume had increased to 3450 mm³. Follow-up X-rays each year showed no further change in the size and shape of the pituitary fossa.

The pretreatment serum prolactin level was 620 μg/l (NIH reagents hPRL VLS 4 and AFP-anti-hPRL 1). The serum level of prolactin had previously been deter-

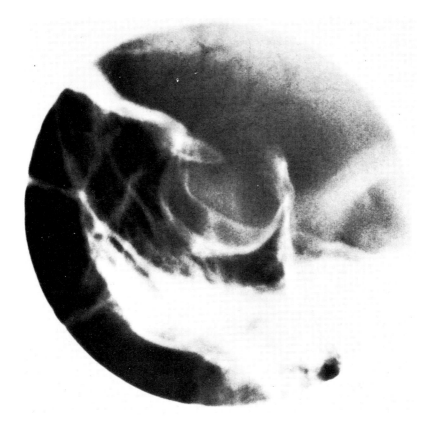

*Fig. 2.* Lateral X-ray of the asymmetric and enlarged pituitary fossa. (From Nillius, S. J., Bergh, T., Lundberg, P. O., Stahle, J., and Wide, L.: Regression of a Prolactin-Secreting Pituitary Tumor During Long-term Treatment With Bromocriptine. Fertil Steril 30: [Dec.] , 1978. Reproduced with the permission of the publisher, *The American Fertility Society*.)

mined in undiluted serum with the use of NIH reagents hPRL VLS 2 and anti-hPRL VLS 3, and found to be more than 200 µg/l (Fig. 1). A high prolactin concentration was also present in frozen serum from 1972. The pretreatment basal gonadotrophin levels were low and so were the gonadotrophin responses to the hypothalamic LH-releasing hormone, LRH (Fig. 3).

During treatment with bromocriptine, the serum prolactin level rapidly decreased towards the upper normal range. The basal levels of FSH and LH gradually increased (Fig. 1). After 18 weeks of treatment, the LH response to LRH was excessive and the FSH response high normal (Fig. 3). An anovulatory bleeding occurred after 40 weeks of treatment, followed by a menstrual cycle with insufficient luteal function (Fig. 1). After that the patient had regular ovulatory menstrual cycles over the next year except for an anovulatory dysfunctional bleeding during treatment week 100 (Fig. 4). The dosage of bromocriptine is shown in Figs 1 and 4.

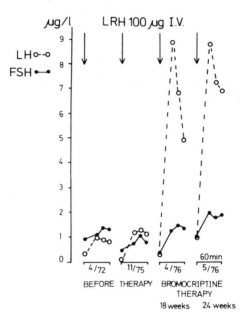

*Fig. 3.* Gonadotrophin responses to LRH before and during bromocriptine therapy. From Bergh *et al.* (1977). Reproduced with permission of the publisher of *Acta Endocrinologica.*

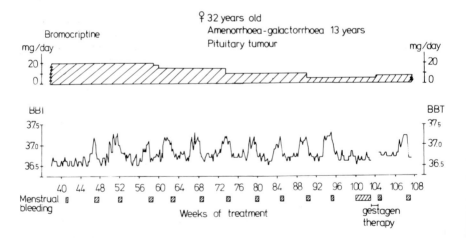

*Fig. 4.* Bromocriptine dosage, basal body temperature and menstrual pattern during the second year of treatment. From Bergh *et al.* (1978b). Reproduced with permission of the publisher of *Acta Endocrinologica.*

After two years of treatment the patient married and wanted to become pregnant. A neuroendocrinological reevaluation was then performed. It included computerized axial tomography, which did not show any suprasellar extension of the tumour. The patient was advised to have her pituitary adenoma surgically removed before attempting a pregnancy.

A transsphenoidal exploration of the pituitary fossa was performed after 27 months of bromocriptine treatment. The left part of the anterior wall and floor of the sella was found to bulge distinctly into the sphenoid sinus as in cases with expanding intrasellar pituitary tumours. The bony wall of the sella turcica was hard and thick in contrast to what is usually found at transsphenoidal removal of large intrasellar tumours. Extradurally there was a 3-4 mm-wide space filled with very loose connective tissue, giving the impression of tumour regression. No pituitary adenoma was identified in the pituitary fossa. Postsurgical reevaluation of the computerized axial tomograms revealed a very slight attenuation of the content of the sella without enhancement after contrast injection.

The bromocriptine treatment was discontinued the day before the operation. The first postoperative ovulation occurred four weeks later at a serum prolactin level of 32 $\mu$g/l (NIH reagents hPRL VLS 4 and AFP-anti-hPRL). The patient conceived after the next ovulation.

## COMMENT

The present case had all the characteristic symptoms and signs of a prolactin-secreting pituitary tumour. She had long-lasting amenorrhoea, galactorrhoea, greatly increased serum prolactin levels and an asymmetrically enlarged pituitary fossa, which had increased in size during the period of amenorrhoea. The serum gonadotrophin levels had gradually decreased and the patient had a severe gonadotrophin deficiency when bromocriptine treatment was instituted.

During the bromocriptine treatment the serum prolactin level decreased and the pituitary gonadotrophin secretion slowly normalized but ovulatory menstrual cycles were regained only after a years treatment with large doses of bromocriptine. Most patients with prolactin-secreting pituitary tumours resume ovulatory function on bromocriptine within 2-3 months (Bergh *et al.*, this volume). After more than two years treatment, evidence suggestive of tumour regression were found in a transsphenoidal exploration of the pituitary fossa.

Further evidence for tumour regression was found at computerized axial tomography (CAT) of the sella turcica. A pituitary tumour may visualize on CAT scan as a mass with an attenuation similar to that of the brain. Contrast usually results in an increase of the attenuation. However, the patient's CAT scan showed a rather low attenuation of the pituitary fossa content without any contrast enhancement.

After discontinuation of bromocriptine in connection with the operation, the patient continued to ovulate spontaneously and later conceived. The clinical and endocrinological responses to the treatment, the findings at operation and in the CAT scan, and the postoperative course strongly suggest that tumour regression occurred during the prolonged bromocriptine treatment.

Other reports on possible anti-tumour effects of bromocriptine in patients with prolactin-secreting pituitary adenomas have recently appeared. Ezrin *et al.* (1978) described tumour regression in a patient with visual field abnormalities due to suprasellar extension of a prolactin-secreting pituitary adenoma. Bromocriptine treatment normalized the visual field defects and repeat pneumoencephalograms after one year of treatment showed shrinkage of the tumour, with air occupying half of the sellar volume. Radiological evidence of partial tumour remission after 13 months of bromocriptine treatment of a patient with a locally invasive prolactin-secreting pituitary tumour was also presented by Sobrinho *et al.* (1978).

The results of these reports need to be confirmed by further studies to decide whether prolonged medical therapy with ergot alkaloid derivatives represents a new possible way to cure patients with prolactin-secreting pituitary tumours.

## REFERENCES

Bergh, T., Nillius, S. J. and Wide, L. (1977). *Acta endocr. (Kbh.)* 86, 683–694.
Bergh, T., Nillius, S. J. and Wide, L. (1978a). *Br. Med. J.* 1, 875–880.
Bergh, T., Nillius, S. J. and Wide, L. (1978b). *In* "The Dopamine Agonist Bromocriptine–Theoretical and Clinical Aspects" (B. Hökfelt and S. J. Nillius, eds) *Acta endocr. (Kbh.)* Suppl. 216, 147–164.
Besser, G. M. (1978). *In* "The Dopamine Agonist Bromocriptine–Theoretical and Clinical Aspects" (B. Hökfelt and S. J. Nillius, eds.) *Acta endocr. (Kbh)* Suppl. 216, 117.
Corenblum, B., Webster, B. R., Mortimer, C. B. and Ezrin, C. (1975). *Clin. Res.* 23, 614A.
Ezrin, C., Kovacs, K. and Horvath, E. (1978). *Med. Clinics North Amer.* 62, 393–408.
Friesen, H. G. and Tolis, G. (1977). *Clin. Endocr.* 6, Suppl., 91s–99s.
Lloyd, H. M., Meares, J. D. and Jacobi, J. (1975). *Nature* 255, 497–498.
MacLeod, R. M. and Lehmeyer, J. E. (1973). *Cancer Res.* 33, 849–855.
Nillius, S. J., Bergh, T., Lundberg, P. O., Stahle, J. and Wide, L. (1979). *Fertil. Steril.* (in press).
Quadri, S. K., Lu, K. H. and Meites, J. (1972). *Science* 176, 417–418.
Sobrinho, L. G., Nunes, M. C. P., Santos, M. A. and Maurício, J. C. (1978). *Lancet* II, 257–258.
Vaidya, R., Aloorkar, A. D., Rege, N. R., Maskati, B. T., Jahangir, R. P., Sheth, A. R. and Pandya, S. K. (1978). *Fertil. Steril.* 29, 632–636.

# REDUCTION IN SIZE OF A PROLACTIN-SECRETING ADENOMA DURING LONG-TERM TREATMENT WITH A DOPAMINE AGONIST (LISURIDE)

P. G. Chiodini[1], A. Liuzzi[1], F. Silvestrini[1], G. Verde[1], R. Cozzi[1], M. T. Marsili[2]
R. Horowski[3], F. Passerini[4], G. Luccarelli[4] and P. G. Borghi[4]

[1] Center of Endocrinology, Ente Ospedaliero, Niguarda, Milano Italy
[2] Department of Ophthalmology, Ente Ospedaliero Niguarda, Milano, Italy
[3] Division of Clinical Research, Schering AG, Berlin, Germany and
[4] Istituto Neurologico C. Besta, Milano, Italy

Dopamine agonists are currently used in the medical treatment of PRL-secreting adenomas owing to their effectiveness in reducing PRL release (Thorner and Besser, 1978; von Werder et al., 1978). However, their place in the therapeutic strategy for this pathological condition is still uncertain because of the lack of a clear-cut demonstration that they can affect tumor growth. The improvement or the normalization of the visual field reported in patients with either GH-(Besser et al., 1978) or PRL-(Thorner and Besser, 1978; Vaidya et al., 1978) secreting adenomas during bromocriptine treatment only suggests an antiproliferative effect of this drug on tumoral cells. In this paper we document by computed axial tomography (CAT) the reduction in size of a PRL-secreting adenoma during a prolonged treatment with a dopamine agonist, lisuride.

## CASE REPORT

A 38-year-old woman sought our help in January 1976 because of secondary amenorrhea lasting for 18 years. Physical examination was normal; galactorrhea was absent, both spontaneously and after breast manipulation. Tests of hypothalamic-pituitary function were performed. Plasma PRL levels about 3000 ng/ml

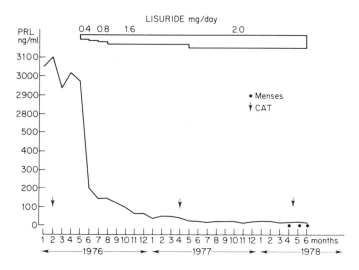

*Fig. 1.* Plasma PRL levels during treatment with lisuride.

were recorded in basal conditions (Fig. 1), without further increase after TRH injection (200 μg, i.v.). Gonadotropin levels were in the normal range but spontaneous fluctuations were absent; after LHRH injection (100 μg, i.v.) a normal rise was recorded. Peak GH values after either arginine infusion (30 g/30 min) or insulin hypoglycemia (0.1 U/kg regular insulin, i.v.) were below 5 ng/ml. Plasma thyroxine, triiodothyronine and TSH levels were normal; TSH increased normally after TRH injection. An enlarged sella turcica was evidenced by skull X-ray; the floor was rounded and eroded, the dorsum sellae was displaced backwards and

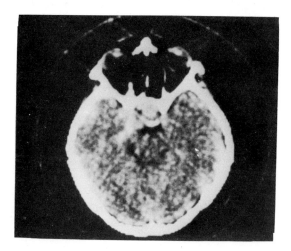

*Fig. 2.* CAT. Plain scan: sella turcica is enlarged and filled with a hyperdense tumor extending on the left side of the sella.

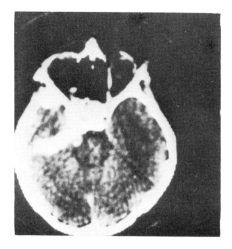

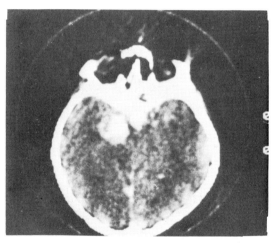

*Fig. 3.* After enhancement the density of the tumor increases. The tumor appears dishomogenous with polylobate borders. The portion of the adenoma evident on the left side of the sella measures approximately 3.5 cm in diameter.

thinned. Thus diagonsis of a PRL-secreting adenoma was made. Left carotid angiography showed vascular changes indicating a parasellar extension of the tumor. CAT showed an enlarged sella turcica filled with a hyperdense tumor extending upwards on the left side of the sella (Figs 2, 3). No visual field defects were demonstrated by either Goldman or Friedman perimetry. As the patient refused to undergo transsphenoidal hypophysectomy, we put her, after informed consent, on lisuride treatment in May 1976. This semisynthetic ergot derivative possesses a long-lasting dopaminergic activity, as shown in experimental (Graf *et al.*, 1976) and in clinical (Liuzzi *et al.*, 1978) studies. The drug was administered orally at doses of 1.6 mg/day given at 0800, 1300, 1800, 2300 h. At this dosage, gradually arrived at from 0.2 mg/day, PRL levels were markedly reduced but not normalized (Fig. 1). After one year of treatment a second CAT was performed: the adenoma appeared to be markedly reduced in size, mainly in its suprasellar portion (Fig. 4). Lisuride dosage was then increased up to 2.0 mg/day and PRL levels ranging between 15 and 25 ng/ml (normal range 2–10 ng/ml) were obtained (Fig. 1). Starting in April 1978, three menses occurred at monthly intervals; progesterone values in the normal range for the luteal phase (5–20 ng/ml) were recorded during the second and the third cycle. In April 1978 a third CAT showed a further reduction in the adenomatous tissue (Fig. 5). Thyroid and adrenal function were reassessed and normal results were again obtained. The GH responses to either

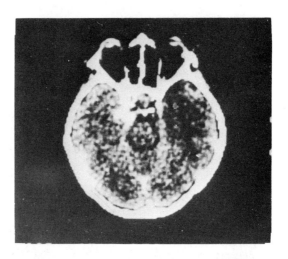

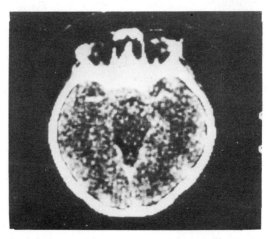

*Fig. 4.* After fourteen months of treatment. CAT by enhancement: the parasellar portion of the adenoma appears markedly reduced in size and with more irregular borders than before therapy.

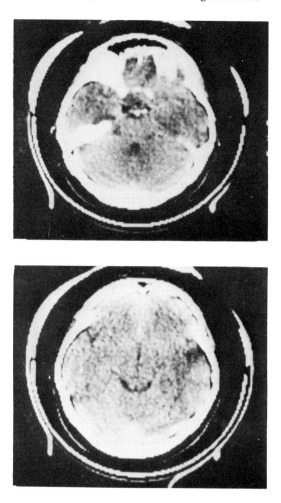

*Fig. 5.* After two years of treatment. CAT by enhancement: a further reduction of the size of the adenoma is evident.

arginine infusion or insulin hypoglycemia were still impaired. Throughout the treatment the visual field, checked at four month intervals, was found to be normal as well as ECG and laboratory tests (complete blood count, serum electrolytes, blood glucose and nitrogen, plasma bilirubin and proteins, urinalysis). The patient complained of mild nausea only at the beginning of the treatment; no other side effects occurred.

Plasma PRL was determined by a double-antibody radioimmunoassay method (kit Biodata-Serono, Rome): 1 ng of the standard employed is equivalent to 1 ng of the NIH standard VLS≠ 1.

The first and the second CAT were performed with EMI MARK 1, the third with EMI CAT 0110.

## DISCUSSION

In this paper the size of a PRL-secreting adenoma is reported to have been markedly reduced during long-term treatment with lisuride. Hypothetically, this reduction might have occurred as the result of pituitary infarction. This seems unlikely, since pituitary infarction is characterized by a dramatic clinical picture which the patient never complained of. In addition, no signs of pituitary insufficiency appeared during the treatment but, when plasma PRL had been lowered by increasing doses of the drug, ovulatory menses appeared after 18 years of amenorrhea. Moreover, CAT did show a gradual reduction in the size of the adenoma without signs of pituitary infarction. Thus, we can suggest that lisuride reduced the tumor size by an antiproliferative effect on the tumoral lactotropic cell replication. This view is reinforced by the demonstration of an inhibitory effect of dopamine agonists on the growth of rat tumor lactotropic cells (MacLeod and Lehmeyer, 1973). Since our patient is still under treatment we cannot say whether she will be cured by lisuride. At present we feel however that patients with large PRL- or GH-secreting adenomas may undergo a therapeutic trial with a dopamine agonist provided that the size of the tumor can be regularly checked by computed axial tomography.

## REFERENCES

Besser, G. M., Wass, J. A. and Thorner, M. O. (1978). *Acta Endocrinol. (Kbh.)* (Suppl) **216**, 187–196.

Graf, K. J., Neumann, F. and Horowski, R. (1976). *Endocrinology* **98**, 598–605.

Liuzzi, A., Chiodini, P. G., Oppizzi, G., Botalla, L., Verde, G., De Stefano, L., Colussi, G., Graf, K. J. and Horowski, R. (1978). *J. Clin. Endocrinol. Metab.* **46**, 196–202.

MacLeod, R. M. and Lehmeyer, J. E. (1973). *Cancer Res.* **33**, 849–853.

Thorner, M. O. and Besser, G. M. (1978). *Acta Endocrinol. (Kbh.)* (Suppl) 216, 131–139.

Vaidya, R. A., Aloorkar, A. D., Rege, N. R., Mascati, B. T., Jahangir, R. P., Shet, A. R. and Pandya, A. K. (1978). *Fertil. Steril.* **29**, 632–637.

von Werder, K., Fahlbusch, R., Landgraf, R., Pickardt, C., Rjosk, H. and Scriba, T. (1978). *J. Endocrinol. Invest.* **1**, 47–58.

# MEDICAL TREATMENT OF AMENORRHEA-GALACTORRHEA: IMPLICATIONS OF GROWTH OF PITUITARY TUMORS DURING PREGNANCY

S. Brem and N. T. Zervas

*Department of Neurosurgery, Massachusetts General Hospital and Harvard Medical School, Boston, Massachusetts, USA*

For women with the syndrome of amenorrhea-galactorrhea, recent advances in pharmacology offer the possibility of control of their disease by medication alone. Recently, bromocriptine has been shown to be an effective dopamine agonist that lowers serum prolactin concentration sufficiently to stop galactorrhea and restore ovulatory cycles in previously infertile women.

Many of these women harbor pituitary adenomas that secrete prolactin, the cause of their amenorrhea-galactorrhea. One group of women have tumors sufficiently large to cause erosion of the sella turcica and/or compress the chiasma leading to visual field defects (Forbes *et al.*, 1954). Another group contains smaller tumors, microadenomas, that cause focal erosion of the sella detected only by sellar polytomes. The incidence of detectable bony deformity in patients with amenorrhea-galactorrhea is approximately 38%. If there is a spectrum of adenomatous hyperplasia, it is reasonable to assume that there is a third group of women with a prolactin-secreting adenoma too small to cause erosion of the sella.

Whatever the size of the tumor, it is well-known that pregnancy may stimulate the rapid enlargement of gland and the tumor, with the severe danger of visual field impairment and possible pituitary apoplexy.

Because of the anticipated widespread use of bromocriptine for induction of pregnancy, it is important to be able to recognize and effectively treat the attendant complications of drugs that restore ovulatory menses in females with large pituitary tumors, microadenomas, or occult pituitary adenomas.

*Table I.* Induced pregnancies complicated by growth of pituitary tumors: clinical summaries, treatment and outcome.

| Pt. # | Author | Induced by | First symptom | Visual symptoms and signs | Treatment | Outcome |
|---|---|---|---|---|---|---|
| 1. | Nelson et al., 1978 | BCT | wk 8: HA and diplopia | OP | tumor removal | Nl. pituitary function. Nl. infant. Nl. vision |
| 2. | Corbey et al., 1977 | BCT | wk 29: visual loss, OD | CC | induced labor | Nl. infant. BCT started post-partum Nl. vision |
| 3. | Van Dalen and Greve, 1977 | ECT | none[a] | CC | tumor removal | Nl. vision. Nl. infant |
| 4. | Thorner et al., 1975 | BCT | none[a] | CC | radiation before pregnancy; induced labor | Nl. vision. Nl. infant |
| 5. | Lamberts et al., 1977 | BCT | none[a] | CC | radiation, $2\frac{1}{2}$ yrs before preg. | Nl. vision. Nl. infant |
| 6. | Wiebe et al., 1977 | 3CT | wk 34: mild DI | none | none | DI cleared within 2 wk post-partum Nl. infant |
| 7. | Bergh et al., 1978 | BCT | 2nd trimester: HA | none | none | Nl. infant |
| 8. | Bergh et al., 1978 | BCT | none[a] | CC | BCT | Post-partum, Nl. vision |
| 9. | Bergh et al., 1978 | BCT | none | none | none | Nl. infant |
| 10. | Bergh et al., 1978 | HMG | decreased vision | CC | none | Nl. vision. Nl. infant |
| 11. | Hervet et al., 1975 | HMG and HCG | wk 24: HA and visual loss | CC | tumor removal | Nl. vision. hormone replacement to mother. Nl. infant |
| 12. | Emperaire et al., 1972 | HMG | 1 month: HA | OP and CC | tumor removal | Nl. vision. Nl. infant |
| 13. | Gemzell, 1975 | HPG and HCG | wk 12: HA | CC | tumor removal | rapid improvement of CC. Nl. twins |
| 14. | Gemzell, 1975 | HPG | wk 32: HA increasing to term | none | induced labor | HA gone after induced labor |

*Table I.* (cont'd)

| Pt. # | Author | Induced by | First symptom | Visual symptoms and signs | Treatment | Outcome |
|---|---|---|---|---|---|---|
| 15. | Gemzell, 1975 | HMG and HCG | wk 8: HA | CC | none | HA gone. Nl. vision. Nl. infant |
| 16. | Gemzell, 1975 | HPG | wk 5: HA and visual loss | CC | none | Nl. twins. Nl. vision. VA |
| 17. | Child et al., 1975 | HMG | within 1st 8 weeks: HA wk 14: blurred vision | CC | Y90 implant pituitary biopsy; induced labor | Nl. infant.? vision |
| 18. | Wolf et al., 1975 | clomiphene | month 4: HA | CC | tumor removal | Nl. twins.? vision |
| 19. | Jewelewicz et al., 1977 | HMG and HCG | wk 22: blurred vision; wk 30: HA and blurred vision | CC | decadron, 12 mg, q.d. | Nl. vision. 9 days post-partum. tumor removal 6 months post-partum with prolactinoma. Nl. triplets |
| 20. | Kajtar and Tomkin, 1971 | HCG | month 2: HA month 7: visual disturbance | CC | tumor removal | Nl. vision. post-op. Nl. infant |
| 21. | Swyer et al., 1971 | HMG and HCG | month 7: cloudy vision, OS | CC | induced labor | vision rapidly returned to Nl. |
| 22. | Burke et al., 1972 | clomiphene | wk 20: HA | none | 90Y implant 1½ yrs before preg. induced labor | HA gone after delivery. triplets (meningomyelocele in 1 child) |
| 23. | Burke et al., 1972 | HMG | first 8 wk: HA wk 14: blurring of vision | CC | 90Y implant, pit bx. | Rapid return of VF after Y90. Nl. infant. |

BCT = bromocriptine; HCG = human chorionic gonadotropin; HMG = human menopausal gonadotropin; HPG = human pituitary gonadotropin; HA = headache; DI = diabetes insipidus; OP = ophthalmoplegia; CC = chiasmal compression; VA = visual acuity; Nl. = normal; OD = right eye; OS = left eye. [a] Asymptomatic visual loss detected by routine exam.

*Table II.*   Peak prolactin levels and radiologic examination of the sella in women
with induced pregnancies complicated by growth of pituitary tumors.

| Pt. # | Peak prolactin level (ng/ml) | Radiologic study of the sella | |
| | | Before pregnancy | During pregnancy |
| --- | --- | --- | --- |
| 1. | 235 | – | A |
| 2. | 185 | A | A |
| 3. | 87 | N | N |
| 4. | 203 | A | – |
| 5. | 68 | A | – |
| 6. | 126 | N | – |
| 7. | 46 | A | A |
| 8. | 72 | A | A |
| 9. | 60 | A | A |
| 10. | 430 | A | A |
| 11. | – | – | A |
| 12. | – | N | A |
| 13. | – | N | A |
| 14. | – | A | A |
| 15. | – | N | A |
| 16. | – | N | A |
| 17. | – | A | A |
| 18. | – | A | A |
| 19. | 900 | N | A |
| 20. | – | A | A |
| 21. | – | N | A |
| 22. | – | – | A |
| 23. | – | A | A |

A = abnormal; N = normal; – = not known or not done.

This report will review the previously recorded instances of tumor growth
occurring during pregnancy of medically-treated females with amenorrhea-
galactorrhea (Tables I and II).

## INCIDENCE

The combined experience of several authors indicates that 6% of all patients
presenting with amenorrhea have a pituitary tumor as evidenced by an abnormal
sella. In those patients with both amenorrhea and hyperprolactinemia, the
figure rises to 38% (Rjosk and Werderk, 1976; Bergh *et al.*, 1977; Franks, 1977).
In 316 patients who presented with galactorrhea, 30% had abnormal sellae
(Gomez *et al.*, 1977; Kleinberg *et al.*, 1977; Nader *et al.*, 1976). In another 315
patients presenting with the amenorrhea-galactorrhea syndrome the possibility
of abnormal sellae was 38% (Fossati *et al.*, 1976; Mroueh and Siler-Khodr,
1977; Spark *et al.*, 1976).

Gemzell (1975) estimated the incidence of visual complications during induced
pregnancy to be approximately 3%. He reported 4 cases in which the sella turcica
increased in size during pregnancy. In addition to Gemzell's 4 cases, there have
been 8 additional cases of tumor growth during gonadotropin-induced pregnancy.

## BROMOCRIPTINE

Bromocriptine is an effective treatment of hyperprolactinemia, and will enable many patients with prolactin-secreting adenomas of the pituitary gland to become fertile. Although it has several side effects (nausea, vertigo, orthostatic hypotension, abdominal cramps, constipation and diarrhea), it is generally well-tolerated (Spark *et al.*, 1976). Bromocriptine-induced pregnancies have been associated with a high rate of spontaneous abortions during the first trimester (Bergh *et al.*, 1978). The drug had been temporarily restricted in the United States because of a feared teratogenic potential. Bergh *et al.* (1978) based on the European experience of 369 bromocriptine-induced childbirths, have unequivocally stated that bromocriptine is non-teratogenic.

The major damage in using bromocriptine to induce ovulation is that it corrects the hormonal imbalance but does not eradicate the tumor mass. Given the physiologic stimulus for the pituitary gland and pituitary adenomas to enlarge, there is a significant risk of catastrophic apoplexy resulting in visual loss.

## SYMPTOMS

In 24 patients with amenorrhea-galactorrhea, the age at time of pregnancy ranged from 21–37, with a mean age of 28 years. There was one case of primary amenorrhea, the others were all secondary with the duration of amenorrhea lasting from 1 to 17 years before pregnancy, with a mean of seven years. Nelson *et al.* (1978), in a briefer review of 12 cases, noted a correlation between the length of the period of amenorrhea and the duration of pregnancy before onset of symptoms. Patients who developed symptoms after the sixth month of pregnancy tended to have longer durations of amenorrhea (10.2 years) than those before the sixth month (3–8 years). The additional cases here would support this general trend. This difference may reflect variation in the growth potential of the tumors. Patients with amenorrhea for many years probably have slower growing tumors, less affected by the stimulus of pregnancy.

The cardinal symptoms of pituitary tumor growth during pregnancy are (1) headaches and (2) visual loss. Fourteen patients presented with a severe headache; four of these patients also had persistent vomiting. Five patients noticed visual deterioration associated with their headaches. Three other patients had visual symptoms without headaches. Ten patients did not complain of visual loss had or developed field cuts and other ocular signs. Thus, a total of 18 of 23 patients had neuroophthalmic complication.

Two patients had extraocular palsies from lateral extension of the tumor. Headache occurred simultaneously with symptoms of visual loss in five patients. The headaches preceded symptoms of visual loss in 5 patients and followed visual loss in one patient. Seven patients showed signs of visual loss without complaining of headache, and in 5 of these patients, the field cuts were detected only by routine examination. Three patients had headache without visual loss. One patient was asymptomatic and had no signs of enlargement but tumor growth was detected by routine skull film. Another woman first had signs of tumor enlargement in the development of diabetes insipidus.

Eleven patients had prolactin levels recorded. The peak prolactin levels ranged from 46 to 900 ng/ml. In women with amenorrhea-galactorrhea, the probability of finding a pituitary tumor correlates with the level of serum prolactin (Frantz, 1978; Boyd *et al.*, 1977; Nader *et al.*, 1976). Boyd *et al.* (1977) suggested a level of 150 as virtually diagnostic of the presence of an adenoma. However, many patients with levels of less than 150 ng/ml will have adenomas. In the present series, 6 of 11 patients with evidence of tumor growth had prolactin levels of less than 150. It is of interest, that none of these 6 women had visual field cuts detected on examination. On the other hand, five patients who complained of visual loss had a mean prolactin level of 391. Those without visual symptoms had a mean prolactin level of 77.

Radiologic evidence of enlargement of the sella was present in 21 (91%) of patients. Six of these patients showed evidence of parasellar or suprasellar extension; all of these patients had either ocular palsies or bitemporal field cuts, respectively.

In each case, vision was satisfactorily restored, although the management varied. Nine patients underwent emergency hypophysectomies (including two patients with $^{90}$Y implants). When the visual field change or sellar erosion was minimal or when tumor growth occurred near the end of the pregnancy, conservative measures were used. These included induction of labor (six patients, three of whom received prior irradiation), and bromocriptine (one patient). Six patients were followed without any surgical or pharmacologic intervention.

Vision rapidly returned to normal following surgical decompression of the sella, or promptly after the pregnancy had been completed. The bony enlargement and erosion of the sella persisted. There were 30 infants, including 5 multiple births. All were normal except for one infant with a meningomyelocele.

A case of particular interest, while not related to pregnancy, has some features which are pertinent to this presentation. The woman in question has had amenorrhea since a single menstruation at age 12. At age 23 skull films of the sella were normal. When she was 25 years of age, Pergonal was administered in an attempt to induce pregnancy. Within a few weeks she developed severe headache, nausea and blurring of vision. Ophthalmologic examination revealed no abnormalities. Subsequently, however, skull films showed asymmetry and erosion of the sella. Biopsy revealed a chromophobe adenoma and radiation therapy was administered (4500 R). The patient was well thereafter, although later she developed mild hypopituitarism requiring replacement therapy. Pergonal was again administered in 1974. Within the first cycle of treatment the patient again developed nausea and vomiting, visual blurring, and this time ptosis of the left lid. An ophthalmologist was unable to detect any evidence of diplopia or visual loss and the patient's symptoms subsided following steroid therapy. Thereafter the patient remained well except for the fact that when prolactin assays became available, her serum level was found to be 1500. This case appears to suggest again that the ovarian stimulation associated with pregnancy will in turn cause enlargement of the contents of the sella due to prolactin stimulation by estrogen.

## DISCUSSION

This analysis of reports of the consequences of pregnancy in patients with small pituitary adenomas suggests that the risk is a small one. Bromocriptine therapy does not appear to be contraindicated for the induction of pregnancy, nor does it appear that patients with small pituitary tumors should be discouraged from carrying forward a pregnancy. Mornex *et al.* (1978) have confirmed the efficacy and safety of bromocriptine therapy in a group of young women with sterility. In most cases recovery of visual function and resolution of headache will occur without any form of treatment whatsoever. A posture of watchful waiting in these patients as the third trimester is spanned can be supported. While some have advocated X-ray therapy in these patients it does not appear that there is sufficient evidence to support that point of view. The indications for hypophysectomy for the removal of a pituitary tumor in these patients have not been established. However, the degree of pituitary enlargement, viz. chiasmal compression, and the level of prolactin should be the basis for this decision. Certainly, progressive visual loss is the prime indication for surgical intervention. From this review of the current literature it does not appear that the hazards of chiasmal compression are so great as to preclude bromocriptine therapy in patients without evidence of suprasellar tumors, but that awareness of the potential problems can lead to their early resolution.

## REFERENCES

Bergh, T., Nillius, S. J. and Wide, L. (1977). *Acta. Endocrinol.* **86**, 683–694.

Bergh, T., Nillius, S. J. and Wide, L. (1978). *Brit. Med. J.* **1**, 875–880.

Boyd, A. E., Reichlin, S. and Turskoy, R. N. (1977). *Ann. Intern. Med.* **87**, 165–175.

Burke, C. W., Joplin, G. F. and Fraser, R. (1972). *Proc. Roy. Soc. Med.* **65**, 486–488.

Child, D. F., Gordon, H., Mashiter, K. *et al.* (1975). *Brit. Med. J.* **4**, 87–89.

Corbey, R. S., Cruysberg, J. R. M. and Rolland, R. (1977). *Obstet. Gynecol.* **50**, (suppl, 1), 69S–71S.

Emperaire, J. C., Riemens, V., Dubecq, J. J. *et al.* (1972). *Bordeau Med.* **15**, 1901–1904.

Forbes, A. P., Henneman, P. H., Griswold, G. C. *et al.* (1954). *J. Clin. Endocrinol. Metab.* **14**, 265–271.

Fossati, P., Strauch, G. and Tournaire, H. (1976). *Nouv. Presse Med.* **5**, 1087–1091.

Franks, S., Jacobs, H. S., Hull, M. G. *et al.* (1977). *Br. J. Obstet. Gynecol.* **84**, 241–253.

Frantz, A. G. (1978). *New Engl. J. Med.* **298**, 201–207.

Gemzell, C. (1975). *Am. J. Obstet, Gynecol.* **121**, 311–315.

Gomez, F., Reyes, F. I. and Faiman, C. (1977). *Am. J. Med.* **62**, 648–660.

Hervet, E., Barrat, J., Pigne, A. *et al.* (1975). *Nouv. Presse Med.* **4**, 2393–2395.

Jewelewicz, R., Zimmerman, E. A. and Carmel, P. W. (1977). *Fertil. Steril.* **28**, 35–40.

Kajtar, T. and Tomkin, G. H. (1971). *Brit. Med. J.* **4**, 88–90.

Kleinberg, D. L., Noel, G. L. and Frantz, A. G. (1977). *New Engl. J. Med.* **296**, 589–600.

Lamberts, S. W. J., Seldenrath, H. G., Kwa, H. G. *et al.* (1977). *J. Clin. Endocrinol. Metab.* **44**, 180–184.

Mornex, R., Orgiazzi, J., Hugues, B. *et al.* (1978). *J. Clin. Endocrinol. Metab.* 290–295.

Mroueh, A. M. and Siler-Khodr, T. M. (1977). *Am. J. Obstet. Gynecol.* **127**, 291–298.

Nader, S., Mashiter, K., Doyle, F. H. *et al.* (1976). *Clin. Endocrin.* **5**, 245–251.

Nelson, P. B., Robinson, A. G., Archer, D. R. *et al.* (1978). *J. Neurosurg.* **49**, 283–287.

Rjosk, H. K. and Werderk, F. R. (1976). *Geburtshilfe Frauenheilkd* **35**, 575–587.

Spark, R. F., Pallotta, J., Naftolin, F. *et al.* (1976) *Ann. Int. Med.* **84**, 532–537.

Swyer, G. I. M., Little, V. and Harries, B. J. (1971). *Brit. Med. J.* **4**, 90–91.

Thorner, M. O., Besser, G. M., Jones, A. *et al.* (1975). *Brit. Med. J.* **4**, 694–679.

Van Dalen, J. T. W. and Greve, E. L. (1977). *Br. J. Ophthalmol.* **61**, 729–733.

Wiebe, R. H., Hammond, C. B. and Handwerger, S. (1977). *Fertil. Steril.* **28**, 426–433.

Wolf, L. M., Houdent, CH., Peugnet, J. P. *et al.* (1975). *Ann d'Endocrinol.* (*Paris*) **36**, 107–108.

# SURGICAL TREATMENT OF GROWTH HORMONE-SECRETING MICROADENOMAS*

M. A. Giovanelli[1], R. Fahlbusch[2], S. M. Gaini[1], G. Faglia[3] and K. v. Werder[4]

[1]*Clinica Neurochirurgica,* [3]*Clinica Medica II, Università di Milano, Milan, Italy*
[2]*Neurochirurgische Klinik Grosshadern,* [4]*Medizinische Klinik Innenstadt,*
*Universität München, Munich, West Germany*

The evaluation of the degree and modalities of variation in the serum levels of the pituitary tropins has introduced a biological standard of reference to assess the activity of a secreting pituitary tumor even in a very early stage. On the other hand, the availability of the transsphenoidal microsurgical technique (Cushing, 1914; Guiot, 1958, 1970, 1973; Hardy, 1969 a, b; Guiot *et al.*, 1971) has made possible the selective excision of very small intrapituitary adenomas, sparing the surrounding normal gland tissue. Such advances have brought about the possibility of treating in an early phase the clinical hyperfunction syndrome due to the tumor while maintaining or even restoring normal functions in the pituitary. Today surgery of small intrapituitary adenomas has changed from a demolitive into a functional outlook and has come to mean the same as extracranial transsphenoidal microsurgical removal of the tiny tumors.

The possibilities of success afforded by this type of treatment are of course related to the different types of adenomas, which possess diverse functional characteristics as well as diverse biological (Landolt, 1975, 1979) and anatomo-topographical features (Hardy, 1976).

In order to verify the actual possibilities of success of this surgery in the treatment of acromegaly and to discuss inherent difficulties as well as failures, we have critically reviewed in a joint study the series of small intrahypophyseal GH secreting adenomas operated in the Neurosurgery Departments of Milan and Munich Universities.

*This work was supported in part by CNR contribution 78.02121.04.115.3936 to M. A. Giovanelli.

427

## PATIENTS AND METHODS

Over the past five years 137 acromegalic patients have been operated on by the transsphenoidal microsurgery technique. Among them 57 had small intrahypophyseal adenomas, 30 were females (52.6%) and 27 males (47.4%).

Age ranged between 23 and 65 years, 6 patients being older than 60. Four cases (Nos 27, 47, 48, 49; see Fig. 2 and following) had previously received external conventional radiotherapy up to 5500 rads one of them (case No. 27) developed ACTH, TSH, LH and FSH deficiency. Tumor size in the 57 patients ranged between 3 and no more than 13 mm, measuring less than 10 mm in diameter in 42 patients and ranging between 10 and no more than 13 mm in the remaining 15 cases (Fig. 1). Actual tumor size has been obtained at operation by comparison with a tool and, in some cases, by filling the post-excision cavity with a small quantity of a gel soaked in contrast medium and then comparing pre- and post-operative roentgenograms.

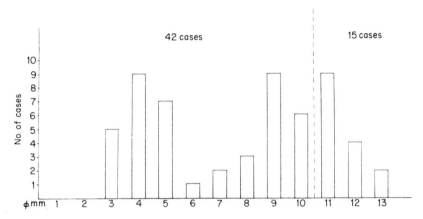

*Fig. 1.* Adenomas size (as determined at the operation) in the overall 57 patients.

Duration of symptoms at the time of operation ranged from 1 to 10 years without a strict correlation to tumor size: in fact tumors of widely differing sizes have been found in cases with brief, as well as very long, histories of acromegalic symptoms.

Radiological assessment of sellar morphology included in all cases plain frontal and lateral skull radiographs and tomograms obtained at 2 mm intervals, either by linear unidirectional or hypocycloidal motion. In all patients sellar floors presented some typical changes corresponding to tumor location verified at operation.

CT scanning with i.v. injection of contrast medium failed to demonstrate the adenoma in the 31 patients who were examined.

Two partial empty sellae (cases No. 41 and 49) were found among the 28 patients who underwent cisterno-encephalography. One was already evident at CT investigation.

### Endocrinological evaluation

In all patients the investigation of endocrine functions has been performed before and after operation.

GH secretion has been evaluated by means of serum hormone assays:

(a)   in basal conditions of morning fast on multiple occasions and at least once during i.v. saline infusion by means of 30 min samples over 4 h;

(b)   after 100 g oral glucose load (OGTT suppression test according to Cryer and Daughaday, 1969; Lawrence and Goldfire, 1970);

(c)   after 200 $\mu$g thyrotropin releasing hormone i.v. injection. (TRH stimulation test according to Faglia *et al.*, 1978.)

Serum GH has been assayed radioimmunologically by HGH-Kit (Dow-Lepetit, Milan) in the series of patients investigated in Milan and employing WHO reagents in the series investigated in Munich. Blind exchange among the two laboratories of serum samples of varying GH content has produced serum GH values closely parallel never exceeding a 5% discrepancy.

Prolactin (PRL) secretion has been investigated assaying the serum hormone levels at morning fast

(a)   in basal conditions (30 min spaced samples) on several occasions and

(b)   after 200$\mu$g TRH i.v. (Faglia *et al.*, 1977).

Serum PRL has been assayed radioimmunologically employing VLS 1 (NIH-NIAMDD) standard in Milan and A71/222 (MRC) in Munich.

Gonadotropic function was determined by radioimmunoassay of plasma luteinizing hormone (LH) and follicle stimulating hormone (FSH) levels in the basal state and after intravenous injection of 25–100 $\mu$g gonadotropin releasing hormone (GnRH). Results were interpreted according to the guidelines suggested by WHO.

Thyroid function has been investigated by means of radioimmunoassay of tyroxine ($T_4$) and tri-iodotyronine ($T_3$) serum concentrations.

In fact thyrotropic response to TRH does not add valuable information in acromegaly (Hall *et al.*, 1972) as a response often lacks also in euthyroid patients.

Adrenocorticotropic function has been assessed by hydroxycorticosteroid (17-OHCS) determination in the basal state and after metyrapone administration and radioimmunoassay of plasma cortisol in basal conditions and following insulin-induced hypoglycemia ($< 40$ mg/100 ml), the results having been interpreted according to Liddle *et al.* (1962) and to Landon *et al.* (1963) respectively.

### Surgical procedures

All patients underwent microsurgical excision of the tumor by the trans-sphenoidal route under fluoroscopic control. Details and variations of surgical technique are reported in the contribution by Fahlbusch *et al.* (1979) in the present volume.

No chemical or physical maneuvre has been used after tumor removal. A graft of fascia lata has been applied in the cases where suprasellar cisternal arachnoid, although intact, protruded through a wide dural ostium.

Light microscopy examination with conventional staining techniques has confirmed a tumor in all cases (eosinophilic in 32 cases and of mixed type in 25).

Immunohistochemical technique has been employed in the last tumors in the series both in Milan and Munich. Ultrastructural investigation has also been performed in the majority of cases.

Hydrocortisone therapy was instituted on the pre-operative day and continued in progressively decreasing doses the four days following operation.

Post-operative antibiotics were routinely prescribed in the Milan group of patients.

The tumor was found an anterolateral location in 31 cases (16 on the right and 15 on the left); in a more lateral location in 9 (7 on the right and 2 on the left); in a paramedian location with some lateral extension in 13; and in a more dorso-lateral location in the last 4 cases.

Tumoral tissue was soft in 52 cases, with haemorragic necrotic patches in 4. In 3 cases we found a tiny cyst containing a yellow fluid. A firm tissue was found in only 2 patients.

In all cases operation was aimed at selective total removal. In 3 cases only, the excision has been purposely wider due to lack of a recognizable border with healthy tissue: 2 of them had undergone a course of radiotherapy several years before operation (cases 27, 49) while the remaining case was one of the "cystic" tumors.

## RESULTS OF TRANSSPHENOIDAL SURGERY

The outcome of operations has been evaluated by repeating all pre-operative tests within three months of surgery. On the basis of post-operative serum GH levels, the patients have been considered:

*normalized* when basal serum GH levels were lower than 5 ng/ml or lower than 10 ng/ml and suppressed under oral glucose load;

*improved* when basal serum GH levels were ranging between 5 and 10 ng/ml, not suppressed under oral glucose load;

*unchanged* when serum GH levels, although lowered in some cases, remained above 10 ng/ml.

As to other pituitary functions, patients have been grouped as follows:

(a) patients with no alterations of pre-operatively normal functions or with return to normal of pre-operatively impaired functions;

(b) patients with no changes or partial improvement of pre-operative defects;

(c) patients with post-operative impairment of previously normal functions.

In the evaluation of the pituitary tropins other than GH, in addition to the serum assays in various conditions as above described, we have closely considered the modifications or the appearance of the clinical signs of hypopituitarism and the necessity of replacement therapy.

### Results on GH

Pre-operative serum GH levels ranged between 4–5 ng/ml to 100 ng/ml. In 41 cases GH normalized immediately. In 6 further cases (No. 6, 11, 15, 20, 39, 40) the attained basal serum GH levels between 7.5 and 5.5 ng/ml were suppressed

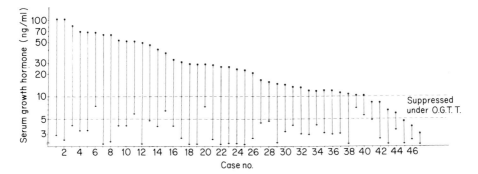

*Fig. 2.* Overall results on serum GH in the 47 normalized patients. Dots (●) indicate pre-operative serum GH levels and arrow-heads (▼) post-operative attained levels in each case. Patients with post-operative GH values between 10 and 5 ng/ml (interrupted horizontal lines) were further supressed under OGTT.

after glucose load. Thus operation can be considered successful in 47 cases (83%) (Fig. 2).

Ten cases were not normalized by surgery (Fig. 3). However in 6 of the latter cases (10%) the post-operative basal serum GH fell to levels between 10 and 5 ng/ml, unsuppressed under OGTT. According to the criteria above defined these 6 patients are considered improved. Overall proportion of patients who are normalized and improved is then 93%. The remaining 4 patients are considered unchanged according to our criteria, although in one of them GH showed a 70% decrease in

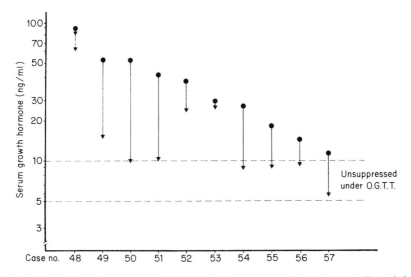

*Fig. 3.* Overall results on serum GH in the 10 non-normalized patients. Dots (●) indicate pre-operative serum GH levels and arrowheads (▼) post-operative attained levels in each case. Patients with post-operative GH values between 10 and 5 ng/ml (interrupted horizontal lines) were not supressed under OGTT.

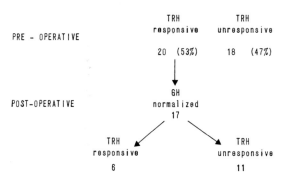

*Fig. 4.* Pattern of TRH response before and after operation in the 38 tested patients.

respect to pre-operative level reaching 15 ng/ml (case No. 49). One of these patients underwent a second more radical operation without success (GH lowered from 85 to 60 ng/ml) (case No. 48). Modification of serum GH levels after TRH administration has been assessed in 38 patients in the present series. Before operation 20 cases (53%) were GH responsive to TRH: among them, serum GH levels fell below 5 ng/ml in 17 patients. Out of these 17 cases, TRH response disappeared in 11 and persisted in 6 (Fig. 4). Results on GH have then been evaluated in relation to tumor size. The 42 cases which fit the definition of microadenoma (Group I) have been considered apart from the 15 cases with diameters between 10 and 13 mm (Group II). Results in the two groups have then been compared. In the 42 patients of Group I (Fig. 5) pre-operative GH serum levels ranged between 4 and 80 ng/ml. After operation in 30 patients GH serum levels were below 5 ng/ml. In 5 other patients the attained GH levels, ranging between 7.5 and 5.5 ng/ml,

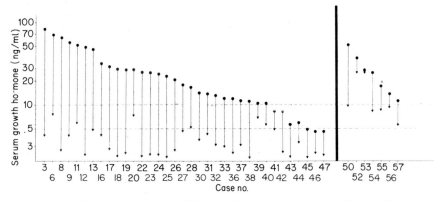

*Fig. 5.* Overall results on serum GH according to adenoma size (Group I). Figure represents pre-operative (●) and post-operative (▼) GH values in adenomas below 10 mm in diameter (42 cases) . Normalized and OGTT supressed cases (35 pts) are found to the left; improved (unsupressed under OGTT) and un-changed cases (7 pts) to the right.

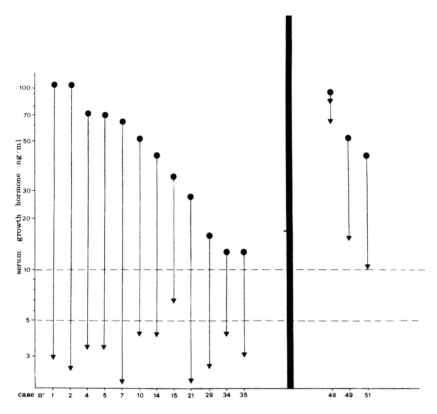

*Fig. 6.*   Overall results on serum GH according to adenoma size (Group II).
Figure represents pre-operative (●) and post-operative (▼) GH values in adenomas
between 10 and 13 mm in diameter (15 cases). Normalized and OGTT supressed
cases (12 pts) are found to the left; improved and unchanged cases (3 pts) to
the right.

were suppressed after oral glucose load. All these patients are considered GH
normalized. Operation failed to normalize 7 patients: 5, with GH levels lowered
to values between 10 and 5 ng/ml, unsuppressed after OGTT, are considered
improved, and the 2 remaining patients are considered unchanged.

In Group II, preoperative GH serum levels ranged between 12 and 100 ng/ml
(Fig. 6). Operation normalized 12 cases: in 11 cases serum GH lowered below 5
ng/ml and in the remaining one, a post-operative GH serum level of 6.5 ng/ml
was suppressed under oral glucose load (case No. 15). Operation failed to normalize 3 patients: one, with a GH level of 10 ng/ml unsuppressed under oral
glucose load, is considered improved while the remaining 2 patients are unchanged.

Surgery has then been successful in normalizing serum GH in about the same
proportion of patients in the two groups: 83.3% of patients in Group I and 80% in
Group II (Fig. 7).

| | GROUP I ($\emptyset < 10$ mm) | | GROUP II ($\emptyset > 10$ mm) | |
|---|---|---|---|---|
| NORMALIZED | 35 | 83.3 % | 12 | 80.0 % |
| IMPROVED | 5 | 12.0 % | 2 | 13.3 % |
| UNCHANGED | 2 | 4.7 % | 1 | 6.7 % |
| total | 42 | | 15 | |

*Fig. 7.* Post-operative serum GH and adenoma size. Results in the two groups are compared in the three outcome-categories and are shown to be roughly equal.

### Effect of surgery on the other pituitary functions:

*(a) In the overall series*

Thirty-six of 57 patients had normal pituitary functions before operation; surgical outcome was optimal in 32, which remained normal while post-operative partial deficit appeared in 4 (3 patients had gonadic deficits and 1 thyroid deficit).

Twenty-one patients presented a pre-operative impairment of one or more tropins beside GH.

A multiple impairment of functions was present in 10 cases; adrenal, gonadal and thyroid functions were impaired in 6 cases; gonadal and thyroid functions in 3 and adrenal and thyroid functions in 1. A single impairment was present in 11 cases: gonadal in 10 and thyroid in 1. Operation produced normalization in 8 of these 21 patients. The remaining 13 cases remained impaired, although 2 patients with multiple impairment before operation normalized in regard to a single function. We have then compared the pre-operative conditions and results of operation on tropins other than GH in the two size groups of tumors.

Before operation, pituitary impairment other than GH was present in 16 cases (38%) in Group I and in 5 cases (33.3) in Group II. Post-operative normalization of impaired tropins was obtained in 6 patients of 16 in Group I and in 2 of 5 in Group II. Partial impairment of pre-operative normal functions was recorded in 3 patients of Group I and in 1 of Group II. Therefore, post-operative results on other tropins maintain the same trend of results consistent in both groups.

*(b) In GH-cured patients*

Considering the pituitary functions other than GH in the 47 patients GH cured, 31 had normal pituitary functions before operation. Post-operatively 28 cases were unchanged in this respect. On the other hand among the 16 cases that before operation showed single or multiple impaired pituitary functions, 5 were normalized after operation.

Thus 33 patients (70.2%) among the 47 GH normalized may be judged normal as to all pituitary functions. In 11 patients (23.4%) the pre-operative impairment was either unchanged (10 cases) or improved (1 case). In 3 patients (6.4%), the operation has cured GH hypersecretion causing deficit of the gonadal function: one patient however regained normal ovulatory cycles one year after operation.

## Glucose tolerance

An impairment of carbohydrate metabolism of varying degree was present in 22 among the overall 57 patients before operation (38.6%). In more detail, 6 patients presented overt diabetes and 16 impaired glucose tolerance. One out of the 6 patients with overt diabetes normalized after surgery, 2 were improved and stopped medical therapy, while 3 were unchanged. Ten out of the 16 cases with impaired glucose tolerance were normalized after operation, 4 improved and 2 remained unchanged.

## Complications

There was no surgical mortality in this series of patients. A single case presented slight CSF rhinorrhea in the eighth post-operative day, that was successfully treated by spino-external CSF shunting over 5 days.

No septic complications have been observed. A transient diabetes insipidus, lasting between 2 and 5 days, appeared in 7 patients.

## DISCUSSION

The pituitary tumors of the present report include, along with a majority of microadenomas (Group I), some small intrapituitary adenomas certainly exceeding the diameter of 10 mm (Group II).

We have included the latter tumors on the basis of the consideration that from the surgical point of view the most important feature of microadenomas is their amenability to selective removal. In fact the functional results of transsphenoidal surgery are conditional on the possibility of radically removing the small adenoma sparing variable amounts of normal pituitary tissue. In order to correctly evaluate the therapeutical possibilities of this type of surgery we have then deemed worthwhile to control whether and to what extent the surgical results obtained in microadenomas diverge from those observed in a group of intrahypophyseal tumors small enough to be likely that a small portion of normal pituitary tissue is present beside the tumor.

In the overall series pre-operative GH serum levels ranged from close to normal to values close to 100 ng/ml.

Three patients with clinical and radiological features consistent with acromegaly had basal serum GH levels close to the upper limits of the normal range. However they were considered to have an active acromegaly on the basis of the persistence of progressive acromegalic changes, and of altered patterns of GH secretion throughout the 24 hours (including the absence of sleep related peaks) and in response to oral glucose load (Cryer and Daughaday, 1969; Lawrence and Goldfire, 1970). Moreover, in these patients positive TRH response has contributed

to confirm the presence of active tumoral tissue (Giovanelli *et al.*, 1976; Faglia
*et al.*, 1978), thus further advising in favour of surgery.

Serum GH levels averaged lower values (23.1 ng/ml) in the smaller tumors
(Group I) compared to the average values met in tumors with diameters ranging
between 10 and 12-13 mm (50.9 ng/ml) (Group II). Extreme values ranged from
4 to 80 ng/ml and from 12 to 100 ng/ml respectively in the 2 groups.

About 76% of tumors in Group I (32 cases) presented serum GH values below
30 ng/ml; however 26.6% of tumors in Group II (4 cases) were in the same range
as well. It is interesting to note how in the smallest microadenomas (up to 8 mm
in diameter) GH serum levels above 30 ng/ml are exceptional (3 cases out of 28),
while microadenomas in the 8-10 mm range in diameter present GH values closely
resembling tumors in Group II. (Fig. 8).

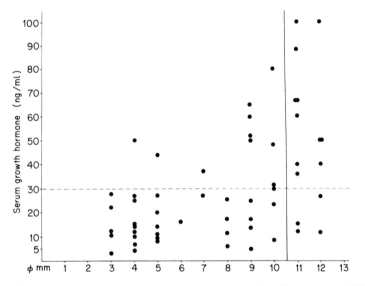

*Fig. 8.*  Pre-operative GH secretion and adenoma size. The figure shows GH
serum values are lower in the smaller adenomas (diameter below 10 mm), and
GH values below 30 ng/ml are very frequent in the adenomas below 8 mm in
diameter while present in only 4 cases larger than 10 mm across.

Removal has been radical and selective in all cases but three where a more
extensive ablation has been performed. Two of the latter cases had been treated
many years before with successive courses of external conventional radiotherapy.
A definite tumor boundary with residual normal pituitary tissue was not recognized,
thus confirming the reported difficulty in being selective in long previously irradiated patients (Hardy *et al.*, 1976). As to results on GH, post-operative serum levels
of the hormone do not show significant differences in the two groups of tumors as
the percentage of GH cured patients is practically the same (83.3% in Group I *vs* 80.0%
in Group II). Thus in the overall 57 patients 82.4% were completely GH cured.

Comparing results with pre-operative GH serum levels, chances of surgical
success appear high in the 35 patients (31 in Group I and 4 in Group II) with pre-

operative GH serum levels below 30 ng/ml: in fact we obtained 30 post-operative normalizations (85.7%). Nonetheless operative results in cases with pre-operative levels below 30 ng/ml do not seem to have a very close relation with tumor size: as a matter of fact all four patients in Group II normalized while all five failures belong to Group I.

Less satisfactory results have been obtained in the 22 patients with pre-operative serum GH above 30 ng/ml: 77.2% of cases (17 patients) were cured. These patients belong in equal numbers to the two groups: eleven in Group I and eleven in Group II. Failures have been respectively two and three cases. Considering that the pre-operative GH values above 30 ng/ml are present in Group I almost only in the larger tumors (between 8 and 10 mm), we may suggest surgical therapy has practically equal possibilities of success in these as in the tumors in Group II. Furthermore, grouping together the adenomas with a diameter between 8 and 13 mm, results seem significantly conditioned by pre-operative GH serum levels; in fact at least in our series and with such tumor sizes, failures ensued wherever pre-operative GH serum levels exceeded 30 ng/ml.

The drop of serum GH values, when present, was apparent in a short time. In fact serum GH assays during operation and in the course of the following 24 hours in a group of acromegalics, showed that in the patients who will subsequently be confirmed normalized, a dramatic GH serum fall is evident during operation and in the immediate subsequent hours. Serum levels obtained in the first 24-48 hours tend to remain stable (Fahlbusch and von Werder, 1974; von Werder and Fahlbusch, 1977). Immediacy of results is certainly a feature of primary importance in the surgical transsphenoidal treatment of acromegaly, if we consider the many progressively debilitating aspects of this disease (Bishop and Briggs, 1958; Bricaire and Strauch, 1970).

In the cases with elevation of both GH and PRL serum levels, surgical results have been exactly parallel, normalization of both being attained in four cases, while in one case GH and PRL levels were post-operatively unchanged.

Results on GH have been evaluated considering a measure of cure the stable attainment of GH values below 5 ng/ml, as well as the attainment of values between 5 and 10 ng/ml suppressed under oral glucose load (Lüdecke *et al.*, 1976; Hardy *et al.*, 1976; Fahlbusch and Marguth, 1978). We however still lack a safe criterion of evaluation in order to consider cured those patients with GH post-operative basal levels below 5 ng/ml. In these patients GH suppressibility to oral glucose load as well as persistence of the paradoxical rise after oral glucose load, do not appear to be safe criteria of evaluation given their scarce specificity (Pelroth *et al.*, 1967; Samaan *et al.*, 1966; Wright *et al.*, 1968) and reproducibility (Liuzzi *et al.*, 1972).

The assessment of GH response to TRH in the responsive subject may represent a valid adjunctive technique (Faglia *et al.*, 1978). In fact in a sizeable proportion of acromegalics (about 50%) a rise of GH serum values following TRH administration is present (Irie and Tsushima, 1972; Faglia *et al.*, 1973) which seems to depend on direct action of TRH on GH secreting adenomatous cells (De Camilli *et al.*, 1978). If post-operative disappearance of a positive response of GH to TRH were to be confirmed a valid sign of a complete adenoma removal and the persistence of a response a sign of incomplete removal (Giovanelli *et al.*, 1976; Faglia *et al.*, 1978), we would possess a definitive yardstick for deciding the level of cure, at least in the TRH responsive patients before operation. However, the percentage of surgical success would be drastically reduced by employing this method. As a matter of fact, among the 17 pre-operatively TRH responsive patients in which operation reduced serum GH values below 5 ng/ml, 6 still show a response to TRH after the operation. This finding has an immediate practical importance as it implies these patients must be kept closely controlled for a possible recurrence.

In the overall series, 36% of cases presented a pre-operative impairment of tropins other than GH, distributed about equally in the two groups with 38% of patients in Group I and 33% of patients in Group II. Post-operative results evaluated by assessment of the other pituitary functions are also practically identical in the two groups.

On the basis of the latter data and the results on GH, it seem reasonable to state there are no substantial differences as to chances of a favorable outcome in our two groups of adenomas, owing to the more or less extensive portion of residual normal pituitary tissue that can be effectively spared in a selective procedure. We then decided to include in our report the Group II tumors, that in an anatomoradiological grading would correctly pertain to the first group of Grade II enclosed adenomas (without suprasellar expansion) in Vezina's classification. (Vezina and Maltais, 1973). It is also quite likely that adenomas slightly larger in size (up to 15 mm in diameter) could occasionally possess the same possibility of surgical therapy (Lüdecke *et al.*, 1976).

As to patients not cured of GH hypersecretion in which GH values fell to levels between 5 and 10 ng/ml, unsuppressed by OGTT, a sensible remission of clinical symptoms (mostly headache, hyperhydrosis, thickness of the soft tissues) has however been observed and patients have likewise been considered improved.

As already described the operation has been performed with a primary goal of radicality along with the intent of selectivity. Nonetheless, as previously reported (Giovanelli *et al.*, 1976) and in accord with other authors (Hardy *et al.*, 1976; Hoi Sang U *et al.*, 1977; Kautzky *et al.*, 1978) we think the cause for failure in these patients lies in the persistence of hypersecreting tissue remnants. This opinion is rooted in the persistence of TRH response in all non-cured cases that before operation showed a positive TRH response.

Whether biopsy of the pituitary tissue bordering the tumor can help in avoiding failures is still an open question. In two failures of ours the bioptic specimens in the neighbouring tissue did not show any tumoral stems. To be valid biopsies should possibly be multiple and sample several sites in the apparently normal tissue. These maneuvres, however, would carry the risk of damaging residual pituitary functions.

Some failures could as well be due to tumoral implants in peripituitary tissue (Landolt, 1979; Wrightson, 1979) that can take place also in very small sized tumors (Landolt, 1979), as seems to be the case in one of our patients (case No. 48) who underwent a second operation with radical ablation of sellar contents without significant fall in GH serum levels (from 88 to 60 ng/ml). Some authors have adopted preventive maneuvres swabbing the operative cavity with chemical agents such as absolute alcohol (Wilson and Dempsey, 1978) and Carnoy solution (Kautsky *et al.*, 1978). Considering the reported frequency in GH secreting adenomas of spontaneously dissociating tumoral cells maintaining secretive activity (Giovanelli *et al.*, 1978), the above mentioned preventive measures would seem to be valuable together with the protracted irrigation of the surgical cavity.

As to care of non-normalized patients we have among the diverse options available (re-operation, irradiation, drugs) chosen to treat 3 patients with medical therapy (CB 154) along with conventional external radiotherapy with $Co^{60}$.

Results after two years have been positive: from a post-operative level of 8.6, 15 and 85 ng/ml, the serum GH levels fell below 5 ng/ml in the first two patients (cases No. 55 and 49) and reached as low as 10 ng/ml in the last patient (case No. 52). However, in one patient this course of therapy resulted in impairment of the other pituitary functions that previously were normal. Therefore, given the likely indiscriminate impairment produced by irradiation, the decision to submit the patient to a second surgical procedure can be taken into consideration in those patients who present evidence of normal pituitary functions other than GH, confirmed by the direct observation of a residual sufficient quantity of apparently normal gland tissue. Thus reoperation could still offer the chance of selectivity. On the other hand, in those patients with post-operative impairment of tropins other than GH and a dubious quantity of left-over pituitary, the choice between a second radical operation and radiotherapy becomes less crucial. In the latter patients the useful role of medical therapy would be to maintain low levels of GH as long as the effects of radiotherapy become evident.

All patients have been followed after discharge. The follow-up period ranges from six months to three years in most cases, while reaching to four and five years in only eight cases. In all GH-cured patients, the operative results have maintained stable. The endocrine condition of other pituitary tropins has tended to be stable, but for one case: a young woman with post-operative impairment of gonadal functions who after one year, without any therapy, has regained her menstrual ovulatory cycles.

Of course analysis of our whole series can allow only partial conclusions on the merits of this type of treatment. Microsurgical transsphenoidal surgery of small intrapituitary GH secreting adenomas is now being demonstrated as a successful therapeutical procedure, at least employing the currently available methods for assessment of cure. However, the introduction of more sophisticated assessment techniques shows a trend towards reduction of the real effectiveness of this surgical procedure. Nonetheless only a longer observation period will allow validation of results obtained thus far.

## ACKNOWLEDGMENTS

The Authors would like to especially thank Drs Enrico D. F. Motti and Giustino Tomei for their invaluable help. Our gratitude goes to Miss Rita Paglino for her many hours devoted to this work.

## REFERENCES

Bishop, P. M. F. and Briggs, J. H. (1958). *Lancet* I, 735.
Bricaire, H. and Strauch, G. (1970). *Presse Med.* **78**, 159–160.
Cryer, P. E. and Daughaday, W. H. (1969). *J Clin. Endocrinol. Metab.* **29**, 386.

Cushing, H. (1914). *J. Amer. Med. Ass.* **63**, 63.

De Camilli, P., Tagliabue, L., Paracchi, A., Faglia, G., Beck-Peccoz, P. and Giovanelli, M. (1978). *In* "Treatment of Pituitary Adenomas" (R. Fahlbusch and K. v. Werder, eds) pp. 172–179. G. Thieme, Stuttgart.

Faglia, G., Beck-Peccoz, P., Ferrari, C. *et al.* (1973). *J. Clin. Endocrinol.* **36**, 1259–1262.

Faglia, G., Beck-Peccoz, P., Travaglini, P., Ambrosi, B., Rondena, M., Paracchi, A., Spada, A., Weber, G., Bara, R. and Bouzin, A. (1977). *In* "Prolactin and Human Reproduction" (P. G. Crosignani and C. Robyn, eds) Vol. 11, 225–238. Academic Press, London and New York.

Faglia, G., Paracchi, A., Ferrari, C. and Beck-Peccoz, P. (1978). *Clin. Endocrinol* **8**, 373–380.

Fahlbusch, R. and Werder, K. v. (1974). *5th Europ. Congr. Neurosurg. (Oxford) Abstracts* **124**, 278–279.

Fahlbusch, R. and Marguth, F. (1978). *Neurosurg. Rev.* **1/2**, 5–13.

Fahlbusch, R., Giovanelli, M., Crosignani, P. G., Faglia, G., Rjosk, H. K. and Werder, K. v. (1979). This volume.

Giovanelli, M. A., Motti, E. D. F., Paracchi, A., Beck-Peccoz, P. Ambrosi, B. and Faglia, G. (1976). *J. Neurosurg.* **44**, 677–686.

Giovanelli, M. A., Gaini, S. M., Tomei, G., Motti, E. D. F., Beck-Peccoz, P., Paracchi, A. and De Camilli, P. (1978). *In* "Treatment of Pituitary Adenomas" (R. Fahlbusch and K. v. Werder, eds) pp. 272–279. G. Thieme, Stuttgart.

Guiot, G. (1958). *In* "Adénomes Hypophysaires" (G. Guiot *et al.*, eds) pp. 165–180. Masson et Cie, Paris.

Guiot, G. (1970). "Corso superiore sui tumori delle ghiandole endocrine", pp. 109–125. Ambrosiana, Milano.

Guiot, G. (1973). *In* "Diagnosis and Treatment of Pituitary Tumors" (P. O. Kohler and G. T. Ross, eds) pp. 159–178. Excerpta Medica American Elsevier, New York.

Guiot, G., Derome, P. and Wislawski, J. (1971). *Neuro-chirurgie* **17**, 1, 5–10.

Hall, R. J., Ormston, B. J., Besser, G. M. Cryer, R. J. and Mc Kendrik, M. (1972). *Lancet* **1**, 759.

Hardy, J. (1969a) *Clin. Neurosurg.* **16**, 185–217.

Hardy, J. (1969b). *In* "Microneurosurgery" (R. W. Rand, ed.) Chap. 8, 224. C. V. Mosby Co., St. Louis, Mo.

Hardy, J., Somma, S. and Vezina, J. L. (1976). *In* "Current Controversies in Neurosurgery" (T. P. Morley, ed.) pp. 377–391. W. B. Saunders Co. Philadelphia.,

Hoi Sang U, Wilson, C. B. and Tyrell J. B. (1977). *J Neurosurg.* **47**, 840–852.

Irie, M and Tsushima, I. (1972). *J. Clin. Endocrinol. Metab.* **35**, 97–100.

Kautzky, R., Lüdecke, D., Novakowski, H., Schader, D., Stahuke, Ch., Solbach, H. G. and Wiegelmann, W. (1978). *In* "Treatment of Pituitary Adenomas" (R. Fahlbusch and K. v. Werder, eds) pp. 219–225. G. Thieme, Stuttgart.

Landolt, M. A. (1975). *Acta Neurochir. Suppl.* **22**, 1–167.

Landolt, M. A. (1979). This volume.

Landon, J., Wynn, V. and James, V. H. T. (1963). *J. Endocrinol.* **27**, 183.

Lawrence, A. M. and Goldfire, I. D. (1970). *J. Clin. Endocrinol. Metab.* **30**, 646.

Liddle, G. W., Island, G. and Meador, C. (1962). *Rec. Prog. Hormone Res.* **18**, 125.

Liuzzi, A., Chiodini, P. G., Botalla, L. *et al.* (1972). *Folia Endocrinol.* **25**, 393–400.

Lüdecke, D., Kautzky, R., Saeger, W. and Schrader, D. (1976). *Acta Neurochir.* **35**, 27–42.

Pelroth, M. G., Tschudy, D. P., Waxmann, A. *et al.* (1967). *Metabolism* **16**, 87–90.

Samaan, R. H., Pearson, O. H., Gonzales, D. *et al.* (1966). *J. Lab. Clin. Med.* **68**, 1011 (Abstract 118).

Vezina, J. L. and Maltais, R. (1973). *Neurochirurgie* **19**, Suppl. 2, 35–56.

Werder, K. v. and Fahlbusch, R. (1977). *Europ. J. Clin. Invest.* **7**, 233.

Wilson, C. B. and Dempsey, L. C. (1978). *J. Neurosurg.* **48**, 13–22.

Wright, A. D., Lowy, C., Fraser, T. R. *et al.* (1968). *Lancet* **2**, 798–800.

Wrightson, P. (1979). This volume.

# DIFFERENTIATED THERAPY OF MICROPROLACTINOMAS:
## SIGNIFICANCE OF TRANSSPHENOIDAL ADENOMECTOMY*

R. Fahlbusch[1], M. Giovanelli[2], P. G. Crosignani[3], G. Faglia[4], H. K. Rjosk[5]
and K. v. Werder[6]

[1] *Neurochirurgische Klinik Grosshadern,*
[5] *I. Frauenklinik,* [6] *Medizinische Klinik Innenstadt,*
*Universität München, Munich, West Germany.*
[2] *Clinica Neurochirurgica,* [3] *Clinica Ostetrica e*
*Ginecologica IV,* [4] *Clinica Medica II,*
*Università di Milano, Milan, Italy*

## INTRODUCTION

The optimal form of treatment in patients with small prolactin-producing adenomas, prolactinomas, is still in discussion. Since these tumors have been diagnosed more and more since the radioimmunological determination of PRL has become available, the management of these patients has varied from no treatment other than observation to medical or surgical therapy.

The present study is based on a similar concept of treatment of microprolactinomas developed in close cooperation between neurosurgeons, endocrinologists and gynecologists in Milan and Munich.

We differentiate between very large adenomas (macroprolactinomas) growing from the sella into the intracranial space and very small adenomas growing inside the sella. In general the tumor size correlates well with the PRL levels (Fahlbusch *et al.*, 1978). Obviously no clear dividing line can be made on the basis of anatomical findings. When we speak about microadenomas in this study we mean those adenomas growing within the pituitary gland, the so-called "enclosed adenomas" of Guiot (1973, 1978), and also those adenomas growing inside the sella and

*Study partially supported by C.N.R. under the special program on Reproductive Biology to P. G. Crosignani and by C.N.R. contribution No. 78.02121.04.115.3936 to M. A. Giovanelli.

displacing the pituitary to the sella periphery. These adenomas have diameters of less than 10 mm, conforming with Hardy's definition (1973), but those of 12 - 14 mm were also included in this study.

There is no dispute that the large adenomas often accompanied by ophthalmological disturbances must be treated surgically (Fahlbusch, 1978; Fahlbusch and Marguth, 1978). Whereas there is still divergence of opinion about a differentiated therapy for microprolactinomas. There is no other type of endocrinologically active or inactive adenoma with such variance of tumor size. In addition these microadenomas seem to occur almost exclusively in women (Fahlbusch, 1978; L'Hermite *et al.*, 1978). In Munich we observed 4 men with intrasellar prolactinomas: the 2 men operated on had PRL levels of 12 000 and 16 000 $\mu$U/ml, but the adenomas were larger than 10 mm in diameter. The other 2 men with only slightly elevated PRL levels and a pathological sella floor were not operated on.

We have evidence that some microprolactinomas proliferate very slowly or not at all. We observed 2 patients with hyperprolactinemic amenorrhea who had unchanged sellar configuration over 10 and 13 years. This may correspond to the occurrence of microscopic adenomas in up to 22.5% of routine autopsies (Costello, 1935a,b) and minor radiological alterations in sella tomograms of normal subjects (Swanson and du Boulay, 1975) and amenorrhoic women with no hyperprolactinemia (Hotton *et al.*, 1976). On the other hand, we observed 5 hyperprolactinemic patients with normal sellar configuration 2 years before who had at the time of operation clear sellar enlargement and further increased prolactin levels. When treating patients with hyperprolactinemic amenorrhea we have to consider the desire for pregnancy in addition to hypogonadism. Hyperprolactinemia itself is no indication for surgical treatment, unlike the ACTH-excess in Cushing's disease or the GH-excess in acromegaly, which cause severe metabolic disturbances.

## METHODS AND PATIENTS

The following concept was applied to 95 patients with microprolactinomas (Table I):

(1) No treatment other than observation of the tendency to proliferation of the prolactinoma, by measuring PRL-levels and X-ray, in 5 patients who had no desire for pregnancy and did not complain of loss of libido.

(2) Treatment with antiprolactinemic agents for hypogonadism, especially for desired pregnancy, in 32 patients.

(3) Selective transsphenoidal adenomectomy in order to normalize or lower elevated PRL-levels, in 58 patients.

*Table I.* Study on 95 patients with microprolactinomas in Milan and Munich.

| No. of patients | |
|---|---|
| 5 | Observation (no treatment) |
| 32 | Bromocriptine only |
| 58 | Transsphenoidal operation |

In all patients, endocrine investigation was performed before and three to six weeks after the operation. PRL was measured by radioimmunoassay. Normal PRL levels in Munich are less than 650 $\mu$U/ml for women and 500 $\mu$U/ml for men. Twenty $\mu$U/ml of the MRC-standard A-71/222 are equal to 1 ng VLS-PRL (NHI). Normal PRL levels in Milan are less than 25 ng/ml for women and less than 15 ng/ml for men. PRL levels were found to be in the same range in both laboratories, in interlaboratory comparison. PRL secretion was tested by i.v. administration of 200 $\mu$g TRH. Gonadal function was investigated by LH-RH stimulation of LH secretion. Thyroid function was examined by determination of $T_3$ and $T_4$ and a TRH test. Adrenal function was tested by the ACTH-test and by the insulin-induced hypoglycemia test (IHT) with serum cortisol as the index. Growth hormone was measured in the IHT. For neuroradiological diagnosis (Table II), X-rays of the skull and 2-3 mm tomograms of the sella antero-posterior and lateral were made by linear and spiral techniques. Most important for the exclusion of

*Table II.* Operation, endocrine follow-up and radiological examination in Milan and Munich

| *Milan* | *A. Operative procedure* | *Munich* |
|---|---|---|
| Nostril | nasal approach paraseptal intrasellar: no Carnoy's or alcoholic solution | sublabial |
| In general nothing or lyodura | sella closure | fascia in larger sella openings no antibiotics |
| antibiotics 48 h | nasal tamponade | 24 (to 48) h |
| | *B. Endocrine follow-up* | |
| 3 weeks 3, 6, 12 months | controls | 1 week, 6–8 weeks 6, 12 months |
| | hormone replacement | |
| 200 mg Hydrocortisone 50 cortisone acetate | during operation day 1–5 | 100 mg Hydrocortisone, reduced to 25 mg or nothing if selective adenomectomy proven |
| | *C. Radiology* | |
| | before operation X-ray of the skull computerized tomogr. no air study in gen. | |
| Linear technique 2 mm | sella tomograms during operation televised x-ray no air study | spiral technique 2–3 mm |

supra- and parasellar tumor extension is computerized tomography (CT) of the skull, performed since 3 years ago in nearly all patients. By this method the tumor is already detectable within the sellar entrance, before a larger suprasellar extension leads to a chiasma syndrome (Fahlbusch et al., 1976; Kazner et al., 1978).

*Table III.*  Summary of results in 58 operated microprolactinomas.

A. *Patients*
   58 women, 17–43 years, mean age: 31.6 years
B. *Endocrinological findings*
   Duration of amenorrhea: 8 months–17 years, mean 5.1 years
   Primary amenorrhea: 3, secondary amenorrhea: 52, oligomenorrhea: 2, galactorrhea: 49
   PROLACTIN LEVELS
      Before operation 2 to 65-fold increases
      After transsphenoidal operation:                                  + Bromocr.
                                        normal    32/58 (=55%)
                                        decreased 26/58 (= 45%)    46/46
   GONADAL FUNCTION
   Menses                                                          46/46
      Op. alone                                         33/58
   Pregnancy                                                         13
      Op. alone                                          10
   OTHER PITUITARY FUNCTIONS

| (PITUITARY INSUFFICIENCY) | before operation | after operation |
|---|---|---|
| GH (IHT) | 15/52 (29%) | 12/39 (30%) |
| LH-RH-test | 11/53 (20%) | 9/47 (19%) |
| Sec. hypothyroidism | 0/58 (0%) | 0/58 (0%) |
| TRH-test | 3/18 (17%) | 2/18 (11%) |
| Cortisol (IHT) | 9/32 (28%) | 6/50 (19%) |
| DIABETES INSIPIDUS | 0/58 (0%) | |
| Transitory, 1–3 days | | 10/58 (17%) |
| Longer than 8 weeks | | 2/58 (3%) |

C. *Operative findings*
   Volume of the adenoma          smaller than 5 mm:       12
                                  between 5 and 10 mm:  36
                                  larger than 10 mm:       10
   Tissue: soft: 52/58   firm 6/58
   Haemorrhages 7/58
   Cysts         2/58
   Complications:  death                      0/58
                   transient rhinorrhea       3/58
                   transient meningitis       1/58
                   sphenoid sinusitis         2/58
D. *Radiological findings*
   Sella enlargement
      slight or normal            45/58
      medium                      13/58
   Pathological configuration     58/58
   Computerized tomography neg  33/36
      (horizontal sections)

With the small adenomas, no carotid angiography is necessary while the air study may be helpful if a cisternal herniation (empty sella) is suspected from the CT (Check *et al.*, 1978; Domingue *et al.*, 1978; Fahlbusch *et al.*, 1976; Wilson and Dempsey, 1978). The smallest adenomas, under 5 mm, were not detectable in horizontal sections in our EMI scanner, the results are questionable in coronal projection (Kazner *et al.*, 1978) but they should probably be visible in sagittal sections.

Of 95 women with hyperprolactinemic amenorrhea, 32 patients were treated with bromocriptine alone. PRL levels were not increased more than 4 - 5 fold (3000 $\mu$U/ml) and only slight sellar alterations were seen. Thirteen women who wished to become pregnant had normal pregnancies. Bromocriptine as the drug of choice is also recommended by some other groups (Bergh *et al.*, 1978; Friesen and Tolis, 1977; Thorner *et al.*, 1974) The Munich results are discussed by von Werder *et al.* (1978) and the follow-up of patients during pregnancy by Rjosk *et al.* (1979). There are no patients with normal sellar configuration and amenorrhea for whom functional hyperprolactinemia has been suggested (Boyar *et al.*, 1974) and who may harbour microprolactinomas which are not demonstrable even by sella tomography in this series.

This paper will concentrate on the 58 patients from whom microadenomas were removed by transsphenoidal operation.

At the time of operation the age of the patients varied from 17 to 43 years, with a mean age of 31.6 years (Table III). Galactorrhea could be observed in 49 of 58 patients. Four patients had primary and 52 had secondary amenorrhea with a mean duration of 5.1 years; in a third of these patients oligomenorrhea had begun several years before. Two patients had oligomenorrhea before the operation. In Munich, we operated by the transsphenoidal approach, with the head in the same position as originally described by Cushing: the surgeon's position is behind the patient's head. We prefer the sublabial, paraseptal-submucosal midline approach to the sphenoid sinus, thus preserving the nasal septum and the submucosa of the other side. The same midline procedure is performed in Milan (Table II), where the positioning described by Guiot (1974) and Hardy (1973) is used. In Milan the transnasal approach is performed via the nostril. In contrast to Munich, antibiotics are generally given in Milan. In both clinics the tamponade remains for 24-48 hours. Carnoy's solution or alcohol were not used in the sella. The sella floor is closed by fascia, but only for the larger adenomas, greater than 5 to 6 mm in diameter.

## RADIOLOGICAL FINDINGS

The sella size on the lateral X-ray of the skull was regarded as still normal or discretely enlarged in 45 of 58 patients (Fig. 1). In all patients unilateral expansion of the sella floor was accompanied by cortical bone thinning. Thirteen patients had a medium enlargement of the sella. The exact localization of the adenoma could be observed in the majority of cases only by sella tomograms, in agreement with Vezina and Sutton (1974) and Hardy's (1973) findings. However in some cases, an estimation of the tumor size did not agree with the intra-operative findings, since cysts and clots, as well as herniations into the cavernous sinus, cannot be taken into considerations.

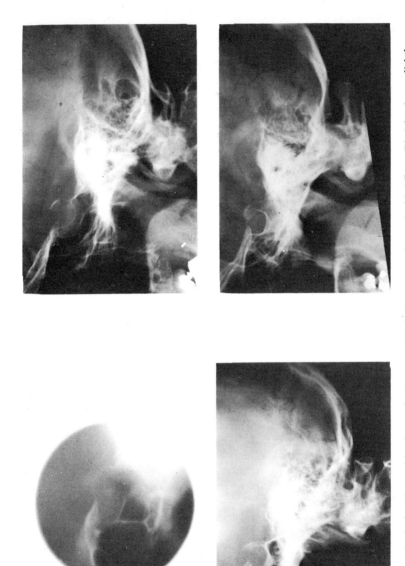

*Fig. 1.* Sella turcica in 4 patients with microprolactinomas; (a) left above: normal size, doubled floor; (b) right above: slightly enlarged, doubled floor; (c) left below: medium-enlarged, unilateral expansion; (d) right below: dorso-lateral bulging of the floor (tomogram).

### OPERATIVE FINDINGS

In all except 4 of 58 patients, the tumor was clearly lateralized, in 2 patients the adenoma was mainly outside the sella, and herniated into the cavernous sinus (Fig. 2). The estimated volume of the tumor, not globular in form in many cases, in 12 patients (= 21%) was smaller than 5 mm in diameter. Eight of these tumors were typically enclosed within the pituitary gland and located medio-posteriorly,

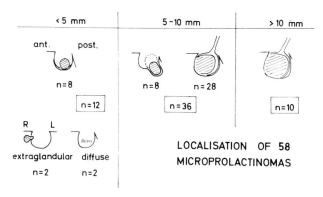

*Fig. 2.*   Localization and sella size of the adenoma in 58 patients.

whereas 2 adenomas were located antero-laterally, were extra-glandular and herniated into the cavernous sinus. Two firm tumors could not be separated clearly from the pituitary. In the larger group of 36 patients (62%) the adenoma size was 5–10 mm. In 8 cases a typical dorsolateral localization with extreme bulging of the posterior sella floor (Fig. 1a) and herniation into the sphenoid sinus was found. In these cases the pituitary was displaced into the anterior and contro-lateral part of the sella, whereas in the majority of cases the adenoma had filled the whole sella and displaced the pituitary to the diaphragm and lateral parts of the sella.

We also have seen 10 other patients (17%) in this series who had intrasellar and well circumscribed adenomas, in which the estimated tumor volume was some millimeters more than 10. In other series (Chang *et al.*, 1977; Hardy *et al.*, 1978; Jaquet *et al.*, 1978; Wilson and Dempsey, 1978) a higher incidence of surgically proven adenomas of less than 5 mm and with PRL levels under 2000 $\mu$U/ml has been found.

In Hardy's *et al.*, series (1978) of 46 women with microprolactinomas (Grade I) half of the patients had PRL levels below 100 ng/ml, and in our series one-fifth.

The tumor tissue was soft-to-fluid in all except five patients, in three of whom PRL levels were normalized, whereas in the two other patients (see above) tumor tissue could not be differentiated from the normal pituitary and no selective removal was possible.

The volume of the microprolactinomas correlated with the PRL levels (Fig. 3). In nine patients with larger tumors and only slightly elevated PRL levels, intra-tumoral haemorrages (*n*=7) and cysts (*n*=2) were found. No secondary hypo-thyroidism or adrenal insufficiency was found.

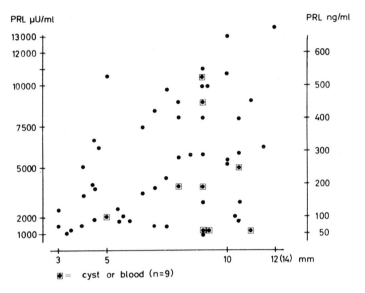

ADENOMA SIZE AND PRL LEVELS IN 58 MICROPROLACTINOMAS

*Fig. 3.* Correlation of PRL-levels and the size of the adenoma in 58 patients.

In three patients the chiasmatic cistern was involved into the sella, in what is known as an "empty sella syndrome". In contrast to other endocrine-active intra-sellar adenomas, no destruction of the sella floor was observed in these 58 patients. Light microscopic examination showed adenomas in all cases, 90% had mixed-type adenomas. Typical PRL-producing adenomas (Hachmeister *et al.*, 1972; Hachmeister, 1973; Kovacs, 1977; Peillon, 1978) were diagnosed in a part of these tumors by electron microscopy. In some adenomas of the Munich series, immunological staining technique was applied by Mashiter and Adam (1979). Biopsies were taken from the tissue adjacent to the adenoma. normal appearing anterior pituitary, in general, was found to be normal pituitary, or, in the case of a larger tumor atrophic pituitary tissue. In one case, hyperplasia of adjacent tissue was seen.

## COMPLICATIONS

No patients were lost in the early or later postoperative phases (Table III). Three patients had slight transient rhinoliquorrhea, occuring in the first days after the operation, cured by lumbar puncture drainage. One patient had a slight menin-gitis cured by antibiotics. No complaints were made during the operative approach. Two patients had mild sinusitis maxillaris, treated symptomatically. The complication rate in all transsphenoidal operations for intrasellar adenomas is about 1%.

## ENDOCRINOLOGICAL RESULTS

In all patients, selective adenomectomy was the aim. An example is given of a 28-year-old woman (Fig. 4), in whom a circumscribed adenoma could be removed selectively, demonstrated by normalized pituitary functions and normoprolactinemia after the operation.

After this operative procedure, PRL levels normalized in 32 of 58 patients (= 55%). In another 26 patients, the PRL levels decreased significantly, in many cases nearly into the normal range (Fig. 5).

The highest PRL level that could be normalized were $10\,043\mu U/ml$ in Munich and 657 ng/ml in Milan. Above these levels, normalization of PRL levels could be reached only by combined therapeutic procedures, performed for all larger adenomas, which usually were growing outside the sella. This has been the experience of other authors also (Chang *et al.*, 1978; Jaquet *et al.*, 1978). The frequency of normalized PRL level is greater in patients with only slightly elevated PRL levels. The best results could be obtained with microprolactinomas less than 5 mm in diameter, located medio- to posterolateral and PRL levels not above $2\,500\ \mu U/$ ml or 125 ng/ml. All the 8 patients had normoprolactinemia (Fig. 6) postoperatively.

Normalization of PRL levels occurred acutely, within hours after the tumor removal, which is shown in 13 patients of our Munich series (Fig. 7). Perioperative

### SELECTIVE ADENOMECTOMY OF A PROLACTINOMA

| B. Sch., ♀ 27 y. | | PRL | LH | GH | TSH | ACTH | ADH |
|---|---|---|---|---|---|---|---|
| PREOPERATIVE | | 9'132 → 9'137 | 1,4 → 5,0 | 0,9 → 7,6 | 1,0 → 8,9 | 9,8→24,5° | n |
| POSTOP. | 1 week | 290 | 1,3 → 11,0 | | 0,5 → 6,9 | 26,3→66,9 | |
| | 2 months | 387 → 688 | 16,3→32,8 | 1,5 →5,2 | 0,9 →12,3 | 9,7→22,4° | n |
| TEST | | TRH | LRH | IHT | TRH | ACTH, IHT° | 17-hours thirst per. |
| NORMAL VALUES | | < 650 µU/ml | ▲30 › 2 ng/ml | ▲ 30' › 7ng/ml | ▲ 30 › 2,7 µU/ ml | plas.cortisol 4 –19 µg% ▲60' › 12 µg% | urine concentr. › 750 mOsm/kg |

*Fig. 4.* Selective adenomectomy in a 28-year-old woman who desired pregnancy, documented by unchanged anterior pituitary functions and normoprolactinemia after the operation.

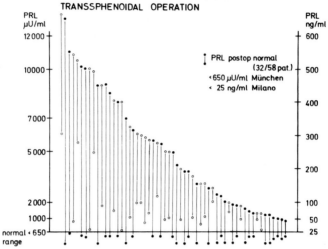

*Fig. 5.* Prolactin-levels before and 3–6 weeks after transsphenoidal selective adenomectomy in 58 patients with microprolactinomas.

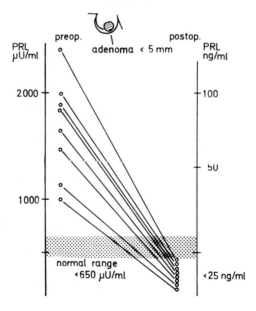

*Fig. 6.* Normalized PRL levels in 8 patients with PRL levels < 2 500 µU/ml and mediolateral prolactinomas < 5 mm.

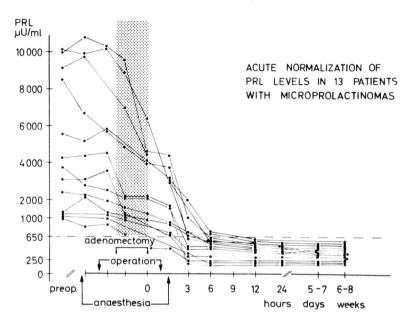

*Fig. 7.* Perioperative PRL levels of 13 patients with microprolactinomas, normalising acutely after adenomectomy.

monitoring of PRL levels in 50 patients with prolactinomas demonstrated that all acutely normalized PRL levels remained normal over periods from 1 to 4 years (Fahlbusch *et al.*, 1977; Fahlbusch, 1978). In the series of macroprolactinomas only, we observed one woman in whom acutely normalized PRL levels, which remained normal over a period of 1 year then increased again, indicating recurrence (v. Werder *et al.*, 1978; v. Werder, 1979). Normalized PRL levels could be stimulated about 100% or more by TRH in half of the patients (7/12).

Normal menses occurred, by the time of the last postoperative control, in 33 of 58 patients, 32 with normal PRL levels (Table III), three of these patients had anovulatory cycle. In 7 patients menses occurred although PRL levels were not clearly in the normal range. After additional bromocriptine therapy of another 13 patients, normal PRL levels and normal ovarian functions had been observed in 46 (of 46) patients. Galactorrhea, which was observed in 83% (48/58) of the patients, disappeared in most of the patients with normoprolactinemia.

No additional partial insufficiency of the anterior lobe occurred which had to be treated with thyroxin or hydrocortisone. No secondary hypothyroidism could be detected before or after the operation. Before operation 28% (9/32) after operation 12% (6/50) had abnormal rises in cortisol during insulin hypoglycemia. Selective adenomectomy could be proved endocrinologically in nearly all patients with normalized PRL levels. Not included in this consideration are the GH secretion, or the LRH- and TRH-induced TSH and LH secretion.

Preoperatively 29% (15/52) had impaired GH secretion, which did not change postoperatively. All adenomas, with exception of three, were more than 8 mm in diameter. Improvement occurred in 6 cases and deterioration in 3. Before the operation, 21% (11/53) of the amenorrhoic patients had an insufficient LH response to LRH, after the adenomectomy 19% (9/47). An insufficient or subnormal TSH response to TRH was found in 11% of the patients.

A slight transitory diabetes insipidus occurred in 17% (10/58) on the first day after the operation. While in these patients only a single injection or no application of antidiuretic hormone was necessary, 2 other patients had to be treated for longer than 8 weeks.

The relatively high rate of diabetes insipidus in intrasellar prolactinomas depends probably on the frequent localization of the adenomas close to the posterior lobe.

## CONCLUSIONS

It remains a question of why, in our microprolactinoma series the PRL levels could be normalized in only 55-60% of the patients. The results were identical in Milan and Munich. Also, why could the same neurosurgeons not achieve with the same microsurgical procedures the results obtained in acromegalic patients (Fahlbusch, 1978; Giovanelli *et al.*, 1979) or in Cushing's disease (Müller and Fahlbusch, 1978)? In those patients with intrasellar adenomas GH-levels or cortisol-levels were normalized in 80-90%.

The classifications of patients with prolactinomas differ so that a valid comparison of operative results is impossible. Yet it seems that Chang *et al.*, (1977), Guitelman *et al.* (1977) and Jaquet *et al.* (1978) have had similar experience. Hardy *et al.* (1978) described normal PRL levels in a higher percentage, in up to 91% in his Grade I patients and in 78% of the intrasellar adenomas in Grade II. All these authors described greater numbers of operated microprolactinomas of smaller size with lower PRL levels on the average, than those in our series.

It is still a question whether the relatively low normalization rate of PRL is due to some special surgical procedure, which should be radical in order to eliminate the adenoma but gentle enough to preserve pituitary function. In addition, the adenomas are often not well separated from residual pituitary tissue and may be atypically located.

In any case, the results show that the "smaller" the microprolactinomas, the greater the possibility to normalize PRL levels by microsurgical procedures.

After more than four years experience, we are extending our operative indications to include patients with smaller adenomas and the patients who became pregnant under bromocriptine. Although no severe complication occurred after microsurgical adenomectomy, the risk of medical therapy with bromocriptine is smaller, especially in places where no competent and experiences neurosurgeon exists. Bromocriptine remains indicated for women with desire of pregnancy who have very small adenomas and PRL levels not greater than 3000-5000μU/ml. In these well-chosen women Rjosk, 1978, 1979) and in other series (Diedrich *et al.*, 1978; Mornex *et al.*, 1978), no complication was observed during pregnancy whereas visual field sequelae and pituitary apoplexy after bromocriptine therapy (Bergh *et al.*, 1978; Van Dalen and Greve, 1977) may occur in patients with larger intrasellar adenomas.

## REFERENCES

Bergh, T., Nillius, S. J. and Wide, L. (1978). *Acta endocr.* **88**, 435–451.

Boyar, R. M., Kapen, S., Finkelstein, J. W., Perlow, M., Sassin, J. F., Fukushima, D. K., Weitzman, E. D. and Hellman, L. (1974). *J. Clin. Invest.* **53**, 1588–1598.

Chang, R. J., Keye, W. R., Young, J. R., Wilson, C. B. and Jaffe, R. B. (1977). *Amer. J. Obstet. Gynecol.* **128**, 356–363.

Check, J. H., Rakoff, A. E., Goldfarb, A. F. and King, L. C. (1978). *Amer. J. Obstet. Gynecol.* **128**, 688–689.

Costello, R. T. (1935a). *Am. J. Path.* **12**, 205.

Costello, R. T. (1935b). *Proc. Mayo Clin.* **10**, 499.

Diedrich, K., Leidenberger, F., Lehmann, F. and Bettendorf, G. (1978). *Geburtsh. v. Frauenh.* **38**, 716–725.

Dominigue, J. N., Wing, S. D. and Wilson, C. B. (1978). *J. Neurosurg.* **48**, 23–28.

Fahlbusch, R. (1978). "Endokrine Funktionstörungen beir cerebralen Prozessein". Thieme-Copythek, Stuttgart.

Fahlbusch, R. and Marguth, F. (1978). *Neurosurg. Rev.* **1/2**, 5–13.

Fahlbusch, R., Grumme, T., Aulich, A., Wende, S., Steinhoff, H., Lanksch, W. and Kazner, E. (1976). *In* "Cranial Computerized Tomography" (W. Lanksch and E. Kazner, eds) pp. 114–127. Springer, Berlin.

Fahlbusch, R., Rjosk, H. K. and Werder, K. v. (1977). *Acta endocr. (Copenhag.)* **208**, 46–47.

Fahlbusch, R., Rjosk, H. K. and Werder, K. v. (1978). *In* "Treatment of Pituitary Adenomas" (R. Fahlbusch and K. v. Werder, eds) pp. 225–237. Thieme, Stuttgart.

Friesen, H. G. and Tolis, G. (1977). *Clin. Endocrinol. Suppl.* **6**, 91–99.

Giovanelli, M., Gaini, S. M., Tomei, G., Motti, E. D. F., Beck-Peccoz, P., Paracchi, A. and De Camilli, P. (1978). *In* "Treatment of Pituitary Adenomas" (R. Fahlbusch and K. v. Werder, eds) pp. 279–372. Thieme, Stuttgart.

Giovanelli, M., Fahlbusch, R. *et al.* (1980). This volume.

Guiot, G. (1973). *In* "Diagnosis and Treatment of Pituitary Tumors" (P. O. Kohler and G. T. Ross, eds) pp. 159–178. Exerpta Medica Amsterdam, American Elsevier, New York.

Guiot, G. (1978). *In* "Treatment of Pituitary Adenomas" (R. Fahlbusch and K. v. Werder, eds) pp. 202–218. Thieme, Stuttgart.

Guitelman, A., Aparicio, N. J., Mancini, A., Encinas, M. T., Levalle, O. and Schally A. v. (1977). *J. Clin. Endocrinol. Metab.* **45**, 810.

Hachmeister, V. (1973). *In* "Modern Aspects of Neurosurgery" (H. Kuhlendahl, M. Brock, D. LeVay, T. J. Weston, eds) Exerpta Medica, Amsterdam. American Elsevier, New York Vol. IV.

Hachmeister, V., Fahlbusch, R. and Werder, K. v. (1972). *Acta endocr. (Copenhag.)* Suppl. **159**, 42.

Hardy, J. (1973). *In* "Diagnosis and Treatment of Pituitary Tumors" (P. O. Kohler and G. T. Ross, eds) pp. 179–194 Excerpta Medica Amsterdam, American Elsevier, New York.

Hardy, J., Beauregard, H. and Robert, F. (1978). *In* "Progress in Prolactin Physiology and Pathology Elsevier" (C. Robyn and N. Harter, eds) pp. 361–370. Biomedical Press, North Holland.

L'Hermite, M., Caufriez, A., Virasoro, E., Stevenaert, A., Copinschi, G. and Robyn, C. (1978). *In* "Treatment of Pituitary Adenomas" (R. Fahlbusch and K. v. Werder, eds) pp. 60–77. Thieme, Stuttgart.

Hotton, F., Kleiner, S., Benchekroun, S. and L'Hermite, M. (1976). *J. Belge Radiol.* **4**, 335.

Jaquet, P., Grisoli, F., Guibout, M., Lissitzky, J.-C. and Carayon, P. (1978). *J. Clin. Endocrinol. Metab.* **46**, 459–466.

Kazner, R., Fahlbusch, R., Lanksch, W., Rothe, R., Scherer, U. Steinhoff, H., Grumme, T., Lange, S., Meese, W., Aulich, A. and Wende, S. (1978). *In* "Treatment of Pituitary Adenomas, 1. European Workshop" (R. Fahlbusch and K. v. Werder, eds) pp. 101–114 Thieme, Stuttgart.

Kovacs, K. (1977). *Clin. Endocrinol. Suppl.* **6**, 71–79.

Mashiter, K. and Adam, E. F. (1979). This volume.

Mornex, R., Orgiazzi, J., Hugues, B., Gagnaire, J. C. and Claustrat, B. (1978). *J. Clin. Endocrinol. Metab.* **47**, 290–295.

Müller, O. A. and Fahlbusch, R. (1978). *Acta endocr. (Copenh.)* Suppl. **215**, 23–24.

Peillon, F., Racadot, J., Noussy, D., Vila-Porcile, E., Oliver, L. and Racadot, O. (1978). *In* "Treatment of pituitary Adenomas" (R. Fahlbusch and K. v. Werder, eds) pp. 114–122 Thieme, Stuttgart.

Rjosk, H. K., Fahlbusch, R., Huber, H. and Werder, K. v. (1978). *In* "Treatment of Pituitary Adenomas" (R. Fahlbusch and K. v. Werder, eds) pp. 395–400. Thieme, Stuttgart.

Rjosk, H. K. *et al.* (1980). This volume.

Saeger. W. (1977). "Die Hypophysentumoren", Vol. 6. Fisher Verlag, Stuttgart.

Swanson, H. A. and du Boulay, G. (1975). *Brit. J. Radiol.* **48**, 366.

Thorner, M. O., Mc Neilly, A. S., Hagen, C. and Besser, G. M. (1974). *Br. Med. J.* **2**, 419.

Tolis, G. (1977). *Clin. Endocrinol. Suppl.* **6**, 81–89.

Van Dalen, J. T. W. Greve, E. L. (1977). *Brit. J. Opthalmol.* **61**, 729–733.

Vezina, J. L. and Sutton, T. J. (1974). *Amer. J. Roentgenol.* **120**, 46–54.

Werder, K. v. and Fahlbusch, R. (1977). *Europ. J. Clin. Invest.* **7**, 233.

Werder, K. v., Fahlbusch, R., Landgraf, R., Pickardt, C. R., Rjosk, H. K. and Scriba, P. C. (1978a). *In* "Treatment of Pituitary Adenomas" (R. Fahlbusch and K. v. Werder, eds) pp. 377–390. Thieme, Stuttgart.

Werder, K. v., Fahlbusch, R., Landgraf, R., Pickardt, C. R., Rjosk, H. K. and Scriba, P. C. (1978). *J. Endocrinol. Invest.* **1**, 47–58.

Werder, K. v. *et al.* (1980). This volume.

Wilson, C. B. and Dempsey, L. C. (1978). *J. Neurosurg.* **48**, 13–22.

# CUSHING'S DISEASE: BELATED
# CONFIRMATION AND MICROSURGICAL TREATMENT*

C. B. Wilson[1], J. B. Tyrrell[2] and P. A. Fitzgerald[2]

[1]*Department of Neurological Surgery and* [2]*Metabolic Research Unit,*
*University of California, San Francisco 94143, USA*

With his characteristic slavish devotion to detail, Harvey Cushing presented and subsequently published his extraordinary study of basophilic pituitary adenomas (Cushing, 1932). Validation of his observations followed long after Cushing's death through the fortunate coincidence of two developments: first, conclusive biochemical definition of pituitary-based hypercortisolism became possible, for the first time differentiating this distinct clinical entity from other causes of hypercortisolism (Liddle and Shute, 1969; Liddle, 1972); and second, the evolution of transsphenoidal microsurgery provided not only an effective means of treating the disease but also permitted unequivocal documentation of ACTH-secreting microadenomas as a distinct entity (Hardy, 1973). Because it is now possible, in one simultaneous maneuver, to detect and remove minute adenomas situated in a pituitary gland of normal dimensions, there has been a revolutionary change in the management of Cushing's disease. Until a superior form of treatment evolves, microsurgical removal of these remarkably occult adenomas offers the highest probability of restoring normal pituitary function to patients affected with the disease.

---

*This investigation was supported in part by grants from the Levi J. and Mary C. Skaggs Foundation of Oakland, CA, the Susan Greenwall Foundation of New York City, and (at the General Clinical Research Center of the University of California, San Francisco) by funds provided by the Division of Research Resources (RR-79), U.S. Public Health Service.

The endocrinologic data from our series of patients were presented separately (Tyrrell *et al.*, 1978), and the subject at hand is the surgical perspective based upon these cases. When faced with a patient carrying the diagnosis of Cushing's disease, the surgeon assumes that the pituitary gland contains an ACTH-secreting adenoma.

## PREOPERATIVE EVALUATION FOR TRANSSPHENOIDAL EXPLORATION

In experienced hands the operation requires two hours of general anesthesia, and to date transsphenoidal exploration has not been rejected as a form of treatment because of a patient's poor general health. Although many are seriously ill in a metabolic sense, most if not all patients can be prepared adequately for an operative procedure of this magnitude.

In order to determine the approximate size of an intrasellar adenoma and to define exactly any extrasellar extension, the surgeon requires hypocycloidal polytomograms of the sella and sphenoid sinus and a pneumoencephalogram with polytomographic sections at 2 mm intervals.

Tomograms of the sella may be normal, in which instance the tumor will be small, in the range of 5 mm or less, and its location can be determined only by exploring the normal gland. If the sella is enlarged, the point of focal expansion indicates the tumor's position. The degree of sellar enlargement, focal and generalized, will provide a reasonable estimate of the tumor's size subject to modification by pneumoencephalographic findings. A suprising number of ACTH-secreting adenomas, small as well as large, penetrate dura and bone to occupy the sphenoid sinus, and although none has extended into the body of the incomplete pneumatized sphenoid, undoubtedly this tumor has the potential to do so. Finally, the surgeon determines the anatomy of the sphenoid sinus and its septations. Because the majority of patients with Cushing's disease have osteoporotic bones as a consequence of long-standing hypercortisolism, even with polytomograms taken at 1 mm intervals the desired detail may not be obtained.

Pneumoencephalography is an unpleasant procedure at best, and at worst it causes headache, vomiting and incapacitation, sometimes continuing for several days. Sharp definition of the subarachnoid cisterns in direct proximity to a tumor's superior surface affords clear visualization of small suprasellar tumor nodules and, less often, extension of the suprasellar cistern in the sella, a finding indicating prior necrosis of the adenoma. Computerized tomographic (CT) scans will demonstrate large suprasellar extensions that deform the subarachnoid cisterns, but the technique does not permit detection of the small and usually eccentric suprasellar extensions more likely to be encountered in Cushing's disease. Recently we have used a newly developed water-soluble iodinated contrast medium instead of air, and the same detailed anatomy can be portrayed with minimal morbidity.

In a few cases we have omitted pneumoencephalography because the sellar tomograms were normal and the patient's general condition was poor. Carotid angiography was performed on all patients early in our experience, but the discomfort and risk were not justified by the information obtained, and angiography has been eliminated as a routine preoperative test.

## OPERATIVE APPROACH FOR TRANSSPHENOIDAL EXPLORATION

The transsphenoidal procedure developed by Hardy has been followed without significant modification (Hardy, 1973). Because the designated subject is the adenoma whose diameter measures less than 10 mm, i.e. microadenoma, removal of larger tumors will not be considered.

At the outset, the surgeon recognizes the difficulties involved when approaching a normal sella. Microadenomas seldom present on the exposed surface of the anterior lobe, and with few exceptions the tumor's location must be determined by entering an apparently normal gland. Adequate exploration for a small tumor requires wide exposure: laterally to the edge of both cavernous sinuses, superiorly to the junction of diaphragma sellae and tuberculum, and inferiorly to the horizontal plane of the sellar floor. In two cases early in our experience, the presence of large dural venous sinuses overlying the gland precluded adequate exploration in a bloodless field, and in both instances the operation was abandoned without opening the dura.

The operative approach is based upon a series of 37 adenomas, with completed postoperative testing and follow-up for 4–56 months after operation. Microadenomas (diameter 9 mm or less) accounted for 31 tumors, 4 of which had extended beyond the sella: 1 perforated the floor of the sella to present in the sphenoid sinus, 1 extended extradurally beneath the cavernous sinus, and 2 had small suprasellar nodules. The majority of microadenomas (20/31) measured 5 mm or less (Table I). Particular difficulty may be encountered in locating adenomas 3 mm and smaller, the size of 10 tumors in this group. The

*Table I.* Size of pituitary adenomas in Cushing's disease.

| Size (mm) | Number of adenomas |
|---|---|
| Microadenomas | |
| 1 | 2 |
| 2 | 5 |
| 3 | 3 |
| 4 | 3 |
| 5 | 7 |
| 6 | 3 |
| 7 | 2 |
| 8 | 3 |
| 9 | 3 |
| | (31) |
| Macroadenomas | |
| 10 | 3 |
| 15 | 1 |
| 20 | 1 |
| 30 | 1 |
| | (6) |
| | 37 |

two smallest tumors, 1.5 and 1 mm, were missed at the time of exploration, and both were identified in serial sections of the totally excised glands.

When the tumor's intrasellar location is known either from tomographic changes or by direct inspection of the exposed anterior lobe, removal follows the technique described by Hardy (Hardy, 1973). With no clue to the tumor's location, the surgeon must make stepwise incisions into the gland. In our series the tumors were distributed almost equally in the lateral lobes and middle of the anterior lobe. Two tumors occupied the pars intermedia and posterior lobe, where the customarily clear delineation of tumor from normal anterior lobe is lacking.

Until an unlocalized tumor is identified, the following steps are carried out in order:

(1)  a horizontal incision is made completely across the mid-portion of the anterior lobe, bisecting the gland, to expose the posterior lobe at the depth of the incision;

(2)  a vertical incision is extended from the gland's upper surface to the sellar floor—first in the midline and then into each lateral lobe;

(3)  the surface of the gland lying against each cavernous sinus and on the floor of the sella is inspected;

(4)  the superior surface of the anterior lobe beneath the diaphragma sellae is visualized if the preoperative pneumoencephalogram did not conclusively exclude a suprasellar nodule;

(5)  with the anterior lobe now divided into eight sections, any of the eight sections that are disproportionately large should be incised; and

(6)  finally, if the patient understands the implications of total hypopy-sectomy and has agreed beforehand, the pituitary stalk is sectioned and the entire pituitary gland is excised and submitted for pathologic examination.

With five exceptions, soft, dull white to grey adenomas have been sharply demarcated from adjacent anterior lobe and dura. Three tumors, all measuring 2 mm, were atypical: the pathologic nature of the tissue was unequivocal, but the appearance suggested a focal area of softening rather than a discrete neoplastic nodule. Two tumors occupied the pars intermedia and posterior lobe, and because of similarities in color as well as texture, these adenomas were removed along with the immediately adjacent posterior lobe.

A curative operation demands strict attention to details. The surgeon must visualize the entire surface of the cavity that remains after gross removal of the adenoma. This may require additional incisions into the overlying anterior lobe, and if the tumor is small and lies posteriorly, adequate visualization often dictates removal of a 2–3 mm wedge of normal anterior lobe. Because of its remarkable resiliency and an apparent capacity to re-establish vascular connect-ions when separated into islands by multiple exploratory incisions, the described maneuvers have not impaired anterior lobe function as determined by post-operative testing.

Thorough inspection of the cavity should be carried out under high magni-fication in a bloodless field. Unless the tumor rests against the cavernous sinus, in which instance the most anterior surface may be obscured by a medial exten-sion of the cavernous sinus across the sella, the tumor's bed can be visualized directly. Mirrors are useful aids in removing macroadenomas, but their use is no substitute for direct inspection.

Frozen sections of grossly normal anterior lobe have not been obtained. The demarcation between anterior lobe and tumor is distinct, and anything beyond token sampling with frozen sections has been considered unnecessary in view of the small number of recurrences in a large series of endocrine-active adenomas. Perhaps a few clonogenic neoplastic cells penetrate the apparently uninvolved anterior lobe, but if so present evidence suggests that they are destroyed by alcohol.

Alcohol is used liberally to destroy cells that almost certainly remain in microscopic clusters or sheets. The only contraindication to the use of alcohol is a wide aperture into the subarachnoid space, but this situation will arise rarely in removing tumors. Alcohol (absolute) is introduced into the cavity with a blunt needle followed by tight packing of the cavity with Gelfoam soaked in alcohol. The latter maneuver restores the cavity to its original size and thereby ensures that the entire surface is exposed to the necrotizing action of alcohol. Irrigation and packing are alternated several times, and finally alcohol-saturated Gelfoam is left within the cavity. Depending upon the size and position of the cavity, and therefore the potential for postoperative cerebrospinal rhinorrhea, fat or muscle may be used to pack the tumor cavity. We have followed Hardy's technique for closing the sella with nasal septal cartilage.

We have detected no clinically significant damage to anterior lobe function as a result of the multiple incisions and prolonged exposure to absolute alcohol during the course of identifying and removing these adenomas. Of 12 patients tested serially following selective removal of microadenomas, 11 have had normal values after conventional pituitary stimulation tests, and the remaining patient had normal values except for a blunted response of growth hormone following L-dopa stimulation. All premenopausal women are menstruating normally, and one became pregnant and delivered a normal child.

## ANALYSIS OF OPERATIVE FAILURE

The two smallest tumors, 1.5 and 1.0 mm, were missed at exploration, and in all probability some tumors of this size will be missed in the future.

Seven tumors were either removed incompletely or recurred after initial correction of hypercortisolism. Three failures (two primary failures and one recurrence) were macroadenomas. The present analysis involves four micro-adenomas.

In two patients, who had undergone what was thought to be complete and selective removal of their 5 mm adenomas, hypercortisolism persisted in the immediate postoperative period. One, a young female, was referred for heavy particle irradiation. The other, a male medical student, was improved, and a year later requested reoperation at which time no additional tumor was identified. Except for mild hypercortisolism he has normal pituitary function and at this point declines further treatment.

The third microadenoma failure was a middle-aged female from whom a 2 mm tumor was removed. She, too, had persisting hypercortisolism in the early postoperative period; because of alarming hypertension she elected to undergo reoperation and, if no addition tumor could be identified and removed selectively, total hypophysectomy. When no tumor could be identified at reoperation, total removal of anterior and posterior lobes was performed. Serial sections through the excised gland failed to disclose either an adenoma or hyperplasia of ACTH-secreting cells, although this secondary procedure corrected the hypercortisolism.

The fourth patient had a microadenoma that extended beneath the right cavernous sinus, and its location precluded removal under direct vision. Complete removal was considered doubtful, and an effort was made to destroy nonvisualized tumor with alcohol. Although hypercortisolism was corrected when tested 4 months after operation, recurrence was documented within one year. In this instance, complete removal was not achieved because of the tumor's position.

## DISCUSSION

Transsphenoidal microsurgical removal of the adenomas that cause Cushing's disease has proved to be a therapeutically successful procedure, although the results to date have not resolved the seminal roles of the hypothalamus and adenohypophysis. However, until more specific or selective therapy becomes available, the described operative approach will replace adrenalectomy for the initial management of this condition. The reported results are good, and with further experience improvement is almost inevitable.

Cushing's disease is an uncommon entity, the diagnosis, treatment and long-term endocrine supervision of which can be, and often are, difficult. The operative identification and removal of the ACTH-secreting adenomas taxes and may exceed the technical virtuosity of experienced surgeons. The preceding factors, namely, the rarity of Cushing's disease and the technical demands of removing the offending microadenomas, argue forcefully for the selective referral of these patients to surgeons who have extensive experience in performing pituitary microsurgery. Obviously, younger surgeons must gain experience in transsphenoidal operations, but that experience can and should be gained in treating the vastly larger number of patients with other endocrine-active and endocrine-inactive pituitary tumors.

The exciting activity in neuroendocrinology and the emerging role of transsphenoidal operations for certain endocrine disorders should be predictive of rapid advances in both fields, and no single group will derive greater benefit than patients affected with Cushing's disease. The state of the art at the time of Cushing's death denied him that satisfaction that comes with confirmation of one's pioneering observations and the honor of eponymic designation.

## REFERENCES

Cushing, H. (1932). *Bull. John Hopkins Hosp.* **50**, 137.
Feldman, J. M. (1975). *New Engl. J. Med.* **293**, 930.
Hardy, J. (1973). *In* "Diagnosis and Treatment of Pituitary Tumors" (P. O.

Kohler and G. T. Ross, eds) pp. 179–194. American Elsevier Publishing Company, New York.

Liddle, G. W. and Shute, A. M. (1969). *Adv. Intern. Med.* **15**, 155.

Liddle, G. W. (1972). *Am. J. Med.* **53**, 638.

Tyrell, J. B., Brooks, R. M., Fitzgerald, P. A., Cofoid, P. B., Forsham, P. H. and Wilson, C. B. (1978). *New Engl. J. Med.* **298**, 753.

# THE LIMITATIONS OF SURGICAL TREATMENT OF PITUITARY MICROADENOMAS

P. Wrightson

*Department of Neurology and Neurosurgery, Auckland Hospital, and Department of Surgery, University of Auckland, Auckland, New Zealand*

## INTRODUCTION

The selective removal of a secreting pituitary adenoma is an elegant and appealing procedure which can cure hormonal excess and leave normal pituitary function. It is now widely practised and series of considerable numbers of patients have been published. The success in correcting the endocrine abnormality is well documented, but though some cases have been followed up for ten years or more (e.g. Hardy *et al.*, 1976 for acromegaly, Carmalt *et al.*, 1977 for Cushing's disease) it is not certain as yet that the result is permanent.

Operative descriptions commonly state that excision leaves a well defined clean walled cavity, and some authors (Hardy, 1973; Velasco *et al.*, 1977) refer to histological check of the completeness of the excision at the time of operation. There is, however, no direct evidence of the completeness of surgical excision. Some useful histological indication can be obtained from careful examination of operative specimens and autopsy material (Wrightson, 1978). In specimens in which the pituitary tissue and tumour are preserved in their normal relationship, it is possible to judge how definite the surgical plane of cleavage would be and where it would lie, and if tumour is present beyond this plane. Where dura mater is in contact with the tumour, it can be examined for invasion (Shaffi and Wrightson, 1975). In autopsy specimens it is possible to search for extension beyond the fossa.

Postal address: Dr. P. Wrightson, Department of Neurology and Neurosurgery, Auckland Hospital, Private Bag, Auckland, New Zealand.

It is important to have at least a provisional answer to this question while waiting for the results of long term follow-up. If it can be shown that conservative excision as now practised is incomplete, it will be necessary to modify the policies of management.

## MATERIALS AND METHODS

Pathological material from 48 cases of acromegaly, 2 cases with amenorrhoea and galactorrhoea and 5 cases of Cushing's disease was studied; in addition sellar *dura mater* from 23 cases of non-secreting adenomas was examined. Sixty-nine specimens were obtained at operation and at autopsy; the autopsy material was from patients who had presented with clinical endocrine disease. Biopsy material consisted of fragments of tumour and normal gland, and, where possible, sellar *dura mater*. Autopsy specimens consisted of the entire sella and cavernous sinuses, decalcified and serially sectioned in the coronal plane.

## RESULTS AND CONCLUSIONS

In 25 cases normal gland tissue was present as well as tumour, and in 14 of these the boundary between tumour and gland was preserved and could be studied. Passing from tumour to normal gland, the boundary was usually marked by a reduction in cellularity and an increase in connective tissue stroma. Gland tissue was often compressed, forming the cells into rows at the junction (Fig. 1). This is the appearance classically described and corresponds to the surgeon's finding of a soft tumour, often diffluent, with the boundary with normal gland marked by a sharp increase in consistency. In 2 of the 14 cases there was a more marked condensation of connective tissue at the junction, forming a capsule which would accentuate the surgical plane. In one this marked the true boundary of the tumour, but in the other, tumour could be seen on the far side.

In 25 cases the density of connective tissue in the tumour and normal gland could be compared. In all, the majority of the tumour was highly cellular, with little stroma. However, in 4 cases there were areas of tumour where stroma was at least as dense as that of the gland, and in 5 cases it was even denser (Fig. 2). Such firm areas occurring at the periphery of the tumour may confuse the plane of excision, so that frozen sections may be needed to come to a decision.

In 14 cases the change in cell morphology could be studied in passing from tumour to gland. In the simplest situation, as in Fig. 1, tumour cells give place to normal gland cells abruptly along a regular line representing the plane of cleavage. In only two cases was this seen in all areas. In 8 cases the general line of the boundary could be seen, but there was considerable interchange of cells across it (Fig. 3). In 3 cases there was no real boundary to be seen, tumour cells and gland intermixing over a wide area (Fig. 4).

The adenomas often extended to the periphery of the gland and lay in contact with dura mater. In 41 cases, dura in contact with tumour was examined, and in 23 definite invasion was seen, classed as gross in 6 cases.

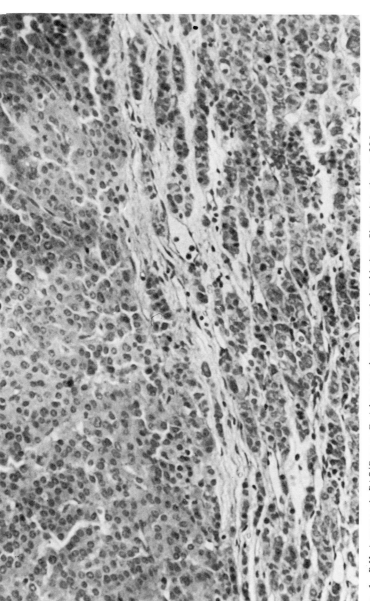

*Fig. 1.* P.H. Acromegaly PAS/Orange G. Adenoma above, normal gland below. Sharp junction. × 285.

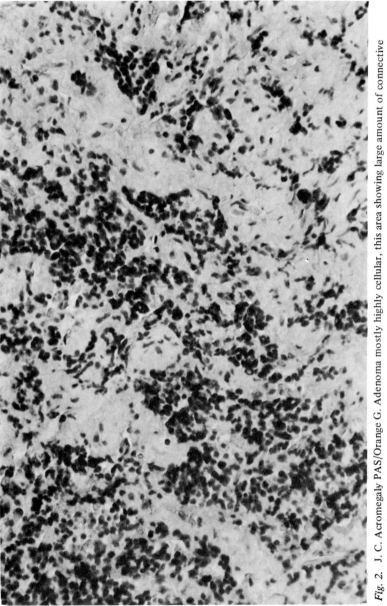

*Fig. 2.* J. C. Acromegaly PAS/Orange G. Adenoma mostly highly cellular, this area showing large amount of connective tissue stroma. × 285.

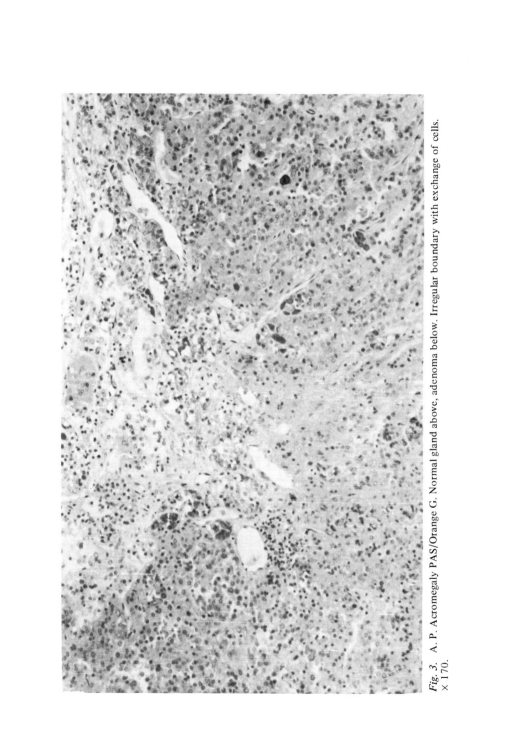

*Fig. 3.* A. P. Acromegaly PAS/Orange G. Normal gland above, adenoma below. Irregular boundary with exchange of cells. × 170.

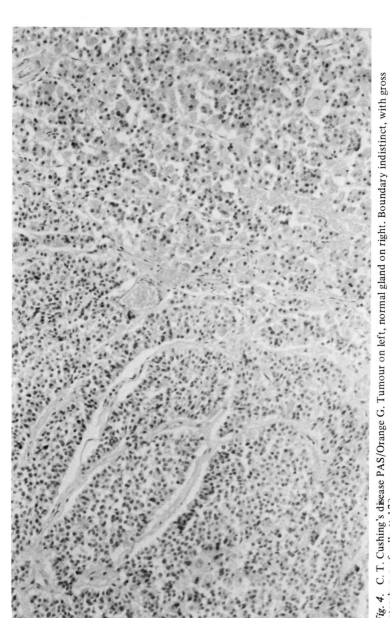

*Fig. 4.* C. T. Cushing's disease PAS/Orange G. Tumour on left, normal gland on right. Boundary indistinct, with gross interchange of cells. × 170.

In one autopsy specimen from a patient with acromegaly who died without treatment, a 10 mm adenoma occupied one side of the sella. The boundary with normal gland appeared sharp. However, posteriorly it had invaded the dorsum sellae and tumour was present in the bone of the posterior clinoid. In a patient with Nelson's syndrome who had died six weeks after clearance of a radiologically normal sella, massive tumour was found in one cavernous sinus. Such extension beyond the sella is commonplace in larger tumours, but plainly can occur in smaller tumours, and especially in Nelson's syndrome.

## DISCUSSION

The histological evidence presented leaves no doubt that though some pituitary microadenomas can be removed completely through a natural plane of separation, this is not always the case, for the following reasons:

(a)   the plane of separation may be confused by areas of adenoma of the consistency of normal gland;
(b)   though there may be a distinct plane, tumour may be present on the gland side of it;
(c)   if there appears to be a capsule around the adenoma, tumour may be present on the outer side;
(d)   there may be no sharp boundary to the tumour;
(e)   dura mater is infiltrated by tumour in over 50% of cases;
(f)   there may be tumour in bone or cavernous sinuses, even when the adenoma is small;

These findings are in conflict with the current impression that most microadenomas have sharply limited boundaries. This impression seems to have arisen in two ways. The term "adenoma" presumes that the tumour is benign; however, as the frequent involvement of dura demonstrates, it has a strong tendency to local invasion. In this it resembles the meningioma, and comparisons may be drawn with the recurrence rate of this tumour. Secondly, conclusions about the anatomy of microadenomas seen clinically have often been drawn from the small "adenomas" found at autopsy (Costello, 1936). These are certainly well localized. However, the age incidence (Kernohan and Sayre, 1956) and the absence of endocrine effects show that these are different entities, and strict comparison is invalid.

In the light of this evidence, it may be advisable to extend the limits of surgical excision, or to cauterize the tumour bed more vigorously. Especially in Cushing's disease, where there may be continued stimulation of the remaining gland, complete sellar clearance may be advisable in some patients. Other methods, such as isotope implantation, may have advantages in this condition (Holdaway *et al.*, 1978).

At present there appears to be a consensus that radiotherapy should not be given unless excision is plainly incomplete, either as seen at operation, or afterwards when hormone levels remain high (Williams *et al.*, 1975; Hardy *et al.*, 1976; Wilson and Dempsey, 1978; Carmalt *et al.*, 1977). It is suggested that post-operative radiotherapy should be the rule rather than the exception. If it is not offered until recurrence is obvious, the patient has returned to his original state;

at that time radiotherapy would not have been expected to cure him.

Whether in the future these histological observations will be found to be important must await long term follow-up. In the meantime, it is prudent to give them considerable weight in deciding on methods of treatment.

## REFERENCES

Carmalt, M. H. B., Dalton, G. A., Fletcher, R. F. and Smith, W. T. (1977). *Q. Jl Med.* **46**, 119–134.
Costello, R. T. (1936). *Am. J. Path.* **12**, 205.
Hardy, J. (1973). *In* "Diagnosis and Treatment of Pituitary Tumours" (P. O. Kohler and G. T. Ross, eds) pp. 179–194. Excerpta Medica Amsterdam, Amsterdam.
Hardy, J., Somma, M. and Vezina, J. L. (1976). *In* "Current Controversies in Neurosurgery" (T. P. Morley, ed) pp. 377–391. W. B. Saunders, Philadelphia.
Holdaway, I. M., Wrightson, P., Frengley, P. A., Scott, D. J. and Ibbertson, H. K. (1978). Proceedings of 6th Asia and Oceania Congress of Endocrinology, pp. 86–91. Singapore.
Kernohan, J. W. and Sayre, G. P., (1956). "Tumours of the Pituitary Gland and Infundibulum" in Atlas of tumour pathology Sect. 10. Fasc. 36, Washington D. C., Armed Forces Institute of Pathology.
Shaffi, O. M. and Wrightson, P. (1975). *N. Z. Med. J.* **81**, 386–390.
Velasco, M. E., Sindely, S. D. and Roessmann, U. (1977). *J. Neurosurg.* **46**, 548–550.
Williams, R. A., Jacobs, M. S., Kurtz, A. B., Millar, J. G. B., Oakley, N. W., Spathis, G. S., Sulway, M. J. and Nabarro, J. D. N. (1975). *Q. Jl Med.* **44**, 79–98.
Wilson, C. B. and Dempsey, L. C. (1978). *J. Neurosurg.* **48**, 13–22.
Wrightson, P. (1978). *J. Neurol. Neurosurg. Psychiat.* **41**, 283–289.

# MICROSURGICAL REMOVAL OF PITUITARY TUMORS WITH "CURE" AND RETENTION OF PITUITARY FUNCTION*

H. St. George Tucker and D. P. Becker

*Departments of Medicine and Surgery, Virginia Commonwealth University,*

*Medical College of Virginia, Richmond, Virginia 23298, USA*

A prospective study was begun in 1972, at the Medical College of Virginia, of patients undergoing transsphenoidal pituitary tumor removal, including detailed pre- and postoperative evaluation of pituitary function in our Clinical Research Center. The hypothesis to be tested was that in the majority of cases tumor could be totally removed with long-term cure, and with retention or even improvement of normal pituitary function. The present report includes all such patients operated on between 1972 and July 1978. Informed written consent was obtained for all studies.

We found a strikingly high rate of reduction of elevated hormone levels to normal (acromegaly 82%, prolactin secreting tumors 64%, Cushing's disease 100%). Loss of pituitary function from surgery was infrequent (acromegaly 16%, prolactin secreting tumors 8%, Cushing's disease 0%).

## MATERIAL AND METHODS

The series included 28 acromegalics, 52 patients with either prolactin secreting or non-secreting adenomas, four patients with Nelson's syndrome and seven with Cushing's disease. Plasma prolactin assay was not available to us until 1974. The 52 patients with prolactin secreting or non-secreting tumors were divided into two groups: 25 women of reproductive age with the galactorrhea-amenorrhea

*Supported by a grant from the National Institutes of Health AMOI RR 65.

syndrome, all of whose tumors were almost surely prolactin secreting, and 27 patients with pressure symptoms only, including six postmenopausal women and 21 men.

All patients had complete preoperative and postoperative evaluation of pituitary endocrine function. This included the measurement of plasma growth hormone, prolactin, TSH and thyroxin, ACTH and cortisol, FSH, LH and testosterone. The reserve secretion of these hormones was tested with insulin-induced hypoglycemia, TRH, oral L-DOPA, and the response of urinary 17-hydroxycorticosteroids to metyrapone. In our laboratory normal plasma prolactin values were up to 50 ng/ml.

All patients had complete neurological examination, including visual fields. All had skull X-rays or coned views of the sella, and anteroposterior and lateral polytomograms. Initially pneumoencephalograms and carotid angiograms were done but these procedures were later replaced by computerized axial tomography with contrast media. Sella size was estimated by the method of DiChiro. Table I lists the degree of sellar enlargement in the various groups of patients, the number in each group showing visual field defects, the number who were hypopituitary before surgery, and the number who had previous treatment.

### Surgical technique

The standard midline sublabial transsphenoidal approach to the sella is used. A wide exposure is emphasized. The anterior wall of the sphenoid sinus is taken down far laterally, and to its superior and inferior margins. The bony anterior wall of the sella is removed to the cavernous sinus dura, to the anterior floor of the skull and to the floor of the sella. The dura is opened widely in stellate fashion, usually beginning inferiorly to avoid the arachnoid. Meticulous scraping of tumor from dura and/or gland is performed, and fixatives such as alcohol are not used. At the end of the procedure it is usual to see the inferior, lateral and posterior smooth walls of the sella, and intact pituitary gland. The stalk is seen only in the unusual situation where the tumor presents superiorly.

Patients were covered with intravenous steroids during surgery. This was discontinued in a few days, except in the Cushing's patients or when the integrity of the remaining pituitary was uncertain. In the latter case, oral maintenance steroids were continued until thyroid function could be monitored at six weeks. If this was normal, cortisone treatment was withdrawn, or in Cushing's disease patients, was gradually tapered off over several months.

Pituitary function was reevaluated two to six months after surgery. After this patients were seen every six months for a year, then once a year. Hormone levels, visual fields and radiological studies were repeated as indicated. Follow-up on the earliest patients now extends to six years.

### RESULTS

### Acromegaly

A pituitary tumor was found in all 28 patients and was removed as completely as possible. Figure 1 shows plasma growth hormone levels before operation, postoperatively, and at the time of the latest follow-up. Pretreatment growth hormone

*Table I.*

| Type of pituitary tumor | Number of patients | Degree of sellar enlargement[a] | | | | | Visual field defects | Preoperative hypopit | Previous treatment |
|---|---|---|---|---|---|---|---|---|---|
| | | Normal | Grade 1 | Grade 2 | Grade 3 | Grade 4 | | | |
| GH-secreting | 28 | 1 | 7 | 8 | 7 | 5 | 4 | 3 | 9 |
| Prolactin secreting or non-secreting | | | | | | | | | |
| Galactorrhea-amenorrhea | 25 | — | 11 | 3 | 3 | 8 | 4 | 1 | 4 |
| Postmenopausal women and males | 27 | — | — | — | 3 | 24 | 22 | 12 | 5 |
| ACTH-secreting | | | | | | | | | |
| Nelson's syndrome | 4 | — | 2 | — | — | 2 | — | — | — |
| Cushing's disease | 7 | 5 | 1 | — | — | 1 | 1 | — | — |

[a] Sellar enlargement: grade 1—erosion c̄ sella size normal or borderline (up to 1200 mm³); grade 2—sella 1200–2000 mm³, usually c̄ erosion; grade 3—sella very large (2000–5000 mm³) but no extrasellar extension; grade 4—extrasellar extension present.

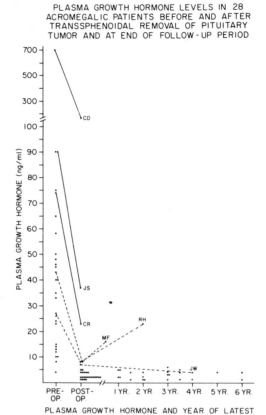

PLASMA GROWTH HORMONE LEVELS IN 28
ACROMEGALIC PATIENTS BEFORE AND AFTER
TRANSSPHENOIDAL REMOVAL OF PITUITARY
TUMOR AND AT END OF FOLLOW-UP PERIOD

PLASMA GROWTH HORMONE AND YEAR OF LATEST
FOLLOW-UP ON EACH PATIENT

*Fig. 1.* For each patient a single dot represents the plasma growth hormone pre-operatively, a few days following surgery, and at the time of the latest follow-up. The solid lines represent those patients whose growth hormone was not reduced to normal. The dashed lines represent those patients whose postoperative plasma growth hormone was between 5 and 10 ng/ml, and indicate their subsequent course. In all other patients postoperative plasma growth hormone was reduced to 5 ng/ml or less, and remained low as shown.

levels ranged from 4–700 ng/ml. Tumor removal reduced plasma growth hormone to 5 ng/ml or less in 22, to between 5 and 10 ng/ml in three, and in three the level remained above 10 ng/ml. All patients whose growth hormone was reduced to 5 ng/ml or less have remained in apparent remission with no subsequent rise in growth hormone. Of the three patients with postoperative growth hormone levels between 5 and 10 ng/ml, one subsequently fell to 4 ng/ml and the patient's acromegaly appears to be in complete remission. The other two patients relapsed, with rises in growth hormone. Thus, acromegaly was apparently cured in 23 of 28 patients but not in five. A second transsphenoidal operation in three of these patients was of little benefit. Patients with persisting elevation of growth hormone were given pituitary irradiation if they had not previously received a maximal amount. Irradiation produced further lowering of growth hormone with no subsequent tendency to rise.

Patients whose growth hormone was reduced to 5 ng/ml or below showed shrinkage of the soft tissue of the hands and feet, lessening of facial furrows and decrease in sweating and oiliness of the skin. Skeletal symptoms improved in most cases, although the bony findings of acromegaly showed no visible change. Diabetes was markedly improved in all of 12 patients. On the other hand hypertension was unaffected by reduction of growth hormone to normal in 9 of 10 patients. Headache was relieved in 14 of 18 patients, even when growth hormone was only partially lowered.

Complications in 31 operations on 28 patients included transient diabetes insipidus in 10, permanent in one. The only serious complication was one spinal fluid leak with *Klebsiella meningitis* which cleared up after intensive intravenous and intraventricular antibiotic treatment.

Four patients with preoperative diminished gonadal function became hypopituitary. All are doing well on replacement hormones. Three patients showed improved gonadal function following surgery. In all other pituitary endocrine function was unchanged by surgery.

### Prolactin secreting or non-secreting tumors

*Galactorrhea-amenorrhea syndrome*

Pituitary adenomas were found and removed as completely as possible in all 25 patients. Plasma prolactin levels before and after surgery are shown in Fig. 2, section A. Preoperatively 20 of the 21 measured plasma prolactins were elevated. Postoperatively 16 of 25 were reduced to normal, nine remaining elevated.

Two patients had second transsphenoidal procedures because of recurrence of headache and a rise in prolactin. Additional tumor was found and removed, with relief of headache but no further reduction of prolactin levels. Pituitary irradiation was given to patients whose plasma prolactins remained above 100 ng/ml, with further reduction and apparent stabilization of prolactin levels. Irradiation was withheld in three patients with prolactin between 50 and 100 ng/ml to try clomiphene treatment, which resulted in pregnancy in two.

Headache was relieved in 11 of 15 patients. Galactorrhea ceased in 13 of 22 patients. Regular menses were resumed in 10 of 22 amenorrheic patients. Four of six married patients has six subsequent pregnancies, making a total of eight pregnancies in six patients. Prolactin levels were no higher following the pregnancies than before. Complications in the 27 operations included transient diabetes insipidus in nine, permanent in one, transient ocular palsies in two, and one spinal fluid leak which was repaired without difficulty.

One patient who was hypopituitary before surgery remained so. Two others became hypopituitary. All are doing well on replacement hormones. There was no other loss of pituitary endocrine function.

*In postmenopausal women and men*

Figure 2, section B shows plasma prolactin levels before and after surgery and following irradiation in six postmenopausal women and in 21 men. Preoperative

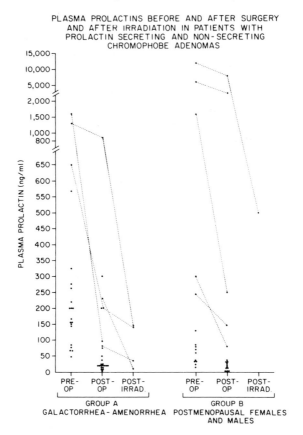

PLASMA PROLACTINS BEFORE AND AFTER SURGERY
AND AFTER IRRADIATION IN PATIENTS WITH
PROLACTIN SECRETING AND NON-SECRETING
CHROMOPHOBE ADENOMAS

*Fig. 2.* For each patient a single dot represents the plasma prolactin preoperatively, following surgery, and in some patients where prolactin remained high, following pituitary irradiation. The dashed lines indicate the sequential prolactin levels in a few patients with the highest initial values.

prolactin levels were elevated in 10 of 15. Postoperatively 13 of 18 were normal, five still elevated. Three of those with still elevated plasma prolactins have received pituitary irradiation with further lowering of prolactin levels.

All these patients had very large tumors. Six had seizures, lethargy, or other neurologic symptoms, and X-rays showed extensive brain invasion by tumor. Four had already had open craniotomy plus irradiation. Transsphenoidal surgery was undertaken with the knowledge that it would be at best only palliative. Four of these patients have subsequently died, two months to two years after surgery, apparently from extension of the tumor. The other two, although hypopituitary, are well and active on replacement hormones, five years and one year after operation.

One 62-year-old woman with a very large tumor with lateral suprasellar extension, appeared well after operation but died one month later from internal carotid artery hemorrhage, almost surely a complication of surgery. Two other patients had spinal fluid leaks with meningitis with recovery. Diabetes insipidus occured in seven, transient in six, and permanent in one. Two patients had transient sixth nerve palsies.

The 12 patients who were hypopituitary before surgery remained so. Two hypogonadal patients became hypopituitary. All are doing well on replacement hormones. Two other hypogonadal patients regained normal gonadal function. All others showed no change in pituitary endocrine function.

Headache was relieved in 13 and 15 patients. Visual field defects returned to normal in three of 19, improved in 11, and were unchanged in five. Of the entire group, 16 feel well and are fully active, while six have minor complaints. Serial plasma prolactin levels, visual fields and skull X-rays have shown no evidence of progression of any remaining tumor.

## ACTH secreting tumors

### Nelson's syndrome

Table II shows plasma ACTH levels in the four patients pre- and postoperatively, and, in the last two, after subsequent irradiation. Patients 1 and 2 had small pituitary tumors which were apparently removed completely. The tumors in patients 3 and 4 had invaded the sphenoid sinus and could not be removed completely. Postoperative irradiation was given. The follow-up period of one year on each is not enough to evaluate the ultimate outcome.

*Table II.* Plasma ACTH levels (pg/ml) in patients with Nelson's syndrome before and after pituitary tumor removal[a].

| Patient | Preop | Postop | One year later | Post-irrad Rx Rx |
|---------|--------|--------|----------------|------------------|
| 1 | 2570 | 514 | | — |
| 2 | 4200 | 850 | 1000 | — |
| 3 | 3500 | 650 | 1000 | 400 |
| 4 | 16,000 | 6200 | | |

[a]All plasma ACTH levels are the average of three or more fasting 8 a.m. levels, 12 hours after last dose of oral cortisone acetate 12.5 mg.

The only complication of surgery was a transient sixth nerve palsy in patient 1. All patients had normal pituitary function other than ACTH, with no change after surgery.

### Cushing's disease

Our first patient with Cushing's disease was a 369 lb woman who had a very large tumor with suprasellar extension and bitemporal hemianopsia. The tumor was apparently successfully removed, but one week later she suffered a massive pulmonary embolism which eventually led to cardiac arrest and death.

The next six patients with Cushing's disease have all had transsphenoidal surgery in the past 16 months. In four the sella was entirely normal by all radiological procedures, and in two the sella was of normal size but with erosion on polytomograms. In every case a pituitary adenoma was removed, apparently completely. The signs and symptoms of Cushing's disease have disappeared over the next six months. Normal menses have returned. One 13-year-old girl and a young man of 22 with Cushing's disease for 10 years had had cessation of growth. It is too early to tell whether relief of hypercortisolism will restore growth in these patients.

Following removal of the ATCH secreting tumor, there is profound suppression of pituitary ACTH secretion and steroid support for six to eight months has been necessary, the dosage being gradually tapered off and then discontinued. The first of these six patients has lost all signs of Cushing's, has been off steroids for eight months, feels fine and is working regularly. All pituitary functions are normal including basal ACTH and adrenal function, but she still shows no response to metyrapone. Two other patients have been off cortisone only a month. The other patients are still on steroid replacement.

Transient diabetes insipidus occurred in four patients. There were no other complications. All other pituitary functions have remained normal.


## DISCUSSION

Our findings suggest that all patients with acromegaly have a growth hormone secreting pituitary adenoma, and that in a high percentage of patients the tumor can be removed successfully by the transsphenoidal approach. A "cure" appears to have been accomplished in 82% of our patients, with plasma growth hormone remaining no more than 5 ng/ml. Patients whose growth hormone has been reduced to this level by surgery have shown no tendency to relapse to date. We consider transsphenoidal tumor removal the treatment of choice in acromegaly. Serious complications occurred in only 7%, and surgical hypopituitarism in only 16%. Hypopituitarism and failure to reduce growth hormone to normal were more likely with the larger tumors. When growth hormone remained elevated, a second transsphenoidal operation was of little benefit. Irradiation, however, further reduced growth hormone levels and appeared to limit further growth of the tumor.

The availability of prolactin assay and sella polytomography have made possible the early diagnosis of prolactin secreting tumors as the cause of amenorrhea or galactorrhea in young women. Such tumors can be diagnosed when they are quite small and amenable to complete removal by transsphenoidal surgery, usually with good preservation of pituitary function. In 64% of our patients elevated prolactin levels were reduced to normal. Regular menses were restored in 45% of our patients, with a high incidence of pregnancy when desired. Amenorrhea persisted in those patients whose prolactin remained elevated and in a few whose prolactin was reduced to normal, probably because of gonadotropin insufficiency. The poor results were mostly in patients with large tumors. Patients with persisting prolactin elevation were not much benefitted by a second transsphenoidal operation. These patients were treated with pituitary irradiation, with further lowering and stabilization of prolactin levels. Two patients with moderately elevated prolactin levels following surgery were not given irradiation but treated with clomiphene with resulting ovulation and pregnancy.

Prolactin secreting or non-secreting pituitary tumors in men and postmenopausal women reached very large sizes before pressure symptoms led to discovery. Eighty-nine per cent showed extrasellar extension, 82% had caused visual field defects, and 44% had produced hypopituitarism. Serum prolactin was elevated in 10 of 15 patients in whom it was measured. Transsphenoidal tumor removal relieved headache in most patients, relieved or improved visual field defects in three-quarters of patients and reduced prolactin to normal in 13 of 18. Tumors with suprasellar extension could often be successfully removed transsphenoidally. Parasellar extension was less accessible, and complete removal was often impossible. Where extensive brain invasion by tumor had occurred, transsphenoidal removal was of limited benefit. Patients with obviously incomplete tumor removal or with persisting hyperprolactinemia were treated with irradiation.

In patients with Nelson's syndrome, if the ACTH secreting tumor can be diagnosed when still small, complete removal by the transsphenoidal route is possible. Such tumors may grow aggressively, and when they are large complete removal may not be possible. If so, postoperative irradiation should be given. Treatment of Cushing's disease by removal of pituitary microadenomas rather than by total adrenalectomy should eliminate the occurence of Nelson's syndrome in the future.

The results of transsphenoidal removal of ACTH secreting microadenomas in patients with Cushing's disease are most encouraging but still preliminary because the follow-up has been short. Pituitary exploration in six patients revealed an adenoma in each, although only two had shown any radiologic evidence of tumor. Removal of the adenoma has led to dramatic reversal of the manifestations of Cushing's disease. Restoration of menses in several women suggests that pituitary function is preserved, but a longer follow-up will be necessary to determine this. Prolonged postoperative ACTH suppression has been seen in every patient. The first three of these patients required cortisone for six months, and the others are still receiving steroids. It should be remembered that all patients with Cushing's disease have increased risk at surgery because of vascular fragility, osteoporotic bones, weakened musculature and connective tissue and poor wound healing.

## CONCLUSION

Transsphenoidal excision of pituitary adenomata, in experiences hands, can result in a high incidence of reduction of elevated hormone levels to normal. A long term cure seems feasible in many patients. Further follow-up is needed to confirm this. Pituitary function can usually be retained and sometimes improved. Surgical technique is critical for obtaining these reported results. At operation, a wide exposure, adequate sella exploration and meticulous curettement of tumor permits excision of tumor and recognition and retention of normal pituitary gland.

# ONE HUNDRED AND TEN PROLACTIN
# SECRETING ADENOMAS:
# RESULTS OF SURGICAL TREATMENT

G. C. Nicola, G. P. Tonnarelli and A. Griner

*Department of Neurosurgery, Legnano General Hospital,
20025 – Legnano, Italy*

From January 1976 to February 1978 we operated on by the transsphenoidal approach 110 patients with prolactin secreting adenomas whose diagnosis was mainly based on endocrinological data, while the radiological studies have rather served as confirmation of an already suspected adenomatous origin of the hyperprolactinemia allowing us to determine its site and its volumetric characteristics. Of course, the endocrinological data have been of major importance in the macroadenomas, when radiological study cannot provide certain data or may even show nothing.

## PATIENTS

One hundred and one patients were women and 9 were men. Seventy of them had adenomas smaller than 10 mm; 40 of them had adenomas larger than 10 mm (24 enclosed, 16 invasive).

Among the group of women patients 69 were microadenomas (Table I) with mean age of 27.5 years and length of disease from 6 months to 15 years (mean 7.6 years). One-hundred per cent of the patients were affected by menstrual troubles, while 95.7% of them were affected by galactorrhea. Twenty-two were enclosed adenomas, and these women had a mean age of 33.5 years and length of disease from 3 months to 12 years (mean 6.9); 81.8% were affected by menstrual troubles and 59% by galactorrhea. Ten were invasive adenomas, with

*Table I.*   General aspects.

|  | No. of cases | Mean age (yr) | Duration of disease (yr) | Menstrual Disorders (%) | Galacto-rrhea |
|---|---|---|---|---|---|
| Microadenomas | 69 | 27.5 | 7.6 | 100 | 95.7 |
| Enclosed adenomas | 22 | 33.5 | 6.9 | 81.8 | 59 |
| Invasive adenomas | 10 | 42.5 | 10.5 | 60 | 50 |

mean age of 42.5 years and length of disease from 1 to 20 years (mean 10.5);
60% were affected by menstrual troubles and 50% by visual defects.

Among the men we found only one microadenoma: it was in a 28 year old
patient, with length of disease of 5 years, galactorrhea and impotence. There were
2 enclosed adenomas, in men with mean age of 31.5 years and length of disease of
6 months and 3 years. Impotence was found in both of the patients. Then there
were 6 invasive adenomas in men, with mean age of 43.6 years and length of
disease from 2 months to 10 years (mean 3 years). In 3 cases there was impotence,
while visual defects were found in 4.

We have observed, as accessory troubles, weight increases in 30%, loss of hair
in 20% and headache in 14.5% of the total cases.

## RESULTS

We think it is worthwhile to present our experience because of its characteristics,
such as the quite large number and the homogeneity of the preoperative studies,
surgical treatment and evaluation of results (controls at 15 days and 6 months at

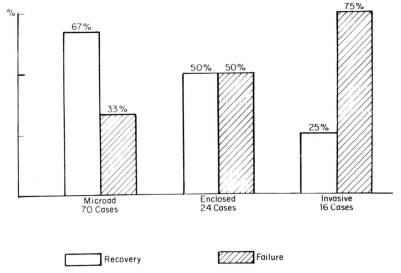

*Fig. 1.*   Interrelationship between surgical results and tumor size.

least after the operation). The evaluation of results took into account the postoperative fall in PRL values to normal levels, as well as the preservation of other hypophyseal functions and regression of preoperative signs and symptoms.

Subdividing our case list according to the Hardy classification, we had the following percentage of successes (Fig. 1): microadenomas, 67%; enclosed adenomas, 50%; invasive adenomas, 25%. These data show that the most favourable results are obtained with the smallest adenomas and that they are worse as soon as the lesion becomes larger and invasive. The high percentage of failure in the microadenoma groups and in the enclosed groups, in contrast with our constant operative impression of radical removal of the adenomas, is not easily explainable.

The clinical and radiological data did not give us anything to justify this outcome. These unsatisfactory results are probably due to histological aspects of these adenomas, that is the lack of real capsule between adenomatous and normal tissue and the tendency of these benign tumors to locally infiltrate the surrounding structures. This fact induced us to modify some technical aspects of the operation, such

*Table II.* Surgical results classified according to the PRL (ng/ml) values (No. of cases).

|  | < 100 | | 100–400 | | > 400 | |
|---|---|---|---|---|---|---|
|  | Recovery | Failure | Recovery | Failure | Recovery | Failure |
| Microadenomas | 25 | – | 14 | 6 | 8 | 17 |
| Enclosed adenomas | 5 | 1 | 4 | 5 | 3 | 6 |
| Invasive adenomas | 4 | 2 | – | 2 | – | 8 |

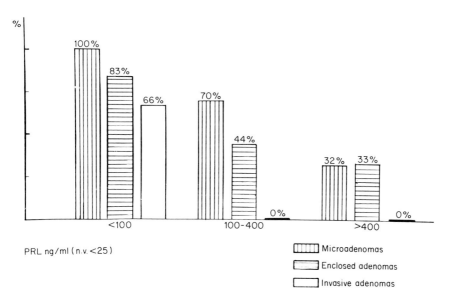

*Fig. 2.* Percentage of cured patients classified according to their basal prolactin levels.

as the use of absolute alcohol instead of Zenker fluid in the tumoral bed and the careful determination of removal of all the tissue that looks suspect under the operating microscope. On the other hand, we tried to evaluate our results by adding to the above-mentioned morphological criteria a functional one, that is, subdividing the adenomas on the basis of the preoperative basal PRL values (Table 2, Fig. 2). The data allowed us to draw some conclusions, influencing us quite strongly towards the surgical treatment of these adenomas. The fundamental fact is that the results obtained in the smallest adenomas with lower basal hormonal values confirms that surgical treatment is always of choice in amenorrhea-galactorrhea syndrome when endocrinological studies have allowed us to diagnose with certainty worse when one passes to groups of larger adenomas with high secreting power and characteristics of invasivity.

This particularly favourable result in the microadenomas with low basal PRL values confirms that surgical treatment is always of choice in amenorrea-galactorrhea syndrome when endocrinological studies have allowed us to diagnose with certainly a prolactinoma. Even when the radiological studies are negative, dopaminergic therapy and a delay of surgical treatment do not seem, in our opinion, to be justified.

In fact, therapy with dopaminergic drugs is very effective in decreasing serum PRL levels and in producing the regression of symptoms; nevertheless its anti-proliferative action is not yet proved and, when it is stopped, we often see an increase over pre-treatment PRL values. A delay in operation can cause not only the transition from a micro-adenomatous to a macro-adenomatous stage, but also the increase of PRL values to less easily curable levels. Both of these occurrences contribute to worsening the final results. It is clear that to avoid the growth of adenomas and to prevent their biological evolution, an early endocrinological diagnosis must be made and, then, an early operative treatment is necessary. The surgical treatment is also suitable for the other volumetric-biological classes: in the group of large invasive adenomas surgery has, of course, a fundamentally decompressive aim and only additionally is followed by biological success. Finally, surgical treatment is also advised for microadenomas and for enclosed adenomas with high PRL values because it allows us to obtain biological recovery in a sufficient percentage of cases and also because it makes easier the subsequent pharmacological treatment, since the serum PRL levels fall constantly in the post-operative period.

# GROWTH HORMONE DEFICIENCY AFTER SELECTIVE REMOVAL OF PITUITARY ADENOMA IN ACROMEGALY

G. Schaison, O. Helal and B. Pertuiset

*Hôpital de La Pitié, 75013-Paris, France*

The pathogenesis of growth hormone (GH) overproduction is still questionable. At present it is uncertain whether acromegaly is due to autonomous GH secretion from a pituitary tumor, or whether the primary defect is an abnormal hypothalamic control of GH secretion. The aim of the present study was to assess GH regulation in the residual pituitary tissue after selective hypophysectomy removing the GH secreting tumor. In some patients successful surgical treatment might be anticipated from the results of preoperative endocrine investigations. Furthermore, in the cured patients postoperative dynamic GH studies indicated that the pituitary tumor was the primary defect and did not arise from an excessive stimulation by hypothalamic growth hormone releasing factor (GHRF).

## PATIENTS AND METHODS

### Patients

Over a four-year period, 14 acromegalic patients (3 males and 11 females), who had never been treated before, underwent transsphenoidal surgical exploration of the pituitary. The mean age was 41.4 years. There were no visual field defects and the surgical decision was based only on the endocrinologic evidence of acromegaly. They were treated by selective removal of histologically confirmed GH secreting tumor.

Patients were divided into two groups according to surgical results. In nine patients, (group I), postoperative plasma GH concentrations fell under 5 ng/ml.

*Table I.* Minimal plasma GH levels (ng/ml) after GTT in 14 acromegalic patients before and after transsphenoidal selective adenomectomy.

| | Patient no. | Radiological classification | GH response to GTT | |
| --- | --- | --- | --- | --- |
| | | | Before surgery | After surgery |
| Group I | 1 | enclosed | 14 | 3.5 |
| | 2 | enclosed | 26 | 3.2 |
| | 3 | enclosed | 43 | 2.1 |
| | 4 | enclosed | 31 | 1.3 |
| | 5 | enclosed | 67 | 1.0 |
| | 6 | enclosed | 51 | 3.7 |
| | 7 | invasive | 28 | 2.7 |
| | 8 | invasive | 17 | 3.3 |
| | 9 | invasive | 73 | 4.1 |
| Group II | 10 | enclosed | 20 | 19.5 |
| | 11 | enclosed | 20 | 14.6 |
| | 12 | enclosed | 32 | 52.0 |
| | 13 | invasive | 71 | 8.7 |
| | 14 | invasive | 84 | 74.0 |

No recurrences were observed over a follow up period from one to three years (Table I). In five patients, (group II), plasma GH levels decreased but remained excessive after resection of the pituitary adenoma (Table I).

In both groups hypocycloidal polytomography and pneumoencephalography were performed in all patients. The pituitary adenoma was enclosed in six cases and invasive in three cases of group I; enclosed and intrasellar in three cases, invasive and/or suprasellar in two cases of group II according to Hardy's classification (Hardy, 1973).

## Methods

Plasma GH was measured by radioimmunoassay using a commercially available anti-hGH antibody (Institut Pasteur, Paris). Accuracy was tested against the NIH-HS/1643 A reference standard. The interassay coefficient of variation was ± 8.3%, and the intraassay ± 5.1%. The diagnosis of acromegaly was established by the non-suppressibility of plasma GH below 5 ng/ml after oral glucose load (GTT).

Dynamic GH studies were as follows. All experiments were performed in the morning after an overnight fast and at least two hours of bed rest. After two baseline samples, glucose was given orally in a dose of 1 g/kg, and blood samples were obtained every 30 minutes therefore, for a five-hour period. Insulin was administered intravenously in a dose of 0.15 iu/kg in order to achieve a blood glucose level of less than 0.50 g/l. The response to TRH and to dopaminergic drugs was also determined 10, 20, 30 and 60 minutes after TRH (200 μg i.v.), 30, 60, 90 and 120 minutes after L-dopa (500 mg orally), and every hour for five hours after a 5 mg oral dose of bromocriptine (CB 154, Sandoz Ltd, Basel, Switzerland).

The other pituitary functions were estimated by evaluating plasma levels of prolactin, TSH, LH, FSH and ACTH determined by radioimmunoassay techniques before and after successive administration of TRH, LHRH (100 μg i.v.) and metyrapone (500 mg/every four hours/six times).

The same endocrinological evaluations and, particularly, dynamic growth hormone studies, were repeated from 15 to 30 days after surgery without any drugs or telecobaltotherapy in between. The nine patients who normalized their postoperative plasma GH levels, were reinvestigated over a one to three years period.

## RESULTS

### Preoperative values

In the nine patients of group I, mean basal GH levels ranged between 14 and 73 ng/ml (Table I). These preoperative serum GH levels were not related to the sellar size. No significant inhibition of plasma GH occurred after glucose load, and one patient even exhibited a paradoxical rise. The individual values varied widely from day to day. Therefore in some acromegalic patients the interpretation of the dynamic tests was often uncertain. However all patients failed to demonstrate any change during the i.v. insulin test. On the other hand a 52–100%

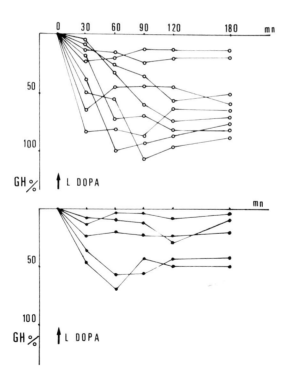

*Fig. 1.* Preoperative GH response to L-dopa (500 mg oral) in group I patients (upper panel), and group II patients (lower panel).

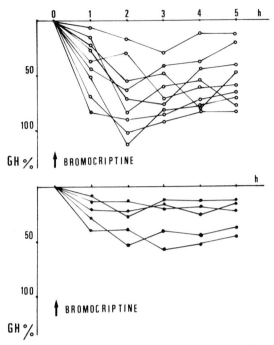

*Fig. 2.* Preoperative plasma GH response to bromocriptine (5 mg oral) in group I patients (upper panel) and group II patients (lower panel) .

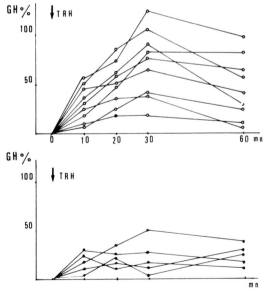

*Fig. 3.* Preoperative plasma GH responses to TRH (200 μg IV) in group I patients (upper panel), and group II patients (lower panel) (GH values are expressed in percentage of basal values).

decrease in GH levels was observed between 30 and 180 minutes after L-dopa (seven patients, Fig. 1) and 120 minutes after bromocriptine (eight patients, Fig. 2). Furthermore, after TRH, GH levels increased by at least 50% in six patients, and the peak occurred at 30 minutes (Fig. 3).

In the five patients of group II, mean preoperative GH levels ranging from 20 to 84 ng/ml, were also not related to the sellar size. In two cases a marked rise in plasma GH occurred after insulin hypoglycemia, and in two other cases paradoxical rises of plasma GH followed glucose administration. After L-dopa or bromocriptine administration the reduction of the GH levels to nearly 50% of basal levels was only found in two patients (Figs 1 and 2). Moreover the elevated GH levels remained unchanged after TRH in all but one patient (Fig. 3).

Before surgery, other pituitary function studies revealed no TSH response to TRH in four group 1 patients, and a high prolactin plasma level which did not increase after TRH in one patient of each of the two groups. In all patients from both groups, gonadotropic and adrenocorticotropic functions were normal after LHRH and metyrapone.

### Postoperative values

All group I patients were apparently cured. Two weeks after surgery they showed a clinical improvement, and their plasma GH concentrations during GTT were less than 5 ng/ml in each sample (Table I). Furthermore these nine patients failed to increase serum GH after all stimulations. The paradoxical GH decrease after L-dopa and bromocriptine was not measurable any more. All patients became GH-unresponsive to TRH and showed impaired GH response to hypoglycemia. Besides, the total and selective removal of the tumor was supported by the lack of demonstrable postoperative endocrine dysfunction which required hormonal replacement. Pituitary functions, and particularly the stimulation of GH secretion were tested after three months and reassessed after one year in eight patients and after three years in four patients. There was no evidence of reacurrence of acromegaly, and the integrity of pituitary functions was maintained. In all patients the stimulation of GH secretion was insignificant or absent. Only two of these patients had a normal GH increase after both insulin-induced hypoglycemia and dopaminergic stimulation three years later, only one after hypoglycemia one year following surgery. Thus in six patients GH deficiency remained over a follow-up period of one to three years.

Two weeks after surgery plasma GH concentrations were higher than 5 ng/ml during the glucose tolerance test in all group II patients (Table I). The mean basal postoperative values decreased, but excessive GH secretion and abnormal response to provocative stimuli remained. Particularly, the paradoxical GH response to TRH in one patient and to bromocriptine in two did not disappear after surgery. Other pituitary functions were found to be unmodified with respect to preoperative values.

### DISCUSSION

Many endocrine studies support the concept that, in acromegaly, the primary defect is an abnormal hypothalamic control of GH secretion. In some cases the normal, exaggerated or paradoxical response to one or more GH modifying stimuli suggests that GH secretion was not autonomous (Cryer and Daughaday, 1969; Lawrence *et al.*, 1970). Furthermore, Hagen *et al.* (1971) reported that acromegalic plasma appeared to contain GH releasing activity not found in normal plasma, and which released GH from monkey pituitary gland *in vitro*. However, in recent years, newly developed microsurgical techniques have verified the efficiency of selective transsphenoidal adenomectomy (Allen *et al.*, 1974; Hoyte and Martin, 1975). The complete reversion to normal GH responsiveness suggested that in certain cases acromegaly is due to pituitary dysfunction alone.

In the first group of patients, the selective removal of the GH secreting tumor resulted in a fall in plasma hormone concentration to under 5 ng/ml. The lack of demonstrable postoperative endocrine dysfunction allowed us the assumption that the normal pituitary and its neural and vascular connections with the hypothalamus were left essentially intact. However, in these patients, postoperative plasma GH did not increase after hypoglycemia, L-dopa, bromocriptine and TRH. This GH deficiency, reinvestigated over a one to three-year period, suggests that the hypothalamus and normal somatotropic cells have been chronically suppressed by pathological secretion of GH. Indeed, it is unlikely that no residual somatotrophs were left after surgery, or that concurrent hypothalamic dysfunction inhibited the effect of the GH secreting stimuli. The absence of response may best be explained by an inhibition of GH-releasing factor secretion or release of somatostatin by the short loop negative feedback system. A study by Sakuma and Knobil (1970) brought convincing evidence that GH acts upon its own regulation, since GH administration prior to hypoglycemia blocked the expected GH discharge in the rhesus monkey. Likewise the pituitary GH concentration was significantly reduced after GH pellet implantation into bovine median eminence (Kats *et al.*, 1969). Thus all the evidence points to the fact that in these patients the primary disorder resided in the pituitary gland. Hypoglycemia in three patients, and bromocriptine in two increased plasma GH levels after six months. But, so far, there has been no recurrence among all the group I patients.

In the group II patients, plasma GH remained excessive after resection of the pituitary adenoma. In these patients, surgical failure may account for sustained abnormal GH secretion. The main reason for that could be that the adenoma was too large to remove, or that residual tissue in the sella turcica, because of limitations of the transsphenoidal approach. There were, as a matter of fact, in this group three enclosed and intrasellar adenomas. There is no doubt, as Hardy (1973) reported in 40 acromegalic patients, that the distinction between a small enclosed adenoma and a larger invasive suprasellar adenoma is one of the criteria for predicting the surgical outcome. But these anatomical findings are not sufficient in themselves to explain the results of transsphenoidal surgery in all cases. It may be that some acromegalic patients have a hypothalamic abnormality, and that other patients have a primary pituitary defect. Perhaps only this last group can be cured by a selective transsphenoidal resection.

In some acromegalic patients, serum GH increases after TRH and the inhibitory action of dopaminergic drugs appear to be mutually correlated (Liuzzi *et al.*, 1974). In others the pharmacologic agents produce little or no effect. The exact cause of this discrepancy remains to be clarified. But it is noteworthy that the group I patients were GH-responsive to bromocriptine in eight cases, to L-dopa in seven, and to TRH in six. This group was clearly characterized by the effectiveness of transsphenoidal surgery in lowering serum GH levels.

The mechanism of the paradoxical effect of TRH in acromegaly remains speculative. It has been suggested that functional disconnection between the central nervous system and the anterior pituitary might explain this response. Udeschini *et al.* (1976) demonstrated that a direct GH-releasing effect of TRH could be obtained in the hypophysectomized rat bearing an ectopic pituitary. Reasoning by analogy, the release of GH which occurred in the group I patients should result from the inhibition of GHRF or the stimulation of somatostatin by the primary GH secretion at the pituitary level. However, somatostatin, which decreases the GH release induced by hypoglycemia, fails to inhibit the paradoxical stimulation by TRH (Giustina *et al.*, 1974). Furthermore, in the group I patients, the GH response to TRH disappeared after surgery, even though there were some normal residual somatotrophs, although they had been rendered inactive by persistent GHRF inhibition. So, the TRH-induced GH release in acromegaly may best be explained by an alteration of membrane receptors of the adenomatous cells and may suggest pituitary dysfunction alone.

The inhibitory effect of dopaminergic drugs on plasma GH in acromegaly may also be mediated by a direct pituitary action. Malarkey and Daughaday (1972) showed that L-dopa and bromocriptine exerted an inhibitory effect on the release of GH by rat pituitary tumor cells. One may therefore postulate that their inhibitory effect in acromegaly may only occur when the non-tumorous GH cells are functionally missing, as observed in the group I patients whose GH deficiency was revealed after surgery.

The group II patients were not cured after removal of the pituitary tumor. In the one case where GH was responsive to TRH, and the two cases where GH was responsive to bromocriptine, the persistence of the paradoxical response undoubtedly indicated some remaining adenomatous tissue. In the three other patients unresponsive to TRH, L-dopa and bromocriptine before surgery, removal of the adenoma was not followed by a period of normal GH secretion or a postoperative hyposomatotropism. This suggests that the hypothalamus and remaining normal GH cells had not been chronically suppressed by pathological GH hypersecretion.

At present it seems that there are several varieties of acromegaly with different primary abnormalties: those with a primary defect in the hypothalamus, and those with a primary defect in the pituitary. Only this last group may be cured by selective transsphenoidal surgery. However, further studies are required to ascertain the usefulness of dynamic tests to establish such distinctions.

## ACKNOWLEDGMENT

We are indebted to Ch. Trolliet for secretarial help.

## REFERENCES

Allen, J. P., Cook, D. M., Greer, M. A., Paxton, H. and Castro, A. (1974). *J. Neurosurg.* **41**, 38–43.
Cryer, P. E., Daughaday, W. H. (1969). *J. Clin. Endocrinol. Metab.* **29**, 386–393.
Giustina, G., Reschini, E., Peracchi, M., Cantalamessa, L., Cavagnini, F., Pinto,M. and Bulgheroni, P. (1974). *J. Clin. Endocrinol. Metabl.* **38**, 906–909.

Hagen, T. C., Lawrence, A. M. and Kirsteins, L. (1971). *J. Clin. Endocrinol. Metab.* **33**, 448–451.

Hardy, J. (1973). Transsphenoidal surgery of hypersecreting pituitary tumors. *In* "Diagnosis and Treatment of Pituitary Tumors" (Kohler, P. O. and Ross, G. T., eds) I.C.S. 303, pp. 179–194. Excerpta Medica, Amsterdam.

Hoyte, K. M. and Martin, J. B. (1975). *J. Clin. Endocrinol. Metab.* **41**, 656–659.

Katz, S. H., Molitch, M. and McCann, S. M. (1969). *Endocrinology*, **85**, 725–734.

Lawrence, A. M., Goldfine, I. D. and Kirsteins, L. (1970). *J. Clin. Endocrinol. Metab.* **31**, 239–247.

Liuzzi, A., Chiodini, P. G., Botalla, L., Silvestrini, F. and Müller, E. E. (1974). *J. Clin. Endocrinol. Metab.* **39**, 871–876.

Malarkey, W. B., Daughaday, W. H. (1972). *Endocrinology*, **91**, 1314–1317.

Sakuma, M. and Knobil, E. (1970). *Endocrinology*, **86**, 890–894.

Udeschini, G., Cocchi, D., Panerai, A. E., Gil-ad, I., Rossi, G. L., Chiodini, P. G., Liuzzi, A. and Müller, E. E. (1976). *Endocrinology*, **98**, 807–814.

# RESIDUAL ADENOHYPOPHYSIAL FUNCTION AFTER TRANSSPHENOIDAL MICROADENOMECTOMY FOR CUSHING'S DISEASE

N. Kageyama, A. Kuwayama, T. Nakane and M. Takanohasi

*Department of Neurosurgery, Nagoya University, School of Medicine, Nagoya, Japan*

Transsphenoidal surgery in the treatment of pituitary adenomas has been improved by Guiot (1973) and Hardy (1969). Its superiority to the intracranial approach is now widely accepted, especially in cases of functional adenomas. Although the primary lesions in the etiology of Cushing's disease are still in dispute, give a high clinical remission rate following a transsphenoidal microadenomectomy has been reported. (Hardy, 1973; Tyrrell *et al.*, 1978; Salassa *et al.*, 1978). However, little information is available on hormonal studies after this operation. In the present paper, we describe the residual pituitary function and postoperative clinical results after transsphenoidal microadenomectomy for Cushing's disease.

## PATIENTS AND METHODS

### Patients

One male and nine female patients with Cushing's disease, ranging in age from 13 to 52 years, underwent transsphenoidal microadenomectomy between January, 1977 and May, 1978 in our department. All patients had endocrinological evidence for pituitary ACTH hypersecretion and roentgenological findings of bilateral adrenal enlargement.

### Neuroradiological studies

Routine radiographs of the skull and hypocycloidal polytomographs of the sella at every 2 mm intervals were obtained for all patients. Bilateral carotid angiography and pneumotomoencephalography were routinely performed. Magnified serial carotid angiography and computed tomography were also carried out for the majority.

### Endocrinological examination

#### *Hypothalamic–pituitary–adrenal axis*

The levels of plasma ACTH and cortisol were measured by radioimmunoassay. Eight consecutive blood collections at 4 hour intervals, starting at midnight, were taken from all patients. The responsiveness of plasma ACTH and cortisol to insulin hypoglycemia (0.1–0.13 U/kg, i.v.) and 8-lysine vasopressin (10 U, i.m.) were also examined in 6 cases. Urinary 17-hydroxycorticosteroids (17-OHCS) were determined by the method of Silber and Porter. The responses of urinary 17-OHCS to dexamethasone (2 mg and 8 mg/day for 2 days each, p.o.) and metyrapone (4.5 g in 6 divided doses, p.o.) were examined in all patients to evaluate hypothalamo-hypophysial responsiveness.

#### *Other anterior pituitary hormones*

The levels of plasma GH, PRL, TSH, LH and FSH were determined by radioimmunoassay. Their responsiveness to insulin hypoglycemia, synthetic TRH (500 µg, i.v.) and synthetic LH-RH (100 µg, i.v.) were obtained. For postoperative studies, the replacement therapy with cortisol was discontinued at least 24 hours before testing, in every case.

## RESULTS

### Neuroradiological findings

Roentgenological examinations revealed slight enlargement of the sella in two patients (Nos. 1 and 2). Four cases including these two had localized expansion of the sella floor on the midline hypocycloidal tomogram, suggesting the existence of a microadenoma. Mild suprasellar expansion was found in one patient (No. 1), but in no other cases by pneumoencephalotomography. Carotid angiograms and computed tomographs were not of diagnostic value, even using their magnification methods.

### Operative findings and clinical results

The sublabial rhinoseptal transsphenoidal approach was applied as described by Guiot (1973) and Hardy (1969). Upon incision of the pituitary dural capsule greyish-white coloured microadenomas were easily found on the surface of the pituitary gland in six cases. In general, these were the large adenomas, ranging from 5 to 10 mm, and in two cases adenomas filled most of the intrasellar space with a minimal residual adenohypophysis beneath the diaphragma sellae. In 4 of 10 cases, the surface of the pituitary gland was seemingly normal and intraparency curettage through a midline vertical incision disclosed the microadenomas. They were the smaller ones, with diameters of less than 5 mm. To ensure complete adenomectomy, grossly normal tissue around the adenomas was partially resected. The tumor bed was soaked with 100% pure alcohol for 3–10 minutes.

During operation no serious complications or side-effects were experienced. Postoperative complications or side-effects were experienced. Postoperative complications were minimal. Only 3 patients had diabetes insipidus, which did not last more than 6 weeks. No CSF rhinorrhea, meningitis and nasal hemorrhage occurred. In all patients, postoperative substitution therapy of glucocorticoids was necessary, but only 3 of them needed continuous support of steroids for more than 3 months.

The successful microadenomectomy was followed by marked clinical improvement in 9 of 10 patients. One who had no such clinical improvement (No. 4) also had no significant decrease in plasma cortisol level. In successful, cases skin pigmentation disappeared completely within 1 or 2 months after surgery. Regular menstrual cycles occurred in all 4 premenopausal patients, who had had amenorrhea preoperatively. Disappearance of the cental obesity or moon face usually took approximately two months after surgery.

### Histological findings

Light microscopic study was obtainable in 8 cases. All adenomas showed that the majority of the adenoma cells were basophilic with a mixture of chromophobic cells. Grossly normal appearing adenohypophyses around the adenomas were studied in the last 5 cases. Typical Crooke's cells were confirmed in all of them, although the numbers of degenerated cells were different in each case. In No. 7 the enzyme-labelled antibody method with anti-ACTH rabbit serum was applied to both adenoma cells and normal tissue. The majority of adenoma cells were diffusely positive to anti-ACTH serum. In the normal tissue, most Crooke's cells showed a positive reaction, but the other cells did not. This would suggest that the largest number of ACTH-secreting cells may undergo Crooke's degenerating processes.

### Endocrine results

*Hypothalamic–pituitary–adrenal axis (Table I)*
(a) Preoperative results: the morning resting levels of plasma ACTH ranged from 59 to 420 pg/ml (mean, 160) and of cortisol from 23 to 53 $\mu$g/ml (mean 32) (Table I). Diurnal rhythmicity of plasma ACTH and cortisol was absent in all patients. A dexamethasone suppression test with the lower dose (2 mg/day for 2 days) resulted in only partial decrease of urinary 17-OHCS excretion. In response to a larger dose (8 mg/day), all patients showed a decrease of more than 50% of the basal value in urinary 17-OHCS excretion. In response to metyrapone administration, urinary 17-OHCS excretion increased in all patients. A test of pituitary-

*Table I.*  Plasma cortisol and ACTH response to insulin-hypoglycemia and lysine-vasopressin before and after transsphenoidal microadenomectomy in patients with Cushing's disease.

| Patients | | | Pre-op / Post-op | Cortisol (μg/dl) | | | | ACTH (pg/ml) | | | |
| No. | Age | Sex | | Insulin | | Vasopressin | | Insulin | | Vasopressin | |
| | | | | Basal | Peak | Basal | Peak | Basal | Peak | Basal | Peak |
| 1 | 27 | F | pre | 24.5 | | | | 158 | | | |
| | | | post | 9.9 | 17.5 | | | 48 | | | |
| 2 | 51 | F | pre | 35.0 | 38.0 | | | 223 | | | |
| | | | post | 6.9 | 11.7 | 7.0 | 12.6 | | | | |
| 3 | 43 | F | pre | 24.0 | | | | 260 | | | |
| | | | post | 14.9 | 14.1 | 11.6 | 37.0 | 68 | 75 | | |
| 4 | 13 | F | pre | 53.0 | 40.0 | 51.0 | 85.0 | 98 | | 68 | 110 |
| | | | post | 28.0 | 39.0 | | | 54 | | | |
| 5 | 52 | F | pre | 30.4 | 20.5 | 20.4 | 31.4 | 92 | 62 | 92 | 170 |
| | | | post | UD | UD | UD | UD | UD | 23 | UD | 14 |
| 6 | 31 | F | pre | 23.0 | 23.5 | 11.8 | | 76 | 70 | | |
| | | | post | UD | 10.9 | 2.8 | 20.5 | UD | 50 | UD | 53 |
| 7 | 50 | F | pre | 29.0 | 28.0 | 23.5 | 41.5 | 110 | 95 | 134 | 730 |
| | | | post | UD | | | | UD | 59 | 24 | 29 |
| 8 | 25 | F | pre | 21.0 | 21.4 | 20.8 | 25.7 | 165 | 210 | 215 | 580 |
| | | | post | 1.9 | 11.2 | 3.2 | 6.5 | UD | 115 | UD | 160 |
| 9 | 34 | F | pre | 23.9 | 23.5 | 19.0 | 45.5 | 59 | 57 | 64 | 305 |
| | | | post | 9.1 | 16.5 | UD | 6.5 | 32 | 76 | 22 | 33 |
| 10 | 32 | M | pre | 37.1 | 33.3 | 39.0 | 61.5 | 115 | 115 | 74 | 280 |
| | | | post | UD | 12.9 | 3.1 | 6.2 | 19 | 53 | 28 | 53 |

UD: Undetectable.

adrenal responsiveness to insulin hypoglycemia in 8 patients resulted in no significant increase of either plasma ACTH or cortisol, as suggested by Krieger and Luria (1977). On the contrary, following an injection of 8 lysine vasopressin (10 U, i.m.) all 6 patients showed remarkable increases in plasma ACTH. The increment in plasma cortisol was also significant, but not so great as that in plasma ACTH.

(b) Postoperative results: plasma ACTH and cortisol levels fell within two hours after microadenomectomy and very often became undetectable (Fig. 1). These subnormal levels of plasma ACTH and cortisol were sustained for the subsequent several months. In most cases diurnal rhythm of plasma ACTH and cortisol has been restored postoperatively, but not completely. In contrast to preoperative results, insulin hypoglycemia significantly increased plasma ACTH and cortisol levels, although not sufficiently in most cases. The preoperative response of plasma ACTH to lysine vasopressin became insignificant in 5 of 6 patients postoperatively (Fig. 2). The follow-up studies are now in progress.

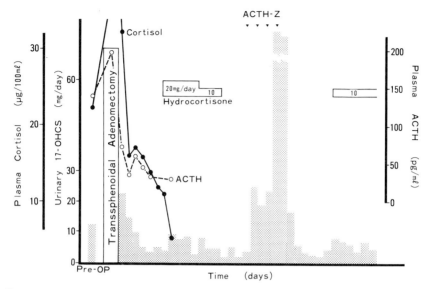

*Fig. 1.* Illustration of the immediate fall in urinary 17-OHCS excretion and plasma ACTH and cortisol levels following the removal of ACTH-secreting microadenomas (Case 1).

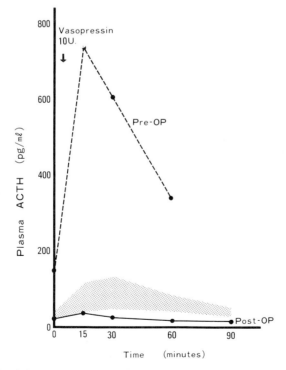

*Fig. 2.* An example of the changes of plasma ACTH-responsiveness to lysine vasopressin before and after surgery (Case 7). The dotted area represents the range of plasma ACTH in 5 normal adults.

Table II. Improvement in pituitary hormone function after transsphenoidal microadenomectomy.

| Patients No. | Pre-op / Post-op | Insulin GH (r.g/ml) | | TRH test TSH (μU/ml) | | PRL (ng/ml) | | LH-RH test LH (mIU/ml) | | FSH (mIU/ml) | |
|---|---|---|---|---|---|---|---|---|---|---|---|
| | | Basal | Peak | Basal | Peak | Basal | Peak | Basal | Peak | Basal | Peak |
| 1 | pre | 0.8 | 0.9 | 5.0 | 8.5 | 11.7 | 30.0 | 6.0 | 10.0 | 10.0 | 13.0 |
| | post | 5.0 | 5.0 | 4.5 | 9.5 | 10.5 | 61.0 | 14.0 | 31.0 | 9.0 | 12.0 |
| 2 | pre | 1.9 | 2.0 | 0.6 | 1.7 | 21.5 | 38.7 | 32.0 | 114.0 | 80.0 | 130.0 |
| | post | 2.7 | 10.6 | 7.0 | 34.5 | | 124.0 | 97.0 | 332.0 | 100.0 | 174.0 |
| 3 | pre | 1.5 | | 5.0 | 10.5 | 22.7 | 51.5 | 5.0 | 7.0 | 8.0 | 8.0 |
| | post | 3.3 | 5.0 | 2.5 | 12.5 | 47.0 | 49.0 | 7.0 | 31.0 | 5.0 | 8.0 |
| 4 | pre | 2.2 | 2.2 | 3.2 | 6.2 | 13.5 | 78.0 | 0.6 | 3.9 | 1.0 | 3.1 |
| | post | 1.4 | 2.7 | 3.0 | 4.0 | 14.5 | 46.0 | 5.0 | 12.0 | 3.0 | 14.0 |
| 5 | pre | 1.2 | 1.3 | 1.0 | 2.5 | 9.3 | 62.0 | 8.3 | 9.8 | 14.1 | 18.4 |
| | post | 1.9 | 3.4 | 1.0 | 4.0 | 22.5 | 111.0 | 44.0 | 128.0 | 45.0 | 65.0 |
| 6 | pre | 1.4 | 2.8 | 1.5 | 10.5 | 22.5 | 83.0 | 3.0 | 81.0 | 14.0 | 38.0 |
| | post | 1.1 | 6.2 | 2.0 | 20.0 | 51.5 | 103.5 | 14.0 | 292.0 | 9.0 | 22.0 |
| 7 | pre | 1.9 | 2.4 | 6.5 | 7.5 | 25.0 | 47.2 | 3.0 | 9.0 | 4.0 | 15.0 |
| | post | 2.4 | 5.3 | 4.5 | 9.0 | 36.1 | 85.0 | 24.0 | 57.0 | 36.0 | 41.0 |
| 8 | pre | 2.8 | 7.5 | UD | 3.0 | 7.3 | 61.0 | 20.0 | 101.4 | 15.8 | 17.7 |
| | post | 3.0 | 14.0 | 3.0 | 11.5 | 27.8 | 84.0 | 14.0 | 52.0 | 10.0 | 13.0 |
| 9 | pre | 0.8 | 3.9 | UD | 4.0 | 15.8 | 53.5 | 4.0 | 31.0 | 10.0 | 27.0 |
| | post | 1.4 | 11.8 | 4.5 | 19.0 | 16.5 | | 15.0 | 42.0 | 17.0 | 27.0 |
| 10 | pre | 1.5 | 1.3 | UD | UD | 19.4 | | 9.4 | 28.3 | 12.6 | 18.4 |
| | post | 1.8 | 11.7 | 4.0 | 11.0 | | | 35.0 | 95.0 | 15.0 | 23.0 |
| Mean ± s.d. | pre-op | 1.6 ± 0.6 | 2.7 ± 1.9 | 2.3 ± 2.3 | 5.4 ± 3.5 | 16.0 ± 6.3 | 56.5 ± 17.3 | 6.9 ± 5.9[a] | 37.5 ± 35.7[a] | 10.2 ± 4.5[a] | 17.9 ± 10.9[a] |
| | post-op | 2.3 ± 1.1 | 7.9 ± 3.9 | 3.6 ± 1.6 | 13.5 ± 8.6 | 26.7 ± 13.2 | 79.7 ± 27.2 | 14.9 ± 9.0[a] | 79.3 ± 90.1[a] | 9.7 ± 4.6[a] | 17.0 ± 6.5[a] |
| P Value | | < 0.35 | < 0.01 | NS | < 0.05 | < 0.02 | NS | < 0.05 | < 0.05 | NS | NS |

UD: undetectable, NS: not significant.
[a]Postmenopausal patients (No. 2, 5, 7) were excluded.

*Other anterior pituitary hormones*

Pre- and postoperative resting levels of plasma GH, TSH, PRL, LH and FSH, with their peak values in the provocative tests, are summarized in Table II. Preoperative morning resting levels of plasma GH were $1.6 \pm 0.6$ ng/ml and only minimal responses to insulin hypoglycemia were obtained ($2.7 \pm 1.9$ ng/ml). No patients showed a peak value of more than 10 ng/ml. Postoperatively, both their basal and peak values became statistically higher ($P < 0.05, 0.01$, respectively). In 4 of 9 patients, GH response was more than 10 ng/ml. The resting levels of plasma TSH were not significantly different pre- and postoperatively. But, postoperative TSH responses to TRH were larger than preoperative responses ($P < 0.05$). The postoperative recovery of pituitary gonadal function was remarkable. Conspicuous improvement of LH responsiveness to LH-RH was observed in all patients, which corresponded to such clinical improvements as the reappearance of regular menstrual cycles. FSH responsiveness was not influenced by this operation in premenopausal patients, but an apparent increase in FSH secretion occurred in all 3 postmenopausal patients.

## DISCUSSION

The reasons why most adenomas in Cushing's disease stay as microadenomas for their full life is still unknown. In fact, positive roentgenological findings cannot be obtained in most cases. Aside from the difficulty of diagnosing them, their favourable aspects can also be pointed out. Total removal is easier with microadenomas than with larger ones and more normal tissue can be preserved.

Besides ACTH, the secretion of other anterior pituitary hormones is affected in most patients with Cushing's disease. The most interesting question is whether the resulting hypercortisolism is reversible or not. Our results clearly show that the hormonal function of residual adenohypophysis in Cushing's disease can be returned to normal by correction of hypercortisolism. Tyrrell *et al.* (1977) reported improved GH responsiveness to insulin hypoglycemia after surgery. Considering these results, transsphenoidal adenomectomy is preferable for the treatment of Cushing's disease.

It is generally accepted that vasopressin increases ACTH secretion by directly acting on the pituitary gland and insulin hypoglycemia acts via the hypothalamus. The fact that positive ACTH responses to hypoglycemia became apparent after correction of hypercortisolism in our patients suggests that the secretion of corticotropin-releasing factors from the hypothalamus might have been impaired before surgery. The influences in the ACTH response to vasopressin before and after surgery argues that the conspicuous preoperative response is caused by adenoma cells. ACTH-secreting cells in the residual tissue seem to have been damaged both functionally and morphologically. Follow-up studies are necessary to clarify whether these dysfunctions are reversible.

Our overall results point out that transsphenoidal adenomectomy has obvious efficacy in the treatment of Cushing's disease. It is also suggested that the primary lesions in Cushing's disease seems to be in the pituitary gland, rather than in the hypothalamus.

## REFERENCES

Guiot, G. (1973). *In* "Diagnosis and Treatment of Pituitary Tumors" (P. O. Kohler and G. T. Ross, eds), pp. 159–178. Elsevier, New York.

Hardy, J. (1969). *Clin. Neurosurg.* **16**, 185–217.

Hardy, J. (1973). *In* "Diagnosis and Treatment of Pituitary Tumors" (P. O. Kohler and G. T. Ross, eds), pp. 179–194.

Krieger, D. T. and Luria, M. (1977). *J. Clin. Endocrinol. Metab.* **44**, 361–368.

Salassa, R. M., Laws, E. R. Jr, Carpenter, P. C. and Northcutt, R. C. (1978). *Mayo Clin. Proc.* **53**, 24–28.

Tyrrell, J. B., Wiener-Kronish, J., Lorenzi, M., Brooks, R. M. and Forsham, P. H. (1977). *J. Clin. Endocrinol. Metab.* **44**, 218–221.

Tyrrell, J. B., Brooks, R. M., Fitzgerald, P. A., Cofoid, P. B., Forsham, P. H. and Wilson, C. B. (1978). *N. Engl. J. Med.* **298**, 753–758.

# CRYOSURGERY OR MICROSURGERY FOR PITUITARY MICROADENOMAS ?

G. Teasdale, I. D. Hay, G. H. Beastall, D. McCruden and K. W. Grossart

*Institute of Neurological Sciences and University Departments of Medicine and Clinical Chemistry, Glasgow, Scotland*

Harvey Cushing advocated, in 1927, "a direct early attack on the adenoma of acromegaly while the sella is still small, in the hope of forestalling the oftentimes disastrous secondary effects".

The size of a pituitary adenoma has an important influence upon the outcome of treatment, whether the method employed is pharmacological, radiotherapeutic or surgical. Indeed, patients with large tumours, with suprasellar extensions, are usually excluded from some forms of therapy, and with other methods the prospects for success are lessened. A comparison of the overall results of cryosurgery and microsurgery in the treatment of acromegaly has been reported previously (Teasdale *et al.*, 1978). In this short communication we have focused upon those patients who had no more than minimal enlargement of the pituitary fossa. By this means we have compared the results of the two methods in patients with small pituitary adenomas.

## PATIENTS AND METHODS

Between 1967 and 1977, 57 patients had transsphenoidal operations for acromegaly or gigantism at the Institute of Neurological Sciences, Glasgow. Stereotactic cryosurgery was employed from 1967 to 1974, and subsequently microsurgical excision.

Cryohypophysectomy was carried out by a stereotactic technique described by Cross (1972) and Grossart (1972). Whenever possible, anterior and posterior bilateral lesions were made, depending on the size of the pituitary gland.

Microsurgical hypophysectomy was performed by a standard sublabial, transseptal, transsphenoidal approach (Hardy, 1971). Usually an attempt was made to preserve some non-adenomatous pituitary, unless the patient had growth hormone excess which was uncontrolled by prior treatment, in which case a "radical" operation was attempted.

For the purposes of this study, one of us (KWG) who did not have knowledge of the patients' pre- and post-operative endocrine states reviewed each patient's skull films. He made an arbitrary distinction between small and large pituitary adenomas on the basis of a sella turcica area of $1.6$ cm$^2$ in the lateral view. This dividing line permits comparison of our results with a large previous report (Levin *et al.*, 1974).

Patients had recently undergone a comprehensive post-operative endocrine assessment, for the purposes of this report. Growth hormone levels were determined by radioimmunoassay. In analysing the results we have calculated the mean of 5 early morning basal samples and 7 samples taken at 2 hour intervals during a day when the patient was allowed unrestricted activity in the ward. A mean level below 10 mU/l was regarded as normal. Basal levels of thyroid, adrenal and gonadal hormones and hormonal responses to hypoglycaemia and pituitary trophic hormones were studied to assess anterior pituitary reserve.

## RESULTS

### Cryosurgery

Seventeen operations were performed on 16 patients (8 males, 8 females; mean age 45; mean duration of disease 4.7 years). Pre-operative HGH levels were obtained in 14 cases and the mean value was 77 mu/l. Thirteen patients (81%) were previously untreated but three had previously received megavoltage irradiation.

The cryosurgical patients were reviewed after a mean period of 58 months (range 4–101). Only 4 patients (25%) had GH levels of $<$ 10 mU/l and in 1 patient this was achieved only at the cost of 2 operations. As a direct consequence of operation 12 patients (75%) required steroid replacement and 10 (63%) required thyroxine therapy. Of the 4 patients whose GH had been normalized, 3 required steroids and 2 thyroxine. The 1 patient with normal anterior pituitary function was 1 of 6 patients in whom only 1 lesion had been made on either side of the gland; the other 3 came from a group of 7 in whom 2 lesions were made bilaterally.

### Microsurgery

Microsurgery was performed on 1 patient with gigantism and 11 acromegalics who had lateral sellar areas of $<$ 1.6 cm$^2$ (3 males, 9 females; mean age 41; mean duration of disease 3 years). The pre-operative GH level was obtained in all patients and the mean level was 52 mU/l. Ten patients (83%) were previously untreated; 1 patient had undergone previous cryosurgery with post-operative irradiation and 1 patient had received prior pituitary irradiation.

The microsurgical cases have been followed on average for 11 months (range 3–24). In 11 cases where exact pre- and post-operative GH levels were available, there was a mean reduction of GH by 92%. At last follow-up, 11 patients (92%) and GH levels of < 10 mU/l.

Anterior pituitary function (adrenal, thyroid, gonad) was intact in 10 patients (83%). The 2 patients who had previously had other treatments had elected to have a deliberately radical procedure; as a consequence both require steroids and 1 has a persisting gonadotrophin deficiency.

### Cryosurgery vs microsurgery

It is clear, from this review of 2 series of patients with small pituitary adenomas that microsurgery has considerable advantages over cryosurgery both in the eradi-cation of HGH excess and in the retention of anterior pituitary trophic function (Tables I and II). It is also associated with less risk of operative morbidity.

After cryosurgery one patient developed a quadrantic field defect. Transient CSF leaks occurred and 2 patients developed meningitis after this procedure. By contrast, microsurgical operation has not led to extraocular muscle palsies or visual impairment, nor has infection occurred.

*Table I.*  Pre-operative features.

|  | Cryosurgical series | Microsurgical series |
|---|---|---|
| Number of operations | 17 | 12 |
| Age of patients (mean) | 45 yr | 41 yr |
| Estimated duration (mean) | 5 yr | 3 yr |
| Growth hormone < 50 mU/l | 8 patients | 7 patients |
| > 50 mU/l | 5 patients | 5 patients |

*Table II.*  Pituitary function after surgery.

|  | Cryosurgery $n = 16$ | Microsurgery $n = 12$ |
|---|---|---|
| Growth hormone < 10 mU/l | 4 patients | 11 patients |
| Adrenal deficiency | 12 patients | 2 patients |
| Thyroid deficiency | 10 patients | 0 |

## DISCUSSION

The favourable results obtained by microsurgery are comparable to those in other recent series (Garcia Uria *et al.*, 1978; U and Wilson, 1977; Ludecke *et al.*, 1976). The reasons for the failure to achieve "normalization" of growth hormone levels by cryosurgery as consistently as have others (Levin *et al.*, 1974; Di Tullo and Rand, 1977) are not clear. It seems unlikely that larger lesions could have been made without incurring even greater loss of normal pituitary function and more "para-sellar" complications.

If the sella is not grossly enlarged, or growth hormone only moderately increased it is almost always possible to achieve a "selective" cure by microsurgery. It seems particularly important to offer young patients the possibility of preserving normal pituitary function. Neither conventional radiotherapy nor bromocriptine treatment lowers growth hormone sufficiently consistently and continuingly to be regarded as ideal in early cases. However, patients with large tumours and very high growth hormone levels may need a combination of surgery, radiotherapy and drug treatment.

The crucial comparison cannot yet be made: which treatment does most to reduce the morbidity and prolong the life of an acromegalic patient? In the short term the level of growth hormone is generally accepted to be the best arbiter of the efficacy of management, even though it does not show a very close parallel with clinical indices of the severity of the disease. Whether a persisting elevated level, despite a good clinical response to operation, carries a bad prognosis is not yet clear. Histological abnormalities may extend beyond the confines of the obviously adenomatous part of the pituitary (Wrightson, 1978) and the possibility of recurrence after surgery exists. Nevertheless this seems to occur rarely when a well-localized tumour was seen at operation and post-operative hormone levels are normal (Ludecke *et al.*, 1976). Accepting even these reservations, transsphenoidal microsurgery comes nearest to achieving Cushing's goal.

## REFERENCES

Cross, J. N., Glynne, A., Grossart, K. W., Jennett, B., Kellett, R. J., Lazarus, J. H., Thomson, J. A. and Webster, M. H. C. (1972). *Lancet* i, 215–217.

Cushing, H. (1927). *Br. Med. J.* 2, 48–55.

Di Tullo, M. V. and Rand, R. W. (1977). *J. Neurosurg.* 46, 1–11.

Garcia-Uria, J., Del Pozo, J. M. and Bravo, G. (1978). *J. Neurosurg.* 49, 36–40.

Grossart, K. W. (1972). *Br. J. Radiol.* 45, 659–663.

Hardy, J. (1971). *J. Neurosurg.* 34, 582–594.

Levin, S. R., Hofeldt, F. O., Schneider, V., Becker, N., Karam, J. H., Seymour, R. J., Adams, J. E. and Forsham, P. H. (1974). *Am. J. Med.* 57, 526–535.

Ludecke, D., Kautzky, R., Saeger, W., Schrader, D. (1976). *Acta Neurochirurgica* 35, 27–42.

Teasdale, G., Grossart, K. W. and Miller, J. D. (1979). Thieme Verlag, Stuttgart (in press).

U, H. S., Wilson, C. B. and Tyrrell, J. B. (1977). *J. Neurosurg.* 47, 840–852.

Wrightson, P. (1978). *J. Neurol. Neurosurg. Psychiat.* 41, 283–289.

# STEREOTACTIC RADIOSURGERY AS TREATMENT IN PITUITARY-DEPENDENT CUSHING'S SYNDROME

M. Thorén[1], T. Rähn[2], K. Hall[1] and E. O. Backund[2]

[1] Department of Endocrinology and [2] Department of Neurosurgery,
Karolinska Hospital, 104 01 Stockholm, Sweden

## INTRODUCTION

The results when treating pituitary-dependent Cushing's syndrome with conventional radiation to the hypophysis have been discouraging. The doses which can be given without damaging the optic tract are limited to 4.5–5.0 krad, which is insufficient to control the syndrome in most patients. When radiation techniques allowing higher doses to be administered became available such as high energy charged particles (Lawrence et al., 1976) and pituitary implants of radioactive gold or yttrium (Burke et al., 1973) the number of remissions increased. Gamma radiation delivered with the stereotactic technique permits greater precision and then higher doses can be given to the hypophysis. We have treated patients with pituitary-dependent Cushing's syndrome by sterotactically-directed gamma radiation from [60]Co and in this report we present the results.

## PATIENTS

Twenty patients have been treated. Sixteen had pituitary dependent-Cushing's syndrome and four had Nelson's syndrome. The diagnosis of Cushing's syndrome was established by clinical signs and symptoms and conventional biochemical tests. The sella turcica was normal in size or only slightly enlarged in all the patients. One patient, however, had a small suprasellar extension of an intraseller tumour but normal visual fields. The patients with Nelson's syndrome had previously been subjected to bilateral adrenalectomy because of Cushing's syndrome and subse-

507

*Table I.* Cushing's syndrome.

| Patient | Age at treatment (yr) | Sex | Disease curation (yr) | Sella X-ray | Pneumoencephalography | Urinary cortisol excretion[a] nmol. $10^3$ per 24 h | Pituitary insufficiency |
|---|---|---|---|---|---|---|---|
| A | 40 | F | $\geqslant 3$ | normal | partially empty sella | 1.0 | none |
| B | 60 | M | $\geqslant 3$ | slightly enlarged | partially empty sella | 1.3 | none |
| C | 56 | F | $\geqslant 10$ | rounded shape | partially empty sella | 0.8 | none |
| D | 44 | F | $\geqslant 1$ | rounded shape | partially empty sella | 1.8 | none |
| E | 36 | F | $\geqslant 4$ | normal size, asymmetry | partially empty sella | 0.5 | none |
| F | 24 | M | $\geqslant 7$ | normal | normal | 1.1 | none |
| G | 31 | F | $\geqslant 3$ | normal | partially empty sella | 0.8 | none |
| H | 41 | F | $\geqslant 5$ | asymmetry | normal | 0.8 | none |
| I | 60 | F | $\geqslant 4$ | normal | small suprasellar tumour | 1.0 | gonadotrophins |
| J | 13 | F | $\geqslant 2$ | normal | normal | 5.7 | none |

[a]Normal range 0.09–0.28 nmol. $10^3$/24 h.

*Table II.* Nelson's syndrome.

| Patient | Age at treatment (yr) | Sex | Time since adrenalectomy (yr) | Sella X-ray | Pneumoencephalography | Hyperpigmentation |
|---|---|---|---|---|---|---|
| K | 53 | F | 7 | normal | partially empty sella | moderate |
| L | 63 | M | 2[a] | normal | — | severe |
| M | 51 | F | 5 | frontal expansion | — | severe |
| N | 54 | F | 19 | asymmetry | suprasellar extension of intrasellar tumour | severe |

[a]X-ray treatment to the pituitary, 5 krad, 0 effect.

quently developed hyperpigmentation concomitant with elevated plasma ACTH levels. All had radiological evidence of a pituitary tumour. One of these patients who had a suprasellar extension of the tumour with slight impairment of the visual fields had refused recommended open surgery.

The patients were re-examined three to four months after therapy. If not in remission at the first re-examination the patients were then re-investigated after another two or four months. They were then observed after one year and then at least every half year at which times tests for cortisol excretion, thyroid and gonadal functions were performed.

Ten of the patients with Cushing's syndrome and all the patients with Nelson's syndrome have follow-up periods of more than seven months. These patients are presented in Table I and II.

## METHODS

### Radiation technique

A modification of the gamma unit described by Leksell (1971) was used for the irradiation. The unit was designed for the purpose of producing minute spherical shaped lesions in the brain to treat tumours and vascular malformations. The lesion is induced by collimated beams from 179 [60]Co sources distributed within a hemispherical sector. The beams are radially directed towards the centre of the

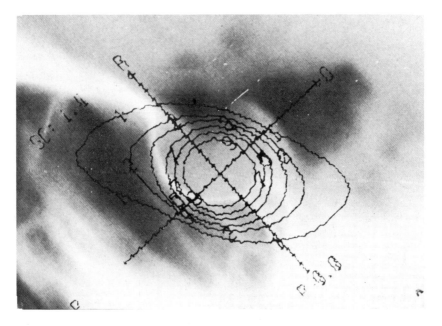

*Fig. 1.* Sagittal dose distribution. The irradiated area is indicated by the 10, 20, 30, 50, 70 and 90% isodose curves (from Thorén *et al.*, 1978a, Fig. 1).

unit at which the target point in the gland has to be positioned. By changing the collimators, the geometric cross-section of each beam can be altered from 8 to 14 mm to match the size and shape of the pituitary.

The irradiation was given in one single session and the individual doses varied between 5 and 10 krad. The irradiation time with this technique was 4-5 min krad. The dose gradient is very steep, permitting a high dose in the target point while the adjacent structures receive much lower doses. The dose to the optic tract is less than 10% of the dose in the target point when it is placed in the centre of the adenohypophysis and a total dose distribution like that shown in Fig. 1 can be obtained. The stereotactic localization of the pituitary, the determination of the coordinates of the target point and the positioning of the patient in the irradiation unit were the same as the corresponding steps during an open stereotactic procedure.

### Hormone determinations

Cortisol in plasma was measured using a fluorimetric method (de Moor *et al.*, 1962). Urinary cortisol (Ruder *et al.*, 1972; Ficher *et al.*, 1973), serum LH, FSH, somatomedin and plasma ACTH were measured by radioimmunoassay (Svensson *et al.*, 1978; Thorén *et al.*, 1978b; Hall *et al.*, 1978).

### RESULTS

No complications occurred during the irradiation or the following three months.

The results for the 10 patients with Cushing's syndrome followed for more than 7 months are summarized in Table III. The observation times for these patients have been 7-34 months.

In all the patients there was a gradual improvement of the clinical symptoms. Six patients gained complete clinical remission accompanied by normal or low urinary cortisol excretion which continued throughout the observation period. The patient (A) with the longest observation time had a normal diurnal rhythm of cortisol after 24 months. Normal cortisol excretion was achieved after different lengths of times, from 3 months to 1 year.

Among the 4 patients without complete remission, 2 (H, J) have been followed for 7 and 10 months, respectively. Both had lower cortisol excretion than before treatment in parallel with clinical improvement. Two patients may be considered not to have been cured by the treatment. One patient (D) who improved considerably still had slightly elevated cortisol excretion after 21 months. She then received additional radiation treatment with 4 krad and the hyperadrenocorticism was controlled by drug treatment using a combination of elipten and metyrapone. The evaluation of the effectiveness of the second radiation has not yet been carried out. The patient (I) who has an intrasellar tumour with suprasellar extension improved initially both clinically and biochemically but after 6 months her symptoms recurred.

One patient (B) developed clinical ACTH insufficiency 7 months after therapy without distinct evidence of insufficiency of any other pituitary hormones. Two

Table III. Cushing's syndrome.

| Patient | Dose received (krad) | Observation time (months) | Clinical Cushing's syndrome | Cortisol normal after months | Cortisol excretion at last assessment | Complications |
|---|---|---|---|---|---|---|
| A | 7 | 34 | remission | 3 | normal | none |
| B | 10 | 29 | remission | 6 | —[a] | ACTH insufficient 7 months |
| C | 10 | 28 | remission | 12 | normal | none |
| D | 7.5 | 28 | improvement | — | slightly elevated | none |
|   | 4.0 | 7 |  |  |  |  |
| E | 7 | 17 | remission | 12 | normal | none |
| F | 7 | 14 | remission | 6 | slightly subnormal | none |
| G | 7 | 12 | remission | 8 | normal | none |
| H | 8 | 10 | improvement | — | slightly elevated | none |
| I | 7 | 9 | unchanged | — | unchanged | none |
| J[b] | 7 | 7 | improvement | — | slight improvement | none |

[a]Cortisol replacement therapy.
[b]Treated while on bromocriptine therapy.

of the patients (A and G) had transitory subnormal cortisol excretion without clinical symptoms. None of the patients acquired any insufficiency of any other pituitary hormone after the treatment. Serum levels of somatomedins remained normal, indicating normal GH production.

In the four patients with Nelson's syndrome there was decreased hyperpigmentation with lower plasma ACTH values than before treatment. However, the patient who had a rather large pituitary tumour with suprasellar extension had bitemporal hemianopsy four months after therapy, but the visual fields improved and were normal two months later.

## DISCUSSION

Stereotactic gamma lesion of the hypophysis has been shown to be a promising therapeutic alternative in treating pituitary-dependent Cushing's syndrome. Six out of 10 patients had complete clinical remission within the first year. In addition 2 patients with shorter observation times improved, indicating a possible cure in the future. All 4 patients with Nelson's syndrome exhibited a clear improvement with decrease of the hyperpigmentation and lower ACTH levels. One patient with Cushing's syndrome who had a small suprasellar extension relapsed after initial improvement. The lack of effect in this case is not surprising because the suprasellar part is outside the irradiated area.

No acute complications of the irradiation were found. However, transient bitemporal hemianopsia occurred 4 months after treatment in 1 patient with Nelson's syndrome, who had a large suprasellar extension of a pituitary tumour. Except for ACTH insufficiency in one patient, no other patient acquired hypophyseal insufficiency after treatment.

Providing the patients with suprasellar extension of the tumour are excluded, the therapy by gamma lesion seems to be both effective and safe. In addition, the treatment can be performed without hospitalization of the patient. It is not yet possible to state whether the cure will be permanent. This doubt is raised because the underlying pathology in pituitary-dependent Cushing's syndrome is not yet clearly defined. The same hesitation is also valid for other forms of treatment directed to the hypophysis, such as surgical enucleation of adenoma or other forms of radiation therapy.

## ACKNOWLEDGEMENT

We thank Drs. Bengt Hallengren, Pavo Hedner, J.-G. Ljunggren, K.-G. Nilsson and A. Widström for help in the follow-up of the patients.

## REFERENCES

Burke, C. W., Doyle, F. H., Joplin, G. F., Arnot, R. N., Macerlean, D. P. and Russell Fraser, R. (1973). *Q. JL Med, New Series* **XLII**, 693–714.
Ficher, M., Curtis, G. C., Fanjam, V. K., Joshlin, L. and Perry, S. (1973). *Clin. Chem.* **19**, 511-518.

Hall, K., Brant, J., Enberg, G. and Fryklund, L. (1979). *J. clin. Endocr. Metab.* (In press).

Lawrence, J. H., Tobias, C. A., Linfoot, J. A., Born, J. L. and Chong, C. Y. (1976). *J. Am. med. Soc.* **235**, 2307–2310.

Leksell, L. (1971). "Stereotaxis and Radiosurgery. An Operative System." Charles C. Thomas, Springfield, Illinois.

de Moor, P., Osinski, P., Deckx, R. and Steno, O. (1962). *Clinica chim. Acta* **7**, 475–480.

Ruder, H. J., Guy, R. L. and Lipsett, M. B. (1972). *J. clin. Endocr. Metab.* **35**, 219–224.

Svensson, J., Eneroth, P., Gustafsson, J.-A., Ritzén, M. and Stenberg, Å. (1978). *J. Endocr.* **76**, 399–409.

Thorén, M., Rähn, T., Hall, K. and Backlund, E. O. (1978a). *Acta endocr., Copenh.* **88**, 7–17.

Thorén, M., Ajne, M. and Hall, K. (1978b). *Acta endocr., Copenh.* submitted for publication.

# ALPHA PARTICLE PITUITARY IRRADIATION IN THE PRIMARY AND POST-SURGICAL MANAGEMENT OF PITUITARY MICROADENOMAS

J. A. Linfoot

*Donner Pavillon, University of California, Berkeley, USA*

Since 1957, helium ions have been used to suppress pituitary function in 796 patients with a variety of neoplastic and metabolic disorders including mammary carcinoma, diabetes complicated by retinopathy and functioning and non-functioning pituitary tumors. This method of treating pituitary tumors has become an internationally recognized therapeutic procedure. The long-term follow-up of these patients has been a unique investigation of the biological properties of the human pituitary. It has provided a valuable source of information regarding acute and long-term effects of localized heavy ions on normal and abnormal pituitary tissue and peptide hormone secretion, as well as neuro-ophthalmological and histopathological data on the immediate and long-term effects of heavy ions on the brain and cranial nerves.

This review presents our experience in the treatment of 429 pituitary tumor patients, both micro- and macroadenomas, using alpha particle pituitary irradiation (APPI). Thirty-two patients with non-functioning tumors will not be discussed at this time. The duration of follow-up in these patients ranges from 6 months to 20 years with the majority of patients having been followed for at least 5–10 years.

## RADIOTHERAPEUTIC TECHNIQUE

Soon after parallel beams of atomic nucleon were available at the Berkeley 184-inch synchrocyclotron, systematic investigations were undertaken in rats and primates under the direction of Lawrence and Tobias (Tobias *et al.*, 1958). These animal studies became the basis for developing dose schedules in our human patients. Using a projected physical dose system with a geometric delivery which limited the volume of extrasellar tissue irradiated by the particle beam, a system for pituitary irradiation was developed (Lawrence, 1957). A pencil-shaped beam is made to fit the contour of the sella turcica. By multiport exposure and a sequential pendulum motion, a dose distribution is achieved that maximizes the particle beam at the center of the pituitary while protecting the basal structures, such as the optic chiasm, brain stem, hypothalamus and the temporal lobes, which receive less than 10% of the central pituitary dose. The doses to skin and peripheral portions of the brain are minimal and no epilation occurs. In most of our patients the beam is passed through the head and is referred to as the plateau or "through and through" technique. An additional property of heavy ions, the Bragg peak, provides a means of more effectively localizing irradiation and increasing the relative biological effect (RBE) through greater linear energy transfer (LET) in tissue. We have limited our use of the Bragg peak to selected patients with large, invasive tumors, but it has been used extensively by others (Kjellberg *et al.*, 1962).

## PATIENT SELECTION CRITERIA

These patient selection criteria have been developed for alpha particle therapy: (1) confirmed presence of a pituitary tumor by neuroradiological or histological examination; (2) demonstrated pituitary hypersecretion with detectable endocrine or metabolic effects; (3) absent history of prior therapeutic irradiation to the pituitary or parasellar structures; (4) absence of major suprasellar extension; (5) cerebrospinal fluid (CSF) growth hormone level $< 1.5$ ng/ml in patients with pituitary gigantism or acromegaly; (6) pituitary tumor size $< 2.5$ cm (7) clearly definable radiological tumor landmarks in the presence of extensive sphenoid extension; (8) adequate localization of the optic chiasm and residual tumor mass in post-surgical patients.

While skull films with sellar tomography, central axial tomography (CAT scan), bilateral carotid angiography and cavernous sinus venography are helpful in the evaluation of patients for pituitary treatment, pneumoencephalography (PEG) is still essential. The use of fractional PEG with hypocycloidal polytomography remains the most sensitive method of demonstrating a small suprasellar extension and an unsuspected empty sella and currently is the only technique that consistently localizes the position of the optic chiasm.

Using the neuroradiological techniques described above, we have recently employed a radiological classification of tumors proposed by Hardy (1973). Using this classification, pituitary tumors can be characterized in the following fashion: Grade I tumors are enclosed microadenomas which measure $< 10$ mm in maximal diameter; Grade II tumors are larger and more invasive, causing obvious sellar distortion and occasionally suprasellar extension. The degree of suprasellar extension may be small and completely asymptomatic: Type A, moderate to massive and Types B and C, causing optic chiasmal symptoms and displacement of the third ventricle. Grade III and IV tumors are the most common in our series and include lesions with marked extension into the sphenoid sinus and usually an indeterminate degree of lateral extension into the cavernous sinus. Grade III and

IV tumors invariably represent difficult therapeutic problems. As suggested by Hardy (1975), we have found this classification of practical value since it correlates with our clinical data and reflects the extent of the APPI field and is predictive of the post-treatment prognosis.

## GOALS OF TREATMENT

We have attempted to achieve four primary therapeutic goals with APPI: (1) control of tumor growth; (2) control of hormonal hypersecretion; and to accomplish the first two goals with (3) acceptable hormonal and (4) minimal central nervous system side effects. Although APPI has been suitable as a primary treatment in the majority of our referred patients, an increasing number of patients have been referred following transfrontal or transsphenoidal surgery. Failure to appreciate multiple microadenomata or adenomatous hyperplasia (Ludecke *et al.*, 1976) and/or inability to completely excise the invasive tumor resulting in inadequate control of hormonal hypersecretion and tumor regrowth has suggested that combined therapy, surgery and APPI, will be necessary for many patients.

Over the past 20 years, it has become apparent that in accomplishing the first two goals of therapy, we produce varying degrees of hypopituitarism in a small but significant number of patients. Neurological complications have been infrequent. Using the data from the original animal studies, and our extensive long-term patient studies, we have established central nervous system radiosensitivity guidelines and can accurately deliver pituitary doses which are free of side effects in nearly all cases.

## TREATMENT OF CUSHING'S DISEASE

Since 1959, we have treated 64 patients with Cushing's disease. Fifty-nine patients have had sellar volumes within the normal range and can be classified as Grade I lesions. The greater effectiveness of pituitary irradiation with conventional photon therapy in juvenile Cushing's has been recently emphasized (Jennings *et al.*, 1977). Our 5 teenage Cushing's, 17–19 years of age, have been cured by APPI without hypopituitarism or central nervous system side effects. These results are superior to those described for photon therapy.

Fifty-nine adult Cushing's, 21–78 years of age, have been treated; 9 patients were subsequently referred for bilateral adrenalectomy (8 cases) or hypophysectomy (1 case) because of either a delayed response or clinical relapse. It is of interest that in the group of Cushing's treated prior to 1972, the cure rate of 22 patients treated with 6000–15000 rad in 6 alternate day treatment fractions was 68%. The majority of our failures or incomplete responses occurred in these patients. Subsequently, of 42 patients treated with 8000–12000 rad administered in 3–4 daily fractions, the cure rate was 95%. This degree of success has not been achieved with photon therapy (Orth and Liddle, 1971). Attempts to achieve comparable results by shortening the treatment course and/or increasing the dose per fraction have occasionally been associated with extensive radionecrosis due to the large volume of parasellar central nervous system tissue (optic chiasm, hypothalamus and temporal lobes), that are necessarily included in the radiation field (Aristizabal *et al.*, 1977).

During the past 19 years we have developed a 5-day "work up" which provides a maximum amount of information and usually confirms: (a) a diagnosis of Cushing's syndrome, (b) excludes primary adrenal neoplasm and (c) excludes ectopic ACTH production from non-adrenal tumors, as causes of hypercortisolism (Linfoot, in press). Figure 1 shows the serial pre- and post-treatment endocrine changes observed in those patients who have been evaluated with this 5-day protocol. The mean urinary fluorogenic cortisol (Mattingly, 1962) in 37 patients

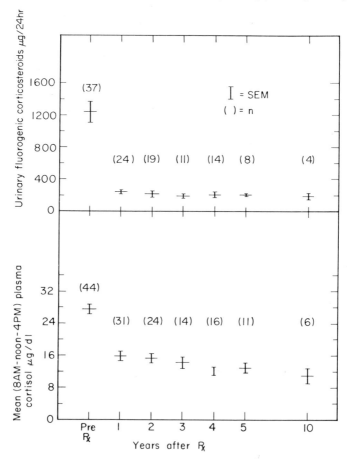

*Fig. 1.*    Results of APPI in Cushing's disease. Pre- and post-treatment changes in the mean (± s. e.) plasma cortisol (lower panel) and urinary fluorogenic corticosteroids (upper panel) are shown. Normal plasma and urinary cortisol values were observed at one year and were maintained for at least 10 years. The number (*n*) of patients studied is indicated in parenthesis.

was 1350 μg/ml which fell to a normal mean level of 200 μg/ml; concomitantly, the average daily plasma cortisol (8 a.m., noon, 4 p.m.) fell from 30 μg/dl to 16 μg/dl. These normal levels have been maintained in patients followed for up to 10 years. The diurnal rhythm also improved to normal in most patients. In spite of the well-known delay in radiation effect, the response to APPI has been relatively prompt. Since the majority of our patients return for follow-up at one year intervals, we have limited data obtained at earlier times. Patients who have florid Cushing's are usually treated with metyrapone (Jeffcoate *et al.*, 1977) and/or aminoglutethimide (Givens *et al.*, 1970) for varying periods while awaiting APPI to suppress pathological adrenocorticotropic function. In retrospect, several of our early patients were referred prematurely for adrenalectomy because the effectiveness of these adrenal blocking agents was not appreciated.

The results of overnight dexamethasone suppression and metyrapone testing are illustrated in Fig. 2. Prior to treatment, cortisol was incompletely suppressed by dexamethasone. Following treatment, the basal levels were lowered and normal suppression to values < 5 μg/dl occurred. The metyrapone responses prior to treatment were variable; many patients are hyper-responsive while some have a normal response. During the first year after treatment, metyrapone responses fell

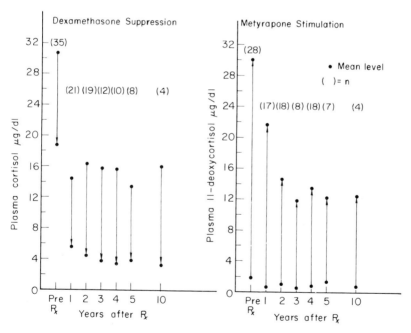

*Fig. 2.* Results of APPI in Cushing's disease. Dexamethasone suppression tests (right panel) and metyrapone stimulation tests (left panel) pre- and post-treatment are shown with arrows depicting the change from baseline levels. Normal plasma cortisol suppression by dexamethasone and plasma 11-deoxycortisol response to metyrapone were observed at one year and persisted for at least 10 years. Relapse is rare and normal ACTH reserve is maintained in most patients.

into the normal range and normal ACTH reserve was maintained in the majority of patients for at least 10 years following treatment.

The endocrine side effects in Cushing's patients have been determined by the use of adrenal, thyroid and gonadal steroid (estrogen or testosterone) replacement data. Using these criteria, the actual incidence of hypopituitarism may be over-estimated due to lack of consistent criteria for the prescription of hormonal replacement especially for thyroid and gonadal steroids. Analysis of patients treated solely with APPI show that 9% require adrenal replacement, 16% thyroid replacement and 11% gonadal steroid replacement.

Neurological side effects have been infrequent in our Cushing's patients. Three patients (5%) may have had minor cranial nerve lesions as a result of treatment. The spontaneous occurrence of third nerve lesions in Cushing's disease is well known (Hsu, 1977). Two early patients developed partial third nerve lesions which cleared spontaneously. A third patient developed visual field cuts three years after treatment. Retrospectively, she had a poor mask fit and inadequate head fixation. Her sella was unusually small and a subsequent PEG (which was not performed prior to treatment) revealed a prefixed chiasm and an empty sella. Currently, visual fields are stable and visual acuity normal.

Other complications in our series include two patients who developed Nelson's syndrome after bilateral adrenalectomy which was performed after inadequate APPI. Nelson's syndrome is uncommon but has occurred after photon as well as APPI therapy (Moore *et al.*, 1976). There have been 2 deaths, one elderly patient died of a cerebral vascular accident within a few months after treatment and a mentally retarded patient who had been confined to a nursing home for most of her life, developed pneumonia and died 3 years after successful treatment of her Cushing's disease.

### TREATMENT OF NELSON'S SYNDROME

We have treated 15 patients with Nelson's syndrome. Nine of these patients were treated solely with APPI while 6 patients had either transfrontal or trans-sphenoidal surgery prior to treatment and were treated because of residual tumor and elevated ACTH levels. Although there has been decreased pigmentation and dramatic fall in ACTH levels in all patients, ACTH levels have rarely returned to normal. Lack of sellar change in all but one patient who had an invasive tumor with suprasellar extension indicates that tumor control has thus far been achieved in these patients.

### TREATMENT OF ACROMEGALY

Two hundred and ninety-nine patients with acromegaly have been treated with APPI. There is general agreement that the optimum therapy in the treatment of acromegaly must produce control of tumor growth as well as adequate lowering of elevated immunoassayable growth hormone (GH) concentrations. Figure 3 shows the fall in hGH of patients treated solely with APPI. Fall in plasma hGH has been associated with striking clinical and metabolic improvement, e.g. improved glucose tolerance, loss of insulin resistance and fall in elevated serum phosphorus levels,

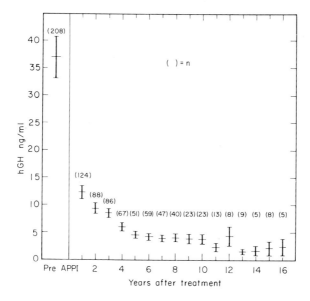

*Fig. 3.*    Results of APPI in acromegaly. Pre- and post-treatment mean (± s. e.) fasting plasma growth hormone (immunoreactive hGH) levels are displayed chronologically in acromegalic patients followed for as long as 16 years. The number (*n*) of patients studied is shown in parenthesis.

and is frequently seen within the first year even before the GH levels fall to < 10 ng/ml. More striking improvement is observed when GH falls to 5-10 ng/ml.

We have treated 65 patients with Grade II-IV lesions who have had previous transfrontal, transsphenoidal or cryogenic surgery. These difficult cases appear to have responded well to APPI albeit more slowly. The growth hormone levels tended to be somewhat higher but the rate of fall was parallel to the *de novo* group. Although we frequently encounter difficulties in fulfilling our selection criteria in these cases, our results (see Fig. 4) are extremely encouraging and support the use of APPI for an increasing number of patients referred after surgical procedures.

To evaluate the results of treatment in acromegalics with microadenomas, we have graded our patients according to sellar volumes (tumor size) as previously described. There was a positive correlation between the sellar volumes and the basal GH levels, confirming the observations made by Wright *et al.* (1969) who employed the area of the sella calculated from measurements from the lateral skull X-ray. Figure 5 chronologically displays the GH fall in the Grade I patients and compares these responses to the combined data from the Grade II-IV patients. Nearly all the microadenoma patients have shown a rapid normalization of GH and it can be anticipated they have an excellent prognosis for cure. The ultimate GH response in the Grade II-IV tumor patients is comparable to the microadenoma patients but delayed. These invasive tumors present difficult therapeutic geometry for APPI and have a less favorable prognosis. However, in many of these cases, the accurate distribution of APPI may have advantages over

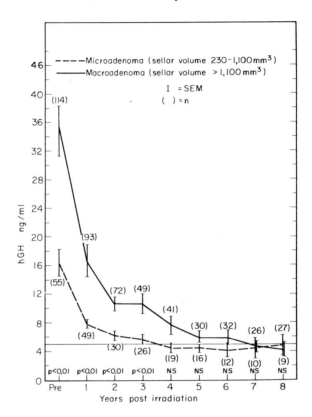

*Fig. 4.*    Results of APPI in acromegaly. Serial fasting plasma growth hormone (immunoreactive (GH) changes (pre- and post-treatment) are shown in Grade I microadenoma patients (dotted lines). Compared to Grade II–IV macroadenoma patients (solid lines). Microadenoma patients have lower GH levels and respond more rapidly. A lower incidence of post-treatment hypopituitarism is observed in these patients (see text).

surgical procedures as *de novo* treatment; but the combined use of surgery and radiation may often be the optimal therapy in many of these difficult cases (Linfoot and Wilson, 1978).

Rarely has the radiation dose selected been the cause of partial response or post-treatment relapse in our patients. The majority of our failures can be traced to inadequate fitting of the aperture and the geometric distribution of the irradiation dose. This was mainly the result of our failure to appreciate the presence of some degree of extrasellar extension. Through retrospective analysis, we have identified 4 major reasons for what we refer to as a "geometric miss". This analysis is depicted in Table I.

The endocrine side effects have been analysed in the acromegalics in the same fashion described previously in our Cushing's patients. Sixty-six per cent of patients treated solely with APPI are on no adrenal replacement, while 34% have been placed on adrenal steroids after irradiation. Similar data were observed for

## ACROMEGALY

COMBINED THERAPY

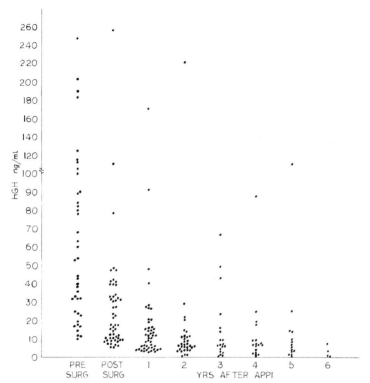

*Fig. 5.* Results of APPI in acromegaly. Serial changes in GH before and after either trans- .- frontal or transsphenoidal microsurgical hypophysectomy followed by APPI. The combined therapeutic approach produced normal GH levels within one to two years in most cases. A combined approach is being utilized in an increasing number of patients referred for APPI.

thyroid replacement. Sixty-one per cent are on no thyroid replacement, 6% were on thyroid prior to APPI and 33% required thyroid after APPI. Seventy-three per cent were on no gonadal steroid replacement, 2% were on replacement prior to APPI and 25% were on gonadal replacement after treatment.

It is difficult to find long-term data on the incidence of post-treatment hypopituitarism since the early studies lacked sufficient data and the newer modalities have been used for insufficient time to determine any long-term hormonal effects. We have generally concluded that the replacement therapy needs are greater than for transsphenoidal surgery (Wilson and Dempsey, 1978) but less than observed after conventional photon therapy (Samaan *et al.,* 1975; Sheline, in press).

The neuro-complications have been largely limited to seven patients who had received previous unsuccessful photon therapy and patients with Grade IV tumors who were treated with the Bragg peak. The incidence of complications in these patients have been summarized in Table II. Two photon patients (29%) had visual field cuts which fortunately did not impair visual acuity and were essentially asymptomatic. Three photon patients (43%) developed unilateral third nerve lesions which partially cleared. Three photon patients (29%) developed temporal lobe epilepsy which was easily controlled with anticonvulsant therapy. As a result of these early complications, since 1961 we have not accepted patients who had

*Table I.*    APPI relapse: acromegaly.

| Patient | Type of tumor extension | | | |
| | 1 | 2 | 3 | 4 |
| --- | --- | --- | --- | --- |
| IB | | | | + |
| JD | + | | | |
| JM | | + | | |
| BS[a] | | + | | |
| HV | | + | | |
| AI | | + | + | |
| BS | | | + | |
| MD | + | | | |
| GC | | | | |
| LP[b] | | | | |
| LL | | + | | |
| MS | + | | | |
| GO | | + | | |
| RM | | + | | |
| PL | | + | + | |
| EW | + | | | |
| Total | 4(25%) | 8(50%) | 3(19%) | 1(6%) |

1. Suprasellar extension
2. Intrasphenoidal extension
3. Posterior–inferior extension
4. Lateral extension

[a]Secondary proton beam therapy.
[b]Secondary photon irradiation.

received prior photon therapy. Only 2 patients treated solely with APPI received higher doses of radiation that we currently use and both developed temporal lobe lesions. They were treated prior to 1961. If one excludes the patients treated with the Bragg peak and those who had had prior photon therapy, the incidence of central nervous system complications has been < 1%.

While we have limited the use of alpha particle Bragg peak therapy, with newer localization techniques, the Bragg peak can be more effectively utilized with little or no morbidity. The recent availability of Bragg peak therapy with heavier ions, e.g. $^{12}$C, from the Bevalac (Tobias, in press) will have additional advantages over currently available protons and alpha particles.

*Table II.*  APPI complications in acromegaly.

| | Central nervous system complications | | |
| --- | --- | --- | --- |
| | II Nerve | III Nerve | Temporal lobe |
| 1. Prior photon therapy (7 patients) | | | |
| VL | — — | — — | + |
| MO | — — | + | + |
| FS | — — | + | + |
| VK[a] | + | — — | — — |
| LT | — — | + | — — |
| MZ[a] | + | — — | — — |
| Total | 2 (29%) | 3 (43%) | 3 (43%) |
| 2. Bragg peak therapy (8 patients) | | | |
| MS | — — | + | — — |
| MaS | — — | + | + |
| PB | + | — — | — — |
| Total | 1 (13%) | 2 (25%) | 1 (13%) |
| 3. Biplanar rotation therapy (283 patients) | | | |
| JJ | — — | — — | + |
| RM | — — | — — | + |
| Total | | | 2 (1%) |
| Total 298 patients | 3 (1%) | 5 (2%) | 6 (2%) |

[a]Empty sella.

## TREATMENT OF PROLACTIN SECRETING TUMORS

Based on prospective and retrospective radioimmunoassay measurements of prolactin (Prl), performed on frozen plasma samples obtained prior to treatment, we have identified 29 patients with hyperprolactinemia in our series. There were 22 females and 7 males. Seventeen patients were treated solely with APPI and 41% had hypophysectomy prior to APPI either because of incomplete surgical resection, persistent clinical symptoms or persistent hyperprolactinemia. Twenty-four patients had sellar volumes < 1100 mm$^3$ and were considered to have microadenomata, the remainder of the patients had larger sellas and were either Grade II lesions with suprasellar extensions or predominantly Grade III-IV lesions.

Figure 6 shows the plasma Prl measurements in the patients prior to and in the years following APPI. The levels varied from 29-4800 ng/ml. Twelve of 21 patients had normal Prl levels one year following treatment. As in the acromegalic patients, those with the higher levels tended to fall more slowly. There was not a clear correlation between the size of the tumors and the elevation of the Prl levels,

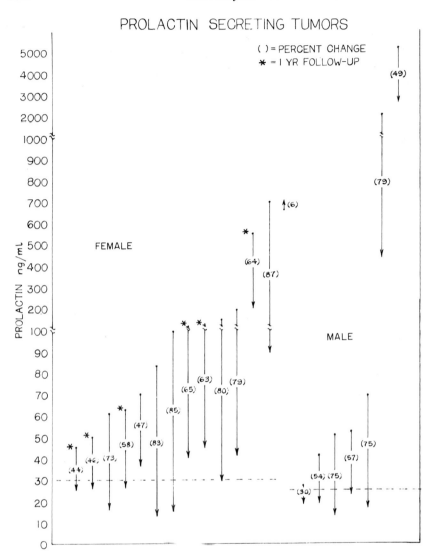

*Fig. 6.* Results of APPI in prolactin secreting tumors. Fasting plasma prolactin levels are shown for pre- and post-treatment in females (left panel) and males (right panel). Arrows indicate the direction of change in prolactin levels after treatment. Twelve patients had normal levels after APPI. A striking fall in prolactin was observed in many patients at one year (indicated by *) post-treatment.

although with the small patient sample size and the frequency of prior surgery in these patients, such a correlation would be difficult to detect.

There is a good deal of variability in the clinical response to the lowering of Prl levels. In patients with secondary amenorrhea, menses often resumed before Prl levels returned completely to normal and usually preceded the cessation of galactorrhea. Although most patients were not treated for infertility, two patients are currently pregnant.

There have not been many endocrine side effects in the Prl-secreting tumor patients. Ten per cent required adrenal replacement, 24% were placed on thyroid and 17% were started on estrogen or testosterone following therapy.

Central nervous system side effects have not occurred in the Grade I microadenomas. One patient with a large tumor with lateral extension developed a transient third nerve lesion 6 months following treatment; this has gradually cleared. Another patient with a huge tumor who had extensive surgical decompression prior to APPI developed a cerebral vascular episode and temporal lobe epilepsy following combined therapy. This patient recovered and returned to work as a physicist.

## SUMMARY

Since 1957, alpha particles (helium ions) have been used to suppress pituitary function in 796 patients with a variety of neoplastic and metabolic disorders including mammary carcinoma, diabetes complicated by retinopathy and functioning and non-functioning pituitary tumors. This method of treating pituitary tumors has become an internationally recognized therapeutic procedure.

Four hundred and twenty-nine pituitary tumor patients including both micro- and macroadenomas with Cushing's disease, acromegaly and hyperprolactinemia have been treated. The duration of follow-up in these patients ranges from 6 months to 20 years with the majority of patients having been followed for at least 5-10 years.

These long-term studies have established that alpha particle pituitary irradiation (APPI) fulfills desired therapeutic goals since pituitary tumor growth and hormonal hypersecretions can be effectively controlled with an acceptable incidence of post-treatment hypopituitarism. With few if any neurological side effects, patients with Grade I microadenomata as well as more invasive Grade II-IV macroadenomas can be effectively treated. The normal response has been shown to occur more rapidly in microadenoma patients and the incidence of hypopituitarism is less that in patients with larger and more invasive tumors.

Eighty-six per cent (95% since 1971) of the 64 patients with Cushing's disease have been cured and the normalization of plasma and urinary cortisol, dexamethasone and metyrapone responses has persisted greater than 10 years. Similarly, 90% of our acromegalic patients have been successfully treated with APPI, resulting in regression of clinical features, normalization of growth hormone and the accompanying improvement of glucose tolerance, insulin resistance and other metabolic parameters. Twenty-nine patients with prolactin-secreting tumors have been treated. While all of these patients have not had microadenomata, lowering of prolactin in all but one patient and normalization of prolactin in half of the patients within one year indicates that APPI is highly effective in the treatment of prolactin-secreting tumors.

In contrast to many forms of therapy currently used in the treatment of pituitary tumors, the long-term effectiveness and late endocrine and central nervous system side effects have been well established. There is no anesthetic or surgical morbidity or mortality and it can be used in difficult cases which have not been effectively treated with the various neurosurgical procedures, photon therapy being an exception. Preliminary studies suggest that combined transfrontal or transsphenoidal hypophysectomy with APPI may be the optimal treatment in many cases.

Because of the overall greater effectiveness, the more rapid endocrine response and the lesser risk of hypopituitarism and radionecrosis, precisely delivered heavy particle therapy (alpha and proton beam) should be used in preference to conventional photon therapy with gamma or X-rays. Microadenomas in Cushing's disease, acromegaly and prolactin-secreting tumors can be effectively treated with APPI. The incidence of hypopituitarism appears to be higher than has been observed in the limited follow-up of micro-surgical cases but less than seen in the long-term follow-up of patients treated with photons.

The recent availability of heavier ions, e.g. carbon ($^{12}$C), newer methods for in vitro monitoring of the Bragg peak should improve the results of pituitary treatment by permitting even more finite localization of radiation in microadenomata and more dense and homogeneous irradiation of large invasive tumors. Hopefully, with this improved dosimetry, the incidence of hypopituitarism can be reduced without sacrificing the control of hormonal hypersecretion and tumor growth.

## ACKNOWLEDGMENTS

This work was supported by the Biology and Medicine Division of the Department of Energy.

Special acknowledgment should be given to my colleagues Joseph Garcia, Claude Chong and John Lyman, and to Jeanette Nakagawa, Ann Yabusaki and Peter Linfoot who helped in the preparation of this manuscript.

## REFERENCES

Aristizabal, S., Caldwell, W. L. and Avila, J. (1977). *Int. J. Radiat. Oncol. Biol. Phys.* **2**, 667–673.

Givens, J. R., Camacho, A. and Paterson, P. (1970). *Metab.* **19**, 818–830.

Hardy, J. (1973). *In* "Diagnosis and Treatment of Pituitary Tumors" (P. O. Kohler and G. T. Ross, eds), pp. 180–194. Elsevier, Amsterdam.

Hardy, J. (1975). *In* "Progress in Neurological Surgery" (H. Krayenbuhl, P. E. Maspes and W. H. Sweet, eds), pp. 200–216. Basel, Switzerland.

Hsu, T. H. (1977). *Arch. Neurol.* **34**, 196–198.

Jeffcoate, W. J., Rees, L. H., Tomlin, S., Jones, A. E., Edwards, C. R. W. and Besser, G. M. (1977). *Br. Med. J.* **2**, 215–217.

Jennings, A. S., Liddle, G. W. and Orth, D. (1977). *N. Engl. J. Med.* **297**, 957–962.

Kjellberg, R. N., Sweet, W. H., Preston, W. M. and Koehler, A. M. (1962). *Trans. Amer. Neurol. Ass.* **87**, 216–218.

Lawrence, J. H. (1957). *Cancer* **10**, 795–798.

Linfoot, J. A. (In press). *In* "Recent Advances in the Diagnosis and Treatment of Pituitary Tumors" (J. A. Linfoot, ed.). Raven Press, New York.

Linfoot, J. A. and Wilson, C. B. (1978). Unpublished data.

Ludecke, D. Kautzky, R., Saeger, W. and Schrader, D. (1976). *Acta Neurochir.* **35**, 27–42.

Mattingly, D. (1962). *J. Clin. Path.* **15**, 374–376.

Moore, T. J., Dluhy, R. G., Williams, G. H. and Cain, J. P. (1976). *Ann. Int. Med.* **85**, 731–734.

Orth, D. N. and Liddle, G. W. (1971). *N. Engl. J. Med.* **285**, 243–247.

Samaan, N. A., Bakdash, M. M., Caderao, J. B., Cangir, A., Jesse, R. H., Jr. and Ballantyne, A. M. (1975). *Ann. Int. Med.* **83**, 771–777.

Sheline, G. E. (In press). *In* "Recent Advances in the Diagnosis and Treatment of Pituitary Tumors" (J. A. Linfoot, ed.). Raven Press, New York.

Tobias, C. A. (In press). *In* "Recent Advances in the Diagnosis and Treatment of Pituitary Tumors" ( J. A. Linfoot, ed.). Raven Press, New York.

Tobias, C. A., Lawrence, J. H., Born, J. L., McCombs, R. K., Roberts, J. E., Anger H. O., Low-Beer, V. B. A. and Higgins, C. (1958). *Cancer Res.* **18**, 121–134.

Wilson, C. B. and Dempsey, L. C. (1978). *J. Neurosurg.* **48**, 13–22.

Wright, A. D., McLachlan, M. S. F., Doyle, F. H. and Fraser R. (1969). *Br. Med. J.* **4**, 582–588.

# PITUITARY MICROADENOMA AND PREGNANCY

D. Weinstein[1], S. Yarkoni[1], A. Sahar[2] and M. Ben-David[3]

[1]*Departments of Obstetrics and Gynecology, Neurosurgery[2] and Pharmacology[3],
Hadassah University Hospital and the Hebrew University-Ḥadassah Medical
School, Jerusalem, Israel*

The success of bromocriptine in inducing ovulation in patients with abnormal pituitary gland and hyperprolactinemia has made the effect of pregnancy on these women increasingly important.

Amenorrhea and sterility with or without galactorrhea have been known to occur in women with clear radiological evidence of a pituitary adenoma, while patients not demonstrating pituitary enlargement have been arbitrarily considered in the past to not have a pituitary adenoma (Forbes *et al.*, 1954). It is still reasonable to assume that in many such instances small adenomas, producing hyperprolactinemia, were the unrecognized cause of the sterility. Using pergonal and clomiphene-citrate, ovulation could be induced without, however, the recognition of the concomitant tumor and hyperprolactinemia.

The treatment of patients with pituitary adenoma is still a highly controversial subject. Should the primary treatment for induction of ovulation be surgical or conservative, e.g. administration of bromocriptine and close follow-up of the patients? The aim of this study is to stress primarily that pregnancy is not contraindicated in hyperprolactinemic anovulatory patients with proved or occult pituitary adenoma. The desire of a woman to become a mother should not be the indication for surgical removal of a pituitary tumor, but rather its size and clinical condition should direct the physician.

Our report is based on 17 selected anovulatory hyperprolactinemic patients who had the following in common: (1) hyperprolactinemia of over 100 ng/ml and galactorrhea; (2) the presence of a pituitary tumor was either confirmed (in 10 patients) or highly suspected (in 2 others) from radiological studies. The remaining 5 patients were suspected to have prolactin-secreting pituitary adenoma on the

531

basis of clinical findings and elevated prolactin values. None showed significant suprasellar extension of the tumor, and all had normal visual fields; (3) ovulation and pregnancy were induced by bromocriptine in all patients without other previous treatment; (4) all patients (except one) had a normal course of pregnancy and maintained normal visual fields, while the radiologic appearance of the pituitary fossa remained almost unchanged.

Elevated serum prolactin levels, ranging from 100-650 ng/ml, were noted in all patients before treatment. After suppression of serum prolactin to the normal range (below 25 ng/ml), ovulation and pregnancy occurred in all patients. During pregnancy, serum prolactin levels rose, reaching values between 224 and 1200 ng/ml. Serum prolactin levels returned either to their pre-pregnancy levels or to values even lower than before pregnancy, which may indicate the return of the pituitary adenoma to its pre-pregnancy condition. Furthermore, on radiologic examination, the adenomas had diminished in size within a few months after delivery, and the elevated prolactin levels seen during pregnancy did not affect the normal course of gestation.

Comparison of serum prolactin levels before treatment with the upper values obtained during pregnancy did not always reveal a positive correlation. Nor was there always a positive correlation between tumor size and pre-treatment prolactin values, or tumor size and highest values during pregnancy. In other words, one cannot draw conclusions as to the behavior of a pituitary adenoma during pregnancy from its size or initial prolactin values. The increase in serum prolactin levels in radiologically non-confirmed patients did not differ from that in the patients with the proved tumor. It is therefore reasonable to assume that an occult microadenoma is present in the former group.

One cannot exclude the diagnosis of a pituitary tumor when the sella appears normal even by the most sophisticated radiologic techniques available (McKenna *et al.*, 1978). Patients with amenorrhea and galactorrhea have been observed to develop abnormalities of the sella after the syndrome has been clinically established. This raised the important question of the frequency of the disorder.

Prediction as to the dose of bromocriptine required cannot be made; the effective doses in our patients were not always related to tumor size or pre-treatment prolactin values.

It should be mentioned that bromocriptine can also be used for shrinkage of the tumor before pregnancy, and for suppression of tumor growth during pregnancy (Corenblum *et al.*, 1975; L'Hermite *et al.*, 1977). This method was used by us in other patients.

We advocate the conservative "wait and see" approach in patients with pituitary adenoma, thereby often preventing unnecessary surgical intervention. Our criteria for choosing conservative treatment or surgery are as follows:

(1) an absolute indication for surgery is evidence of suprasellar extension with optic tract compression. If such findings are observed during pregnancy, they should be treated independent of the stage of pregnancy but without interrupting the pregnancy;

(2) in cases with an enlarged sella turcica with no clinical or ophthalmologic evidence of suprasellar extension, further radiologic studies should be performed. Minor suprasellar extensions do not require surgical or radiologic treatment before induction of ovulation;

(3) clinical and radiologically proved cases with intrasellar adenomas, or suspected cases having hyperprolactinemia with radiologically confirmed adenomas, do not receive treatment directed towards the adenoma itself.

This policy may be critized for being too conservative and arbitrary, and therefore the following points need to be stressed.

The decision to operate on a patient with suprasellar extension and visual field defects should be guided by the condition of the tumor, regardless of the patient's endocrinological situation. An adenoma with no evidence of suprasellar extension is not a threat to the patient's general health.

The morbidity related to surgical resection of the pituitary gland did not increase when performed during pregnancy, and the outcome for mother and child was good (Kaplan, 1961). Surgery for adenoma carries its risks, including the possibility of life-long supportive hormone therapy, and a need for additional bromocriptine treatment. The eventual further growth of the residual tumor has, as yet, not been excluded.

On the other hand, adenomas have been known to regress spontaneously, and some cases diagnosed as adenoma could not be confirmed histologically (Keye *et al.*, 1977).

Advances in medicine, such as screening patients for pituitary adenoma by means of radioimmunoassay for serum prolactin determination, improved radiologic techniques such as computerized axial tomography, and the successful use of bromocriptine should all be employed to the advantage of the patient, facilitating the restoration of ovarian function by means of conservative management with maximal precautions. The surgical option should be retained as a last resort to avoid unnecessary operative risks and its sequelae.

## REFERENCES

Corenblum, B. R., Webster, C. B., Mortimer, C. *et al.* (1975). *Clin. Res.* 23, 614A.

Forbes, A. P., Henneman, P. H., Griswold, G. C. *et al.* (1954). *J. Clin. Endocrinol. Metab.* 14, 265–271.

Kaplan, N. M. (1961). *J. Clin. Endocrinol. Metab.* 21, 1139–1145.

Keye, W. R., Chang, J. R. R. and Jaffe, R. B. (1977). *Obstet, Gynecol. Survey* 32, 727–738.

L'Hermite, M., Caufriez, A. and Robyn, C. (1977). *Fertil. Steril.* 28, 346.

McKenna, T. J., Glick, A. D., Cobb, C. A. *et al.* (1978). *Acta Endocrinol.* 87, 225–233.

# GROWTH OF PROLACTINOMAS DURING PREGNANCY

H. K. Rjosk[1], R. Fahlbusch, H. Huber and K. von Werder

*I. Frauenklinik, Neurochirurgische Klinik und Medizinische, Klinik Innenstadt, University of Munich, W. Germany*

[1]*I. Frauenklinik d. Universität. Maistrasse 11, D 8000 München 2*

With an incidence of 15-20%, hyperprolactinemia is one of the most frequent causes of menstrual disturbances and represents an important factor in female sterility (Rjosk *et al.*, 1976). Whereas in 30% of all hyperprolactinemic patients a pituitary tumor can be diagnosed, the cause of hyperprolactinemia in the other patients remains open. However, even in patients with a normal sella turcica, a microprolactinoma is probable, if other causes of hyperprolactinemia have been excluded (Vezina and Sutton, 1974). Regardless of the cause of hyperprolactinemia, it will respond to bromocriptine and after normalization of the prolactin levels, normal ovulatory cycles occur. HMG/HCG-therapy may also be effective, but it is much more difficult to perform and is associated with well-known risks.

Problems may be encountered in patients with hyperprolactinemia who want to become pregnant. During pregnancy the pituitary gland increases by 70% on account of an increase in the prolactin-producing cells, leading rarely to suprasellar swelling of the pituitary gland, which can lead to compression of the optic chiasma and to visual field defects. This danger arises particularly if a lactotrophic tumor was present before pregnancy. Thus complications have been described and various methods of treatment have been proposed prior to induction of ovulation and pregnancy in hyperprolactinemic patients (Kajtar and Tomkin, 1971; Swyer *et al.*, 1971; Child *et al.*, 1975; Thorner *et al.*, 1975; Gemzell, 1975; Falconer and Stafford-Bell, 1975; Husami *et al.*, 1977; Jewelewicz *et al.*, 1977; Lamberts *et al.*, 1977; Burry *et al.*, 1978; Bergh *et al.*, 1978).

Pretreatment with radiotherapy with 4,500 rad from a 15 MeV linear accelerator (Besser *et al.*, 1977) or Yttrium 90 implantation (Child *et al.*, 1975) are recommended. However, visual field defects cannot always be prevented by radiotherapy (Thorner *et al.*, 1975; Lamberts *et al.*, 1977). In addition, complications such as pituitary insufficiency, visual complications (Harris and Levene, 1976), brain necrosis (Almquist *et al.*, 1964) or CSF fistulas have been reported. Operative removal of microadenomas by trans-sphenoidal microsurgery, often results in normalization of prolactin levels (Hardy *et al.*, 1978; Fahlbusch *et al.*, 1979). However, even with extremely careful technique, hypopituitarism (Franks *et al.*, 1977), CSF fistula (Nicola *et al.*, 1978), hemorrhage and meningitis can occur.

In view of this situation, we prefer a differentiated treatment of sterility in patients with prolactin-producing adenomas (von Werder *et al.*, 1978; Rjosk *et al.*, 1979). The decision about the mode of treatment is made in each case in collaboration by neurosurgeons, internists and gynecologists.

Large adenomas or microadenomas with prolactin levels exceeding 5,000 $\mu U/ml$ are treated operatively. If normalization of prolactin levels is achieved by operation, normal menstrual cycles occur without further treatment.

In operated patients with persisting hyperprolactinemia and in those without the above-mentioned criteria for operative treatment, we use bromocriptine alone after the exclusion of suprasellar tumor growth by cerebral computer tomography.

The dose of bromocriptine is adjusted according to the response in lowering prolactin levels. As soon as the Pregnosticon-test is positive, bromocriptine therapy is stopped. Since the enlargement of the pituitary during pregnancy is almost exclusively due to hypertrophy and hyperplasia of the lactotrophic cells, induced by raised estrogen levels, we use the serum prolactin levels as marker of the growth of the lactotrophic tissue. Prolactin levels during pregnancy of hyperprolactinemic patients do not derive only from the prolactinoma but they are also influenced by the normal prolactin-producing cells, which are stimulated by estrogens. Regardless of which, as in non-pregnant women with prolactinomas, a rapid increase of the prolactin level indicates an increase of the volume of the pituitary gland. In these cases a control by computer tomography may be indicated.

## RESULTS

### Pregnancies in patients after selective adenomectomy

Completely removed prolactinoma ($n = 2$).

After normalization of the prolactin levels by operative treatment, normal ovulatory menstrual cycles occurred. In contrast to the normal rise in prolactin levels during pregnancy, there was no alteration in serum prolactin levels in these patients. From the 20th week of pregnancy, prolactin was below the normal range. After delivery, the prolactin levels remained unaltered and normal ovulatory cycles occurred.

**Pregnancies (*n* = 8) in patients (*n* = 6) with persisting hyperprolactinemia after adenomectomy and treatment with bromocriptine**

After withdrawal of bromocriptine the prolactin levels returned to their post-operative range. In 2 patients, the prolactin levels decreased during pregnancy to 800 µU/ml and 1000 µU/ml at term. After delivery, both patients had normal prolactin levels associated with spontaneous ovulatory cycles, (Fig. 1). In 2 patients a continuous steep increase in the prolactin levels was found. At term, 16000 µU/ml (postoperative range 8000 µU/ml) and 35000 µU/ml (postoperative range 4000 µU/ml) were found. There was no evidence of suprasellar extension of the pituitary by computer tomography performed in the 32nd week of pregnancy in these patients. After delivery one patient was treated with bromo-criptine (5 mg/d), after which the prolactin level fell within 10 days from 20 000 µU/ml to 550 µU/ml.

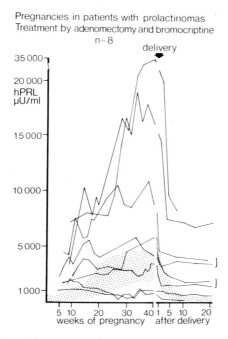

Pregnancies in patients with prolactinomas
Treatment by adenomectomy and bromocriptine
n = 8

*Fig. 1.* Prolactin (hPRL) levels during 8 pregnancies in 6 patients with prolactinomas. (Treatment: adenomectomy and bromocriptine) (dotted area: normal range).

Six patients of this group have conceived twice as a result of this treatment. In 2 patients, both pregnancies have come to term. The prolactin levels during the first pregnancies in both patients were in the normal range and decreased post-partum to the postoperative levels. After treatment with the same dose of bromocriptine, the patients became pregnant again. During the second pregnancies, prolactin levels increased mo e steeply, up to 4500 μU/ml and 9000 μU/ml at delivery. However, 4 weeks post-partum the original values were found.

**Pregnancies in patients with prolactinomas, treated with bromocriptine (*n* = 6) (Fig. 2)**

There is no difference in the pattern of prolactin concentrations as compared with the operated patients. Subnormal levels (twins), normal and highly elevated prolactin levels all occurred. Computerized tomography was performed in the 2 patients with the very high prolactin levels. No evidence for suprasellar growth of the pituitary was found.

With the exception of one patient, the prolactin levels decreased to the pretreatment levels after delivery. However, in one patient with a pretreatment prolactin concentration of 2000 μU/ml, the prolactin level remained at 6000 μU/ml even 4 months after delivery. For this reason, adenoma growth during pregnancy was probable and the patient was therefore adenomectomized. A cystic tumor 1 cm in diameter was removed.

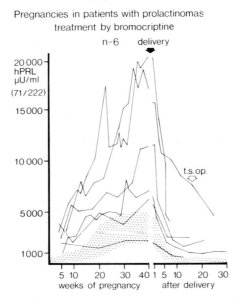

*Fig. 2.* Prolactin (PRL) levels during 6 pregnancies in 6 patients with prolactinomas. (Treatment: bromocriptine) (dotted area: normal range).

The course of treatment of this patient is demonstrated in detail in Fig. 3. After the first pregnancy and trans-sphenoidal adenomectomy, the patient conceived again after treatment with 2.5 mg/day bromocriptine. In the 10th week of pregnancy a hydatidiform mole had to be evacuated. Because of engorgement of the mammary glands, bromocriptine therapy was started again. After 9 months

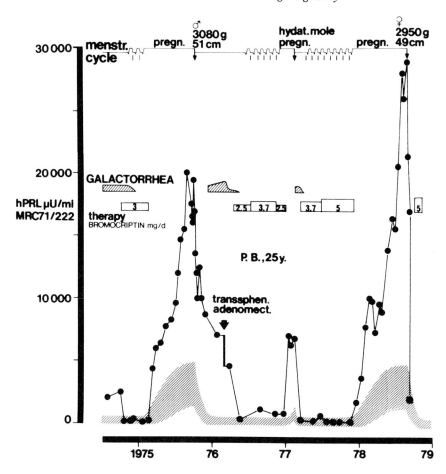

*Fig. 3.* Course of treatment of a patient with prolactinoma (P.B., 25yr). (Shaded area = normal range.)

with negative serum hCG levels, local contraception was terminated. During the first ovulation the patient became pregnant. A very steep increase in prolactin levels was found. This may indicate that incomplete adenomectomy does not prevent complications due to adenoma growth during pregnancy.

## Pregnancies in hyperprolactinemic patients with normal sella turcica (*n* = 21) (Fig. 4)

A normal sella turcica does not exclude the presence of a microadenoma which has not affected the osseous structure of the sella turcica (Vezina and Sutton, 1974). In fact, the patterns of prolactin levels during the pregnancies in this group were not different from those of the other groups. Thus, in 2 patients prolactin decreased, in 12 normal and in 7 patients higher than normal pregnancy prolactin levels were found. In all patients, 3 months after delivery the prolactin levels were within or below the pretreatment range.

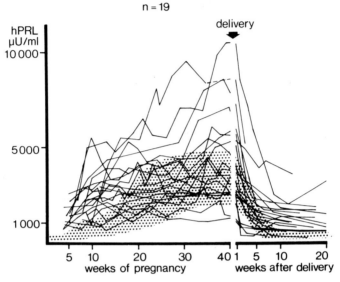

*Fig. 4.* Prolactin levels (PRL) during 19 pregnancies in hyperprolactinemic patients with normal sella. (Treatment with bromocriptine) (dotted area = normal range).

## CONCLUSION

There was no significant correlation between the pretreatment prolactin levels and the prolactin concentrations at time of delivery.

However, with the exception of one, by three months after delivery all patients

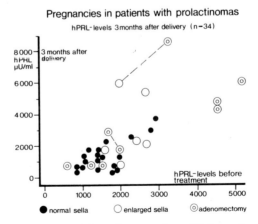

*Fig. 5.* PRL levels 3 months after delivery in comparison with the pretreatment hPRL levels (34 pregnancies in 31 patients with hyperprolactinemia).

had prolactin levels within the pretreatment range (Fig. 5). This finding indicates that elevated estrogen levels during pregnancy do not necessarily induce a permanent enlargement of the prolactinoma, but the tumor cells seem to act like normal lactotropic cells.

In view of these results, it seems justified to use a therapy as conservative as possible in patients with prolactinomas who want to become pregnant. However, the preconditions are an exact diagnosis of the anatomical situation in the sella area and careful control during pregnancy.

## REFERENCES

Almquist, S., Dahlgren, S., Notter, G. and Sundbom, L. (1964). *Acta radiologica* **2**, 179.

Bergh, T., Nillius, S. J. and Wide, L. (1978). *Brit. Med. J.* **1**, 875–880.

Besser, G. M., Thorner, M. O. and Wass, J. A. H. (1977). *In* "Endocrinology" (V. H. T. James, ed.) Vol. 2, 353–357. Excerpta Medica, Amsterdam.

Burry, K. A., Schiller, H. S., Mills, R., Harris, B. and Heinrichs, L. (1978). *Obstet. Gynecol.* **52**, 1 (Suppl), 19s–22s.

Child, D. F., Gordon, H., Mashiter, K. and Joplin, G. F. (1975). *Brit. Med. J.* **4**, 87–89.

Fahlbusch, R., Giovanelli, M., Crosignani, P. G., Faglia, G., Rjosk, H. K. and von Werder, K. (1979). This volume.

Falconer, M. A. and Stafford-Bell, M. A. (1975). *J. Neurol. Neurosurg. Psychiat.* **38**, 919–930.

Franks, S., Jacobs, H. S., Hull, M. G. R., Steele, S. J. and Nabarro, J. D. N. (1977). *Brit. J. Obstet. Gynec.* **84**, 241–253.

Gemzell, C. (1975). *Am. J. Obstet. Gynecol.* **121**, 311–315.

Hardy, J., Beauregard, H. and Robert, F. (1978). *In* "Progress in Prolactin Physiology and Pathology". (C. Robyn and M. Harter, eds), pp. 361–370. Elsevier/North Holland Biomedical Press, Amsterdam, New York.

Harris, J. R. and Levene, M. B. (1976). *Radiology* **120**, 167–171.

Husami, N., Jewelewicz, R. and Vande Wiele, R. L. (1977). *Fertil. Steril.* **28**, 920–925.

Jewelewicz, R., Zimmerman, E. A. and Carmel, P. W. (1977). *Fertil. Steril.* **28**, 35–40.

Kajtar, T. and Tomkin, G. H. (1971). *Brit. Med. J.* **4**, 88–90.

Lamberts, S. W. J., Seldenrath, H. J., Kwa, H. G. and Birkenhäger, J. C. (1977). *J. Clin. Endocr.* **44**, 180–184.

Nicola, G. C., Tonnarelli, G. P. and Griner, A. (1978). *In* "Treatment of Pituitary Adenomas". (R. Fahlbusch and K. von Werder, eds), pp. 287–292. Georg Thieme Publishers, Stuttgart.

Rjosk, H. K., von Werder, K. and Fahlbusch, R. (1976). *Geburtsh. u. Frauenheilk.* **36**, 575–587.

Rjosk, H. K., Fahlbusch, R. and von Werder, K. (1979). *Arch Gynäk.* (In press).

Swyer, G. I. M., Little, V. and Harries, B. J. (1971). *Brit. Med. J.* **4**, 90–91.

Thorner, M. O., Besser, G. M., Jones, A., Dacie, J. and Jones, A. E. (1975). *Brit. Med. J.* **4**, 694–697.

Vezina, J. L. and Sutton, T. J. (1974). *Amer. J. of Roentg. Radiother.* **120**, 46–54.

von Werder, K., Fahlbusch, R., Landgraf, R., Pickardt, C. R., Rjosk, H. K. and Scriba, P. C. (1978). *J. Endocrinol. Invest.* **1**, 47–58.

# TUMOUR ENLARGEMENT DURING PREGNANCY IN AMENORRHOEIC WOMEN WITH PROLACTIN-SECRETING PITUITARY ADENOMAS

T. Bergh, S. J. Nillius and L. Wide

*Departments of Obstetrics, Gynaecology and Clinical Chemistry,
University Hospital, Uppsala, Sweden*

It has previously been described that pituitary adenomas may rapidly enlarge and give rise to tumour complications during pregnancies induced by human gonadotrophins (Gemzell, 1975). Here we report on the clinical course and outcome of 33 pregnancies in amenorrhoeic women with hyperprolactinaemia and radiological evidence of a pituitary tumour. Most of the pregnancies followed treatment with bromocriptine. Only one of the women was treated by surgery and irradiation before induction of ovulation.

## PATIENTS AND METHODS

Nineteen women, aged 22–37 years, with hyperprolactinaemia and radiological signs of pituitary tumour were treated with bromocriptine. Detailed results from 16 of these women have previously been described elsewhere (Bergh *et al.*, 1978, 1979). Two of the women had primary amenorrhoea and the others secondary amenorrhoea of 3–14 years duration. Galactorrhoea, defined as any secretion from the breast, spontaneously or on compression, was detected in all but one of the 19 women. All the patients had an asymmetrical and/or enlarged pituitary fossa, which in combination with amenorrhoea and hyperprolactinaemia was taken as evidence of a pituitary tumour. One of the women had received primary tumour treatment by surgery, later followed by irradiation but hyperprolactinaemia (845 $\mu$g/l) persisted. The visual fields were normal in all the women.

The serum prolactin concentrations ranged between 34–845 $\mu$g/l (mean 85 $\mu$g/l,

NIH hPRL VLS 3). The normal range for healthy women was 2–15 μg/l (mean 6.5 μg/l).

The radiological examination of the skull and pituitary fossa included coned lateral and antero-posterior view of the sella turcica and polytomography. Six of the women had an asymmetrical but normal-sized sella (Grade I abnormality, according to Vezina, 1978). The other 12 women with untreated pituitary tumours had more pronounced sellar changes (Grade II, Vezina, 1978). All the women were re-examined with a pituitary fossa X-ray after delivery.

## CLINICAL COURSE AND OUTCOME OF PREGNANCIES

All but one of the 32 pregnancies occurred after ovulation-inducing treatment. One uneventful pregnancy occurred during a temporary pause in oestrogen substitution therapy of a 32-year-old woman who had amenorrhoea-galactorrhoea for 10 years. After the pregnancy, hyperprolactinaemia was diagnosed and she resumed ovulatory function on bromocriptine therapy.

### Gonadotrophin-induced pregnancies

Human gonadotrophin therapy resulted in 12 pregnancies in 7 of the patients. Eight of these went to term, while 4 ended in early abortion. There were no symptoms or signs of tumour growth during or after 10 of the 12 pregnancies.

A tumour complication occurred in a 34-year-old woman with 5 years of amenorrhoea and galactorrhoea. She developed bitemporal visual field defects during the 28th week of her first pregnancy. The field defects did not progress and the pregnancy could continue until term. The pituitary fossa X-ray showed pronounced enlargement of her asymmetric sella and there was a slight suprasellar extension of the pituitary tumour in an air encephalogram postpartum. After the delivery the visual fields rapidly became normal. A second gonadotrophin-induced pregnancy two years later went uneventfully to term with no further enlargement of the pituitary fossa (Gemzell, 1975; Bergh *et al.,* 1978).

Radiological evidence of tumour growth during a gonadotrophin-induced pregnancy was also obtained in a 27-year-old woman, despite the fact that she had previously had a chromophobe adenoma removed trans-sphenoidally. She had also been treated with irradiation. During pregnancy, this patient had no symptoms or signs of tumour growth but the postpartum X-ray showed that destruction of the dorsum sellae had occurred (Bergh *et al.,* 1979).

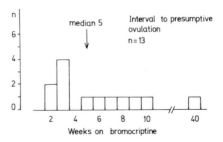

*Fig. 1.*    Time interval to resumption of presumptive ovulation during bromocriptine treatment of 13 infertile women with evidence of a prolactin-secreting tumour.

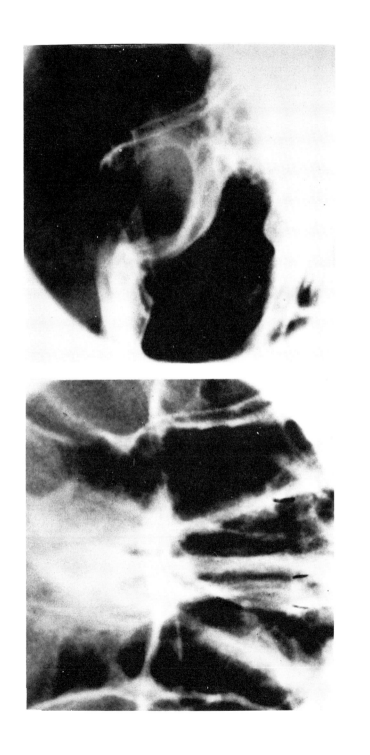

*Fig. 2.* The asymmetrically enlarged pituitary fossa of a 25-year-old hyperprolactinaemic woman with 3 years of amenorrhoea-galactorrhoea. During a bromocriptine-induced pregnancy this patient developed reversible visual field defects and destruction of the sella turcica.

## Bromocriptine-induced pregnancies

Bromocriptine was given to 13 infertile women with prolactin-secreting pituitary tumours. During therapy the prolactin levels decreased to normal and all 13 women resumed normal ovulatory function after 5 weeks of treatment, on the average (range 2–40 weeks) (Fig. 1). Eleven of the women responded to daily bromocriptine doses of 2.5–7.5 mg, while 2 patients received 10 and 15 mg daily, respectively. Treatment was discontinued as soon as pregnancy was suspected, i.e. 1–20 days (median 8) after the expected date of menstruation. During pregnancy the patients were monitored with monthly visual field examinations.

The bromocriptine therapy resulted in 19 pregnancies in the 13 women. Thirteen of the pregnancies went to term, resulting in 14 healthy children while 5 pregnancies ended in abortion (one induced). One patient had one early and one

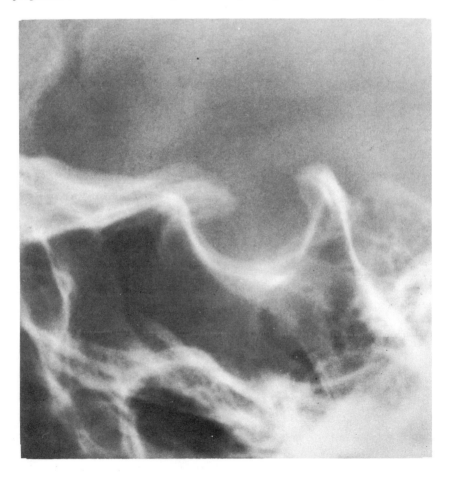

*Fig. 3.* The asymmetrical and enlarged (1700 mm$^3$) pituitary fossa of a 23-year-old hyperprolactinaemic woman with 5 years of amenorrhoea. This patient had a completely uneventful bromocriptine-induced twin pregnancy.

late spontaneous abortion, but is now in week 33 of her third bromocriptine-induced pregnancy.

Tumour complications occurred during 2 of the 19 pregnancies. Visual field defects during pregnancy were experienced by a 25-year-old woman with 3 years of amenorrhoea-galactorrhoea, hyperprolactinaemia (72 μg/l) and a pronounced asymmetrical enlargement of the pituitary fossa (Fig. 2). Bromocriptine therapy resulted in improvement of the visual impairment and the pregnancy could continue until term. After delivery, the visual fields returned to normal but X-ray examination showed destruction of the pituitary fossa (Bergh *et al.*, 1978).

Symptoms of tumour enlargement during pregnancy also occurred in a 25-year-old woman with primary amenorrhoea, hyperprolactinaemia (46 μg/l) and a slightly asymmetrical sella of normal size. She complained of headache from the second trimester of pregnancy but her visual fields remained normal. After delivery the headache rapidly disappeared. The X-ray examination showed enlargement and a more pronounced asymmetry of the sella. Radiological signs of tumour enlargement during pregnancy were also found in a 28-year-old woman with 6 years of amenorrhoea, hyperprolactinaemia (60 μg/l) and an asymmetrically enlarged sella. However, she had no symptoms or signs of tumour growth during her bromocriptine-induced pregnancy (Bergh *et al.*, 1978).

In none of the other bromocriptine-induced pregnancies were there any symptoms or signs of tumour enlargement either during or after pregnancy. The pituitary fossa was markedly asymmetrical and enlarged in many of these women (Fig. 3).

## DISCUSSION

It is evident from our study that patients with prolactin-secreting pituitary adenomas run a risk of developing tumour complications during pregnancy. It has therefore been recommended that patients with such tumours should be pretreated with irradiation or surgery before attempting a pregnancy (Child *et al.*, 1975; Thorner *et al.*, 1975; Franks *et al.*, 1977). However, such pretreatment does not seem to completely prevent the risk of tumour complications during pregnancy. The only one of our 19 patients who had received prior treatment by not only surgery but also irradiation, had evidence of tumour growth (destruction of dorsum sellae) during pregnancy. Visual field abnormalities during pregnancy have previously been described in pituitary tumour patients pretreated with irradiation (Thorner *et al.*, 1975; Lamberts *et al.*, 1977).

Most of our patients had not been pretreated with surgery or irradiation before induction of ovulation and pregnancy. Two of these 18 patients, both with pituitary macroadenomas, developed visual field defects which rapidly regressed after delivery. Another 2 women had radiological evidence of tumour enlargement during pregnancy. However, 14 of the 18 previously untreated tumour patients had completely uneventful pregnancies with no signs of tumour growth in postpartum X-rays. No fewer than 9 of these women had pituitary macroadenomas. In another recent study, Mornex *et al.* (1978) found no tumour complications during pregnancy in 8 hyperprolactinaemic patients with sellar abnormalities.

If visual complications occur during pregnancy in patients with prolactin-secreting pituitary tumours, bromocriptine therapy may be the best primary treatment. The visual field defects in one of our patients regressed when bromocriptine treatment was re-instituted during pregnancy. Improvement of visual field defects on bromocriptine treatment has previously been reported in non-pregnant patients with pituitary tumours (Corenblum *et al.,* 1975; Friesen and Tolis, 1977; Vaidya *et al.,* 1978). If the bromocriptine should fail, alternative treatments have proved to be successful in preventing irreversible visual impairment (see Bergh *et al.,* 1978, for references).

The bromocriptine therapy was discontinued in all our patients as soon as pregnancy was suspected. During a normal pregnancy, the prolactin levels markedly increase and high levels are present both in mother and foetus at term (Aubert *et al.,* 1977). The role of prolactin during pregnancy is unknown. It has been suggested that prolactin is of importance for salt and water balance (Josimovich, 1977; Leontic and Tyson, 1977) and for foetal lung maturation (Hauth *et al.,* 1978). Until more is known about the function of prolactin for foetal development, bromocriptine should not be given prophylactically throughout pregnancy in an attempt to prevent tumour enlargement. However, if serious tumour complications develop, the treatment of choice is probably re-institution of bromocriptine.

Thus, there is a definite risk of tumour enlargement during pregnancy in patients with prolactin-secreting pituitary adenomas. However, the tumour enlargement seldom leads to serious irreversible complications. Infertile women with prolactin-secreting microadenomas, and possibly also some with pituitary macroadenomas, may therefore be treated with bromocriptine alone, provided that they are monitored during pregnancy with repeated visual field examinations for the earliest possible detection of tumour complications. The risk of severe irreversible visual impairment seems to be very small in carefully supervised patients. It is possible that infertile women with prolactin-secreting pituitary adenomas may benefit from prolonged bromocriptine therapy before attempting a pregnancy since recent evidence suggests that such treatment may induce tumour regression (see Nillius *et al.,* this book).

## REFERENCES

Aubert, M. L., Sizonenko, P. C., Kaplan, S. L. and Grumbach, M. M. (1977). *In* "Prolactin and Human Reproduction" (P. G. Crosignani and C. Robyn, eds) pp. 9–20. Academic Press, London and New York.

Bergh, T., Nillius, S. J. and Wide, L. (1978). *Br. Med. J.* **1,** 875–880.

Bergh, T., Nillius, S. J. and Wide, L. (1980). *Clin. Endocr.* (In press).

Child, D. F., Gordon, H., Mashiter, K. and Joplin, G. F. (1975). *Br. Med. J.* **4,** 87–89.

Corenblum, B., Webster, B. R., Mortimer, C. B. and Ezrin, C. (1975). *Clin. Res.* **23,** 614A.

Franks, S., Jacobs, H. S., Hull, M. G. R., Steele, S. J. and Nabarro, J. D. N. (1977). *Br. J. Obst. Gynaec.* **84,** 241–253.

Friesen, H. G. and Tolis, G. (1977). *Clin. Endocr.* **6,** Suppl., 91s–99s.

Gemzell, C. (1975). *Am. J. Obstet. Gynecol.* **121,** 311–315.

Hauth, J. C., Parker, C. R. Jr., MacDonald, P. C., Porter, J. C. and Johnston, J. M. (1978). *Obstet. Gynecol.* **51**, 516–517.

Josimovich, J. B. (1977). *In* "Prolactin and Human Reproduction" (P. G. Crosignani and C. Robyn, eds) pp. 27–36. Academic Press, London and New York.

Lamberts, S. W. J., Seldenrath, H. J., Kwa, H. G. and Birkenhäger, J. C. (1977). *J. Clin. Endocr. Metab.* **44**, 180–185.

Leontic, E. A. and Tyson, J. E. (1977). *In* "Prolactin and Human Reproduction" (P. G. Crosignani and C. Robyn, eds) pp. 37–45. Academic Press, London and New York.

Mornex, R., Orgiazzi, J., Hugues, B., Gagnaire, J-C. and Claustrat, B. (1978). *J. Clin. Endocr. Metab.* **47**, 290–295.

Thorner, M. O., Besser, G. M., Jones, A., Dacie, J. and Jones. A. E. (1975). *Br. Med. J.* **4**, 694–697.

Vaidya, R. A., Aloorkar, S. D., Rege, N. R., Maskati, B. T., Jahangir. R. P., Sheth, A. R. and Pandya, S. K. (1978). *Fertil. & Steril.* **29**, 632–636.

Vezina, J. L. (1978). *In* "Progress in Prolactin Physiology and Pathology" (C. Robyn and M. Harter, eds) pp. 351–360. Biomedical Press, Elsevier/North-Holland, Amsterdam.

# AUTHOR INDEX

# SUBJECT INDEX

## A

Acidophilic stem cell adenoma, 130–132

Acromegaly
  *see* growth hormone-secreting adenomas

ACTH
  secretion
    effects of cyproheptadine *in vitro*, 154–156
    effects of cyproheptadine *in vivo*, 392–393
    effects of ergocryptine *in vitro*, 154–156
    effects of ergocryptine *in vivo*, 393–394
    effects of LVP *in vitro*, 190–193
    monoaminergic control, 16–19, 32–34
    noradrenaline turnover, 33

ACTH-secreting adenomas
  ACTH plasma levels 173–179, 189, 497–498
    after medical treatment, 393
    after α-particle irradiation, 518–519
    after surgery, 498–499
  bromocriptine treatment, 393–394
  carotid angiography, 496
  cortisol plasma levels, 189, 497–498
    after medical treatment, 393
    after α-particle irradiation, 518–519

ACTH-secreting adenomas (*contd.*)
  cortisol plasma levels (*contd.*)
    after surgery, 498–499
    cortisol urinary levels, 508
    after cryosurgery, 512
  cyproheptadine treatment, 392–393
  dexamethasone test, 497–519
  gonadotropic function, 280–288, 497–501
    after surgery, 280, 461, 497–501
  GH plasma levels, 285–286
  hypothalamic origin, 183–184, 191–192, 392
  immunohistochemistry, 95, 141, 195–204
  insulin test, 497
  localization, 10, 92–94, 459–460
  lysinvasopressin test, 497
  medical treatment, 391, 395
    *see* bromocriptine, cyproheptadine
  metyrapone test, 497
  microsurgical treatment, 457–463, 479–480, 495–502
  MSH, 95, 173–179, 195–204
  pneumoencephalography, 496
  PRL plasma levels, 394, 500–501
    after surgery, 500–501
  radiological findings, 9, 314–319, 338, 458, 496
  stereotactic radiosurgery, 507–514
  structure
    at electron microscopy, 94, 111–114, 140, 196–200

555